Innovation in Chinese Medicine

In the West ideas about Chinese medicine are commonly associated with traditional therapies and ancient practices which have been in place, unchanging, since time immemorial.
This volume, edited by Elisabeth Hsu, demonstrates that this is far from the reality. In a
series of pioneering case studies, twelve contributors, from a range of disciplines, explore
the history of Chinese medicine and the transformations that have taken place during the
course of that history from the fourth century BC to the present day. Topics of discussion
cover diagnostic and therapeutic techniques, pharmacotherapy, the creation of new genres
of medical writing and schools of doctrine. Given the growing interest in Chinese medicine,
the volume promises to make a valuable and innovative contribution. Its interdisciplinarity,
a hallmark of the field, will ensure a wide readership amongst scholars and practitioners.

ELISABETH HSU is a lecturer in medical anthropology at the Institute of Social and Cultural
Anthropology, University of Oxford. Her publications include *The Transmission of
Chinese Medicine* (1999).

NEEDHAM RESEARCH INSTITUTE STUDIES • 3

The Needham Research Institute Studies series publishes important and original new work on East Asian culture and science which develops or links in with the publication of the *Science and Civilisation in China* series. The series is under the editorial control of the Publications Board of the Needham Research Institute.

1 Christopher Cullen, *Astronomy and Mathematics in Ancient China: The 'Zhou Bi Suan Jing'*
ISBN 0 521 55089 0

2 Robert Wardy, *Aristotle in China: Language, Categories and Translation*
ISBN 0 521 77118 8

Innovation in Chinese Medicine

Edited by

Elisabeth Hsu

University of Oxford

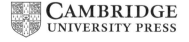

CAMBRIDGE UNIVERSITY PRESS

PUBLISHED BY THE PRESS SYNDICATE OF THE UNIVERSITY OF CAMBRIDGE
The Pitt Building, Trumpington Street, Cambridge, United Kingdom

CAMBRIDGE UNIVERSITY PRESS
The Edinburgh Building, Cambridge CB2 2RU, UK
40 West 20th Street, New York NY 10011–4211, USA
10 Stamford Road, Oakleigh, VIC 3166, Australia
Ruiz de Alarcón 13, 28014 Madrid, Spain
Dock House, The Waterfront, Cape Town 8001, South Africa

http://www.cambridge.org

First published 2001

Printed in the United Kingdom at the University Press, Cambridge

Typeface in Times 11/14.25pt   [GC]

A catalogue record for this book is available from the British Library

Library of Congress cataloguing in publication data

Innovation in Chinese medicine/edited by Elisabeth Hsu.
p. cm. – (Needham Research Institute Studies; 3)
Includes bibliographical references and index.
ISBN 0 521 80068 4 (hardback)
1. Medicine, Chinese.   I. Hsu, Elisabeth.   II. Series.
R601 .I566 2001
610′.951 – dc21

ISBN 0 521 80068 4 hardback

In memoriam Lu Gwei-Djen
(1904–1991)

Contents

Notes on contributors

BRIDIE ANDREWS is Assistant Professor of the History of Science at Harvard University. She is author of *The Making of Modern Chinese Medicine*, forthcoming, and co-editor of *Western Medicine as Contested Knowledge*, 1996.

CHRISTOPHER CULLEN is Senior Lecturer in the History of Chinese Science and Medicine, and Director of Research of the Centre for the History and Culture of Medicine at the School of Oriental and African Studies (SOAS), University of London. He has published *Astronomy and Mathematics in Ancient China*, 1996, and is general editor of the **Science and Civilisation in China** series.

CATHERINE DESPEUX is Professor at INALCO (Institut National des Langues et Civilisations Orientales). She is author of *Taoïsme et corps humain*, 1994, and co-editor of *La maladie dans la Chine médiévale: La toux*, 1997.

UTE ENGELHARDT is Lecturer at the Institute of East Asian Studies, University of Munich, vice-president of the international association of Chinese Medicine (SMS) and editor-in-chief of the journal *Chinese Medicine*. She is co-author of *Chinesische Diätetik*, 1997.

MARTA HANSON is Assistant Professor of History, Department of History, University of California, San Diego. She is co-editor of 'Empires of hygiene', *Positions: East Asia Cultures Critique* 6.3, 1998.

DONALD HARPER is Professor at the Department of East Asian Languages and Civilisations, University of Chicago. He is editor of the journal *Early China* and author of *Early Chinese Medical Literature: the Mawangdui Medical Manuscripts*, 1998.

ELISABETH HSU is Lecturer at the Institute of Social and Cultural Anthropology, University of Oxford. She is author of *The Transmission of Chinese Medicine*, 1999, and co-editor of *Naxi and Moso Ethnography*, 1998.

VIVIENNE LO is Wellcome Trust Research Fellow at the Centre for the History and Culture of Medicine at SOAS, University of London. She is author of *The Zhangjiashan Medical Manuscripts*, forthcoming.

GEORGES MÉTAILIÉ is Directeur de Recherche, at the CNRS and member of Centre Alexandre Koyré – Histoire des Sciences et des Techniques, Paris. He is author of various papers on the history of botanical knowledge in China and Japan before the twentieth century.

FRÉDÉRIC OBRINGER is Chargé de Recherche at the CNRS in Paris. He is author of *L'aconit et l'orpiment: Drogues et poisons en Chine ancienne et médiévale*, 1997.

VOLKER SCHEID is Wellcome Trust Research Fellow at the Centre for the History and Culture of Medicine at SOAS, University of London. He is author of *Contemporary Chinese Medicine: Plurality and Synthesis*, forthcoming.

KIM TAYLOR is Wellcome Trust Research Fellow at the Needham Research Institute, Cambridge. She wrote a PhD thesis entitled 'Chinese Medicine in Early Communist China (1945–1963)'.

Series editor's preface

This book is a collective production, for which credit must be shared amongst a number of scholars, some of whose names do not appear in the contents list. Most of all, thanks are due to Elisabeth Hsu, who has worked over the last five years to edit all the components of this text together to create a coherent whole constituting a major contribution to this field of learning. Without her dedication and thoroughness there would simply be no book at all.

The book has its origin in a workshop meeting that was held at the Needham Research Institute in Cambridge from 8–11 March 1995. One aim of that workshop was to commemorate the life and work of Lu Gwei-djen, who for many years was Joseph Needham's principal collaborator on the *Science and Civilisation in China* project. She was in fact the 'principal evocator' of this immense work through the inspiration she gave, dating from well before the time Needham first visited China. Joseph Needham took part in the workshop, but died a fortnight later. This was therefore, very fittingly, the last scholarly activity to which he contributed in a long and productive life.

The workshop was generously supported by a number of bodies, including the Lu Gwei-djen Memorial Charitable Trust (who also supported the editorial work on this book), the Wellcome Trust, the British Academy, and Robinson College (where Lu Gwei-djen had been an honorary fellow). To these bodies we offer our sincere gratitude for having made this work possible.

As well as those who have contributed their writing to this book, there were others whose participation in the workshop and subsequent advice helped to shape it and to give it direction: Francesca Bray (University of California, Santa Barbara), Judith Farquhar (University of North Carolina, Chapel Hill), T. J. Hinrichs and Lowell Skar, at that time both US National Science Foundation Fellows at the NRI, Francoise Sabban (Ecole des Hautes Etudes en Sciences Sociales, Paris), Sidney White (Temple University, Philadelphia), and also Gregory Blue (University of Victoria). We hope they will be pleased to see what they have helped to bring to fruition. No less than three anonymous academic readers contributed advice on the content and structure of the volume in draft: we hope that the value of their careful checking and criticism will be evident to them from the present appearance of this book.

Throughout the editing of the book, invaluable advice came from a number of scholars whose advice the editor sought on many occasions: David McMullen, Mark Lewis, Geoffrey Lloyd, Michael Loewe, and also Ho Peng-Yoke. Penelope Herbert acted as English style consultant for a volume whose contributors came from a very varied linguistic background. On matters Chinese researchers at the Needham Research Institute helped in many ways; among them are Li Lisha, Guo Shirong, Wang Qianjin, and also Zhao Hongjun and Ma Boying. In the editor's tasks of bibliographic and other background research, much help came from Charles Aylmer of Cambridge University Library and from John Moffett, Librarian of the Needham Research Institute with the assistance of Gao Chuan and Sally Church. As successive secretaries of the Institute, Angela King and Susan Bennett helped manage a complex network of contacts and information flows. Of course none of those who helped in all these varied ways bears responsibility for any errors of commission or omission that may remain uncorrected in the final text.

This book is not in any conventional sense a *Festschrift*. It exists in its own right as a carefully planned and executed collective contribution to a vigorously growing field of learning. But given the field with which it deals, and the occasion which gave rise to the project from which it stems, I hope that it will be taken as a tribute to the life and work of Lu Gwei-djen, whose arrival in Cambridge so long ago led to so much that has increased the understanding and mutual knowledge of China and the West.

Christopher Cullen

Chinese dynasties

Shang dynasty	16th–11th century BC		Sui dynasty	581–618
Zhou dynasty	11th century–221 BC		Tang dynasty	618–907
Western Zhou dynasty	11th century–771			
Eastern Zhou dynasty	770–256		Five dynasties	907–960
Spring and Autumn Period	770–476		Later Liang	907–923
Warring States	475–221		Later Tang	923–936
			Later Jin	936–946
Qin dynasty	221–207 BC		Later Han	947–950
			Later Zhou	951–960
Han dynasty	206 BC–AD 220			
Western Han dynasty	206 BC–AD 24		Song dynasty	960–1127
Eastern Han dynasty	25–220		Northern Song dynasty	960–1127
			Southern Song	1127–1279
Three Kingdoms	220–280			
Wei	220–265		Liao dynasty	916–1125
Shu	221–263			
Wu	222–280		Jin dynasty	1115–1234
Western Jin dynasty	265–316		Yuan dynasty	1271–1368
Eastern Jin dynasty	317–420		Ming dynasty	1368–1644
Northern and Southern dynasties	420–581		Qing dynasty	1644–1911
Southern Song	420–479			
Southern Qi	479–502		Republic of China	1191–1949
Liang	502–557			
Chen	557–589		People's Republic of China	1949–
Northern Wei	386–534			
Eastern Wei	534–550			
Northern Qi	550–577			
Western Wei	535–556			
Northern Zhou	557–581			

Introduction

ELISABETH HSU

Innovation expresses a belief in progress, an investment in the future. Change is equated with improvement; the present is better than the past, and the future will be better still. This view of time is not that of premodern China. Scholars and doctors looked back to a Golden Age in the past. Morals were declining and, for them, time went downhill. If there was any hope for improvement, it lay in a more sophisticated understanding of ancient knowledge. Even today practitioners intent on modernising Chinese medicine declare allegiance to the canonical tradition that links them in a direct line to the legendary figure of the Yellow Emperor. So why devote a book on Chinese medicine to the topic of 'innovation'? Why discuss the many strands of an 'ancient art of healing' from the perspective of a concept that alludes to the strife of modern science and technology?[1]

The contributions to this volume were written to commemorate the initiator of a scholarly project[2] designed expressly to challenge the orientalising view of China as the exotic and remote, good for the connoisseur of art and poetry, but not for the researcher interested in the sciences and technologies that have shaped modern society so decisively. Following the lead of *Science and Civilisation in China,* this volume in memory of Lu Gwei-djen is meant to demonstrate how much is to be gained by using a broader view of science: it presents recent applications of the notion of science to comparable forms of knowledge before and outside post-Renaissance Europe, asking the same serious questions of other histories that we ask of our own.

If difference is construed in hierarchical terms, as so often in cross-cultural comparisons of intellectual, material, or social history, then of course terms like 'technological innovation' which are closely connected in our minds with our own 'scientific revolution'

---

[1] I am indebted to Francesca Bray for extensive work on an earlier draft. I would also like to thank my colleagues at the Needham Research Institute for their valuable comments on a more recent version.

[2] Needham, Joseph et al. (1954–). *Science and Civilisation in China*, Cambridge University Press, Cambridge (abbreviated as *SCC*).

may simply blind us to the nature of the changes that took place in other societies.[3] We cannot expect that all societies follow the same historical trajectory, nor that a theme of research that is illuminating in one society will inevitably prove fruitful in studying another. Yet certain historical processes, in spite of their uniqueness, can have striking cross-cultural similarities. Even though the worldviews of the Chinese past differ greatly from those of the industrialised northern hemisphere in the early twenty-first century, the admittedly culture-specific concept of 'innovation', used with circumspection, opens up interesting ways of thinking about the history of medicine in China. Vice versa, the application of this concept to a premodern and non-western society can enrich our understanding of 'innovation' and the complex processes it involves.

'Innovation' was a topic central to the 'Needham question' of why modern science originated only in Europe when in fact significant technological inventions had been made much earlier in China.[4] At the end of his life, Joseph Needham stressed that Lu Gwei-djen, formerly a research student of his first wife Dorothy Needham, had been 'the dominant influence that caused him to change from being a regular research scientist . . . to becoming a historian of science in China'. Apparently, 'she worked out with Needham the subjects for a book to seek to provide an answer to the great puzzle worrying him'.[5] Among researchers in the field, Lu Gwei-djen is furthermore remembered for her contributions to the history of medicine in publications that were, however, always co-authored.[6] The one exception to this was an article on the great scholar-physician and natural historian of the Ming dynasty, Li Shizhen,[7] whose work continues

---

[3] Sivin, Nathan (1981), 'Why the Scientific Revolution did not take place in China – Or didn't it?' *Chinese Science* 5, 45–66.

[4] Joseph Needham is commonly known for having shown that the three technological inventions that Francis Bacon made responsible for the rise of modernity – the compass, gunpowder, and the printing press – had been invented by the Chinese already in antiquity and mediaeval times.

[5] Goldsmith, Maurice (1995), *Joseph Needham: 20th Century Renaissance Man*, Profiles UNESCO, Paris, 71.

[6] Three of these publications are in book form, namely Lu Gwei-djen and Joseph Needham (1980), *Celestial Lancets: a History and Rationale of Acupuncture and Moxa*, Cambridge University Press, Cambridge; Needham, Joseph (with Lu Gwei-djen) (1983), *Science and Civilisation in China*, vol. V: *Chemistry and Chemical Technology*, part 5: *Spagyrical Discovery and Invention: Physiological Alchemy*, Cambridge University Press, Cambridge; Needham, Joseph (with Lu Gwei-djen) (1986), *Science and Civilisation in China*, vol. VI: *Biology and Biological Technology*, part 1: *Botany*, Cambridge University Press, Cambridge. Three co-authored articles are in Needham, Joseph et al. (1970), *Clerks and Craftsmen in China and the West*, Cambridge University Press, Cambridge. For a posthumously published and updated version of five earlier publications on medicine, see Needham, Joseph (with Lu Gwei-djen), edited by Sivin, Nathan (2000), *Science and Civilisation in China*, vol. VI: *Biology and Biological Technology*, part 6: *Medicine*. Cambridge University Press, Cambridge.

[7] Lu Gwei-djen (1966), 'China's Greatest Naturalist: a Brief Biography of Li Shih-Chen', *Physis* 8 (4), 383–92.

to be celebrated in modern China and who must have been an important figure in her youth – she was the daughter of a distinguished Nanjing pharmacist.

Needham's history of the Chinese sciences is marked by a comparative cross-cultural stance with a tendency to attribute to China what Europe was not, often in idealised ways, and medicine maintained a very special place in his writings. In an article outlining an oecumenical vision of world sciences, he characterised medicine as one of the most progressive Chinese sciences.[8] He had both great awe and belief in it, and perhaps for this reason he could not terminate his researches on its history in his lifetime. This *Festschrift* in memory of his lifelong Chinese collaborator and second wife, which appears approximately at the same time as the posthumously published *SCC* volume on medicine, represents an attempt to focus on developments in medicine in their own right, without, however, entirely forestalling comparisons with the West.

Despite extensive historical research in East Asia and the West, many practitioners and large sections of the public still hold onto the illusion that 'Traditional Chinese Medicine' is five thousand years old, and that this elaborate edifice of mysticism has remained 'essentially the same' throughout millennia to the present day. Admittedly, there is written evidence of medical concerns which can be traced back thousands of years; inscriptions on oracle bones from the 14th to the 11th century BC, for instance, have been identified with Chinese characters that later appear as part of the medical vocabulary in scholarly treatises. No doubt 'medicine in China', which embraces a great variety of different therapeutic practices, is as old as 'China' itself;[9] but 'medicine in China' is not to be confused with 'Traditional Chinese Medicine'.[10] Needless to say, medical knowledge and practice, like any other aspect of society, have been subject to change.

'Innovation' is a concept more specific than 'change'. As a theme of research for more than half a century now, it has the advantage of providing researchers and readers with a well-known set of questions and reasonably differentiated problems arising from the study of science and technology in Western cultures. Even if the transposition of this

---

[8] Needham, Joseph (1970), 'The Roles of Europe and China in the Evolution of Oecumenical Science', in *Clerks and Craftsmen,* 396–418.

[9] Unschuld, Paul U. (1985), *Medicine in China: a History of Ideas*, University of California Press, Berkeley.

[10] The term 'Traditional Chinese Medicine' (TCM) generally refers to Chinese medicine today. Some authors consider it to reify differences between Western and Chinese but a more recent definition of TCM as the 'revived Chinese medicine that has been promoted by the government of the PRC from the late fifties onwards' overcomes this problem. For a book-length monograph on it, see Farquhar, Judith (1994), *Knowing Practice: the Clinical Encounter of Chinese Medicine*, Westview, Boulder. For the above definition, see Hsu, Elisabeth (1999), *The Transmission of Chinese Medicine*, Cambridge University Press, Cambridge, 9 and 168–223.

concept from one culture to another and from modern to premodern times poses problems, they are not insurmountable. This transposition is moreover facilitated through recent developments within the history of Western post-Renaissance science, and alternative ways of accounting for artefacts and events generally considered as 'innovative' are now outlined by historians – some of them known as 'anthropologists of science' – who study 'innovation' but barely mention the term.[11]

Innovation

Historiography that explains historical changes by indicating solely the conditioning or causal factors, particularly demographic and economic ones, has long been found too simplistic. It was in the course of criticising such a view of history that Schumpeter gave the frequently cited definition of innovation as 'the doing of new things or the doing of things that are already being done in a new way'.[12] He pointed out that there were 'different kinds of reaction to changes in "condition" ' and proposed to distinguish between 'adaptive responses' and 'creative responses', the latter being responses that led to innovation.

The 'creative response', according to Schumpeter, had 'three essential characteristics': it could be understood only *ex post* and practically never *ex ante*; it would shape the course of subsequent events and their long-term outcome; and, admittedly to varying degrees, it depended on the quality of available personnel and individual decisions, actions, and patterns of behaviour. Schumpeter invoked the notion of innovation in the light of historical processes that one recognised as such only in retrospect and could not explain by the usual procedure of searching for conditioning or causal factors. It was a historian's concept for processes that the actors themselves might have phrased in a different vocabulary, an analytic tool of the outside observer. So, regardless of whether or not the historian is interested in the insiders' viewpoint, according to Schumpeter, certain historical processes can be described as the 'creative response' that gives rise to innovation.

As important as Schumpeter's notion of 'innovation' has remained, its flaws have long been apparent. Innovation has as its defining characteristic 'the new', and for Schumpeter 'the new' had a positive value. But people are often ambivalent towards 'the new' and in some historical periods or cultural contexts this may turn into an

[11] See for instance Shapin, Steven and Schaffer, Simon (1985), *Leviathan and the Air-Pump. Hobbes, Boyle, and Experimental Life*, Princeton University Press, Princeton.
[12] Schumpeter, Joseph A. (1947), 'The Creative Response in Economic History', *The Journal of Economic History* 7 (2), 149–59; citation from p. 151.

outright resistance to anything considered 'new'. Particularly in premodern societies 'the new' was usually not advertised as 'new'. Protagonists like Galen in the Hellenistic occident or Sima Qian in Han dynasty China – and on the medical front his spokesman Chunyu Yi – did not present their writings as innovative. They claimed adherence to tradition, and yet to a historian their writings are strikingly 'new', both in style and content. Galen, who presented himself as a commentator of the Hippocratic writings, built a scholarly edifice that was to dominate large parts of the mediaeval world and Sima Qian, who indirectly alluded to Confucius' words 'I transmit and do not create',[13] created the model for the dynastic histories of the following two thousand years. While advocating 'the old' they set the basis for 'the new'.

Schumpeter saw in the 'creative response' a change of social and economic situations 'from which there is no bridge to those situations that might have emerged in its absence'.[14] His article distinguished between the inventor and the copyist, mystified the creativity of the former as inexplicable and held imitation as something mindless and straightforward. Such an understanding of innovation is often grounded in the assumption that, due to their intrinsic superiority, inventions effortlessly diffuse into their surroundings. It postulates that some changes are qualitatively different from others, involving quantum leaps that lead to radically altered conditions; and these conditions are, in turn, often depicted as more stable than they actually are.

None of the contributions to this volume reports on an 'innovation' of that kind, and a historian of modern Western science might want to conclude that the apparent 'lack' of quantum-leap-like innovations arises from the peculiarity of the object of research: medicine in premodern China. Such a historian might take this finding as evidence for the incapacity of Chinese physicians to produce generally accepted 'paradigms' that remained stable over a certain period of time, and thereby explain the lack of 'paradigm shifts'. It is more likely, however, that this volume on innovation contains no recordings of 'innovation' in the above sense because of the contributors' scholarly attitude to time and change, and their style of writing medical history.

Convention and controversy

The view of 'medicine in the making' that many of the articles in this book present relates to the social background, technological premises, and conventional knowledge at certain time periods, and to the kind of controversies medical practitioners and

---

[13] Durrant, Stephen W. (1995), *The Cloudy Mirror: Tension and Conflict in the Writings of Sima Qian*, State University of New York Press, Albany, 11.

[14] Schumpeter (1947), 150.

scholars engaged in which eventually led to the changes in medical practice and doctrine that are here offered as examples of innovation in Chinese medicine. The changes described may have been gradual or sudden, they may concern an entire system of thought and medical practice or a single artefact, they may have been instigated by a single individual or they may have happened without there being a known initiator. They concern a wide range of medical endeavour, and include changes in diagnostic methods and techniques, therapeutic practices, pharmaceutical artefacts, philosophical and medical concepts, perceptions of the body, and canonical doctrine as well as other genres of medical writing.

By conceiving of medical innovation as an interplay between convention and controversy the historian stresses the importance of social processes for technological advancement. Innovation in this sense is seen not merely as knowledge production, 'discovery', or invention. Rather, problems related to the validation of newly produced knowledge are emphasised. Since the new is not by definition better, its spread is no more viewed as a natural process of diffusion along a gradient of unequal advancement in technology, and the question is raised of why people are prepared to adopt practices with which they are unacquainted. The acceptance of new ideas and the reproduction of novel artefacts are now viewed as processes that represent a challenge; they are not intrinsically superior. Individuals and social groups receive the new in an active and selective process and they reproduce it more often than not by translation and re-invention. Exact replication has been shown to pose considerable problems; it is not the natural outcome of mindless 'copyists'. Research is thus directed away from the intellectual achievements of heroic individuals and towards institutional settings, state policies, environmental factors, economic incentive; in short, the interests of mutually interacting social groups.

The medical writings investigated in this volume are often technical and particular to a lineage of scholarship, but the nature of the material permitted investigation of the interests of the social groups who produced the medical writings. The information on the authors of the texts discussed in this volume is limited and sometimes scarce, but often it was possible to identify their social standing. A careful reading of their texts has made possible inferences of who the targeted audiences of these texts were, and who the adversaries. Even in the case of unknown authorship, attempts have been made to situate the texts within the social landscape of the period. Generally speaking, the authors of the texts discussed in this volume came from a literate elite. As a consequence, we specify that the texts in this book reflect less the history of 'medicine in China' than that of the medicine of the elite in Imperial times: the history of 'Chinese medicine'. Yet, as we shall see, this elite was diverse with regard to lineage tradition and personal experience, functionary roles and loyalties within and towards the Imperial court, and its interests varied not only geographically but also over time.[15]

The structure of the book

This book is divided into six parts, each comprising two articles on a related theme. These articles are arranged in the order of the events discussed. They are best read as detailed case studies that analyse important aspects of the complex history of Chinese medicine, but they do not aspire to present this history in any comprehensive way. By highlighting given conventions and controversies over them, each article addresses a change in medical doctrine and/or practice that can be viewed as innovative; 'innovation' being treated here as an overarching theme for new approaches to writing history of a premodern science.

Part I describes '*mai* 脈 and *qi* 氣' as two of the most central notions that laid the foundations for Chinese medical reasoning among the medical elite in Imperial times. Even though their meanings varied with place and changed over time, and although in more recent history attempts were made to do away with these two concepts altogether, they deserve particular attention. Vivienne Lo and Elisabeth Hsu emphasise that they came to refer to subtle movements and changes imperceptible to the non-initiated, and although the two articles deal with geographically distant traditions, they both point out common aspects of a body conception in terms of the subtle *mai* and *qi*, findings which implicitly suggest that this opened up the field for medical speculation.

Numerology provides in many traditional sciences a schema for ordering knowledge and a device for speculations about the future. Correlative thinking was not specific to the science of Chinese medicine. It was, as the articles in part II of the book, on 'Correlative cosmologies', show, already prevalent among 'gentlemen with formulae', *fangshi* 方士, who predated the elite doctors in Imperial times, *yi* 醫, by several centuries and later rivalled them, not least over clientele. Donald Harper focuses on some numerological considerations in iatromantic texts on the art of prognosticating the outcome of illness and how they became integrated into medical doctrine. This highlights aspects of how the first imposition of numerology onto Chinese medical reasoning led to the

---

[15] 'Chinese medicine', as a term in the singular, has the danger of invoking a unity of medical practice and doctrine when this term actually refers to a host of practices that first emerged among the elite in the Western Han and can be traced to the present day in numerous lineages of knowledge transmission. Aware of the plurality of different traditions that the term refers to and the controversies between them, one may be tempted to speak of 'Chinese medicines'.

predominance of Five Phase doctrine in Han medical writings which gave rise to what is
commonly known as the 'medicine of systematic correspondences'. Catherine Despeux
discusses a second important event involving a numerological reorganisation in the history of canonical medical doctrine: it had its roots in the Tang dynasty and was in its
full-blown form promulgated by the Song Imperial court, and led to what is known
as the doctrine of the five circulatory phases and six seasonal influences (*wuyun liuqi*
五運六氣) or 'phase energetics'.[16]

   Whereas the concepts *mai* and *qi* developed in the context of cautery and needling
therapy and cleared the ground for medical authority to establish itself through numero-
logically dominated speculation, drug therapy did not play an important role in the
formulation of the canonical Chinese medical doctrine and is considered for many
centuries to have continued to be grounded primarily in empiricism.[17] Part III, on
'Dietetics and pharmacotherapy', contains contributions that discuss innovations within the *materia medica* (*bencao* 本草), the third of the three main traditions of medical
writing in addition to those on medical doctrine (*benjing* 本經) and formulae (*fangji*
方劑). These two contributions on *bencao* literature complement each other insofar as
Ute Engelhardt discusses the categorisation of foodstuffs – waterchestnut and horse
liver – and Frédéric Obringer focuses on a variety of rather toxic substances – arsenic
compounds – and the innovative but short-lived technique used to produce them. Their
juxtaposition highlights the general ambivalence that Chinese physicians had to drugs
(*yao* 藥) and alchemical traditions of drug intake.

   In Late Imperial China the era of the Han was often appraised as that of the genuine
and original doctrine of Chinese medicine, and later writings were degraded to mere
amendments. The two articles on 'The canons revisited' in part IV show that the reap-
praisal of canonical works in fact consisted of virulently innovative scholarship.
The posthumously published *Bencao gangmu* 本草綱目 (Hierarchically Classified
Materia Medica) (1596) by Li Shizhen 李時珍 (1518–93) represents the pinnacle of
the Chinese *bencao* literature. While this text is firmly grounded within the medical
tradition, Georges Métailié has repeatedly stressed its importance for the emergence
of Chinese studies in natural history and the article in this volume provides ample
evidence to corroborate his claim. Similarly, the *Shanghan zabing lun* 傷寒雜病論
(Treatise on Cold Damage and Miscellaneous Disorders) written by Zhang Ji 張機
in the Eastern Han is still today considered the most important work of the formulae

---

[16] Term used by Porkert, Manfred (1974), *The Theoretical Foundations of Chinese Medicine: Systems of
Correspondence*, MIT Press, Cambridge, Mass., 55–106.
[17] According to Unschuld, Paul U. (1986), *Medicine in China: a History of Pharmaceutics,* University of
California Press, Berkeley, 112, the first 'pharmacology of systematic correspondences' dates to the
Song.

tradition of medical writing. It was lost but reconstituted in the Song and, as Marta Hanson shows, its reappropriation by scholar–physicians of the Jiangnan area in the Ming and Qing led to the formulation of the medical doctrine of warmth factor illnesses (*wenbing xue* 溫病學) that ever since has rivalled the pre-eminence of the cold damage tradition.

Whereas the two articles on the canonical *grands oeuvres* required extensive discussion, thereby reflecting the enormous wealth and complexity of knowledge they dealt with, part V, on 'Medical case histories', consists of articles of remarkable brevity and conciseness, by Christopher Cullen and Bridie Andrews. These two articles discuss Chinese physicians who themselves were much concerned with clarity in knowledge presentation and who outlined new ways of structuring information derived from the clinical encounter. Endeavours of this kind, which in the Ming gave rise to a new medical genre, are followed up through the Qing to the Republican period, where the adjustment to Western biomedical practice resulted in interesting modifications. While they have indeed led to a more direct integration of knowledge from treatment of individual cases, they are also shown to provide a standard schema for recording experience in medical practice.

The book ends with a section on 'Medical rationale in the People's Republic', part VI, which not only points out adjustments to a new political style but also indicates much diversity of current medical practice. Kim Taylor's article focuses on a politically motived Western medical doctor who epitomised the movement of 'new acumoxa' (*xin zhenjiu* 新針灸) in the late 1940s and early 1950s and Volker Scheid compares two Chinese medical doctors and their prescriptions for treating dizziness (*touyun* 頭暈 and *xuanyun* 眩暈 respectively) on the basis of ethnographic fieldwork in the mid-1990s. The controversies over Chinese medical practice that these two articles address are strikingly different. Where Taylor highlights unification through political indoctrination, Scheid emphasises pluralism in government-run institutions; where Taylor mentions application of the Soviet sciences, Scheid stresses adaptation of Western medicine; and where Taylor shows how canonical knowledge was done away with, Scheid delves into tracing medical lineages and establishes genealogies of drug prescriptions. These changes of recent decades involve an accentuation of those of the previous two millennia.

Innovation, convention, and controversy

The student interested in the history of science may wonder what can be learnt from this inquiry into a premodern non-Western medical science. It is futile to try to summarise the multilayered articles of this volume in one final paragraph, for the changes identified as 'innovation' are rather diverse in kind. Nevertheless we may note that one of the most frequently encountered innovations discussed in this volume arises from combining knowledge from different traditions of learning. This combination of knowledge sometimes led to the emergence of a novel doctrine or a new literary genre. Another kind of medical innovation consisted of the reordering and reinterpreting of existent medical knowledge that gave rise to entirely new fields of inquiry. It could also involve a formulaic structure for presenting already existent knowledge, an aspect characteristic of medical case histories. Numerological systematisation was yet another form of such formulaic knowledge presentation, and the two chapters treating innovations of numerological systematisation (in part II) discuss two of the most important and long-lived innovations in Chinese medical doctrine. Notably, most of the articles are concerned with innovation in 'literary technology' and only one deals with a technical invention. Given that some of the articles point to the self-awareness of the actors that they were doing something new, while others identify an innovation, often on structural grounds, without having any information of the actors' attitude at all, we acknowledge that in this book the notion of innovation has been applied to a premodern science, regardless of whether the innovation was proclaimed as such or not.

Editor's note

This book brings together research on Chinese medicine from fairly different strands. Given the variety of translations of Chinese medical terminology – most notably by Manfred Porkert, Paul Unschuld, and Nathan Sivin – and the continuing search for adequate translation, I promised from the very start not to impose adherence to a particular terminology throughout the book. For the reader this means that the same Chinese medical term may be approximated in translation by a whole variety of different English words. Therefore great editorial effort was directed at giving a Chinese medical term both in the official transcription system *pinyin* (also in citations originally given in other transcription systems) and in Chinese characters. This should allow the reader to recognise the same term even when its translation varies in different articles.

I also refrained from standardising the translation of book titles and from imposing use of particular editions of the Chinese works – it is a regrettable but dire reality for researchers on Chinese medicine that some of the best editions of canonical works are not widely available. Dates of composition, compilation, or publication are similarly difficult to standardise, and I have adopted the dates given by the individual authors. Book and chapter titles are therefore consistently referred to by their Chinese names, and only well-known works, such as the *Yellow Emperor's Inner Canon* (*Huangdi neijing*) and the like, are first mentioned in English.

The articles deal with a wide range of distinct aspects of Chinese medical knowledge and practice and references are therefore listed at the end of each article; their thematic presentation should enhance clarity and also encourage entry into this burgeoning field of study. They are generally divided into two sections: the first section contains pre-modern Chinese and Japanese works and the second section contains modern works in any language, listed alphabetically by their authors' names. Recently unearthed manuscripts are generally found in the second section under the name of the research group or individual researcher who annotated and transcribed them.

At the beginning of each of the six parts, the two articles of the section are summarised and contextualised. These part introductions are primarily intended to tease out and highlight those processes discussed in the articles that gave rise to the innovations in question.

PART I

Mai and *qi* in the Western Han

Introduction

In the late Warring States a literate elite had established itself in various localities, including as geographically disparate areas as those of present-day Hunan and Shandong provinces, where the medical texts presented in this part come from. Modern scholarship has drawn a vivid picture of the intellectual activities of the nobility and their retainers, their beliefs and convictions, art and technology, and also their daily life.[1] In this milieu the two concepts *mai* 脈 and *qi* 氣 were combined to form the foundations of the elaborate system of Chinese medical doctrine.

In chapter 1, Vivienne Lo asks how it was that the notion of *qi* came to be seen as the basic vital substance that it is in the Chinese 'medical canons' (such as the *Yellow Emperor's Inner Canon* (Huangdi neijing 黃帝內經) and subsequent medical works). In this context she also inquires why names of acumoxa *loci* (*xuewei* 穴位), in contrast to channel (*mai*) names, often convey a strong metaphoric imagery that transposes geographic, architectural, and social landmarks onto the body.

Mai figures as a prominent term among what Lo calls 'acumoxa-related writings'. For instance, in the so-called 'Cauterisation Canons' or 'vessel texts', which were unearthed from a tomb in Mawangdui closed in 168 BC, *mai* are conveyed as routes around the body. Their course is described with verbs of motion, referring to a movement along or through an anatomical location. The description of their course generally begins at the extremities and ends in the body's trunk or head, without further specification of internal structures and functions. *Mai* are in general differentiated from each other depending on whether they run along the upper or lower extremities (arms or legs), and in terms of *yin* 陰 and *yang* 陽. Their names refer to qualities of *yin* and *yang* that express a gradation which remains difficult to interpret, from the *yangming* 陽明 to the *taiyang* 太陽 to the *shaoyang* 少陽 and from the *taiyin* 太陰 to the *shaoyin* 少陰 to the *jueyin* 厥陰.[2]

---

[1] See for instance Harper, Donald (1998). *Early Chinese Medical Literature: the Mawangdui Medical Manuscripts*. Routledge, London, 3–183.

[2] Since only eleven *mai* (and not the twelve canonical ones, namely three *yin* and three *yang* of feet and arms) are described, one of these qualities is not mentioned, the *jueyin* in the arm.

Thematically, these texts consist of two parts. The first informs on the course of the *mai*, and the second part attributes to each *mai* a series of illness conditions that are said to be alleviated by cauterising the *mai*.[3] In these 'acumoxa-related writings' the *mai* thus have a primarily classificatory function for therapeutic intervention.

Vivienne Lo's chapter builds on the recognition that the Mawangdui medical manuscripts – which were found in the same lacquer box and probably intended for the same readership – include various genres. She distinguishes between the above genre of 'acumoxa-related writings' and another genre that she calls 'nurturing life literature'. These two genres anticipate the categories of *zhenjiu* 針灸 (acupuncture and moxibustion, or acumoxa for short) and *yangsheng* 養生 (nurturing life), common in later literature but not attested in the Mawangdui medical corpus. However, regardless of their naming, Lo convinces the reader that the literary styles of the two genres differ significantly. She points out that the 'Cauterisation Canons' give a dispassionate view of the body, and that their descriptions of the body are primarily visual. She contrasts this view of the body with that in one of the works belonging to the 'nurturing life literature', a text on the sexual arts entitled 'Harmonising *yin* and *yang*' (He yinyang 合陰陽), which portrays human sensuality with a poetic lyricism that depicts the body as a landscape of mountains, rivers, surging seas, and other metaphors of the natural and human world as it was conceived at the time.

There is no mention of acumoxa *loci* in the 'Cauterisation Canons', and Lo suggests that the metaphors designating body parts in the sexual arts texts were later incorporated, as names of acumoxa *loci*, into medical writing. They figure in 'medical canons' that were compiled a few centuries later and have been transmitted to us in extant works that have continued to the present day to be regarded as canonical. In the medical canons the visually perceived *mai* from the Mawangdui acumoxa-related writings are littered with *loci* with names reminiscent of the subjectively felt sensuality recorded in the Mawangdui nurturing life literature. The innovation that Lo discusses thus arises from a conflation of two different genres of body description.

Lo furthermore points out that the notion *qi*, which is generally not mentioned in the acumoxa-related writings,[4] is frequently encountered in the 'nurturing life literature'. In texts on the sexual arts 'the extension of *qi*' (*zhang qi* 張氣) describes the sensations of the woman during her orgasm, 'the arrival of *qi*' (*qi zhi* 氣至) the sensation of the

---

[3] This is so according to one but not the other edition of the 'Cauterisation Canons', the 'Foot-Arm Eleven Vessels Cauterisation Canon' (Zubi shiyimai jiujing 足臂十一脈灸經).

[4] There is one exception, a sentence in the 'Document of the Mai' (Maishu 脈書), which interrelates *mai* and *qi* in the context of discussing therapeutic techniques, and Lo takes it as the earliest extant evidence of acumoxa therapy, which she defines as the therapeutic application of needling in order to manipulate *qi*.

man in that moment;[5] and what she calls augmenting and strengthening *qi* are presented as a common principle of proper sexual conduct and breathing techniques. In the nurturing life literature, *qi*, which was later to become one of the predominant concepts of medical discourse, refers to subjectively felt sensations in the body. Lo suggests that this language of subjective experience, developed in the genre of nurturing life literature, was transferred to that of describing the body in terms of *mai*, and in the process made possible more sophisticated ways of medical reasoning.

For the full-blown system of Chinese medical doctrine to emerge the person had to be seen as a whole and medical language had to have a means to account for both the body in anatomical terms and the subjective sensual experience of the individual. Elisabeth Hsu, in chapter 2, comes to the same conclusion: she noticed that the twenty-five medical case histories in the biography of a Western Han doctor, Chunyu Yi 淳于意, recorded in the *Shiji* 史記 (Records of the Historian) (*ca* 90 BC), invariably concerned illness designated by the term *bing* 病 rather than the more commonly used word *ji* 疾 of contemporaneous non-medical writings. Her systematic investigation of *bing* (disorder) in the *Zuo zhuan* 左傳 (Zuo Tradition) revealed that, apart from other meanings, *bing* frequently referred to the emotional state of a person who is aggrieved, often as a result of a previous dispute. On these grounds she suggests that *bing* in the *Shiji* case histories reflects an understanding of illness with regard to a person as a mind–emotion–body complex.

This 'holistic' view of personhood is often stressed as one of the characteristics of Chinese medicine, but because of the uncritical ways in which it is currently used, the term 'holistic' has become meaningless. The finding that medical language included words for expressing subjective sensual experience and emotional distress is better interpreted from a different angle. Considering that the Mawangdui medical manuscripts were found in a tomb of the nobility in the Han kingdom of Chu 楚, and that the medical cases in the *Shiji* were recorded by a doctor sought by the nobility of mostly the kingdom of Qi 齊, we may conclude that it was within the social stratum of the elite that this language began to be cultivated. Insofar as terms like *qi* and *bing* reflected an increased attention to cognitive and emotional processes, we may say that the vocabulary of this language had 'psychologising' tendencies.

In a similar vein, we observe a transformation of the notion *mai* from a term for somatic structure to a more subtle concept. The *mai*, with their clearly demarcated routes, that according to Lo were visually perceived, appear to be anatomical entities in the Mawangdui vessel texts, but in the medical case histories of the *Shiji*, they are more difficult to define: the doctor examines the *mai* and as a result senses different qualities

---

[5] In later acumoxa texts *qi zhi* indicates that needling has been successful.

of *qi*. Hsu therefore proposes to render *mai* in translation as 'vessel-pulses' or as 'pulses' (*nota bene*, not the kind of pulses that biomedicine recognises). Compared with the above understanding of *qi* and *bing*, the notion *mai* is probably less psychologised, while it has a newly acquired sense of 'impulsion' and 'movement' that goes beyond the purely anatomical and alludes to a reality of bodily processes for which a materialist worldview has neither recognition nor vocabulary.

The *Shiji* medical case histories contain the first textual evidence to date of a repeatedly endorsed and systemic interrelating of *mai* and *qi*, which in Hsu's analysis was done with the intention of determining the names of different *bing*. Hsu therefore proposes to regard this text as the earliest extant account of Chinese pulse diagnostics. The notion of *qi*, as already said, is not mentioned in the Mawangdui vessel texts, and this is corroborated by the finding that *qi* in the *Shiji* is never put in correlation with any of the Mawangdui designations of *mai* in terms of *taiyang* or *jueyin* and the like. Hsu observes that by contrast *qi* is often related to the standard five viscera of the medical canons, namely the liver (*gan* 肝), the heart (*xin* 心), the spleen (*pi* 脾), the lungs (*fei* 肺), and the kidneys (*shen* 腎).

The finding that in the *Shiji* chapter 105.2 it is mostly the *qi* that correlates with the five viscera which are detected in the *mai* deserves further attention. It may well indicate that *qi* and the five viscera were first in correlation with each other, and that the viscera were correlated with the *mai* only in a second step. Hsu's article, together with ongoing unpublished research on the first five chapters of the book called *Plain Questions* (Suwen 素問), which constitutes the first book of the *Yellow Emperor's Inner Canon*, suggests that it was only after correlating the viscera with the *mai* that *qi* started to flow in the *mai*. She proposes to view the diagnostic procedure of examining *mai* to detect qualities of *qi* as laying the foundations for a systemic correlation between the five *zang* viscera and the *mai* vessel-pulses. According to Bridgman,[6] the correlations differed from those given in the later medical canons, with their *locus classicus* in chapter 10 of the *Divine Pivot* (Lingshu 靈樞), the second book in the *Yellow Emperor's Inner Canon*; but Hsu's preliminary evidence contests Bridgman.

Medical authority had reached a stage of self-assertion that degraded the patient's perception of pain and illness to unspecific ailments and superficial complaints. Now it was the physician who had the knowledge and authority to detect the underlying condition. In Chunyu Yi's medical case histories *qi* did not only have the sense of subjectively felt 'breath', but figured also in cosmological discourse: the person as a microcosm was linked through the intermediary of *qi* to external workings in the

---

[6] Bridgman, R. F. (1955), 'La Médicine dans la Chine Antique', *Mélanges Chinois et Bouddhiques* 10, 141–5.

macrocosm. The elaborate system of Chinese medical reasoning was made possible not only by psychologising the medical conditions of a person, but also by embedding the person in the environment and taking account of the seasons, the climate, and the ecology.

Hsu points out that these case histories had a highly formulaic structure, similar to the structure of 'models' for jurisdiction in Qin law which prescribed how an official should record individual cases, and she suggests that the recording of each unique case within such a general matrix made it possible to account for illness (*bing*) in a multi-faceted and systemic way. Within a schema identified through linguistic markers Chunyu Yi is shown consistently to provide a name, a cause, and a justification for naming a client's illness.[7] The justification for naming specific *bing*, which implies, as Hsu emphasises, a sophisticated notion of illness, is couched in the terminology of the elusive concepts *mai* and *qi*. Medical authority asserts itself by claiming to have access to esoteric knowledge that gives it the capacity to recognise subtle changes, imperceptible to the non-initiated, in a systemic way.

In this context it is worth mentioning that from the very beginning the medical authority of the elite did not present itself as a homogenous unity; *Shiji* 105.2 mentions adversaries, both internal and external. The external ones Yi dismissively refers to as the 'common doctors' (*zhong yi* 眾醫), and he accuses them in seven cases of misdiagnosis, and in one even of iatrogenic illness. In two cases Yi refers to adversaries who have name and position, and seem to have a degree of medical learning similar to his own. In both cases the application of textual knowledge to the particular case in question becomes a matter of controversy. As the articles in the following parts will show, controversies of this kind continued in the centuries to come.

---

[7] Yi concomitantly mentions his clients' complaints and his own observations of what we would nowadays call 'symptoms', but these observations are not reported within that schema.

1

The influence of nurturing life culture on the development of Western Han acumoxa therapy

VIVIENNE LO

When tomb no. 3 at Changsha 長沙 Mawangdui 馬王堆, a burial mound outside the capital of the old Han kingdom of Chu 楚, was first opened in the early 1970s, scholars could hardly have predicted the degree to which its contents would revolutionise the history of Chinese medicine.[1] Nearly thirty years later the silk and bamboo manuscripts, which the tomb had preserved since its closure in 168 BC, still provide a rich resource for lively debate and new insights into the state of the heavens, the earth, and human society during the early Western Han period. Archaeologists have opened numerous tombs in Chu and elsewhere which have offered up further material for comparison. This study will focus on the texts excavated at Mawangdui and at one other tomb (no. 247) at Jiangling 江陵 Zhangjiashan 張家山.[2]

Evidence from Mawangdui has filled gaps in our knowledge of the relationship of spirit mediums or shamans and their magical practices and incantations to early Chinese medicine.[3] Recipe texts such as 'Wushi'er bingfang' 五十二病方 (Recipes for Fifty-two Illnesses), the largest text of the medical finds, give detailed instructions of how to prepare treatments for specific, named illnesses.[4] Remedies might include

---

[1] The Mawangdui burial mound is located in the northeastern section of Changsha, Hunan. It contains three tombs. Tombs no. 1 and no. 2 belonged to the Lord of Dai 軑, Li Cang 利蒼, and his wife (who was buried in tomb no. 1). Tomb no. 3, from which the manuscripts were excavated, was occupied by one of their sons, who died in 168 BC at the age of about 30. For the excavation report see Hunansheng bowuguan and Zhongguo kexueyuan kaogu yanjiusuo (1974). Details of the find are also in the introduction to Mawangdui Han mu boshu zhengli xiaozu (1980).

[2] On the dating of the Zhangjiashan tomb in Hubei and the identity of its occupant, see Zhangjiashan Han mu zhujian zhengli xiaozu (1985). See also Gao Dalun (1995), 3–7, and Shi Yunzi (1994). It seems that the earliest date for the closure of the tomb is 186 BC with a latest date of 156 BC.

[3] In a number of articles Harper introduces the magical aspects of Warring States medical practice. See for instance Harper (1985). His findings are collected together in *Early Chinese Medical Literature* (1998), 42–68 and 148–83.

[4] The texts did not originally bear titles. I use those given by Mawangdui Han mu boshu zhengli xiaozu (1985).

cautery, the preparation of herbs and animal substances, often selected for their magical properties. Many specify incantations and exorcism of the kind that would require the help or tuition of a specialist intermediary. Among the Mawangdui medical manuscripts there is also important evidence of a new medicine in its infancy – a medicine related to correlative cosmology and its theories of *yinyang*. Central to the new medicine are texts which conceptualise the body in *mai* 脈 (channels)[5] and an examination of the mode of construction of this concept of *mai* is the basic task of this chapter.

Both tombs, at Mawangdui and Zhangjiashan, have provided manuscripts that change our understanding of the *mai*,[6] which were fundamental to the development of classical medical theory first formulated in Han times. Their titles and descriptions bear similarities to the *jingmai* 經脈 (conduits, circulation tracts) of later acumoxa theory and the texts are therefore early examples of a textual genre that we can trace to later compilations such as *Huangdi neijing Lingshu* 黃帝內經靈樞 (Yellow Emperor's Inner Canon: the Numinous Pivot).[7] The Mawangdui medical manuscripts include two such

---

[5] Mawangdui Han mu boshu zhengli xiaozu (1985) contains the official transcription of the Mawangdui medical manuscripts as well as photographs of the originals. Ma Jixing (1992) also provides a transcription and full commentary for all of the medical texts (for many of the texts a modern Chinese rendering is also supplied). The texts are thought to be no earlier than the third century BC. See Ma Jixing (1992), 92. A translation of the entire corpus of the Mawangdui medical manuscripts is in Harper (1998).

[6] The word *mai* is difficult to translate. Harper (1982) translates 'vessel', which draws out the early association with the arteriovenous system. I prefer to follow the contemporary analogy with channel (*du* 瀆) or 'canal' found in the 'Maishu' 脈書 (Channel Document). See Jiangling Zhangjiashan Han jian zhengli xiaozu (1989), 74 (hereafter, 'Maishu' shiwen). The translation 'channel' also serves to emphasise the relationship of the *mai* to the superficial anatomical channels as defined by muscle and bone, as they were understood before the more elaborate theories of the *jingluo* and *jingmai* found in *Huangdi neijing* 黃帝內經 (Yellow Emperor's Inner Canon). *Jingluo* or *jingmai* has been variously translated as 'conduit', 'meridian', 'circulation tract', etc. As the focus of this paper is the excavated medical writing from Hubei and Hunan, which is representative of an earlier period, it is not necessary to commit to a definitive translation of the terms at present. See Sivin (1987), 34, 122 note 11; and Unschuld (1985), 75, 81–3.

[7] *Huangdi neijing* is a corpus now extant in three recensions, the *Taisu* (太素 Great Basis), the *Suwen* (素問 Basic Questions), and the *Lingshu* (靈樞 Numinous Pivot). See Sivin (1993). Each of these is a compilation of small texts dealing with separate topics which may reflect the thinking in a distinct medical lineage. It is thought that the earliest texts were set down during the first or at the earliest the second century BC. Collectively they represent the kind of debate through which classical medical concepts matured. In this respect they act as a convenient marker against which to assess the form and content of the excavated texts. For an extended discussion of the development of medical theories in China based on a clarification of the formation of the *Huangdi neijing*, see Yamada (1979); for a reassessment of the origins of acumoxa, see Unschuld (1985), 93–9. Since the discovery of the excavated manuscripts, most medical historians now agree that an essential fusion of the technical and theoretical elements at the foundation of acumoxa therapy could not have happened much before the first two centuries BC. See Sivin (1993) and Yamada (1979). The canons of acumoxa must also include Huangfu Mi's *Zhenjiu jiayijing* 針灸甲乙經 (AB Canon of Acumoxa) (AD 256–82) and the *Nanjing* 難經 (Canon of Difficulties) (first or second century AD), the latter of which is translated in Unschuld (1986).

texts; their Chinese editors have given one of the texts the title of 'Zubi shiyimai jiujing' 足臂十一脈灸經 (Cauterisation Canon of the Eleven Foot and Arm Channels; hereafter, 'Zubi jiujing') and the other they have called 'Yinyang shiyimai jiujing' 陰陽十一脈灸經 (Cauterisation Canon of the Eleven *yin* and *yang* Channels; hereafter, 'Yinyang jiujing'). Two editions of this latter text were found at Mawangdui, yet another edition was found at Zhangjiashan as part of a compilation titled 'Maishu' 脈書 (Channel Document). 'Maishu', I shall argue, is the earliest treatise to set down explicitly the theory and practice of acumoxa.

Among the manuscripts which were folded together in a rectangular lacquer box at Mawangdui there was a significant amount of writing that set out the philosophy and techniques of nurturing life (*yangsheng* 養生). I use the term 'nurturing life' to refer to those techniques broadly aimed at physical cultivation and longevity which formed a part of elite culture during the Western Han period. The *yangsheng* practices documented in the Mawangdui and Zhangjiashan medical manuscripts include therapeutic gymnastics, dietetics, breath- and sexual-cultivation. The Zhangjiashan manual of therapeutic gymnastics (*daoyin* 導引 literally 'guiding and pulling'), known as 'Yinshu' 引書[8] (Pulling Document), and parts of the Mawangdui manual 'Shiwen' 十問 (Ten Questions) are of particular significance to this study.

Both 'Shiwen' and two further works from Mawangdui that I shall cite, the 'Tianxia zhi dao tan' 天下至道談 (Discussion of the Highest Way Under Heaven) and 'He yinyang' 合陰陽 (Harmonising *yin* and *yang*), specialise in sexual-cultivation. In these three texts sexual-cultivation practice is often combined with elements of breath-cultivation,[9] a combination which later Daoist and medical literature preserves alongside other *yangsheng* practices.[10] *Yangsheng* focuses on preserving and strengthening the body, and the Mawangdui texts give fine detail of technique and practice. It is therefore a significant branch of medicine and was viewed as such by the book collectors who placed *yangsheng* literature together with other texts that concentrated

---

[8] 'Yinshu' transcript can be found in Zhangjiashan Han jian zhengli zu (1990), (hereafter, 'Yinshu' shiwen), accompanied by a detailed analysis by Peng Hao (1990). For a general introduction and annotated transcript see Gao Dalun (1995).

[9] Mawangdui Han mu boshu zhengli xiaozu (1985) 155–6, 163–7, and 146–8. Breath-cultivation involves specific breathing techniques thought to adjust favourably the internal environment of the body by balancing temperature and dryness/humidity in order to build up and store vital essences.

[10] *Beiji qianjin yaofang* 備急千金要方 (Essential Prescriptions Worth a Thousand, for Urgent Need), *juan* 27, 489, is titled 'Yangxing' 養性 (Nurturing Nature). The chapter includes instructions on massage, adjusting the *qi*, breathing exercises, and the sexual arts. The most comprehensive account in English of nurturing life practice can be found in a collection of articles in Kohn (1989).

more specifically on the treatment of illness. The full range of medical practices represented in the Mawangdui medical manuscripts is also reflected in the 'Recipes and Techniques' (*fangji* 方技) section of the 'Yiwen zhi' 藝文志 (Record of Literary Pursuits), the bibliographical treatise in the *Han shu* 漢書 (Document of the Han) (AD 32–92).[11]

A comparison of language and concepts evident in early descriptions of the *mai* with the body as it is revealed in *yangsheng* literature will demonstrate the differences between these two genres of medical literature. At a time when literature describing the *mai* barely recognised an organised movement of *qi* 氣 through the body, when it made no clear reference to acumoxa points, when correspondences with *yin* and *yang* were barely elaborated, the *yangsheng* literature reveals all of this and more. Can we then see a link between *yangsheng* culture of the late Warring States to the early Imperial period and the medical theory and practice found in the acumoxa canons?[12] To answer this question I shall refer extensively to the *Huangdi neijing* compilation, the title most famous for its exposition of classical acumoxa theories.

This paper, for the first time, will begin to explore the contribution that the observation and recording of a phenomenological experience of 'own' body, unique to *yangsheng* literature, made to classical Chinese medical thought. Observations about the body in *yangsheng* literature reflect a realm of human experience that, for obvious reasons, is not evident in medical literature that describes the illness and cure of other bodies. Where the eyes cease to organise and control their environment, visualisation may free our physical space through the practice of meditation. Breath-cultivation may bring increased vitality and a clarity of the spirit, feelings elicited in sexual arts may landscape the body with mountains, rivers, and spurting seas. In this liminal world the body may become a universe, a temple, or a continent.[13] An elaborate code which could at once embrace the body in its spiritual, physical, geographic, and political dimensions was to become a recurring device throughout Daoist literature.

A *yangsheng* culture

In describing the body in its relationship with the macrocosmos, early Chinese *yangsheng* literature brings a metaphysical language into the realm of human physical experience. With its focus on longevity rather than pathology, it sets down a standard physiology of the internal environment of the body. *Yangsheng* techniques, then, describe many ways to assert control over this physiological process. The primary

---

[11] The *Han shu* 'Yiwen zhi', *juan* 30, 1776–80, lists books contained in the Han court library around the end of the first century BC. It is taken from the lost catalogue of Liu Xin 劉歆 (46 BC–AD 23).
[12] See note 7.   [13] Schipper (1993), 100–12.

object of the present study is to examine the dynamic between the medical fields of *yangsheng* and the newly emerging medical models of the body based upon the *mai*.

The criteria for defining exactly which kind of activity came under the umbrella of nurturing life varies according to the period. By the time of the tenth-century Japanese medical work *Ishinpō* 醫心方 (Recipes at the Heart of Medicine), a compilation that preserves a great deal of early Chinese material, the 'Yangsheng' chapter includes such diverse topics as sleep, clothing, and propriety of language. Five of the practices listed in the *Ishinpō* are already represented in the literature of Mawangdui and Zhangjiashan.[14] Mawangdui practices also include the daily ingestion and application of mineral drugs, ingestion of talismans, and ritual interdiction. Recognised as coming under the general rubric of *yangsheng* are contemporary callisthenic exercises in revived form such as *taiji quan* (太極拳) and *qigong* (氣功), the therapeutic movement practised by young and old in Chinese city parks in the morning.

The preponderance of nurturing life texts among the burial goods in the tombs at Zhangjiashan and Mawangdui suggests that the courtly elite of Chu were familiar with the way of life advocated in the texts. I argue elsewhere that a figurine, buried five hundred miles away in south-west China, also testifies to the more general spread of nurturing life culture.[15] Burial goods were similar in design and quality, so it seems likely that the rich culture in the Chu tombs, which was once thought to be exclusive to the southern kingdom, is representative of the central core of elite society in the provincial courts and military outposts of the empire in the early Western Han period.

Despite the fact that *yangsheng* is an evolving category during the Warring States period and does not, by itself, refer to all the practices it later embraces, it is still relevant to consider the emergence of different types of physical activities for enhancing life as a distinctive trend. The above mentioned 'Record of Literary Pursuits' (Yiwen zhi) in the *Han shu* lists eight sexual-cultivation works which testify that they formed a significant part of mainstream medical literature.

Many Warring States writers also seem to know practices akin to nurturing life culture. Breath-cultivation and meditation are particularly common. References to nurturing life practice emerge incidentally in comment or as a more conscious part of a health care regime. The references are not always complimentary. *Zhuangzi* 莊子

---

[14] *Ishinpō*, *juan* 27, 449–59. For some remarks on the sources of the nurturing life material, see Barrett (1980). The five practices are breath-cultivation (*yongqi* 用氣, *shiqi* 食氣), sexual-cultivation (*fangnei* 房內), therapeutic gymnastics (*daoyin* 導引), regulated sleep (*woqi* 臥起), and dietetics (*tiaoshi* 調食).

[15] The figurine is made of black lacquered wood and has red lines which run from head to foot. An analysis of the lines and how they relate to the channels of acumoxa theory as well as other medical practices such as *yangsheng* can be found in He Zhiguo and Lo (1996).

(fourth – second centuries BC) criticises people who nurture the body (*yangxing* 養形) as falling short of the true *dao* 道 (the way):

> To huff and puff, exhale and inhale, blow out the old and draw in the new, do the 'bear-hang' and the 'bird-stretch', interested only in long life – such are the tastes of the practitioners of 'guide-and-pull' exercises, the nurturers of the body, Grandfather Peng's ripe-old-agers.[16]

His is a transcendent, less physical approach to life that is reminiscent of the cults of immortality. We can, perhaps, view immortality cults as an extreme extension of *yang-sheng* culture.[17] Elsewhere, in an obvious reference to the practice of breath-cultivation, *Zhuangzi* says that 'the realised man breathes with his heels'.[18] *Mengzi* 孟子 (late fourth century BC) differentiates between the benefits of breathing *qi* of the morning and that of the evening in nurturing man's original heavenly nature. *Mengzi* sees this practice as inseparable from cultivating moral character. Cultivating courage and rightness comes through nourishing the flood-like *qi* (*haoran zhi qi* 浩然之氣).[19]

Early descriptions of these life-enhancing practices show the development of a subjectivising of philosophical thought which had begun with ideas attributed to Yang Zhu 楊朱 (fl. late fourth century BC). Yang Zhu, or the Yangists, suggested that it is our primary responsibility to protect and nourish our heaven-given nature so that we can live out the time decreed to us. For his followers, prioritising a more subjective, inner experience of life is part of their aim to free judgement from the artifice of an external social morality. Other writers simply described ways of strengthening and nourishing human nature. Perhaps this was to attune themselves to the qualities of heaven, to still the heart in meditation – and in doing so they created a language for the internal environment of the body and simultaneously opened up a new dimension to philosophy. Immediate human experience became a vehicle for understanding the external world and, through the principle of resonance, a mode through which one could exert influence upon it.

This belief in resonance was the fundamental principle of a theory of rulership that can be detected in *Lunyu* 論語 (Analects) (third – second centuries BC) of Confucius (traditional dates: 551–479):

> The Master said, 'If a man is correct in his own person, then there will be obedience without orders being given; but if he is not correct in his own person, there will not be obedience even though orders are given.'[20]

[16] *Zhuangzi, juan* 6, *pian* 15, 1; transl. Graham (1981), 265.   [17] Harper (1998), 114.
[18] *Zhuangzi, juan* 6, *pian* 15, 2.   [19] *Mengzi, juan* 6, 58; tr. Lau (1970), 77.
[20] *Lunyu* 論語, *pian* 13, *zhang* 6, 143; tr. Lau (1979), 199. See also Legge (1935), 266.

Once the ruler behaved correctly, a civilising effect would spontaneously radiate from his very person through the administrative structure. *Lunyu* describes a form of self-cultivation through study and an attendance to social propriety. But the theory that in government a good ruler should concentrate on perfecting his personal actions, patterning his behaviour after heaven, whilst leaving practical administration delegated throughout the bureaucracy achieves full elaboration in *Lüshi chunqiu* 呂氏春秋 (Mr Lü's Spring and Autumn) (*ca* 239 BC):

> One able to nourish what Heaven generates and not interfere with it is called 'Son of Heaven' . . . This is why officials are established; the establishment of officials is to keep life intact.[21]

In many different philosophic and political works, the influence of the conduct of the ruler is understood to be critical to harmony in the environment. Even the *Han Fei zi* (韓非子) (third century BC) suggests that focus and simplicity combined with the principle of non action (*wuwei* 無為) are the desired qualities for effective authority.

> Authority should not be seen, in simplicity with no action. With business in the four quarters, remain at the centre. The sage holds to the essential principles and the four quarters come to serve him. In emptiness he awaits them and they spontaneously do what is needed.[22]

Only Mo Di 墨翟 (fl. late fifth century BC), possibly a carpenter and therefore the only artisan amongst the philosophers,[23] does not refer to nurturing life practices. He is singularly unconcerned about the distinction between the gentleman and the common man. His philosophy does not elevate culture and tradition, the trappings of the elite, but honours utility, the virtue of a craft. This exception suggests that cultivating bodily *qi* in the pursuit of long life was exclusively a part of the lifestyle of an educated elite.

Self-cultivation was a gentlemanly pursuit but it was sometimes at variance with the demands of court society. Zhang Liang 張良 (d. 187 BC), the strategist and military advisor to Liu Bang 劉邦, first emperor of the Han dynasty (reigned 202–195 BC), was a famous self-cultivator. After recurrent illness he took to practising *daoyin* and dietary techniques, leaving society to live as a recluse in company with the immortal, Master Red Pine 赤松子.[24]

Some scholars in the early Western Han period might have opposed ideas of ruling through attention to the kind of self-cultivation that focused on the body, rather than

---

[21] *Lüshi chunqiu, juan* 1, *pian* 2, 136. [22] *Han Fei zi, juan* 2, *pian* 8, 8b.

[23] For a discussion of Mo Di's social position, see Graham (1989), 31–6; for the other Warring States philosophers, see Graham (1989), 3.

[24] *Shiji, juan* 55, 2048.

moral and ritual behaviour or studying classical literature. But the two approaches were
not necessarily in contradiction. Both provided the *literati* with tools for self determination; as guardians of a written history which described the emperor as the pivot between
heaven and earth they were indispensable to the throne. By developing self-help techniques for enhancing and lengthening life, they both freed their bodies from the calamities of ghosts and demons and, at the same time, strengthened themselves against the
vicissitudes of heaven (the influence of the weather). Their lifestyle, as well as their
learning, both distinguished them from the common people and empowered them at the
expense of other practitioners.

'Yinshu' begins with a text which sets out an appropriate seasonal lifestyle in great
detail. It describes a regime for personal hygiene, diet, breath-cultivation, exercise, and
sexual practice in great detail. This is the prescription for life in summer and autumn.

> On summer days wash the hair more frequently and bathe less; do not sleep late.
> Eat more vegetables. Get up early and after passing water, wash and rinse the
> mouth with water, pick the teeth, loosen the hair and pace slowly in front of the
> house. After a while drink a cup of water. Enter the chamber[25] between dusk and
> midnight (when it is time to) cease. Increasing it will harm the *qi*.

> On autumn days bathe and wash the hair frequently; in drinking and eating your
> fill indulge the body's desires. Enter the chamber whenever the body is nourished
> and derives comfort from it. This is the way of benefit.[26]

> 夏日，數沐，希浴，毋莫〔起〕，多食采（菜），蚤（早）起，棄水之后，
> 用水澡澈（漱），疏齒，被（披）發，步足堂下，有閑而飲水一桮（杯）。
> 入宮從昏到夜半止，益之傷氣。秋日，數浴沐，歙（飲）食饑飽次（恣）
> 身所浴。入宮，以身所利安，此利道也。

The concluding passages of 'Yinshu' are a statement about the value of breath-
cultivation and *daoyin* in distinguishing class. In the spirit of the philosophy attributed
to Yang Zhu, the nobility moderate their behaviour through physical training to protect
themselves and preserve their vitality. But the behaviour itself also sets them apart from
the ignorant masses.

> The reason that nobility get illness is that they do not harmonise their joys and
> passions. If they are joyful then the *yangqi* is in excess. If they are angry then the
> *yinqi* is in excess. On account of this, if those that follow the Way are joyful then
> they quickly exhale (warm breath) (*xu* 呴), and if they become angry they increas-
> ingly puff out (moist breath) (*chui* 吹), in order to harmonise it.[27] They breathe in
> the quintessential *qi* of heaven and earth to make *yin* substantial, hence they will

[25] 'Enter the chamber' (*ru fang* 入房) is a euphemism for sexual activity.
[26] 'Yinshu' shiwen (1990), 82.
[27] Ma Jixing (1992), 826 note 17, discusses different techniques of breathing.

be able to avoid illness. The reason that lowly people become ill is exhaustion
from their labour, hunger and thirst; when the hundred sweats cease, they plunge
themselves into water and then lie down in a cold and empty place. They don't
know to put on more clothes and so they become ill from it. Also they do not
know to expel air and breathe out (dry breath) to get rid of it. On account of this
they have many illnesses and die easily.[28]

貴人之所以得病者，以其喜怒之不和也。喜則陽氣多，怒則陰（陰）氣
多，是以道者喜則急昫（呴），怒則劇炊（吹），以和之。吸天地之精氣，
實其陰，故能毋病。賤人之所以得病者，勞卷（倦）饑渴，白汗夬
（絕），自入水中，及臥寒突之地，不智（知）收衣，故得病焉，有（又）
弗智（知）昫（呴）虖（呼）而除去之，是以多病而易死。

Having established that members of elite society in late Warring States, Qin and
Western Han society were at least familiar with *yangsheng* culture, whether they
approved of it or not, I shall turn now to those texts that describe *mai* that were preserved
alongside the Mawangdui and Zhangjiashan *yangsheng* literature.

'Maishu'

The newly excavated Western Han textual sources that describe the *mai* have already
altered our perception of the early development of acumoxa's channel theory. Physiological speculation is primitive when compared to received medical literature.
The excavated texts do not reveal the network of channels systematically associated
with the internal organs or a network of acumoxa points that we know as the mature acumoxa system. Their channels proceed in more parallel fashion along the limbs to the
torso and head. They sometimes cross, but they do not join at the ends to form a contin-
uous ring. The practice of lancing the body is mainly associated in these texts with
abscess bursting, and the principles of practice related to the channels are extremely
basic. These early texts document a first systematic attempt at the kind of physiological
speculation that we see in later medical literature. When we come, for example, to
examine references to *qi* in the excavated texts, we shall see that the authors of the early
acumoxa texts did not conceive of a complex circulation or physiology of *qi*.

'Maishu', a manuscript excavated at the Zhangjiashan burial site, is the most complete and comprehensive of the works that describe the *mai* and is, in my view, the earliest extant treatise to set out theories and practice of acupuncture, wherein an implement
is used to pierce the skin in order to influence the movement of *qi* in the body. It
comprises 65 slips. Harper divides the document into six core texts which he describes
as 'Ailment List', 'Eleven Vessels', 'Five Signs of Death', 'Care of the Body', 'Six

---

[28] 'Yinshu' shiwen (1990), 86.

Constituents', and 'Vessels and Vapor'. Three of these – 'Eleven Vessels'; 'Five Signs of Death'; and 'Vessels and Vapor' – are editions of texts in the Mawangdui medical manuscripts. Harper's titles indicate well the content of each text. I shall adopt his divisions, numbering the texts (1)–(6). Gao Dalun 高大倫, using a different schema, conflates the last three.[29]

'Maishu' (1) is a lexicon of illnesses and illness characteristics. It is organised by superficial anatomy listing sixty-seven illnesses beginning from the head and moving down to the soles of the feet. In part, the text constitutes an early attempt at differential diagnosis which bears a relationship to some of the categories worked out in the recipe text 'Wushi'er bingfang'. It does not define the illnesses according to the kind of physiology that we will see in the remaining 'Maishu' texts.

'Maishu' (2) is an edition of the Mawangdui 'Yinyang shiyimai jiujing'. It describes the course of eleven different channels that run between the extremities and the head. The route of each channel is followed by a list of symptoms associated with a pathology of that channel.

'Maishu' (3) is an edition of the Mawangdui 'Yinyang mai sihou' 陰陽脈死侯 (Death Signs of *yin* and *yang* Vessels). It differentiates between *yin* and *yang* pathology in recognising terminal conditions.

'Maishu' (4), 'Care of the Body', recommends movement and moderation as the secret to long life. This suggests the same philosophy evident in 'Yinshu's *daoyin* regimen. It is a statement which is repeated in *Lüshi chunqiu*.[30]

> Now flowing water does not stagnate, when the door pivots there will be no woodworm because of their movement. When there is movement then it fills the four limbs and empties the five viscera, when the five viscera are empty then the jade body will be benefited. Now one who rides in a carriage and eats meat, must fast and purify themselves in spring and autumn. If they do not fast and purify themselves then the *mai* will rot and cause death.

'Maishu' (5) is peculiar to Zhangjiashan. It provides early analogies for six different parts of the body: bone (*gu* 骨), sinew (*jin* 筋), blood (*xue* 血), channel (*mai* 脈), flesh (*rou* 肉), and *qi*. It follows by attributing a particular quality of pain to each part. Pain indicates the onset of serious physical decline and this text serves as a warning to those who do not take positive action to counteract this deterioration.

'Maishu' (6) is a complex piece of writing that may constitute three separate texts. The first part describes the movement of *qi* and how to influence its flow. This is followed by a very practical guide to abscess lancing. 'Maishu' ends with the earliest

---

[29] Gao Dalun (1992).   [30] *Lüshi chunqiu, juan* 3, *pian* 2, 136.

extant record of pulse taking. Together these elements add up to the most basic principles of acumoxa practice.

Harper concludes that the combination of these final texts in 'Maishu' is indicative of the influence of macrobiotic hygiene (i.e. *yangsheng* nurturing life practice) in the development of vessel (i.e. channel) theory.[31] The aim of the present study is to test this hypothesis using source material from 'Maishu' and the *yangsheng* manuscripts from Mawangdui.

The following passage from 'Maishu' (6) will form the key extract upon which I identify the incidence of acupuncture in the excavated texts.[32] Another edition of this passage exists among the Mawangdui medical manuscripts and has been assigned the title of 'Maifa'. But key lacunae in the 'Maifa' obscure the meaning of the passage which in its recovered state refers to 'cautery' and not to body piercing. In the following extract we will find the most sophisticated of physiological ideas represented in 'Maishu' and the earliest extant treatise to document a link between body piercing and a formal movement of *qi*. For the first time, a text describes *qi* as a medical phenomenon subject to control by another.[33]

> The channels are valued by the sages. As for *qi*, it benefits the lower body and harms the upper; follows heat and distances coolness. So, the sages cool the head and warm the feet.[34] Those who treat illness take the surplus and supplement the insufficiency. So if *qi* goes up, not down, then when you see the channel that has over-reached itself, apply one cauterisation where it meets the articulation.[35] When the illness is intense then apply another cauterisation at a place two *cun*

[31] Harper (1998), 32.
[32] I differentiate 'acupuncture' from blood-letting and other minor surgery by the target of medical intervention. Acupuncture, as I define it, is the act of piercing the body with the intention of moving *qi* in the channels.
[33] 'Maishu' shiwen, 74.
[34] This sentence could also mean that 'the sages have cool heads and warm feet', and if they practise what they preach indeed they should have. However, the focus of this section appears to be on the principles of therapy and so we have translated as if it were a therapeutic situation.
[35] The recurrence of *huan* 環 in the next sentence after the preposition *yu* 於 suggests that *huan* 環 could not be a verb. Harper (1998), 214, translates as 'ring' and speculates that *huan* refers to the waist. My view is that the 'ring' is the articulation of the joints. The very next sentence suggests that the intervention is made at the joints, by specifying treatment at the place where the *qi* comes out at the elbow or knee creases. By applying cauterisation around the joints one can expect to change the direction of movement of *qi* in the body. In this treatment a stone lancet is used to remedy the situation. Once the points for acumoxa were standardised it is easy to see that the point distribution was concentrated around the joints. One can imagine that a natural articulation which at the same time was a narrowing of the body could be considered a significant impediment to a movement of *qi* through the body. The *qi* might be visualised as becoming squeezed and obstructed at this point, just as water swirls backwards when it meets a lock. See note 40.

above the articulation. When the *qi* rises at one moment and falls in the next pierce it with a stone lancet at the back of the knee and the elbow.

> 夫脈者，聖人之所以貴殹。氣者，利下而害上，從煖而去清，故聖人寒頭
> 而煖足。治病者取有徐（餘）而益不足，故氣上而不下則視有過之脈，當環
> 而久之。病甚而上於環二寸益為一久。氣一上一下，當骹與腑之脈而砭
> 之。

On the evidence of the excavated texts alone there is very little to suggest that *qi* in the body is present only in the channels, let alone that it travels in a particular direction along only those channels.

In this passage from 'Maishu' (6), *qi* is understood to move downwards and to the extremities and this is borne out in contemporary texts that describe the practices of breath-cultivation and *daoyin*.[36] The following exercises taken from 'Yinshu' demonstrate this principle in *daoyin*.[37]

> Ailing from *lao li* 醪（瘳）醴（癉）*liquor*.[38] The prescription for pulling is: grasp a staff in the right hand, face a wall, do not breathe, tread on the wall with the left foot, and rest when tired; likewise grasp the staff in the left hand, tread on the wall with the right foot, and rest when tired. When the *qi* of the head flows downwards, the foot will not be immobile and numb, the head will not swell, and the nose will not be stuffed up.

> 病瘳癉，引之之方，右手把丈（杖），鄉（向）壁毋息，左足跮壁，卷
> （倦）而休，亦左手把丈（杖），右足跮壁，亦卷（倦）而休。頭氣下流，
> 足不痿？首不踵鼽毋事恆服之。

Similarly *qi* can be projected into the arms:

> When suffering with there being less *qi* in the two hands, both the arms cannot be raised equally and the tips of the fingers, like rushing water, tend to numbness. Pretend that the two elbows are bound to the sides, and vigorously swing them. In the morning, middle of the day and middle of the night. Do it altogether one thousand times. Stop after ten days.

> 苦兩手少氣，舉之不鈴（鈞），指端湍湍善畀（痹），賈（假）縛兩肘於兩
> 胠，而力揮之，朝，日中，夜半皆為千，句而已。

Downward movement of *qi* is not a feature of the 'Jingmai' treatise of the *Lingshu* where *qi* travels through the channels in the direction of the anatomical references

---

[36] See, for example, the Yellow Emperor's conversations with Rong Cheng 容成 in the 'Shiwen' (Mawangdui Han mu boshu zhengli xiaozu (1985), 146–7).

[37] 'Yinshu' shiwen (1990), 83; Gao Dalun (1995), 122–3.

[38] The symptom is identified as 瘳癉. 癉 is an unattested character. 瘳, read *chou*, can simply be rendered 'ill' or 'to recover'. However, in 'Yinshu' the word must be part of a compound name for an illness. I suspect that this is an illness associated with *lao* 醪 'liquor with sediment' and *li* 醴 'new sweet liquor'.

which are arranged in an order that forms a circuit.[39] No such circuit is evident in the way the channels are formed in 'Zubi jiujing' and 'Yinyang jiujing', the excavated channel texts, where the anatomical references are given in an order that begins at the extremities and travels to the head. If *qi* were travelling in this direction it would be contrary to the natural movement given in 'Maishu' (6) quoted above. On the evidence of this passage and 'Maishu' (2), the text that contains descriptions of the route and direction of the channels, we can, therefore, dismiss the concept of circulation as a feature of the excavated texts.

Classical medical writings

From *Huangdi neijing* we can see that within two centuries following the closure of the Western Han tombs, the body was conceived as a complete microcosm of the external environment. A regulated flow of *qi*, the vital substance of life, was as basic to physical health as it was to the harmony of heaven and earth, and the channels through which it flowed were as carefully mapped as the waterways of the empire.[40] The *yin* and *yang* viscera or the solid and hollow organs of the body (*zangfu* 臟腑), were also described as officials of state with responsibility for the various ministries – for economy, for planning, and for upright judgements.[41]

In *Huangdi neijing* correspondences with *yin* and *yang* have transcended the basic sequence of opposites of light and shade, heaven and earth to become fundamental principles in human physiology, as well as in the classification of different physical substances and conditions, both normal and pathological. Stages in *yinyang* transformation explain states of health as well as the aetiology of disease. The acumoxa channels themselves even have acupoints that reflect the construction of the universe, the structure of the Empire, the Imperial palace, and the geography of China in their names. Amongst the acupoints are the heavenly pivot (*tianshu* 天樞), body pillar (*shenzhu* 身柱), sun and moon (*riyue* 日月), spirit hall (*shenting* 神庭), and illuminated sea (*zhaohai* 照海).

---

[39] *Lingshu, juan* 3, *pian* 10, 1–9.

[40] In *The Way of Water*, Allan (1997), 39–40, describes how, in Chinese mythology, 'directing water' was the first step to a civilised world. Channelling *qi* into routes around the body, like digging irrigation ditches and flood control canals, marks a significant stage in bringing the body, conceived as natural process, under human control. In *Lingshu* 12 the rivers and streams of the body reflect the natural, rather than man-made, waterways of China, see n. 52. Once the analogy between the channels and man-made water courses has been made, all the qualities and techniques of directing and controlling water can then be applied to the movement of bodily *qi*.

[41] *Suwen* 8, *juan* 2, *pian* 8, 1–2. Is the *locus classicus* for a representation of the body as a reflection of the Imperial structure, 'the spleen and the stomach are the officers in charge of the granaries, the five flavours emerge from the large intestine who is the officer of the passage ways . . .' Unschuld (1985), 79–83, sets out some of these ideas. See also Chiu (1986), 73–7.

The body is an intricately mapped out mirror of the macrocosm.[42] But how did this come about? How did the body begin to embrace the greater construction of the universe?

A creative tension

How does the *yangsheng* literature relate to the medical texts that describe how to manage illness in other people? As all the literature came out of the same lacquer box at Mawangdui, we can assume their physical proximity means that all the manuscripts enjoyed a similar readership.[43] But do the ideas that the different genres of medical writings express emerge at the same time, in the same social context? To answer this question we must consider the dynamic nature of technical and conceptual developments and their reflection in literature during the early Imperial period. At a cursory glance it is easy to see that such concepts as *yin* 陰, *yang* 陽, essence (*jing* 精), spirit (*shen* 神), and *qi* 氣 are more prevalent in some of the texts and barely appear in others. Cosmological explanations, for example, are not a significant feature of the pharmacological texts, but are ubiquitous in the descriptions of breath-cultivation in 'Shiwen'.[44]

Rather than list the similarities between the assumptions of the *yangsheng* and the evolving acumoxa literature, it is more fruitful to investigate the differences between the two genres, before the medical synthesis of the ensuing centuries. Such a comparison will serve to emphasise that, for example, in exploring a language to express sexual relationships such texts as 'He yinyang' contributed a unique dimension to the development of later medical concepts. In fact there is a great deal of evidence to show that in the Western Han dynasty medical concepts were in the process of being worked out through the medium of different disciplines.[45] Some contemporary attempts at categorisation were destined for extinction.[46]

---

[42] Unschuld (1985), 51–100.

[43] Nurturing life texts are kept or catalogued next to the medical texts and in later works certainly refer to the same body of knowledge.

[44] Wile (1992), 19–23, lists many points of similarity between the medical texts and those on the sexual arts. He concludes that much is *borrowed* from medicine. My concern in this paper is what is *borrowed back*, what the special focus of, for example, the sexual practices eventually contributes to medicine.

[45] In later nurturing life literature there are many different constructions of the body that utilise terms and concepts which reflect the imperatives of the particular practice for which they were created. In the sexual arts the gate of life (命門 *mingmen*) will relate directly to the reproductive organs and be located deep inside the body. The same terminology in later acumoxa treatises refers to a point just beneath the skin between lumbar vertebrae two and three which can easily be penetrated with a needle, or affected by the heat of moxa, without damaging the tissue of the body.

[46] In a text that attributes the various stages of fetal development to wood, fire, earth, metal, and water, the Five Agents (*wuxing* 五行), one stage is also attributed to stone (*shi* 石), apparently the sixth. This sixth agent was not to be adopted into later tables of correspondence. See Mawangdui Han mu boshu zhengli xiaozu (1985), 136.

It is not my thesis that the authors of what came to be viewed as classical medical treatises took on ideas from *yangsheng* culture wholesale, but that in the construction of the acumoxa body,[47] they selectively adopted some of the perspectives that had been refined through the older *yangsheng* studies. In order to understand the mode of construction of the classical medical body it is necessary to explore the dynamic between representations in such canons as *Huangdi neijing* and representations taken from earlier Western Han medical cultures found in the excavated texts. In particular, to demonstrate the priority of important features of classical Chinese medicine in *yangsheng* literature, I will compare the lyrical descriptions of the surface of the body found in sexual-cultivation with more mundane representations of the exterior of the body in 'Maishu', where we find the earliest extant treatise on acumoxa theory and practice. The second task of this chapter will be to identify the influence of *yangsheng* culture, and in particular breath-cultivation, on the concept of a formalised movement of *qi* in the body. Included in the discussion will be an examination of early methods of influencing the movement of *qi* and how they had a bearing on the critical transition from the perception of *qi* as an independent external phenomenon, to the idea that it filled the body and was amenable to human intervention. In these two stages I will provide ample evidence to identify the influence of *yangsheng* on the development of classical medical theory.

Landscaping the body

By comparing 'Maishu' (2) and 'He Yinyang' we can begin to see how images of the social world were first brought to the surface of the body. In 'Maishu' (2) the body is described in simple terms inspired by superficial anatomy. In contrast, the lyrical descriptions of the sexual arts landscape the body with images of the natural and human world, with mountains and seas, bowls and stoves. The same perception of the body can be traced to the names of the acumoxa points in later medical classics such as *Huangdi neijing Lingshu* or *Zhenjiu jiayi jing* 針灸甲乙經(AB Canon of Acumoxa) (AD 256– 82). I do not intend to privilege a knowledge of acupoints in interpreting the position or meaning of any of the anatomical locations in the excavated texts. I simply wish to demonstrate that a metaphorical language for describing the exterior body developed first within the context of a culture of self-cultivation and that its imagery was retained in classical medical theory by the authors of the acupoints who invoked a similar landscape for the body.

---

[47] i.e. a body delineated by channels through which *qi* moves and on which are points where *qi* can be influenced.

The description of each channel in 'Maishu' (2) begins with a title such as 'Forearm great *yin* channel' (*bi juyin zhi mai* 臂鉅陰之脈) or 'Foot great *yang* channel' (*zu juyang zhi mai* 足鉅陽之脈) followed by a description of the somatographic space occupied by the channel. Each location is linked by verbs of movement. The channel moves in a number of ways. It can go up (*shang* 上), down (*xia* 下), come out (*chu* 出), enter (*ru* 入), pierce (*guan* 貫), among similar verbs. Each verb is then followed by an anatomical location. Two lists of symptoms then follow each of the channel descriptions. The edition known as 'Zubi jiujing' rounds up with the simple directive to cauterise it (*jiu zhi* 久(灸)之).

On the routes around the body taken in 'Yinyang jiujing', all the anatomical terms are visible structures on the surface of the body, except the great *yin* channel, which travels to the stomach, and the forearm lesser *yin* channel, which passes to the heart.[48] Most of the graphs contain radicals of the physical body, such as flesh (*rou* 肉), foot (*zu* 足), bone (*gu* 骨), or eye (*mu* 目):

> The shoulder channel arises behind the ear, descends the shoulder, comes out at the inner surface of the elbow, comes out on the wrist at the outer surface of the forearm, and mounts the back of the hand.[49]

> 肩脈，起於耳後，下肩，出肘內廉，出臂外館上，乘手北。

The nomenclature for the channels themselves, foot and arm, greater and lesser *yang* and *yin*, *yang* illumination and ceasing *yin* signifies the dark and light anatomical planes of the body i.e. an inner/outer, upper/lower distinction – meanings associated with the earliest known references of *yin* 陰 'the dark side of the hill' and *yang* 陽 'the sunny side of the hill'.[50] A few exceptions such as the fish thigh (*yugu* 魚股), a location that appears to be a more lyrical and less visual representation of the body, in fact only describe shape – in this case the fish-like shape of the quadriceps above the knee. And this simple rationale is retained in the names of a number of acupoints described, for example, in *Zhenjiu jiayi jing*.[51] Prostrate hare (*futu* 伏兔) is still the name of an acupoint on the stomach channel known in modern acumoxa theory as stomach 32. Its location is given as, '6 *cun* (寸) above the knee on the anterior prominent muscle of the thigh'. Seen from

---

[48] Although the routes of the channels are superficial to the body, illnesses of the channels commonly include symptoms of the alimentary tract and urinary system.

[49] 'Maishu' shiwen (1989), 73.

[50] See Granet (1934), 361–88.

[51] A comprehensive list of acupoints is in *The Location of Acupoints* by Anon. (1990), which also provides historical sources for both names and locations. See *Zhenjiu jiayi jing, juan* 3, 576, 683, and 685, for the classical sources of names and locations given in this paragraph.

a lateral angle the acupoint is on the eye of a prostrate hare that is formed by the seams of the muscles of the lateral, anterior thigh. An acupoint on the central anterior channel, known as *ren* (任) 15 in modern acumoxa theory, was also first seen named dove tail (*jiuwei* 鳩尾). Its location is given as '0.5 *cun* below the xiphoid process'. This is the end of a bone structure which, taking in the rib cage and the sternum gives a skeletal impression of a spreading dove's tail. Calf nose (*dubi* 犢鼻), later known as stomach 35, is 'on the border of the patella in the depression beside the large ligament'. When the knee is bent and seen from an anterior view the acupoint forms the calf's nostril.

The authors of the channel descriptions in 'Maishu' (2) privileged a visual knowledge of the external body. A handful of visual clues in 'Maishu', like the *yugu*, only hint at the vividly described microcosm conjured up by the classical acupoint names. The names of the acupoints landscape the whole of the body's surface. There are *yin* articulations (*yinxi* 陰郄), *yin* valleys (*yingu* 陰谷), *yang* valleys (*yanggu* 陽谷), *yang* ponds (*yangchi* 陽池), and the like. The metaphor of water which constantly informs us about the movement of *qi* also gains full maturity in the acupoint body where seas and oceans swell in the abdomen and fill the knees and elbows. Further on down the limbs there are rivers, springs, streams, and wells as the *qi* flows in different shapes and speeds towards the extremities.[52]

'Maishu' does not provide many leads towards understanding the development of a body landscaped with acupoints – nor does it link its channels systematically with movements of *qi*. In contrast 'He yinyang' (Harmonising *yin* and *yang*) begins with a kind of pre-coital massage which is couched in lyrical verse about the surface of a woman's body. The text proceeds in parallel form, mostly beginning with verbal instructions to take actions that end in particular locations of the body. Each anatomical landmark is represented by the kind of two-graph term used later in the names of the acupoints.

I do not intend to translate the text or to attempt to determine definitively which parts of the body are massaged. That has been adequately accomplished both in English and in modern Chinese.[53] Where there appears to be confusion it is useful to refer to Li Ling and Keith McMahon who survey anatomical terminology in the whole of the Mawangdui sexual-cultivation corpus, making a critical study of existing interpretations.[54] I include massage at this point to build up a broad picture of the exterior body

---

[52] The *locus classicus* for an analogy of the circulation tracts with the waterways is *Lingshu, juan* 3, *pian* 12, 11–13, which matches rivers to the channels of the body. The rivers can be matched to those on maps of the early Han period. See for example Tan Qixiang (1982), 19–20.

[53] Harper (1998), 412–22. Wile (1992), 51–73. Ma Jixing (1992), 977.

[54] Li and McMahon (1992), 145–85.

in self-cultivation culture, a culture which prepares the ground for a new medical view of body topography.

Although the various translators often disagree, enough common ground can be found between the interpretations to begin and end the massage although, in the middle section, the exact anatomical locations become a little vague and cannot be conclusively determined. The massage begins on the *yang* 'light', or back side of the hand. It proceeds to the elbows and then to the armpits. Each of the locations so far has been designated with two graphs, one of which relates to a commonly used anatomical term. After these three unremarkable terms, the texts start using names that are far more lyrical.

The massage proceeds upward to a part of the body known as the stove net-rope (*zaogang* 灶綱), follows through to the neck region (*xiangxiang* 項鄉), and then to *chengkuang* (拯匡), variously interpreted as receiving canister (*chengkuang* 承筐)[55] and identified as the female pelvis or as receiving light (*chengguang* 承光), a name which later refers to the acupoint located on the bladder channel on the top of the head.[56] Thereafter there is a direction to cover (*fu* 彿) the encircling rings (*zhouhuan* 周環) – perhaps the eye sockets, the breasts, or the belly.[57]

After covering the 'encircling rings' the massage moves downwards to the broken bowl (*quepen* 缺盆), a term listed in *Shiji* as the clavicle,[58] but in *Suwen* adopted as the name of an acupoint on the stomach channel which nestles in the depression located above the centre of the clavicle.[59] In *Zhenjiu jiayi jing* we have another utensil, heavenly cauldron (*tianding* 天鼎) located close to the 'broken bowl'.[60] Both these acupoints are sitting on top of the thoracic cage which suggests that the chest cavity might have been conceived as a stove within which a fire burnt. This might then explain the position of the stove net-rope, *zaogang*. Harper reads *zaojiong* (灶炯) and translates 'stove trivet'. He refers to the numerous metal trivets for holding cooking utensils over an open fire that have been excavated from Han burial sites.[61] Alchemical imagery cannot be

[55] Harper (1987), 571–2. Harper makes a strong argument that the canister is the 'osseous basket' that holds the female genitals. He cites examples in *Shijing* and *Yijing* where the canister refers directly to female sexuality.
[56] Ma Jixing (1992), 979 n. 9, and *Zhenjiu jiayi jing*, juan 3, 476.
[57] Harper identifies the *zhouhuan* as the waist, Li and McMahon the breasts. 'Maishu' refers to the idiom, 'the eyes are ringed, the look engraved' (*muhuan shidiao* 目圜視雕), as the fatal sign of blood pathology. Perhaps *zhouhuan* refers to the rings of the eye sockets and covering the woman's eye is a part of sexual foreplay.
[58] *Shiji, juan* 105, 2811.   [59] *Suwen, juan* 15, *pian* 59, 13.
[60] *Zhenjiu jiayi jing, juan* 3, 547.   [61] Harper (1998), 412–13.

ignored. Meditation texts also use the same kind of images to describe the process of refining *qi*, essence, and spirit in the body.[62]

Returning to 'He yinyang' 's massage procedure, the guiding rope of a net (*gang* 綱) of the term stove net-rope (*zaogang*) may be compared with another acupoint, *yang net-rope* (*yanggang* 陽綱) which can be located at either side of the spine between thoracic vertebrae ten and eleven. There are many acupoints along the spine with names that also suggest the line of support for a larger structure, for instance, heavenly column (*tianzhu* 天柱), body column (*shenzhu* 身柱), spirit way (*shendao* 神道). Given the many, essentially similar images that we know to be simultaneously superimposed upon the body, a woven net spreading out from the spine would seem to have the same inherent qualities. Another resonant image is suggested by the term warp (*jing* 經), the thread of the net, which later becomes standardised for the channels of acumoxa therapy.

Continuing downwards from the clavicle, the movement travels over the syrupy liquor ford (*lijin* 醴津) perhaps the way through the fluid streaming down from syrupy liquor spring (*liquan* 醴泉)[63] which arises under the tongue or at the navel, alternatively, or perhaps simultaneously, the cleavage between lactating breasts[64] to two more locations before the final instruction to enter the dark gate (*xuanmen* 玄門), a euphemism for the vagina.

The first of the two intermediate massage locations, the spurting sea (*bohai* 浡海) and the second, mount constancy (*changshan* 常山), are both sites referred to in *Shanhai jing* 山海經 (Canon of Mountains and Lakes), possibly another text local to the region of Chu.[65] Harper maps the lakes and mountains onto the body and sets out the arguments for specific identification with anatomical locations.

Neither 'mount constancy' nor 'dark gate' are attested in the acumoxa canons, but by the time of *Zhenjiu jiayi jing* and *Lingshu* the body is littered with gates and mountains. Below the navel, at the probable location of the spurting sea (*bohai*) comes sea of *qi* (*qihai* 氣海) which is also called *boyang* 脖胦. *Bo* 脖 (neck), the first graph, is homophonous with *bo* 浡 (spurting) which suggests that the name may be a graphic variation.[66] Outside of the external malleolus of the ankle are the Kunlun mountains 崑崙山, the stairway to Heaven.[67] There are gates of dumbness and numerous palace

---

[62] See for example Robinet (1989). Robinet, discussing inner alchemy, explores the many different levels at which the image of the furnace and the crucible can be simultaneously understood.

[63] Wile (1992), 222 n. 8.

[64] Harper (1987), 576–7 describes the geographic locations of the *liquan* as they are given in Han sources. He identifies the *liquan* with a manifestation of the cosmic axis which joins heaven and earth.

[65] See Fracasso (1993).   [66] *Zhenjiu jiayi jing, juan 3,* 582.   [67] Major (1993), 46–67.

gates, not to speak of the gates of the various spirits and souls associated with human life, the *hun* 魂, the *shen* 神, and the door of the *po* 魄.[68]

For the purposes of this article it is not necessary to attempt to resolve the controversies in meaning and translation of the locations in 'He yinyang'. It is enough to note that although all these terms clearly refer to physical locations, not one of them is a common anatomical term. Each is a metaphoric representation and can only be understood by appealing to literary allusion or analogous structures in contemporary society.

Some of the analogies relating to the natural and social worlds introduced here in the massage procedure are matched in the exercises described in 'Yinshu'. In 'Yinshu' we find raising the body up on to the ball of the foot conveyed through the image of looking down from the battlements (*bini* 埤堄), perhaps peering over the crenellations of a castle wall:

> With feet together leave the flat position, rocking thirty times. This is called working the toes. Extend the lower leg and straighten to the heels. With feet together rock thirty times. This is called looking down from the battlements.
>
> 傅（附）足离翕（合），㢮（䠊）三十，曰金指。信（伸）胻直踵，并㢮（䠊）三十，曰埤堄.

Waving the arms mimics the action of the *fuche*, thought to be equivalent to a *fanche*, a vehicle for trapping birds and rabbits:

> Covering the cart.[69] With two arms parallel, wave them high to left and right, and then bring them down straight and wave them.
>
> 復車者，并兩臂，左右危揮，下正揮之。

'Maishu', 'Yinshu', and 'He yinyang' are educational treatises on the body. The former is devoted to the interpretation and treatment of symptoms, the second is a *daoyin* manual, and the latter a treatise on health-promoting sexual practice. Together they may

---

[68] *Lingshu*, *juan* 2, *pian* 8, 7b–9. 'Benshen' 本神 (rooting in the spirit), describes the relationship between the internal organs, emotion, and other aspects of the human consciousness and entities that we might approximate to spirit and souls. The *hun* 魂 and the *po* 魄, for example, are aspects of a human being that come to be paired in life and separated at death. New research into early references to these concepts has shown that *hun/po* dualism is not at the foundation of Han burial practice. Brashier (1996), 125–58 shows how the pair are related to medical states of anxiety. In *Lingshu* 8 the *hun* is said to reside in the blood, the *po* in the lungs. The will (*zhi* 志) resides in the kidneys. The *shen* 神 (originally a term for 'spirit' entities external to the body – and, in the *Lingshu*, a somatisation of the qualities of brightness and spontaneous perception that the spirits represented) is said to reside in the channels (*mai*).

[69] 'Yinshu' shiwen (1990), 83, and Gao Dalun (1995), 114. I take *fu* 復 as a graphic variant of *fu* 覆 (to cover). The movement could be a mime of throwing and shaking a soft covering over a cart.

all represent the activities of the same social class, but the nature of the human relation-ships between observer and observed revealed by each text is different. The descrip-tions of the exterior of the body in 'Maishu' (2) are records of the body observed. But they are limited by the distance inevitably imposed by the activity of one person record-ing the symptoms of another by means of visual perception.

'Yinshu' begins to release perceptions of the external body from the limitations of the eye alone and introduces models of animal movement, such as the bear warp (*xiongjing* 熊經), dragon rising (*longxing* 帶興), or mandarin duck bathing (*fuwo* 鳧沃), as an aid to train and strengthen the body. The record in 'He yinyang' uses a language which bridges the visual with a richer multi-dimensional experience of the body. Because of the nature of the activity the authors are intimately involved with the subject. We could consider the involvement to be purely imaginative, undertaken in the isolation of a study, or even to be the records of sexual encounter, but the imagery springing from the realms of visualisation leads to a marriage of imagination, the senses, and the forms that meet the eye. This subject blurs any distinction between the interior and exterior of the body.

The massage procedure provides an early model for elaborate constructions of the body which we can find in later medical, meditation, and alchemical literature, each with the imagery and specific anatomical locations moulded by their respective discip-lines. This massage text produces a representation of the body which pre-dates and therefore, in its method of describing the body in metaphorical terms, anticipates the acupoints. It only refers to the surface of the body – or just below the surface in the case of the acupoints. We have to look elsewhere to find descriptions of the inner landscape of the body.

Referring effect in the body

'Maishu' accounts of body piercing are fairly primitive in relation to later accounts of the potential of acumoxa treatments. No profound effect on the inner body is expected where 'Maishu' implies minor surgery. But in the short passage that links body piercing with *qi*, 'Maishu' begins to attribute a greater potency to body piercing. And once the channels are described as penetrating more deeply into the body and are systematically associated with the internal organs, with the circulation of *qi* and the elaborated system of *yinyang* and Five Phase correspondences of canonical acumoxa literature, acupunc-ture needle or cautery with moxibustion have radically extended spheres of influence. Producing a distal effect through the medium of any of these systems by stimulating the body at a point on or just below its surface is what I will label 'referring effect'. To what extent can we see this kind of distal stimulation in the medicines in the excavated texts?

Most contemporary schools which claim to sustain traditional Chinese medical methods still teach, as a fundamental skill of acumoxa therapy, referral of the benefit from points on the surface to the inside of the body and through to any of the many bodies circumscribed within the *yinyang* and five phase correlative system. Acupoints are stimulated with the intention of influencing another more distal place along the channel, an associated internal organ, bodily function, or emotional body. Success or failure of the intervention may be determined by the patient's ability to 'feel' the movements of *qi* as a change in the condition of the inner body, whether that be experienced as numbness, tingling, immediate change in the quality of pain or discomfort, an alleviation of oppressive emotional states, or an increased feeling of calm or lightness.

From the excavated texts we can identify a range of activities that involve referring effect around the body from strategic points upon its surface. Understanding the transference and alleviation of pain is an obvious starting point to identifying referred effect in the body of another. I have described elsewhere how 'tracking the pain' from the extremities to the inside of the body was one way of determining the course of the channel.[70] The concentration of effort expended by both 'Yinshu' and 'Maishu' on siting pain helps us to envisage the kind of empirical activity that could have established fundamental principles of where to make an intervention to best effect pain relief. Observations made by Lu and Needham in the 'Lore of Vital Spots' about how pain disappears when pressure is applied to strategic body points take on new relevance.[71]

In later periods it is easy to see a more general culture of strategic body points. Lu and Needham go some way towards establishing the contexts within which one person may make observations of referred effect in the bodies of others. For example, they match the development of strategic damage points through the practice of martial arts to the thirteenth-century charts of early Chinese forensic scientists.[72] These charts demonstrate a sophisticated knowledge of anatomy and the devastating effect of violence to small areas of the body. But 'Maishu' or parallel texts at Mawangdui make no mention of specific acupoints and none are definitively revealed in the biographies of medical doctors in *Shiji* 105 or on the medical figurine excavated at Yongxing 永興 in Mianyang 綿陽 district of Sichuan,[73] so there is no evidence to show that stimulating the channel network via a mature acupoint system was a feature of the therapy during the second to third centuries BC. The acupoints which seem to exist in the excavated texts are in fact simply anatomical locations. We have seen that the broken bowl (*quepen* 缺盆) is a term used in pre-coital massage to refer to the area of the clavicle, and I shall show that the

---

[70] Lo (1998), 240–66.   [71] Lu and Needham (1980), 303–18.   [72] See McKnight (1981).
[73] See He Zhiguo and Lo (1996), 81–123, for an extensive discussion of the figurine.

middle extremity (*zhongji* 中極) is clearly an important anatomical location from which sensation refers, without yet being the name and location for the acupoint on the anterior, central channel known in modern acumoxa theory as *ren* 3 that it eventually becomes.

The lone reference of 'Maishu' (6) to influencing the movement of *qi* by piercing the body seems to be the exception that establishes the rule for the period. Intervention may be specified where the *qi* circles around (*huan* 環) in this one isolated discussion, but 'Maishu' (6) also gives us strong evidence to confirm that the body piercing was predominantly localised needling or minor surgery. How then can we understand the development of a medical activity based upon stimulating distal reaction from strategic points on the surface of the body?

Manipulating *qi* in sexual-cultivation

Daoyin and breath-cultivation literature show us how an individual's activities can influence their own *qi*. So it follows to look at the self-cultivation techniques which involve two people in order to understand how the same effects can be stimulated in another. Augmenting and strengthening *qi* are already common principles in refined sexual conduct. One section of 'Tianxia zhi dao tan' states '*qi* has eight (signs of) increase' (*qiyou bayi* 氣有八益). The eight signs of increase are contrasted with seven signs of diminishing (*qisun* 七損) and once again relate to ways of storing, moving, and absorbing *qi*, specifically that of the sage and gentleman, through sequences of sexual activity that variously involve diet and breath-cultivation. The outcome can also be compared with the outcome of breath-cultivation. Without paying attention to regulated sexual-cultivation, medical intervention is fruitless.

> If he penetrates inside quickly, it cannot be guided. He becomes ill, perspires and pants. He becomes distressed at the centre and his *qi* is out of order so it cannot be treated. When internal heat is generated, he drinks pharmacological infusions and applies moxibustion to improve his *qi*; he takes tonic medicines to help his exterior. However, if he over-exerts himself (in sexual activity), (illness) cannot be guided, pustules are produced and the testicles swell.[74]

> 疾使內，不能道，產病出汗楯（喘）息，中煩氣亂，弗能治，產內熱，飲藥約（灼）灸以致其氣，服司以輔其外，強用之，不能道，產痤（腫）橐。

Evidently therapy must be appropriate to the location of the illness; the location may be determined as an internal or external site or in the body as it manifests as a

---

[74] Mawangdui Han mu boshu zhengli xiaozu (1985), 164.

thermostatic entity or as a mass of *qi*.[75] Heat is resolved with pharmacology, tonics relate to the exterior of the body. Moxibustion, like regulated sex, improves the *qi*. Other passages in 'He yinyang' and 'Tianxia zhi dao tan' which refer to eliciting responses in the woman's body can be closely compared to the aims of intervention with moxibustion and body piercing, and are of most interest at this point in my argument.

Sections of 'He yinyang' and 'Tianxia zhi dao tan' are devoted to observation of the signs of female sexual arousal. The signs are an anticipated sequence of physical responses to actions taken by the man and provide the cue for the next step in a formal procedure. In the pre-coital massage sequence the aim is to stimulate the woman by stroking her body along a course concentrated on strategic points. Completing this stage in the procedure alone is said to lead to nourishment and joy for both male and female bodies. Both works then document the moment when penetration is prescribed.

> When the *qi* rises and her face becomes hot, slowly exhale (warm) breath. When her nipples become hard and her nose perspires, slowly embrace her. When her tongue spreads and becomes slippery, slowly press her. When below secretions moisten her thighs, slowly hold her. When her throat becomes dry and she swallows saliva, slowly rock her. These are called the 'five signs', these are called the 'five desires'. When all the signs are ready then mount.[76]

> 氣上面熱，徐呴（呴），乳堅鼻汗，徐葆（抱），舌薄而滑，徐傅，下夕（液）股濕，徐操，益（嗌）乾因（咽）唾，徐緘（撼），此謂五微（徵），此謂五欲，微（徵）備乃上。

In 'He yinyang' the same moment is described as when 'the signs of the five desires' manifest. We can see that actions like holding (*cao* 操), pressing (*fu* 傅), and rocking (緘 (*han* 撼))[77] deliberately stimulate the next prescribed response in the woman's body. Interpreting the condition of inner body *qi* is one guide to action. With sexual arousal, rising *qi* and heat are, exceptionally, not signs of pathology, but simply an anticipated stage in the whole sequence. Ways of moving and distributing *qi* at the moment when it accumulates are also specified in the next passage, which clearly anticipates the language of needle technique common to later acumoxa therapy.

[75] See Zhangjiashan Han jian zhenglizu (1990), 82. 'Maishu' (5) also lists bone, *qi*, muscles, flesh, and blood as the primary location of fatal pathology.
[76] Mawangdui Han mu boshu zhengli xiaozu (1985), 166. A similar passage is Mawangdui Han mu boshu zhengli xiaozu (1985), 155.
[77] I follow the editorial amendments in Mawangdui Han mu boshu zhengli xiaozu (1985), 166.

Stab upwards but do not penetrate in order to stimulate *qi*, when the *qi* arrives (*qizhi* 氣至) penetrate deeply and thrust upward in order to distribute the heat. Now once again withdraw so as not to cause its *qi* to dissipate and for her to become exhausted.[78]

上揣而勿內，以致其氣。氣至，深而內上撅之，以抒其熱，因復下反之，毋使其氣歇，而女乃大竭。

Of the sets of principles to follow in sexual union, the eight ways (*badao* 八道) detail eight different movements of the penis to respond to different states of female arousal. We cannot ignore the recurring motif of penetration in the care taken with thrusting the penis and the manipulation of the needle as ways to reveal change in the inner body. Harper has already drawn an analogy between the use of the burning wooden poker to crack the tortoise's plastron in the pyromantic arts and the use of cauterisation and needle on the mature acumoxa system. He gives good philological evidence to substantiate the association.[79] Each of these activities assumes that the act of penetration and/or heating of the surface of a thing will reveal its underlying nature, and therefore render it, or the situation it represents, amenable to further intervention.

Chunyu Yi 淳于意, a Western Han doctor, states that stone and cauter cause the arrival of *qi* (*jiqi* 及氣).[80] The 'arrival of *qi*' in acumoxa literature is an indication of successful intervention with the needle. This technique is described in detail in *Lingshu* 9 which frequently states:

As for the method of needling . . . when the *qi* arrives, stop.[81]

凡刺之道，氣至乃休。

and *Lingshu* 1:

If you pierce the body yet the *qi* does not arrive do not question the number (of insertions); if you pierce the body and the *qi* arrives, then take it away and do not needle again . . . the essentials of needling are that the *qi* arrives and there is an effect.[82]

刺之而氣不至，無問其數，刺之而氣至，乃去之，勿復針 . . . 刺之要，氣至而有效。

---

[78] See 'He yinyang' in Mawangdui Han mu boshu zhengli xiaozu (1985), 155.
[79] Harper (1982), 271–4. Harper finds that the link between divinatory cauterisation and medical cauterisation suggests that early somatological theories developed within the practice of cautery.
[80] *Shiji*, *juan* 105, 2816.   [81] *Lingshu, juan 2, pian 9*, 10–11.
[82] *Lingshu, juan 1, pian 1*, 3.

Qizhi and a similar expression, obtaining *qi* (*deqi* 得氣)[83] are still essential features of modern acupuncture needling. They describe a range of sensations that accompany successful needle technique and confirm that the *qi* has moved in the manner intended. Here is a description of the arrival of *qi* from a modern text book:

> Signs of the arrival of *qi*: When the patient feels soreness, numbness, heaviness and distension around the point, or their transmission upward and downward along the meridians, it is a sign of the arrival of *qi*. Meanwhile, the operator should feel tenseness around the needle.[84]

The common feature of all these references to the 'arrival' or 'obtaining' of *qi* is certainly the climax of a change in inner body sensation, whether pain, pleasure, or even the alleviation of pain. In fact pain and pleasure are the two experiences that most inspire metaphors of macrocosm in the body.[85]

Breath-cultivation literature also describes beneficial effects of working on *qi*. The overall aim of the retention of semen, the skill of successful sexual-cultivation for the male, can also be compared with adjusting the *qi*. In one stage of the sexual procedure ten movements (*shidong* 十動) are described:

> If there is no orgasm in the first movement, the ears and eyes will become keen and bright, with the second the voice becomes clear, with the third the skin gleams, with the fourth the back and flanks are strengthened, with the fifth the buttocks and thighs become sturdy, with the sixth the waterways flow freely, with the seventh one becomes sturdy with strength, with the eighth the patterns of the skin shine, with the ninth one gets through to an illumination of the spirit, with the tenth the body endures: these are called the ten movements.[86]

> 一動毋決，耳目蔥（聰）明，再而音聲（章），三而皮革光，四而脊脅強，五而尻脾（髀）方，六而水道行，七而至堅以強，八而奏（腠）理光，九而通神明，十而為身常，此胃（謂）十動。

We can also compare these very medical fruits of sexual-cultivation with a passage in *Lingshu* 9 which describes the aim of acupuncture needling:

---

[83] *deqi* 得氣 is an expression used in 'Maishu' to describe a positive sensation that heralds amelioration of bowel obstruction by *qi* masses (*qijia* 氣叚). See 'Maishu' shiwen, 72.

[84] Cheng Xinnong (1990), 326.

[85] In 'Maishu' we have seen pain differentiated in relation to different parts of the body: 'Now the bones are the supporting column, the tendons are the bundle, the blood is fluid, the channels are the canal, the flesh sticks on and the *qi* twists and turns' (夫骨者柱叚 筋者束叚 血者濡叚脈者瀆叚 肉者附叚 氣者胊叚). The pain associated with the channels for example 'flows' like the canal. See 'Maishu' shiwen, 74.

[86] Mawangdui Han mu boshu zhengli xiaozu (1985), 155.

In all cases the way of needling entails stopping when the *qi* is adjusted: tonify the *yin* and sedate the *yang*, the voice and *qi* become increasingly clear, the ear and the eye become keen and bright, if one goes against this, the blood and the *qi* will not flow freely. What is meant by the arrival of the *qi* (*qizhi*) and obtaining of effect is with sedation the emptiness is increased.[87]

凡刺之道，氣調而止，補陰瀉陽，音氣益章，耳目聰明。反此者，血氣不行。所謂氣至有效，瀉則益虛。

At the culmination of 'He yinyang', we find a sequence that continues a description of the woman's body as she approaches and achieves orgasm. The passage is unusual in that self-cultivation literature is written for the empowerment of educated men as was most written work of this period. But the description is certainly a continuation of a sequence that records physical responses of the female body.[88] Orgasm is completed at the point when *qi* extends throughout the body bringing the now familiar inner transformation:

The symptoms of the great death (grand finale) are: the nose sweats, lips are white, the hands and feet all move, the buttocks do not touch the mat, rise and withdraw, if it becomes flaccid then there will be weakness. At this point the *qi* extends from the middle extremity (*zhong ji* 中極), the essence and spirit enter the viscera and an illumination of the spirit is born.[89]

大卒之徵，鼻汗脣白，手足皆作，尻不傅席，起而去，成死為薄。當此之時，中極氣張，精神入臟（藏），乃生神明。

In the culmination of 'He yinyang' we come across the image of the middle extremity *zhongji* in its incarnation as the uterus. Eventually the same terminology is used for the acupoint on the anterior, central channel known today as *ren* 3, located just below the skin on the lower abdomen – an acupoint which has a powerful effect on acute urogenital

[87] *Lingshu, juan* 2, *pian* 9, 10b.
[88] The philological arguments that discuss whether the orgasm is male or female (including Harper's argument) are conveniently set out in Wile (1992), 225 n. 29. I follow Harper's analysis. This sequence in 'He yinyang' is unequivocally a discussion of female response. See Mawangdui Han mu boshu zhengli xiaozu (1985), 74.
[89] Mawangdui Han mu boshu zhengli xiaozu (1985), 156. Some contemporary explanations of natural phenomena also use similar terms. Earthquakes, as a macrocosmic model for momentous sensation, provide an early model for the workings of *qi* in the channels of the inner body and for dynamic movement arising from the interaction of *yin* and *yang*. See *Guoyu* 國語, *juan* 1, *pian* 6, 15. *Qi* seems to be the universal medium through which pressure created by the interrupted and pathological interaction of its *yin* and *yang* aspects can lead to violent eruptions. See also *Guoyu* 國語, *juan* 1, *pian* 10, 22–7. The *Guoyu* text sets a precedent for the idea that *qi* travels through *mai*, in this case the fault lines of an earthquake, but later, as we have seen, one of the terms to be adopted for the courses or channels for acumoxa therapy.

problems. But at this earlier time, or at least in the particular medium of the sexual-cultivation literature, it is either the womb itself or a physical source in either male or female, where sensation accumulates and then radiates around the body in the form of *qi*. Here we also have an early description of how the movement of *qi* influences the capacity of the viscera to store essence and spirit – an important theme in the medical canons.

Conclusion

For some time it has been assumed that *yangsheng* practices and classical Chinese medical acumoxa theory emerged within the same social and intellectual milieu. To some extent this was true and in the absence of conflicting material it was a fair enough assumption. But since the discovery of the tomb manuscripts there has been plenty of resource material to begin to unravel the creative processes behind acumoxa therapy. A simple comparison of anatomical terminology in two of the excavated texts has served to highlight how much the naming of the acumoxa points owes to the early sexual-cultivation literature.

The Western Han descriptions of channels and channel pathology in 'Maishu' present a view of the body that is geared towards explanation of physical symptoms. Descriptions of the body are primarily visual. From related texts, we can see descriptions of *qi* beginning to give the body a wider, more universal resonance, but these descriptions are still embryonic in comparison to the sophistication of similar treatments a couple of centuries later.

In contrast we have seen that body representations in 'He yinyang' are far more elaborate. The body is described in a way that transcends the language inspired by the eyes alone. It is a language that weaves physical sensation and visual features into a landscape mirroring the natural topography of the known world. *Yin*, *yang*, and *qi* were commonly used to explain phenomena of the perceived patterns of heaven and earth; it is mainly in the *yangsheng* literature that these concepts have already begun to penetrate the body and provide a model for the landscaping of the internal environment – a landscape that becomes a familiar feature of later Daoist and medical practice. It is in these texts that we can see the earliest evidence of an important transition that was made between Western Han and the first century AD: *qi*, from being a term that referred to climatic conditions and the external stuff of the universe, became the life-giving vitality that circulated around the body, a vitality that could eventually be influenced and benefited by the intervention of a physician.

The most obvious distinction between the early acumoxa and prescriptive literature and the *yangsheng* literature is that the latter focused on the individual and the elevation of personal health, rather than being directed towards the illness of a third party, the patient. The influence of *yangsheng* literature brings first-hand experience of health to the otherwise dispassionate clinical observation witnessed in 'Maishu' (1). Sensations of pleasure, pain, and simply good health form the experience through which the cosmological explanations of *qi*, *yin*, and *yang* became part of the physiology of the inner body and eventually became the foundation of medical theory. Once we have recognised the influence of personal records of the body on ideas such as *yin*, *yang*, and *qi* it is a very short step to appreciate how, in the elaboration of medical correspondences, the authors of classical medical theory also described physical experience of emotion, joy, rage, fear, and grief in the same terms. In this way they prevented any radical disintegration of human being into mind and body in Chinese medical thought. Through subjective descriptions of the experience of sex, of breathing and of other health-related activities, classical Chinese medical thought gained a language and cosmology based on the attainment of a radiant *sense* of well-being rather than merely a state of health defined by the absence of the symptoms of sickness.

References to premodern Chinese and Japanese works

Beiji qianjin yaofang 備急千金要方 (Essential Prescriptions worth a Thousand, for Urgent Need). Tang, 650–9. Sun Simiao 孫思邈. Renmin weisheng chubanshe, Beijing, 1955.

Guoyu 國語 (The Sayings of the States). Zhou, 5th to 2nd centuries BC. Anon. Shanghai guji chubanshe, Shanghai, 1978.

Han Fei zi 韓非子. Zhou, 3rd century BC. *SBBY*.

Han shu 漢書 (Document of the Han). Han, 32–92 AD. Ban Gu 班固. Zhonghua shuju chubanshe, Beijing, 1975.

Huangdi neijing 黃帝內經 (The Yellow Emperor's Inner Canon). Zhou, Qin, Han, to 1st century AD. *SBBY*.

Ishinpō 醫心方 (Remedies at the Heart of Medicine). 982 AD. Tambano Yasuyori 丹波康賴. Huaxia chubanshe, Beijing, 1993.

Laozi 老子. Warring States, 3rd century BC. References to *Laozi xiaogu*. Annotated by Ma Xulun 馬敘倫. Guji chubanshe, Shanghai, 1956.

Lingshu 靈樞 (Divine Pivot). See *Huangdi neijing*.

Lüshi chunqiu 呂氏春秋 (Mr Lü's Spring & Autumn). Zhou, 3rd century BC. References to *Lüshi chunqiu jiaoshi*. Annotated by Chen Qiyou 陳奇猷. Xuelin chubanshe, Shanghai, 1984.

Lunyu 論語 (The Analects). Zhou, 3rd century BC. References to *Lunyu yizhu*. Annotated by Yang Bojun 楊伯峻. Zhonghua shuju, Beijing, 1958. Transl. by D.C. Lau 1979, and James Legge (1893) 1935.

Mengzi 孟子 (Mencius). Zhou, 4th century BC. *SBBY*. Transl. by D.C. Lau.

SBBY: *Sibu beiyao* 四部備要 (Complete Essentials of the Four Divisions of Literature). 1927–35. Zhonghua shuju, Shanghai.

Shiji 史記 (Records of the Historian). Han, *ca* 100 BC. Sima Qian 司馬遷. Zhonghua shuju, Beijing, 1975.

Shuowen jiezi 說文解字 (Discussing Patterns and Explaining Words). Han, *ca* 55–149 AD. Xu Shen 許慎. References to *Shuowen jiezi zhu*. Qing, 1776–1807. Commentated by Duan Yucai 段玉裁. Shanghai guji chubanshe, Shanghai, 1981.

Suwen 素問 (Basic Questions). See *Huangdi neijing*.

Zhenjiu jiayi jing 針灸甲乙經 (AB Canon of Acumoxa). Wu, Jin, 256–82 AD. Huangfu Mi 皇甫謐. References to *Zhenjiu jiayi jing jiaozhu*. Annotated by Zhang Can'ga 張燦玾 and Xu Guoqian 徐國仟. Renmin weisheng chubanshe, Beijing.

Zhuangzi 莊子. Zhou, Qin, Han, 4th to 2nd centuries BC. *SBBY*.

References to modern works

Allan, Sarah 1997. *The Way of Water and Sprouts of Virtue*. State University of New York Press, Albany.

Anon. 1990. *Location of Acupoints*. Foreign Languages Press, Beijing.

Barrett, Timothy 1980. 'On the Transmission of the *Shen Tzu* and of the *Yang-Sheng Yao-Chi*'. *Journal of the Royal Asiatic Society* 2, 168–76.

Brashier, Kenneth E. 1996. 'Han Thanatology and the Division of "Souls"'. *Early China* 21, 125–58.

Cheng Xinnong 1990. *Chinese Acupuncture and Moxibustion*. Foreign Languages Press, Beijing.

Chiu, Martha 1986. 'Mind, Body and Illness in a Chinese Medical Tradition'. PhD thesis in History and East Asian Languages, Harvard University.

Fracasso, Riccardo 1993. 'Shan hai ching'. In Loewe, 359–61.

Gao Dalun 高大倫 1992. *Zhangjiashan Han jian 'Maishu' jiaoshi* 張家山漢簡脈書校釋 (Explanation of the 'Channel Document' on Han Dynasty Bamboo Slips from Zhangjiashan). Chengdu chubanshe, Chengdu.

1995. *Zhangjiashan Han jian 'Yinshu' yanjiu* 張家山漢簡引書研究 (Research into the 'Pulling Document' on Han Dynasty Bamboo Slips from Zhangjiashan). Bashu shushe, Chengdu.

Graham, Angus C. 1981. *Chuang-tzu: the Inner Chapters*. Allen and Unwin, London.

1989. *Disputers of the Tao: Philosophical Argument in Ancient China*. Open Court, La Salle, Ill.

Granet, Marcel 1934. *La Pensée Chinoise*. La Renaissance du Livre, Paris.

Harper, Donald 1982. 'The Wu Shi Erh Ping Fang: Translation and Prolegomena'. PhD thesis in Oriental Languages, University of California, Berkeley.

1985. 'A Chinese Demonography of the Third Century BC'. *Harvard Journal of Asiatic Studies* 45, 459–541.

1987. 'The Sexual Arts of Ancient China as Described in a Manuscript of the Second Century BC'. *Harvard Journal of Asiatic Studies* 47, 539–93.

1998. *Early Chinese Medical Literature: the Mawangdui Medical Manuscripts*. Kegan Paul, London.

He Zhiguo 何志國 and Vivienne Lo 1996. 'The Channels: a Preliminary Examination of a Lacquered Figurine from the Western Han Period'. *Early China* 21, 81–124.

Hunansheng bowuguan and Zhongguo kexueyuan kaogu yanjiusuo 湖南省博物館，中國科學院考古研究所 1974. 'Changsha Mawangdui er, sanhao Hanmu fajue jianbao' 長沙馬王堆二，三號漢墓發掘簡報 (Excavation Report of Han Tomb nos. 2 and 3 at Changsha, Mawangdui). *Wenwu* 7, 39–48.

Jiangling Zhangjiashan Han jian zhengli xiaozu 江陵張家山漢簡整理小組 (eds.) 1989. 'Jiangling
    Zhangjiashan Han jian "Maishu" shiwen' 江陵張家山漢簡《脈書》釋文 (Transcript of the
    'Maishu' on Bamboo Slips from Jiangling Zhangjiashan). *Wenwu* 7, 72–4.
Keegan, David 1986. 'The *Huang-ti nei-ching*: the Structure of the Compilation: the Significance of the
    Structure'. PhD thesis in History, University of California, Berkeley.
Kohn, Livia (ed.) 1989. *Taoist Meditation and Longevity Techniques*. Center for Chinese Studies,
    University of Michigan, Ann Arbor.
Lau, D. C. 1970. *Mencius*. Penguin, Harmondsworth.
    1979. *Confucius, The Analects*. Penguin, Harmondsworth.
Legge, James 1935. *The Chinese Classics*, vol. I. *Confucian Analects, the Great Learning, and Analects
    of the Mean*. Reprint of last edition of Oxford University Press, Jinxue shuju, Taibei.
Li Ling and McMahon, Keith 1992. 'The Contents and Terminology of the Mawangdui Texts on the Arts
    of the Bedchamber'. *Early China* 17, 145–85.
Lo, Vivienne 1998. 'The Influence of Yangsheng Culture on Early Chinese Medical Theory'. PhD thesis
    in History, School of Oriental and African Studies, University of London.
Loewe, Michael (ed.) 1993. *Early Chinese Texts: a Bibliographical Guide*. Institute of East Asian
    Studies, University of California, Berkeley.
Lu Gwei-djen and Needham, Joseph. 1980. *Celestial Lancets: a History and Rationale of Acupuncture
    and Moxa*. Cambridge University Press, Cambridge.
Ma Jixing 馬繼興 (ed.) 1992. *Mawangdui guyishu kaoshi* 馬王堆古醫書考釋 (Explanation of Ancient
    Medical Documents from Mawangdui). Hunan kexue jishu chubanshe, Changsha.
'Maishu' shiwen (1989), see Jiangling Zhangjiashan Han jian zhengli xiaozu.
Major, John 1993. *Heaven and Earth in Early Han Thought: Chapters Three, Four and Five of the
    Huainanzi*. State University of New York Press, Albany.
Mawangdui Hanmu boshu zhengli xiaozu 馬王堆漢墓帛書整理小組 (eds.) 1980. *Mawangdui Hanmu
    boshu* 馬王堆漢墓帛書 (The Silk Documents from a Han Tomb at Mawangdui), vol. I. Wenwu
    chubanshe, Beijing.
    (eds.) 1985. *Mawangdui Hanmu boshu* 馬王堆漢墓帛書 (The Silk Documents from a Han Tomb at
    Mawangdui), vol. IV. Wenwu chubanshe, Beijing.
McKnight, Brian E. 1981. *The Washing Away of Wrongs – Song Ji*. Center for Chinese Studies, University
    of Michigan, Ann Arbor.
Peng Hao 彭浩 1990. 'Zhangjiashan Han jian "Yinshu" chutan' 張家山漢簡引書初探 (Preliminary
    Investigation of The Han Dynasty Bamboo Slips from Zhangjiashan). *Wenwu* 10, 87–91.
Robinet, Isabelle 1989. 'Original Contributions of *Neidan*'. In Kohn, 325–8.
Schipper, Kristofer 1993. *The Taoist Body*. University of California Press, Berkeley.
Shi Yunzi 石雲子 1994. 'Jiekai Zhangjiashan Han mu muzhu zhi mi' 揭開張家山漢墓墓主之謎
    (Solving the Mystery of the Owner of the Han Dynasty Tomb at Zhangjiashan). *Zhongguo wen-
    wubao* 14, 3.
Sivin, Nathan 1987. *Traditional Medicine in Contemporary China*. A Partial Translation of *Revised
    Outline of Chinese Medicine* (1972) with an Introductory Study on Change in Present-day and Early
    Medicine. Center for Chinese Studies, University of Michigan, Ann Arbor.
    1993. 'Huang ti nei ching'. In Loewe, 196–215.
Tan Qixiang 譚其驤 1982. *Zhongguo lishi dituji* 中國歷史地圖集 (Collection of Historical Chinese
    Maps). Ditu chubanshe, Beijing.
Unschuld, Paul U. 1985. *Medicine in China: a History of Ideas*. University of California Press, Berkeley.
    1986. *Nan-Ching: the Classic of Difficult Issues*. University of California, Berkeley.
Wile, Douglas 1992. *The Art of the Bedchamber: the Chinese Sexual Yoga Classics Including Women's
    Solo Meditation Techniques*. State University of New York Press, Albany.

Yamada Keiji 1979. 'The Formation of the Huang-ti Nei-ching', *Acta Asiatica* 36, 67–89.

'Yinshu' shiwen (1990), see Zhangjiashan Han jian zhenglizu.

Zhangjiashan Han jian zhenglizu 張家山漢簡整理組 (eds.) 1990. 'Zhangjiashan Han jian "Yinshu" shi-wen' 張家山漢簡《引書》釋文 (Transcription of the Zhangjiashan 'Yinshu' on Han Dynasty Bamboo Slips). *Wenwu* 10, 82–6.

Zhangjiashan Han mu zhujian zhengli xiaozu 張家山漢墓竹簡整理小組 (eds.) 1985. 'Jiangling Zhangjiashan Han jian gaishu' 江陵張家山漢簡概述 (An Overview of the Bamboo Slips from Jiangling Zhangjiashan). *Wenwu* 1, 9–15.

2

Pulse diagnostics in the Western Han: how *mai* and *qi* determine *bing*

ELISABETH HSU

This chapter explores an early text on pulse diagnostics. This text is, in fact, the earliest relatively comprehensive account still extant, and since it predates the literature on canonical medical doctrine, it is not easy to understand. It contains twenty-five medical case histories and this study focuses on the key concepts of the pulse diagnostics which are contained in them. The analysis proposes that the text interrelates the notions *bing* 病 (disorder), *mai* 脈 (vessel-pulses), and *qi* 氣 (vapour-impulsions) in ways not recorded in earlier writings: the doctor examines the *mai* and thereby detects the qualities of *qi* on the grounds of which he determines the name of a disorder (*bing*).

The first part of the study will examine the structure of the text and context in which it is embedded, and with an excerpt it will point out the style of medical reasoning particular to this text. The second and main part of the study explores the concepts *bing*, *mai*, and *qi*. The third and concluding part compares their meaning in this text with that found in earlier medical texts. The chapter documents 'a change of the way of doing things' in Chinese medicine which, from an outsider's viewpoint, is tantamount to an 'innovation'.

The main protagonist of the text did not see himself as an innovator. Nor did he consider his methods of diagnostics innovative. He did, however, present his skills as superior to those of other doctors. As will be shown below, he reasoned within a conceptual framework more sophisticated than theirs: his notion of *bing* systematically accounted for several facets of the patient's condition, including the name, the cause, and what I propose to call the 'quality' of the disorder. This quality of the disorder which, as put forward here, belongs among the crucial factors for determining the name of the disorder (*bing*), was assessed by interrelating *mai* and *qi* in new ways.[1]

---

[1] This article summarises ongoing research for a comparativist project on medical case histories in antiquity, jointly undertaken with Sir Geoffrey Lloyd. It is based on an earlier study (Hsu 1987) and a preliminary translation of the 'Canggong zhuan' completed with help from Mark Lewis and Michael Loewe, and with comments by Catherine Despeux and Robert Gassmann. An earlier draft of this article was discussed in Mark Lewis' study group with Kenneth Brashier and Roel Sterckx.

I: Introduction

The 'Canggong zhuan'

What is here called the 'Canggong zhuan' 倉公傳 (Memoir of the Master of the Granary) forms the latter part of chapter 105 in the *Shiji* 史記 (Records of the Historian).[2] It is probably based on a document that was written, after 164 BC and before 153 BC, in response to an Imperial decree (*zhao* 召) and was presumably edited, by 90 BC, for inclusion among the Memoirs (*liezhuan* 列傳).[3] The Memoirs constituted a new genre in Chinese historiography: in them, the narrative was clustered around the lives of particular individuals. This innovation in historiography arose during the Han dynasty when the Grand Historian (*taishiling* 太史令) Sima Qian 司馬遷 (?145–86 BC) was confronted with the difficult task of accounting for the complexities of local histories in the newly installed empire.[4] He addressed the problem by creating different text genres for different aspects of the empire's history which structured the *Shiji* into five parts: the Basic Annals (*benji* 本記), the Chronological Tables (*biao* 表), the Treatises (*shu* 書), the Hereditary Houses (*shijia* 世家), and the Memoirs.[5] The Annals were modelled on former histories of the Zhou and focused on politically central figures, while the newly created genre of Memoirs accounted for more peripheral personages. With seventy chapters, they constituted by far the most voluminous part of the *Shiji.*

The Memoirs discussed men of letters, thinkers, generals, wives of politically important persons, statesmen of the principalities, great financers, famous inventors, pioneers, barbarians, outlaws, and specific groups of people such as ethnic groups or people with similar talents.[6] 'The intense focus on a few great heroes was replaced by a multitude of short biographies of the merely eminent or exemplary.'[7] These personages were often discussed in pairs within one Memoir, though they did not necessarily have geographic

---

[2] This study is primarily based on the *Shiki kaichū kōshō* 史記會注考證, *juan* 105, 16–62, edited by Takigawa Kametarō 瀧川龜太郎. For an early translation into German, see Hübotter (1927); for an annotated translation into French, see Bridgman (1955). These translations by Western medical doctors represent a remarkable achievement but necessarily have limitations, given that the Mawangdui manuscripts have since been unearthed and the history of Chinese medicine has since become a recognised field of scholarly inquiry.

[3] Loewe (1997).

[4] Twitchett (1961), 96, points out that the Memoirs elaborated on an aspect of the 'tradition' (*zhuan* 傳), especially that known as the *Zuo zhuan* 左傳 (Zuo Tradition) which had already extended 'the field of history far from the dry chronicle of court ritual centered on the king which is presented by the Spring and Autumn Annals'.

[5] Watson (1958), 104–7.   [6] Chavannes (1895), vol. I, clxxix–clxxx.   [7] Johnson (1981), 271.

or chronological affinities. In the Memoirs, the Grand Historian is considered to have recorded theme-oriented 'connected events', this in complementarity to the first part of the *magnum opus*, the Basic Annals, which were chronologically organised.[8]

Chinese historians have categorised the two main protagonists of the 45th Memoir, Bian Que 扁鵲 and Canggong 倉公 as medical doctors (*yi* 醫) who both belonged to the same 'lineage' or 'tradition of learning' (*xue pai* 學派) noted for its pulse diagnostics.[9] But Loewe remarks: 'If the chapter is to be regarded as an account of a particular profession or group, its title does not reflect that aim, as do titles of other chapters.'[10] In support of this one notes that the chapter's concluding remark draws attention to a common moral pattern of the two doctors' lives, rather than to a common professional concern: 'Hence Laozi says: "Beauty and goodness are the instruments for [attracting] the inauspicious." Isn't he speaking about Bian Que's and others' calamities? As for Canggong, one can say that he was close to them' (故老子曰：《美好者，不祥之器》. 豈謂扁鵲 等邪？若倉公者，可謂近之矣.).[11] The quote attributed to the legendary author of the *Daode jing* 道德經 (Canon of the Way and its Power), which cannot be located in its extant versions, seems to say that the Memoir is concerned with a moral issue: two personages of outstanding talent were, rather than being honoured, precisely because of their talent treated unfairly. The title and the conclusion of the Memoir contain no allusion to medicine as the chapter's theme.

Leaving aside the difficult question of what in fact was the intention of the Grand Historian for composing the 'Bian Que Canggong liezhuan' 扁鵲倉公列傳 (Memoir of Bian Que and the Master of the Granary), this study concentrates on the textual material that makes up most of the chapter and informs us about medicine. The medicine presented refers indeed in both biographies to *mai* as a means of diagnostics. In the 'Bian Que zhuan' 扁鵲傳,[12] the protagonist's skills in 'examining the *mai*' (*zhen mai* 診脈) are mentioned in the opening paragraph, but their diagnostic use in most of the following narrative is minor, if not outrightly denied. In the 'Canggong zhuan', by contrast, 'examining the *mai*' is an important constituent of medical reasoning.

The 'Bian Que zhuan' and 'Canggong zhuan' are, in fact, so different that their juxtaposition in one Memoir invites comment. The contrast is already marked by the appellations rendered in the chapter title: Bian Que, the name by which Qin Yueren 秦越人 is indicated, refers to a feathered and winged being.[13] Taicanggong 太倉公, the title of

---

[8] Watson (1958), 120–34.   [9] Li Bocong (1990).   [10] Loewe (1997), 304.
[11] *Shiki kaichū kōshō, juan* 105, 62.   [12] *Shiki kaichū kōshō, juan* 105, 2–19.
[13] 'The expression Bian Que could perhaps be interpreted as meaning "by the sign of a Magpie", deriving from a placard of the device that Qin Yueren was thought to have adopted to display his professional activities.' See Loewe (1997), 304.

Chunyu Yi 淳于意, indicates a government position: Yi was an official of Qi 齊 during the early Western Han, the Director of the Great Granary (*taicangzhang* 太倉長).[14] These designations alone, which may well be the protagonist's terms of self-reference, seem to announce that two opposing facets of medicine are to be presented: the miraculous and fabulous in the first account, the meticulous and formulaic in the second.

The activities of Bian Que span a period of several generations during the Eastern Zhou, located at times in Qi 齊 and at times in Zhao 趙. The historicity of this personage is evidently questionable.[15] Canggong, by contrast, can in all probability be related to a historical figure who came from Linzi 臨菑 (in the modern province Shandong). He was active as a doctor in the middle of the second century BC and had a clientele that lived in Qi and in neighbouring kingdoms, identifiable in a historical atlas.[16]

Bian Que had extraordinary faculties of clairvoyance which he absorbed by drinking over thirty days a potion given to him by an 'unusual person' (*fei chang ren* 非常人), the gentleman (*jun* 君) Zhang Sang 長桑. Chunyu Yi, by contrast, actively sought the guidance of more than one master.[17] For three long years he endured learning texts he had received from his most revered teacher Yang Qing 陽慶 and their subsequent application to medical practice until they proved effective. Even if reported in a guarded fashion, Bian Que's deeds were known for bordering on the fantastic – he was held to bring the dead back to life – and he was, at least on one occasion, highly esteemed. Canggong, however, was not a famous, feared, or admired doctor. He was accused in front of the magistrate because there were clients he had refused to treat. But in the end Bian Que was killed due to a mighty and envious rival, while Canggong was set free thanks to the pleas of his fifth daughter, the weakest of the weak.[18]

The two narratives also differ in their styles of writing. Bian Que's biography often has the flow and rhythm of a folk tale, while Canggong's report is punctilious and rich in technical terminology. The accounts were not written at the same time: aspects of their

---

[14] Loewe (1997) points out that *gong* may be used by way of self-reference among officials, e.g. Sima Qian who held the post of a *taishiling* (Grand Historian) and referred to himself as *taishigong* 太史公. Taicanggong may, like Bian Que, indicate the name by which the personage referred to himself.

[15] For an extensive study on Bian Que and his biography, see Yamada (1988).

[16] Tan Qixiang (1982), 15–16, 19–20. For the controversy over Chunyu Yi's exact life dates, see Wilbur (1943), 288–9, whom Loewe (1997) follows, and Bridgman (1955), 66.

[17] For the transmission of medical knowledge in the 'Canggong zhuan' as recorded in the introductory and closing section of the text, see Sivin (1995).

[18] The episode is also recorded in *Shiji, juan* 10, 427–8, and *Han shu* 漢書 *juan* 23, 1097–8, in the thirteenth year of Emperor Wen 文 (167 BC). Based on this, Yi's fifth daughter Chunyu Tiying 淳于緹縈 is praised for skills in argumentation in the *Lienü zhuan* 列女傳 (79–78 BC). See *SBBY*, 6.13b–6.14b.

contents, like medical idioms,[19] indicate that at least parts of Bian Que's biography are more recent than Canggong's.[20] This raises the question of why the more recent text should be presented first. One could guess that, despite the above comments, the order of the texts reflects chronology. But reasons of rhetoric are more compelling: the contrast to the narrative of Bian Que's deeds that border on the legendary heightens the emphasis on method and detailed observation in Canggong's account. In what follows we shall focus on the latter.

Text excerpt: the 'heat disorder' of the envoy who in winter fell into cold water

From a historical and philological viewpoint, the 'Canggong zhuan' may be divided into two parts: an introductory summary rendered in the voice of the historian and the main part of the chapter which is given in the voice of a subject answering to an Imperial decree. This decree was issued to the person(s) 'who had experience and success in treating illnesses and [recognising imminent] death or life' (*suo wei zhi bing si sheng yan zhe* 所為治病死生驗者).[21] Since it is not mentioned in the Annals, it was probably intended for limited circulation or possibly even restricted to a particular individual.[22] The questions in the decree are spelt out in the beginning of the second and main part of the biography. There then follows a more comprehensive account of Canggong's personal history and medical learning, twenty-five case histories, and eight interview questions and answers.

From a structural and thematic viewpoint, Canggong's biography, like Bian Que's, is divided into three parts. The introductory part provides a summary of the protagonists' names and places of origin, their inclinations in their youth, and their ways of learning medicine. The main part consists of individual case histories: three in the 'Bian Que zhuan' and twenty-five in the 'Canggong zhuan'. The third part, where comparison between the two biographies is more difficult, contains more generalised statements: where the 'Bian Que zhuan' summarises the six conditions where a doctor is not to treat an illness – generally cited as the earliest statement of Chinese medical ethics, the 'Canggong zhuan' ends with eight questions and their respective answers.

---

[19] The triple *jiao* (*sanjiao* 三焦), for instance, is mentioned in the 'Bian Que zhuan', but not in the 'Canggong zhuan'. See *Shiki kaichū kōshō, juan* 105, 13–14.

[20] Bridgman (1955), 14, suggests that the 'Bian Que zhuan' was written in 90 BC, sixty years later than the 'Canggong zhuan'.

[21] *Shiki kaichū kōshō, juan* 105, 21.

[22] Loewe (1997). There is some controversy over the reasons why the decree was issued, see Sivin (1995) and Cullen (this volume).

The following analysis of the three key concepts *bing*, *mai*, and *qi* is based on a systematic investigation of the twenty-five case histories which constitute, from a structural and thematic viewpoint, the second part of the 'Canggong zhuan'. Before embarking on it, one of these case histories is presented in its entirety (case 4):[23]

1. Xin 信, the chief of the palace wardrobe of Qi, fell ill (*bing*).[24]
2. I entered [his room] to examine his *mai* and reported:
3. 'It is the *qi* of a heat disorder.[25]
4. It is like in summer heat that you sweat.[26]
5. The *mai* is slightly weakened.
6. You will not die.
7. This illness is contracted when actually bathing in running water when it is very cold, and once it is over, getting hot.'
8. Xin said: 'Yes, so it is.
9. Last winter season, I was sent as an envoy of the king to Chu 楚.
10. When I got to the Yangzhou 陽周 river in Ju 莒 county,[27] the planks of the bridge were partly broken.
11. I then seized the shaft of the carriage;
12. I did not yet intend to cross.
13. The horses became frightened and they promptly fell.
14. I was immersed in water, I almost died.
15. Some officers immediately came to save me and pulled me out of the water.
16. My clothes were completely soaked.
17. After a short time I felt cold.
18. When this was over, I felt hot like a fire.
19. Up to today, I cannot stand the cold.'
20. Your servant, Yi 意, immediately made for him the liquid *huoji* 火齊 to drive away the heat.[28]

---

[23] *Shiki kaichū kōshō*, *juan* 105, 30–1. In what follows, the twenty-five cases are the units of reference, page numbers being given only for citations.

[24] *zhongyu fuzhang* 中御府長 (chief of the palace wardrobe), see Bielenstein (1980), 188 n. 126.

[25] *rebing qi* 熱病氣 (the *qi* of a heat disorder), not *rebing* 熱病. Although *re* refers in all likelihood to fever, the literal translation of *re* as heat is adopted here.

[26] *ran* 然 (this so being) is translated as *ru zhi* 如之 (like it), see Pulleyblank (1995), 180. Evidently, profuse sweating was a characteristic of summer heat.

[27] Ju 莒 was in the kingdom of Chengyang 成陽國, see *Han shu*, *juan* 28B, 1635. It was located on 35.3°N and 118.5° E, see Tan Qixiang (1991), 19–20.

[28] *yetang huoji* 液湯火齊 (lit. the liquid broth [called] fire regulation). The compound word *yetang* is unusual; *tangye* occurs in titles of various books as for instance the *tangye jingfa* 湯液經法 in *Han shu*, *juan* 30, 1777.

21. After drinking the first dose, the sweating came to an end.
22. After drinking the second, the heat left.
23. After drinking the third, the illness subsided.
24. I then made him apply medicines.[29]
25. After about twenty days, he did not have any illness.
26. The means whereby I recognised Xin's illness were that at the time when I took his *mai*, there was a joined *yin*.[30]
27. The 'Model of the Vessel-pulses' (Maifa 脈法) says:
28. 'If in the case of a heat disorder, *yin* 陰 and *yang* 陽 intermingle, one dies.'
29. When I took [the *mai*], there was no intermingling, but a joined *yin*.
30. In cases of the joined *yin*, the *mai* is smooth, clear, and well.[31]
31. Although his heat had not yet come to an end, he was still going to live.
32. The *qi* of the kidneys was sometimes for a moment muddled,
33. when it was at the opening of the *taiyin mai* 太陰脈, however, it was scarce.[32]
34. This is because of water *qi*.[33]
35. As long as the kidneys are firm [and strong], they control the water.[34]
36. By means of this I knew it.
37. Had I neglected to treat [the illness] instantly, then it would have turned into a coldness and heat.[35]

1. 齊中御府長信病。
2. 臣意入診其脈，告曰：
3. 熱病氣也。
4. 然暑汗。
5. 脈少衰。
6. 不死。
7. 此病得之當浴流水而寒甚，已則熱。
8. 信曰：唯然。

---

[29] *fu yao* 服藥 (to apply medicines), often refers to an external application in early medical texts, see Ma Jixing (1992), 429, 432, 566, 568, but there are exceptions, see Harper (1982), 407, and Ma Jixing (1992), 500.
[30] *bingyin* 并陰 (double *yin*). Not attested in the received literature.
[31] *shun qing er yu* 順清而愈; the alternative reading is, 'being smooth and clear, one is healthy'.
[32] *taiyin* 太陰 (major *yin*), one of the six classificatory qualities of *mai*, already recorded in the Mawangdui vessel texts and standard in canonical doctrine, enumerated on p. 83.
[33] *shuiqi* 水氣 (lit. water *qi*). Not mentioned in *Lingshu* but frequent in *Suwen*.
[34] *shen gu zhu shui* 腎固主水 has as alternative reading: 'the kidneys certainly control the water'.
[35] *hanre* 寒熱 ([intermittent] coldness and heat). Frequently mentioned in the *Suwen* and *Lingshu*.

9. 往冬時，為王使於楚，
10. 至莒縣陽周水而莒橋粱頗壞。
11. 信則攬車轅，
12. 未欲渡也。
13. 馬驚即墮。
14. 信身入水中，幾死。
15. 吏即來救信，出之水中。
16. 衣盡濡。
17. 有閒而身寒，
18. 已熱如火。
19. 至今不可以見寒。
20. 臣意即為之液湯火齊，逐熱。
21. 一飲汗盡。
22. 再飲熱去，
23. 三飲病已。
24. 即使服藥。
25. 出入二十日，身無病者。
26. 所以知信之病者，切其脈時并陰。
27. 脈法曰：
28. 熱病陰陽交者死。
29. 切之不交，并陰。
30. 并陰者，脈順清而愈。
31. 其熱雖未盡，猶活也。
32. 腎氣有時閒濁，
33. 在太陰脈口而希，
34. 是水氣也。
35. 腎固主水。
36. 以此知之。
37. 失治一時，即轉為寒熱。

The medical reasoning in this case history relates in a fairly comprehensive way to the occurrence of an illness in an individual. It identifies the name of the client's condition (line 3), gives the concomitant signs and symptoms (lines 4–5), a prognostic statement (line 6), an announcement of the cause of the illness (line 7), a prolonged account of the onset of the illness (lines 8–19), information on treatment and its effect on the course of the illness (lines 20–5), medical speculation in terms of *mai* and *qi*, *yin*, and *yang* (lines 26–36), and a statement about an alternative progression of the illness if no therapeutic steps had been taken (line 37).

Compared with episodes of illness described in the *Zuo zhuan* 左傳 (Zuo Tradition) from the Warring States period, those in the 105th chapter of the *Shiji* are more comprehensive, but less transparent. Medical speculation is expounded in a highly technical vocabulary which is comparable to that in early medical manuscripts unearthed from tombs closed in 168 BC in Mawangdui 馬王堆 and in at the earliest 186 BC or at the latest 156 BC in Zhangjiashan 張家山.[36]

The 'Canggong zhuan' combines descriptive narrative, as known from the *Zuo zhuan*, with elaborate medical speculation, as known from early medical manuscripts with a distinct technical vocabulary.[37] It can be regarded as innovative insofar as it is the first known text to record medical reasoning in the form of individual case histories. The fact that doctors started writing *zhenji* 診籍 (consultation records),[38] as Chunyu Yi calls them, is in itself worth investigation. For what purpose were they written and what effect did they have on medical reasoning? Given the scarcity of documentation, it is difficult to discern the effect that writing case histories had on medical reasoning. There is no doubt, however, that the medical reasoning in Chunyu Yi's case histories is highly sophisticated and more systematic and systemic than in any other early medical text.[39]

There are several possible ways of interpreting ancient case histories: one can try to elucidate them in terms of modern medical practice, an undertaking which can be justified by arguing that both ancient and modern medical practice are interested in assessing and influencing processes that are to a certain extent biological and hence in many respects similar, cross-culturally and diachronically. This is naturally a difficult undertaking, fraught with the dangers of comparing and contrasting different culturally specific conceptual frameworks and, more recently, historians have much preferred text-critical studies into the literature of the same time period. I have made use of (a) interpretations in terms of Western biomedicine, (b) contemporary Chinese medicine, (c) the philological method of tracing the same word in different texts of the late Zhou and the Han, and (d) a linguistically informed method that I propose to call 'structural

---

[36] For official transcription of the Mawangdui medical manuscripts, volume IV, see Mawangdui Han mu boshu zhengli xiaozu (1985). For translation of all Mawangdui medical texts, see Harper (1998). For an earlier translation of the 'Wushi'erbing fang', see Harper (1982). For discussion of how the Mawangdui vessel texts interweave with *Lingshu* 10, and the translation of these three texts, see Keegan (1988), chapter 3, 114–66, and appendix 2, 265–344. For an edited, richly annotated and indexed text of the medical Mawangdui manuscripts, see Ma Jixing (1992). For the Zhangjiashan 'Maishu' 脈書, see Gao Dalun (1992) and Jiangling Zhangjiashan Han jian zhengli xiaozu 1985.

[37] The vocabulary is technical, but does not represent a technical terminology characteristic of the modern sciences. For explorations of the purpose of the case histories, see Lloyd.

[38] *Shiki kaichū kōshō, juan* 105, 53.

[39] By 'systemic' I mean 'within a system of medical terms'. Reasoning in Chinese medical treatises is generally systemic rather than systematic.

analytic'. Though each of these methods has its limitations, each was useful for clarifying the case histories.

Any retrospective diagnosis calls for a note of caution, but Chunyu Yi's description of individual cases is so detailed that it is difficult to resist biomedical speculation. In his interpretation of the above case history, Bridgman[40] diagnoses malaria on the grounds of the names given for the client's condition – a heat disorder (*rebing* 熱病) that is about to become a coldness and heat (*hanre* 寒 熱). He explains that Xin must have contracted the malaria before falling into the water and considers Chunyu Yi to have mistaken the true cause of the illness. *Hanre*, often synonymous with *nüe* 瘧 (intermittent heat and coldness), is indeed generally considered to refer to the intermittent fevers characteristic of malaria.[41] However, rather than imputing an error to the ancient doctor, today's researchers are well advised to admit our own serious limitations regarding ancient medical knowledge: *hanre* can refer to many conditions other than malaria.

Lu Gwei-djen and Joseph Needham affirm, without any further explanation, that Xin's condition was 'surely bronchitis or pneumonia'.[42] If it were bronchitis, one would expect the patient to complain of coughing or of chest pain. But it is possible that the hypothermia that Xin suffered after falling into the water in winter may indeed have given rise to pneumonia, or any kind of infection for that matter.[43] Sweating (reported in line 4) and fear of the cold (reported in line 19) can be a reaction to hypothermia, but given that the doctor anticipates that the condition would turn into a coldness and heat (in line 37), which from a Western medical viewpoint must refer to chills, the sweating and fear of the cold are best taken as symptoms of a fever, possibly a fever due to an infection. The name of the disorder refers to heat which also indicates fever. In the case of a fever, one would expect a rapid pulse, but the pulse is (in line 5) reported to be only slightly weakened (*mai shao shuai* 脈少衰). This may mean, in a rather general way, that the patient has not been much affected by the pathological condition.

The effect of the treatment, given in lines 20–5, is understood from a Western medical viewpoint to mean that the high fever was first lowered, which stopped the sweating, and that the residual lowered temperature was soon normalised. The doctor's insistence on treating the patient with externally applied medicines for another twenty days was certainly the appropriate thing to do in the case of an infection before the advent of antibiotics. European folk medicine, for instance, prescribed long term hot fomentation (potato, onion, or cabbage fomentation).

---

[40] Bridgman (1955), 73.   [41] Yu Yunxiu (1953), 235.   [42] Lu and Needham (1967), 231.
[43] Dr Dorin Ritzmann, MD, p.c., who provided also the following Western medical interpretation of this case.

The above attempt at a biomedical interpretation of Xin's case history highlights two important points: firstly, it shows that this case history is not completely nonsensical; at least in parts a biomedical doctor can relate to it. If it were a satire or travesty, as has been suggested in the light of the difficulties that the interpretation of the medical rationale in these case histories poses, their author must have understood something of the nature of illnesses and their course. Secondly, we observe that the Western biomedical diagnosis is based on information about signs and symptoms as well as reports of the onset and course of the illness: when it comes to pulse diagnostics (lines 26–36), biomedical doctors can only shrug their shoulders.

A consultation with practitioners of Traditional Chinese Medicine well versed in pulse diagnostics revealed that with the exception of the quotation from the 'Maifa' (line 28), Chunyu Yi's reasoning in terms of *mai* and *qi* is hard to interpret. The final part of the 'Maifa' citation, saying that the intermingling of *yin* and *yang* leads to death, is commonplace in contemporary Chinese medicine.[44] Reasoning as recorded in the 'Maifa' has evidently been handed down to the present day – often in a surprisingly unaltered form – not only from this case history, but also from several others. In the 'Maifa', and in the subsequent medical literature we know of, there is generally no explicit reporting on the interrelations between *mai* and *qi*. This aspect of Yi's pulse diagnostics does not seem to have survived in the verbally explicit form in which it is recorded in some of these case histories (e.g. lines 32–6 in case 4). This suggests that Yi must have engaged in a form of pulse diagnostics that was related to and yet distinct from that recorded in the 'Maifa'. He must have combined knowledge of pulse diagnostics from different and possibly quite distinct strands of medicine. We will return to this conjecture of mine later, at the end of section II, when attempting to elucidate lines 32–6.

The philologist's method of comparing the same term in different texts from roughly the same time period proved most useful for interpreting some of the key terms. In the above case they are *rebing* 熱病 (heat disorder), *hanre* 寒熱 (coldness and heat), and *yinyang jiao* 陰陽交 (*yin* and *yang* intermingle). With this method I found in respect to *rebing* that in the Mawangdui vessel texts there is a condition called 'heat expels sweat' (*re chu han* 熱出汗), which belongs among the illnesses generated on the *yangming mai* 陽明脈 (*yang* brightness vessel).[45] In the *Huangdi neijing* 黃帝內經 (Yellow Emperor's Inner Canon), *rebing* is often mentioned in the text and there are even chapter titles referring to it, such as those of *Suwen* 素問 31 and 33 (Basic Questions) and *Lingshu* 靈樞 23 (Divine Pivot). Among the conditions described in those chapters, there is one in

---

[44] See Hsu (1999), 83.   [45] Mawangdui Han mu boshu zhengli xiaozu (1985), 4.

Suwen 31 which has traits similar to Xin's: 'If a person is harmed by the cold, then the illness he gets is hot; and even if the heat is severe, he will not die' (人之傷於寒也 則為病熱　熱雖甚不死).[46]

The condition of *hanre* is not mentioned in the Mawangdui medical texts, while it frequently occurs throughout the *Inner Canon*: *Lingshu* 21 is entitled *hanre bing* and *Lingshu* 70 has the title *hanre*, but the conditions described there do not directly apply to this case.[47] Considering that Xin must have suffered from fevers over some time and that fevers do weaken the body, it is quite possible that *hanre* indicates in this case a condition of shivering due to general exhaustion. This means that *hanre* does not always refer to intermittent fevers but that it can occur as an end stage to a previous, possibly chronic condition. *Hanre* would then designate a general state of exhaustion, and would not refer to an intermittent fever.

One may have been inclined to view *yinyang jiao* as mentioned in the 'Maifa' quotation, as referring to *hanre*, but there are several reasons for taking account of the description of *yinyang jiao* in *Suwen* 33, which is a chapter not on *hanre* but on *rebing*.[48] There, *yinyang jiao* delimits a state of delirium due to high fever. Given that Xin's condition is called *rebing qi*, it seems reasonable to interpret Yi's citation from the 'Maifa' accordingly.

This is just about as far as conventional methods of interpreting the above case history can bring us. The Western biomedical interpretation was based on the events and symptoms the patient reported on lines 3–25 and on the doctor's consideration given on line 37; contemporary Chinese medicine highlighted the fact that some of the knowledge recorded in line 28 is still considered valid today – this in contrast to the description of *mai* in lines 32–6; and the analysis of selected terms in different contexts threw some light on the notions of *rebing*, *hanre*, and *yinyang jiao*. Since parallels to Xin's condition were found in the extant canonical medical literature, we can safely confirm that Chunyu Yi's medical practice was partly informed by traditions of medicine that were later canonised.

The descriptions of *rebing* and *hanre* vary greatly in the received literature and the condition described in this case correlates with only a few of them (cited above). Medicine was clearly not a monolithic edifice of scholarship but there must have been, two thousand years ago just as now, a multiplicity of points of view.[49] One may be inclined to emphasise that there was rivalry between competing traditions of medicine,

---

[46] *Suwen, juan* 9, *pian* 31, 92. See also *Suwen, juan* 16, *pian* 61, 166, last few sentences.

[47] A condition called *hanre* in *Suwen, juan* 12, *pian* 42, 92, comes, however, closest to this case.

[48] *Suwen, juan* 9, *pian* 33, 96. For a more detailed analysis of this case, see Hsu (2001).

[49] Farquhar (1995).

but the key to the case histories lies in the recognition that Chunyu Yi did not merely emphasise the distinctiveness of his own practice. As will become more obvious below, he was innovative in that his case histories bring different strands of medical knowledge together.

II: Structural analysis of the case histories

Apart from a few sentences in the Mawangdui 'Maifa' and Zhangjiashan 'Maishu' (see section III), medical literature prior to the 'Canggong zhuan' contains hardly any reference to pulse diagnostics. In the later medical literature consulted, it has been very difficult to find parallels to some of the technical terms used here which establish the interrelation of *bing*, *mai*, and *qi*. To explore these interrelationships requires a structural analysis of all the case histories. In the following section I will first establish that Chunyu Yi had a medical specialist's understanding of *bing*.[50] With this sophisticated conception of *bing* in mind, he accounted in a formulaic fashion for various aspects of the illness experience.

The notion of bing

The opening statement in almost every case history is that a certain person is ill (*bing*). Usually, the doctor reports that so and so was ill and then adds that he was summoned to examine this person. Sometimes this opening statement is made specific in terms of the patient's subjective complaint: once the client was ill with a headache (case 1), once he was ill with pain in the lesser abdomen (case 7), and once he was reported to be 'ill' with a bad tooth (case 13).[51] Sometimes the condition of the illness is modified and said to be serious (*bing shen* 病甚), regardless of whether it is lethal (case 23) or can be cured (case 19).[52]

The opening sentence of each case history is still more informative: the person who fell ill is usually named (adult men and women of rank, but not their slaves or children) and identified by status and place (titles of nobility, mostly from the kingdom of Qi).

[50] The term 'medical specialist' is used here because the terminology in early texts that are nowadays considered medical is relatively technical. The term 'specialist' (e.g. ritual specialist) commonly used in anthropology is not used in the sense of the 'specialist' in the modern sciences.

[51] In case 11, the wetnurse herself complains of heat in the feet, but not of an illness (*bing*); however, Yi says that it is an illness (*bing*) and names it, see table 2.1. In case 20, the client considers himself ill (*bing*), but it is uncertain as to whether or not Yi considers the condition an illness; see footnote 61, 68.

[52] In two cases (case 11, 14), the term *bing* is not mentioned in the introductory sentence, but from the context it becomes clear that the condition described does refer to *bing*, see footnote 63.

This was a standard way of identifying subjects during the Han dynasty, particularly in the legal context, as is evident from the twenty-five 'Models for Sealing and Investigating' (Fengzhen shi 封診式) in the *Remnants of Ch'in Law*.[53] Those twenty-five legal case records have a similar formulaic structure, and are intriguing for the detailed style of recording individual cases according to a general schema. They are, however, written in the format of hypothetical actors: they represent models for case records rather than case histories. Moreover, they deal with a large spectrum of different crimes, while Chunyu Yi's case histories centre on one theme: *bing*.

Bing is the common term for designating illness in the case histories, and this contrasts with non-medical pre-Han texts like the *Zuo zhuan*. In the *Zuo zhuan*, *bing* is often used to designate a condition of general disorder, impoverishment, famine, or difficulty of a kingdom (*guo* 國) or city (*yi* 邑), or also of a people (*min* 民 and/or *ren* 人), rather than of an individual. In this sense, it is also used as a causative with the meaning 'to cause trouble or general disaster'. With regard to a person, *ji* is the usual term for designating illness and *ji bing* for referring to a serious illness, while *bing* frequently refers to the emotional state of a person who is aggrieved, often as a result of a previous dispute. In the one text passage where *bing* refers to an illness, it is glossed to mean that the illness is very serious and designates a lethal condition.[54] This interpretation coincides with the definition of *bing* in the *Shuowen jiezi* 説文解字 (Analytic Dictionary of Chinese Characters): '*Bing* is *ji* and more' (病疾加也),[55] which, in turn, is reinforced by Bao Xian's 苞咸 comment on *Lunyu* 9 論語 (Analects): 'If the *ji*-illness is serious, you call it *bing*' (疾甚曰病).[56]

In the case histories under discussion, *bing* is not used in the sense of a pathological condition that is more serious than *ji*. Though in later medical texts often used interchangeably with *ji*, *Shiji* 105.2 in one particular text passage of case 22 distinguishes between *bing* and *ji*: 'The *judgement* says: if a *yang* pathological condition resides inside and a *yin* form resonates on the outside, do not apply violent drugs and stone needles' (論曰：陽疾處內，陰形應外者，不加悍藥及針石).[57] In this sentence, a *yangji* 陽疾 (pathological condition) inside the body is opposed to a *yinxing* 陰形 (form or appearance) on its surface. *Ji* refers, in this case, to a latent pathological condition inside the body, impossible to detect.

[53] Hulsewé (1985), 185–207 and McLeod and Yates (1981). For the four cases of forensic medicine, see also Bodde (1982).
[54] *Zuo zhuan* 3.1046. The above survey of *bing* in the *Zuo zhuan* accounts for all entries in Lau and Chen (1995). I am indebted to Bill Jenner, John Moffett, and Robert Neather for help in working out the meaning of *bing* in the over sixty text passages studied. For detailed discussion, see Hsu (forthcoming).
[55] *Shuowen jiezi, pian* 7, 348.   [56] *Lunyu, pian* 9, *zhang* 12, 341.   [57] *Shiki kaichū kōshō, juan* 105, 50.

Harper makes an observation that is strikingly similar to the above. In the iatromantic Shuihudi 睡虎地 manuscripts that he discusses, *ji* is associated with one of the Five Phases (*wuxing* 五行), say Wood, and becomes *bing* when, for instance, Wood conquers Earth (*mu ke tu* 木克土). Harper comments: '*Ji* is the point of origin of a morbid condition . . . the morbid condition [*ji*] attached to the sign Wood becomes a manifest ailment [*bing*] on the days when Wood conquers Earth.'[58] In the Shuihudi manuscripts, just as in case 22, *ji* refers to an invisible condition that corresponds to a manifest and visible one. Since the Five Phases are associated with certain days in the Shuihudi manuscripts, one could be inclined to emphasise the temporal order between *ji* and *bing*: *ji* is the latent point of origin that eventually develops into the visible pathological condition *bing*. Harper's carefully chosen circumscription of *ji* as 'point of origin' allows one, however, to view *ji* as a latent condition that is located in time and space. Case 22 certainly emphasises the spatial order: *ji* is the latent condition inside the body that is contrasted with *xing* 形 (form) on the outside.[59]

The notion of *bing* in the case histories is superordinate to *ji* and *xing*. It comprises both invisible, postulated processes inside the body, and the manifest aspects of an illness. It may relate to a latent condition, but it can be detected by the doctor using diagnostic means such as, for instance, the quality of the vessel-pulse (*mai* 脈) or the complexion (*se* 色). In some cases, whether the condition described in the case history constitutes a *bing* or not appears controversial.[60]

The translation of *bing* as 'ailment', as suggested for the Shuihudi manuscripts, would be inadequate for the case histories insofar as the term 'ailment' not only implies in most cases superficial manifestations of a morbid condition, but also conveys a sense of subjectively perceived, undefined conditions of unease. *Bing* in the case histories of the 'Canggong zhuan' is not an unspecific entity but has several aspects which a modern reader may identify as name, symptoms, causes, diagnostic signs or qualities and processes that are postulated to take place inside the body. Some of those aspects are systematically recorded, others are mentioned concomitantly. In other words, Yi's notion of *bing* implies a relatively sophisticated conception of illness.

This suggests that *bing* primarily designates a medical specialist's notion of disease as opposed to the experience of illness of the non-specialist. In the case histories, however, there are instances where a layperson uses the word *bing* too, even though *bing* predominantly belongs to the vocabulary of the doctor. In case 15, the opposition

---

[58] Harper (this volume), p. 112.

[59] The latent, the immanent, or potential is located in a time–space continuum, ordered into rubrics that comprise both dimensions. See Granet (1934), 86–114.

[60] See for instance case 19, and the interpretation of *raojia wei bing* 蟯瘕為病 in Hsu (2001).

between the doctor's notion of *bing* that comprises conditions that are latent but apparent to the specialist and that of the layperson, who associates *bing* with consciously felt pain, becomes a matter of dispute. In case 20, the client is reported to be ill (*bing*) and another doctor also considers him ill (*bing*), while Yi distinguishes between *bing* (to be ill) and the condition of this client which he calls *dang bing* 當病 (to match an illness).[61] These episodes show that Yi has a specialist's conception of *bing*, while the word *bing* can be used in a more general sense than that of the medical specialist.

The marked aspects of bing

If one accepts that in the case histories *bing* refers mostly to the medical specialist's understanding of illness, which aspects mattered for identifying *bing* and distinguishing between different *bing*? In order to find the category-determining aspects of *bing*, I examined instances in which Chunyu Yi used the same wording. The method relied on imputing meaning into differences of expression in language, not on the level of syntax which without further specifications would be problematic, but in respect to the repeated use of the same figure of speech. By exploring those aspects that the author of the text explicitly marked, I tried to avoid imposing my own conceptions of illness onto this ancient Chinese text.

Systematically repeated phrases included:

1. a statement in the beginning of each case following the word *yue* (I said); see table 2.1 in appendix
2. a statement following the phrase *bing de zhi* (the illness is contracted by); see table 2.2 in appendix
3. statements introduced by the phrase *suo yi zhi x bing zhe* (the means whereby I recognised x's illness were . . .); see table 2.3 in appendix

These repetitive phrases made the reading of the case histories fairly formulaic and allowed me to explore the meaning of words not only in a syntagmatic way as one usually does when reading a text, but also in a paradigmatic way: by comparing one of the three above-mentioned aspects of an illness with twenty-four others. I refer to aspect (a) as 'the name of the disorder', to (b) as 'the cause of the disorder', and to (c) as 'the name-determining quality of the disorder'. The following analysis includes separate discussion of each of these three marked aspects of the illness episodes and ends with an attempt to interrelate them. The 'quality of the disorder' rather than the 'cause of the

---

[61] From the context, it seems reasonable to assume that Yi means that the condition will turn into an illness in the future if it is not treated, see footnotes 51, 68.

disorder' will be shown to belong among the main factors determining the 'name of the disorder'. This finding will allow interpretation of the as yet unexplained lines 32–6 of the envoy Xin's condition that concern the interrelations between different *mai* and *qi*.

The name of the disorder

After stating in the opening sentence that the case history concerns the *bing* of an individual x with title y from place z, Yi states in the second sentence that he examined the patient. He then announces (*yue* 曰) the name of the patient's condition (see table 2.1 in appendix).[62] The only conditions that are not named are those of a client who complained to be ill with a bad tooth (case 13) and a pregnant woman whose breasts did not grow as they should (case 14), it being clear from the context that the doctor considered both conditions *bing*.[63]

The names of the disorders are quite technical and render their identification in terms of biomedicine impossible. They represent an aspect of a conceptual framework that is systemic in character, but very different from the biomedical one. The constituents which make up the compound words that represent names,[64] include heat (*re* 熱), coldness (*han* 寒), numbness or inversion (*jue* 蹶), wind (*feng* 風), and *qi*, which for reasons given below is here perhaps more accurately approximated as 'vapour-impulsion' (*qi* 氣). They also include notions that indicate that the normal flows and fluxes in the body are disturbed by blocking off (*ge* 鬲) or accumulations (*ji* 積), amassments (*shan* 疝), conglomerates (*jia* 瘕), and obstructions (*bi* 痹). Harm (*shang* 傷) is mentioned either in the sense of injury (of the lungs in case 21) or of an invisible and probably functional damage (of the spleen in cases 12 and 15). It designates in all three cases a lethal condition. Pathogenic processes, which are not differentiated from pathological ones, include striking the centre (*zhong* 中), lodging (*ke* 客), penetrating (*dong* 迵), rising (*shang* 上), gushing (*yong* 湧), wasting (*xiao* 消), leaking (*yi* 遺), being inverted or numb (*jue* 蹶), and being sluggish (*ta* 沓). The body parts mentioned in the names comprise the internal parts (*nei* 內), the bladder (*pao* 脬 or *pang guang* 膀胱), the lungs (*fei* 肺), the spleen (*pi* 脾), and the kidneys (*shen* 腎).

---

[62] The ending of the clauses that followed the word *yue* 曰 (I said) could not always be determined by structural criteria. The number of constituents that make up the names are therefore not structurally defined and, at this research stage, they have been arbitrarily determined.

[63] In case 13, Yi says that the illness ceased (*bing yi* 病已) after five to six days of treatment; in case 14, Yi mentions, after applying medicines which restore the breasts, a lingering illness (*yubing* 餘病). These statements imply that the doctor considered the condition a *bing*.

[64] According to Cruse (1986), 25 f., 'any constituent part of a sentence that bears meaning . . . will be termed a semantic constituent'. Compound words are composed of constituents.

Qi, which is notoriously difficult to translate, has shades of meaning in this text that differ from those in later medical texts. It is mentioned four times as a constituent of the name of the disorder. In case 2 *qige bing* 氣鬲病 indicates that *qi* is being blocked and in case 10 *qishan* 氣疝 probably refers to a *qi* amassment. In the cases where Yi states *rebing qi* 熱病氣 (case 4) and *shangpi qi* 傷脾氣 (case 15), *qi* figures as a categoriser.[65] The interpretation of *qi* as a categoriser in the name of the disorder is particularly difficult. There must be a reason why Yi does not simply call these conditions *rebing* or *shangpi*. There is, of course, the possibility that Yi refers here, in an unsystematic manner, to the quality of *qi* that he senses when taking the *mai*. However, the qualities that are mentioned after the formula 'the means whereby I recognised that x was . . .' are very different in kind and generally are not compound words (see table 2.3), which makes this irregularity in the use of *qi* unlikely to result from negligence on the part of Yi.

Some of the names are ideogrammatically marked and are written with the illness-radical (no. 104), namely, an abscess (*ju* 疽), a conglomerate (*jia* 瘕), an amassment (*shan* 疝), a so-called exhaustion-heat (*dan* 癉), and an obstruction (*bi* 痹). Only Chunyu Yi, and no other doctor that he mentions, refers to disease names that are written with the 104th radical. Yi is also unique in referring in the name of a disorder to body parts in terms of the five depositories and *qi*.[66] In comparison with other doctors, he clearly has a more sophisticated concept of disease.

In seven cases Yi refers to an anonymous crowd of other doctors.[67] These doctors clearly do not have as elaborate a medical system as Yi. The constituents of their names for the disorders include only coldness (*han*), heat (*re*), numbness (*jue*), and wind (*feng*). The only body part affected is an unspecified centre (*zhong*). Pathogenic and pathological processes are designated by verbs like enter (*ru* 入) and strike the centre (*zhong*). The names by which the other doctors label the disorder provide further evidence that Yi's conception of *bing* was new, and in this sense innovative, when compared to that of other doctors whom Yi speaks of most dismissively as if they had a lower standing.

There are, however, two cases where Yi disagrees with another doctor, the doctors both being named. These two doctors, Xin 信 (case 20) and Sui 遂 (case 22), seem to be just as learned as Yi, but fail to apply their knowledge correctly. Xin diagnoses a

---

[65] Constituents at the word ending are called categorisers, according to Cruse (1986), 25 ff.

[66] The *bing* that are named in early medical manuscripts are in transcription often rendered with the 104th radical but, with few debatable exceptions, they do not refer to body parts in terms of the five depositories and *qi*.

[67] Listed in table 2.1: cases 3, 8, 10, 15, 18, 19, 23. *Zhong yi* 眾醫 probably means 'the common doctors' (alternative reading: all the many doctors). Compare with Epler (1988), 9, on the preface to *Shanghan lun*: he translates the term *fan yi* 凡醫 (lit. all the doctors) as 'common physicians'.

penetrating wind (*dongfeng* 洞風) and predicts death, but Yi contradicts and, implying that the penetrating wind has not yet arisen, says that the patient suffers from a condition which matches (*dang* 當) a penetrating wind, a condition which he can cure.[68] Sui, who is himself ill, gets into a heated dispute with Yi about his condition.[69] Yi and Sui refer to the same medical authorities, but interpret them differently. Xin, Sui, and Yi seem to be familiar with the same technical vocabulary and from this it may be surmised that they belonged to the same tradition of medical learning, one that was, possibly in opposition to that of 'the common doctors', text-based.

If one views the sickness labels that Yi identifies as 'names' of disorders, the process Yi engaged in can be considered diagnostic, although Yi did not examine signs and symptoms for setting up a modern differential diagnosis.[70] While these names scarcely give us a clue about the disease in biomedical terms, they clearly indicate that Yi's conceptualisation of disorders was relatively sophisticated. The question is now whether the names correlated with other aspects of the client's condition? And if so, to what extent?

The cause of the disorder

The formula 'the illness is contracted by . . .' (*bing de zhi* 病得之) introduces statements referring to an aspect of illness best approximated by calling it 'the cause of the disorder', although Yi himself does not use a term which means in translation 'cause'; *de* literally means 'to get, to attain'. In a first attempt to understand what Yi means, it seems reasonable to analyse his statements in respect to categories of biomedicine like 'pathogenesis' and 'disease etiology'. Frake defines pathogenesis as a 'mechanism that produces or aggravates the illness' and contrasts it with etiology, which in turn is defined as 'the [long-term] circumstances that lead a particular patient to contract an illness'.[71]

In the case histories, two cases report on an accident and, therefore, they certainly do not account for the disease etiology. In case 4, presented above, Xin contracts the illness because he 'actually was immersed in running water when it was very cold, and once this was over, he felt very hot'. Yi diagnoses '*qi* of a heat disorder' and says that this

---

[68] Compare with footnotes 51 and 61.

[69] This case 22, and also case 6, represent cases of a doctor's malpractice aggravating the patient's condition.

[70] Dictionary definitions of 'diagnosis' emphasise the importance of *naming* the pathological condition.

[71] Frake (1961), 125. Etiology is often understood in a wider sense, but for distinctions made in the following analysis, Frake's definition is useful. 'Aetiopathogeny' (p. 147) embraces both the etiology and the pathogenesis of a disorder.

condition is on the verge of turning into a 'coldness and heat'. One may suggest that the principle that 'like effects like' is to be seen as the 'the agent or mechanism that produces or aggravates the illness', but such a semantic stretch of the notion 'pathogenesis' obscures rather than clarifies the processes described. In case 21, the lungs were injured by 'falling from a horse and, thereby, falling supine onto a rock' (*duo ma jiang shi shang* 墮馬僵石上). Yi speaks of *bing*, but a biomedical doctor would probably rather speak of an injury, and not of a disease that has a pathogenesis. This shows that in two of the twenty-five cases, the rubric introduced by the phrase 'the illness is contracted by . . .' does not refer to the etiology of a disease, nor can one comfortably say that it relates the pathogenesis of a disease, without stretching the meaning of the biomedical notion of pathogenesis beyond sensible limits.

In the twenty-three other cases, Yi can be considered to refer to the etiology of the illness, namely the long-term circumstances that facilitate the emergence of a disorder. Yi refers to habits such as drinking 'alcoholic beverages' (*jiu* 酒) and indulging in 'sexual intercourse' (*nei* 內) in ten of the twenty-five cases. Notably, the client who suffered from an obstruction in case 17 contracted the illness because 'he was fond of picking up heavy things' (*hao chi zhong* 好持重), and not because of a single incident where he accidentally 'picked up heavy things'.[72] Yi obviously had a long-term condition in mind and was not interested in the one incident that resulted in an injury. However, just as one hesitates to apply the biomedical notion of pathogenesis to Yi's reports, the modern notion of disease etiology seems to miss Yi's own viewpoint.

Here recourse to the discussion of other ancient nosologies proves insightful. The modern word etiology is derived from the Greek word *aitia*: 'Thus before *aitia* came to be used generally in the sense of "cause", it meant responsibility or blame, and the meaning of *to aition* is equivalent to "that which is responsible".'[73] Lloyd points out that terms of physical causation are 'derived from the sphere of human responsibility'. To view Yi's statements as referring to 'that which is responsible' for the condition he diagnoses makes much more sense than trying to force them into the modern categories of pathogenesis and etiology, grounded in a completely different worldview and understanding of bodily processes. This understanding of 'cause' applies to all twenty-five case histories; Yi invariably makes the behaviour and general conduct of his clients responsible for their conditions.[74]

---

[72] *Shiki kaichū kōshō, juan* 105, 44.   [73] Lloyd ((1950) 1983), 29.
[74] *bing rao de zhi yu hanshi* 病蟯得之於寒濕 could be translated as follows, in order to account for behaviour: 'The illness, i.e. the worms, are contracted from *dwelling* in the cold and damp', see *Shiki kaichū kōshō, juan* 105, 46; *yu* 於 could be a verb referring to a behaviour, 'dwelling'.

Wind (*feng*),[75] for instance, is in three cases made responsible for the patient's condition, and always in combination with other causes related to the client's behaviour: in case 13, where wind effects a bad tooth (caries), it could enter the body because the person kept the mouth wide open. Notably Yi adds mention of the behaviour, 'eating and not rinsing the mouth' (*shi er bu sou* 食而不嗽), which is from a modern scientific viewpoint considered responsible for caries. In case 24, the '*qi* of wind' or 'wind and *qi*' (*fengqi* 風氣) are mentioned as cause, but combined with indulgence in drinking alcohol. Case 15 is remarkable because the second statement can be understood as an explanatory comment on the first. The first clause explains the immediate cause, namely that the slave would sweat profusely when he went outside, the second specifies the circumstances under which the slave was sweating, namely after having roasted by the fire.[76] The great winds he exposed himself to are made responsible for the illness, but again wind is not the sole cause, being mentioned in combination with behaviour.

Sweating (*han* 汗) is mentioned four times as cause for the illness. This fact surprises a modern reader: why should sweating be regarded as a behaviour for which the client is made responsible? Moreover, a modern reader considers sweating to be a symptom of a pathological condition rather than its cause. It would, however, be wrong to maintain that the ancient doctor confused cause and symptom. In case 25, sweating is obviously mentioned as a symptom: it follows physical exertion. However, even in this case, sweating is conceptualised as a consequence of deviant behaviour – overindulgence in a ballgame – and even here sweating figures as a cause of another bodily process: it triggers vomiting blood which, in turn, leads to death.

Sweating seems to designate an aspect of behaviour or, rather, misbehaviour. Paradigmatic reading of the case histories revealed that sweating is often associated with sexual intercourse. In case 9, Yi explains that the king of Jibei who suffers from a wind inversion (*fengjue* 風蹶) had excessively many ejaculations. 'Sweating and lying prostrate on the ground' (*han chu fu di* 汗出伏地) quite unambiguously hints at sexual intercourse as the cause of the disorder. In case 12, the slave called Shu 豎, a name of abuse in Han China, was in all likelihood skilled in the sexual arts. 'Profuse sweating' (*liu han* 流汗) is the behaviour made responsible for her illness. 'Profuse sweating'

---

[75] For wind (*feng*) in the Warring States period and the Han dynasty, see Lewis (1990), 214–21, and Kuriyama (1995).

[76] This specification of sweating seems to be necessary to avoid misunderstandings because of the connotations sweating has in other case histories (see below).

in case 5 indicates in all likelihood a deviant behaviour of sexual overindulgence as well.[77]

Reasoning about disease was not usually monocausal. Frequently, two coinciding aspects of the same event or activity were made responsible for the illness (linked by the conjuction *er* 而). Exceptions are alcoholic beverages alone being made responsible for the condition of a 'penetrating wind' in case 8 and the above-mentioned habit of being fond of picking up heavy things in case 17. Sexual intercourse is mentioned as sole cause in cases 3, 23, and 25, but apart from these few incidences, an illness is considered to arise from several factors in combination.

To summarise, the cause of a disorder does, quite often, correlate with the name of the disorder. It also correlates with many concomitantly mentioned complaints and manifestations of the illness. In several cases, the interrelations are tenuous, in others they can be made only indirectly by identifying the conditions mentioned in the case histories with others in later medical writings. Since overindulgence in alcoholic and sexual pleasures, including those indicated by sweating, occurs in thirteen of the twenty-five cases, and since the name of the disorder in these thirteen cases is not identical, but different in each case, the illness cause is clearly not interrelated with the name in the same way as a pathogen with the diagnosis of disease. It must therefore be conceded that the cause cannot be the name-determining factor of the disorders identified in the case histories.

The quality of the disorder

Apart from the name and cause of the disorder, there is a third aspect of *bing* that is marked by a recurrent clause. It concerns the 'quality' of the disorder. This aspect of the disorder is introduced by the standard phrase: 'the means whereby I recognised x's illness were that . . .' (*suoyi zhi x bing zhe* 所以知 x 病者), and this phrase is almost always followed by variations of the statement: 'when I examined the vessel-pulse . . .' (*zhen qi mai* 診其脈) (in cases 1–10, 18–21, and 24–5). In cases 15 and 17, the phrase 'the means whereby I recognised . . .' is followed by a statement about the complexion and in case 23, Yi says he examined the client but does not specify whether he examined the vessel-pulse or the complexion, or whether he engaged in any other kind of

---

[77] Sweating may be an euphemism for excessive sexual intercourse. Notice that sweating is mentioned in respect to clients with a fairly high position: case 9 concerns a king, case 12 the slave of the king mentioned in case 9, and case 5 a queen dowager. Sweating during sexual intercourse was considered pathological, at least according to the Mawangdui text on sexual techniques 'Tianxia zhi dao tan' 天下至道談. See Mawangdui Ha mu boshu zhengli xiaozu (1985), 164, and also Pfister (1992), 89.

diagnostic procedure. Thus in all the cases where Yi cares to present an explanation for the client's condition introduced by the above clause, he refers to *mai*, with only three exceptions (cases 15, 17, and 23). Evidently, in the case histories, Yi's discussion of pulse diagnostics is introduced with a recurrent formula. His insistence on the same formula could be taken as further evidence that the diagnostic method related to *mai* is innovative.[78]

The formula 'the means whereby I recognised the illness of x were ...' opens up the second part of the case history, which is often lengthier than the first. For the purposes of this chapter, the explanation is considered to end in four recurrent patterns,[79] leaving the structurally determined statements listed in table 2.3. At first glance, this list of statements does not appear systematic to a modern reader. For instance, the phrase that follows the standard formula 'the means whereby ...' shows much variation for no apparent factual reason. Other variations, which from a scientific viewpoint are more meaningful, concern the verbs in these phrases: *zhen* 診 (to examine), *qie* 切 (to palpate or to rub), and *xun* 循 (to stroke). *Zhen* is always mentioned in a clause preceding the clause in which *qie* is mentioned and *qie* before *xun*. *Zhen* may well be a more general and vague term than *qie* and *qie* a more general term than *xun*.[80]

Mai is in translation sometimes rendered as a pulse or pulses (*mai*1), sometimes as the study of the pulses (*mai*2), sometimes as a vessel or vessels (*mai*3), and sometimes it has a meaning comparable to *qi* (*mai*4). *Mai* often seems to imply simultaneously the meaning of pulse and vessel, hence the proposal to approximate it in translation as 'vessel-pulse'. The term is for a Western person vague because we distinguish, in the case of pulse and vessel, between the contents (or the movement) in an object and the object itself.[81]

Mai in the sense of vessel-pulse or vessel-pulses is not to be confused with the modern notion of pulse that reflects the heartbeat and the movement of the vessel walls. Yi

---

[78] The above does not imply that all the conditions rendered in terms of *mai* and *qi* are given in the marked statements: in cases 12 and 14, for instance, Yi explicitly refers to the condition of the *mai* but without marking his explanation with the above clause. It should be noted that the examination of *mai* is closely related to that of *se*. See cases 15 and 17.

[79] These patterns are identified by the four different manners in which the text continues, given in table 2.3. The present analysis of *mai* and *qi* is largely based on the information rendered in these marked statements that have the formula 'the means whereby I recognised the illness of x were ...' as opening and the four above patterns as closure. A more extensive analysis of *mai* is beyond the scope of this article.

[80] *xun*, in all probability, refers to stroking the surface of the skin (see case 19).

[81] *mai* as an object are not defined by their physical structure but by their course that is derived, as Epler (1980) puts it, from the observation of 'surface anatomy'. See also Vivienne Lo (chapter 1, this volume). On pulse diagnostics, East and West, see Kuriyama (1999).

may have *qie mai* at the wrist, at the place where the pulse (in its modern sense) is very distinctive, but he may have *qie mai* at other areas of the body surface as well. It is unclear what exactly Yi did when he said that he *qie mai*. It may have included rubbing the surface of the *mai*, as in case 19, but it also seems to refer to the activity of sensing the movements and other qualities inside the *mai*. In some cases, Yi specifies the exact location at which he rubbed: the opening of a *mai*.[82] He sometimes names the *mai* in the same way as they are named in the Mawangdui vessel texts, for instance in case 4, as *taiyin*.

After stating that he examined *mai*, Yi described the sensations he had: in some cases (cases 1, 21, and 25), he explicitly says that he 'got the *qi* from the liver' (*de ganqi* 得肝氣), he got *yinqi* from the lungs or *qi* from the lungs which are *yin* (*de feiyinqi* 得肺陰氣),[83] or he got the reversed [or spreading] *yang* (*de fan* [*bo*]*yang* 得番[播]陽). In others (cases 10 and 28), he refers to 'a coming of the *mai*' (*mai lai* 脈來) which he modifies with various adjectives, like difficult (*nan* 難) or slippery (*hua* 滑). Other adjectives with which he characterises the *mai* are, for instance, large and frequent (*da er shuo* 大而數), damp (*shi* 濕), large and full (*da er shi* 大而實), deep, small, and soft (*shen, xiao, ruo* 深小弱).[84]

Yi uses similar and sometimes identical adjectives to modify *qi* as in case 1, where he explicitly says that *qi* [coming] from the liver was murky but still (*zhuo er jing* 濁而靜) or in case 2, where we can assume by implication that he refers to *qi* [coming] from the heart and describes it as murky and hurried, yet transient (*zhuo zao er jing* 濁躁而經). In case 3, *qi* was taut (*ji* 急). In case 6, the *qi* from the lungs was hot (*re* 熱). Case 21 seems to imply that the coming that was dispersed (*san* 散) refers to the *qi* [coming] from the lungs, but it might equally refer to the coming of the *mai*, mentioned earlier. This suggests that the adjectives and verbs modifying *mai* and *qi* can be used interchangeably.

Yi's use of the same adjectives for modifying the condition of *mai* and of *qi* coincides with the observation that Yi seems to use the characters *mai* and *qi* in some contexts interchangeably: in case 9, he sensed that *mai*, rather than *qi*, [coming] from the heart was murky; in case 18, he again sensed *mai*, rather than *qi*, [coming] from the kidneys. In other cases, however, Yi makes a clear distinction between *mai* and *qi*, for

---

[82] In the Mawangdui vessel texts, the course of the *mai* generally goes from the extremities to the internal parts of the body. If Yi conceived of the course of the *mai* similarly, the opening of the *mai* was on the extremities.

[83] Consider a possible parallel to the phrasing *fei shou taiyin mai* 肺手太陰脈 (the vessel-pulse of the lungs that are categorised as the hand's *taiyin*) in *Lingshu*, *pian* 10, 299.

[84] In case 4, Yi refers to *bingyin* 并陰 (joined *yin*), in case 25, to *fanyang* 番[播]陽 (reversed [spreading] *yang*). It is unclear whether Yi refers to the sensation he had when examining *mai* or whether *bingyin* and *fanyang* refer to conditions that he deduces from his sensation of the *mai*.

instance, when he says that *mai* did not have the *qi* [coming] from the five depositories (*mai wu wuzang qi* 脈無五藏氣).

In case 1, which is one of the longest case histories, Yi states the interrelation between *mai* and *qi* most clearly: he palpates or rubs the *mai*, he senses the *qi* coming from a depository, and he characterises the qualities of this *qi* with different adjectives. This seems to imply that Yi's pulse diagnostics are directed at identifying (a) from where the *qi* comes and (b) what kind of qualities it has. As will be shown below, these qualities of *qi* are category-determining when Yi names the disorder. Even when *mai* and *qi* are used interchangeably, I suggest interpreting the text along the lines of the fuller description of the diagnostic process as given in cases 1 and 2.

Yi's examination of *mai* yields many problems of interpretation, in particular in respect to the adjectives which designate the qualities of *mai*. The following discussion is limited to the interrelation between *mai* and *qi* which the case histories for the first time record in a systemic way. In the marked statements, Yi mentions the *qi* [coming] from the liver (case 1), the heart (case 2), none of the five depositories (case 3), the wind (cases 5 and 9), the lungs (case 6), and the lungs that are *yin* (case 21). In the unmarked statements, he additionally mentions *qi* [coming] from the kidneys (case 4), the water (case 4), the bladder (case 5), the spleen (case 7), conglomerates (case 7), and internal wind (case 8). It is unclear what exactly the interrelation between *qi* and the five depositories, the bladder, wind and water, and the conglomerates is: *qi* may be an aspect of, belong to, or come from them.[85]

It is also unclear what exactly Yi perceived when he said that he 'got the *qi*' (*de qi* 得氣). Here a comparison with Yi's statement in case 10 proves illuminating: he first describes the quality of *mai* with a set of different adjectives and then explains that this quality of *mai* was indicative of the *dong* 動 of the *jueyin* 蹶陰: *dong* is in this context best approximated by notions like impulse, impulsion, motion, movement, agitation, or irritation. Possibly, like *dong*, *qi* designates a kind of movement or motion, impulse, or change in the *mai*, hence the proposal to approximate *qi* in Chunyu Yi's case histories as 'vapour-impulsion'.

Yi does not combine the categoriser *qi* with the notion of *jueyin* or any other of the categories according to which the vessels are named in the Mawangdui manuscripts.[86] This finding nicely parallels the observation that *qi* is not mentioned in the Mawangdui

---

[85] Since Yi considers *mai* 'to come', it is possible that he also conceives of *qi* 'coming', hence the here proposed translation of *ganqi* as '*qi* [coming] from the liver'.

[86] In case 5, Yi says: 'When your servant, Yi, examined her pulse and took it at the opening of the *taiyin*, it was damp, this being so, there was a wind *qi*' (切其太陰之口溼然風氣也). This could be taken as counterevidence for the above statement. My point is that Yi does not speak of *taiyin zhi qi* '*qi* [coming] from the *taiyin*'.

vessel texts. In the Mawangdui vessel texts, disorders (*bing*) are either produced by the *mai* (*suo chan bing* 所產病) or they arise from an irritation of the *mai* (*shi dong ze bing* 是動則病). In case 10, when Yi refers to the motion (*dong*) of the *jueyin*, he uses the word *dong* in the same sense as it occurs in the Mawangdui vessel texts.[87]

The above observations suggest that the vessels that are classified according to their *yinyang* qualities can be aroused and start into motion (*dong*), this in contrast to the five depositories, the bladder, conglomerates, and wind and water, which correlate with *qi*.[88] In particular, the close interrelation between *qi* and the five depositories should be stressed: the sensation of *qi* that Yi gets when he rubs the *mai* informs him about the condition of the five depositories inside the body, information he would otherwise be unable to obtain.

However, *qi* figures also as a categoriser of wind (*fengqi*) and water (*shuiqi*) as well as of certain conditions of disease such as, for instance, a heat disorder (*rebing qi*) or a damaged spleen (*shangpi qi*). It does not exclusively inform us about the state of depositories but can also be used in collocation with notions that refer to the ecological environment and disease names. *Qi* is a categoriser of several variables, but within a restricted range. In the *Shiji* case histories, *qi* does not seem to designate that all-encompassing 'stuff' which constitutes and permeates the universe, as in later medical texts.[89] Moreover, there is no evidence that *qi* circulates in *mai* which formed a circulation system.

It is quite probable that the use of the concept *qi* in interrelation with *mai* was new to medical practice. Why otherwise would Yi consider it necessary to explain what he meant by *qi* in the third part of the biography: 'As for the so-called *qi*, one ought to harmonise drink and food, and choose clear days for coach rides and walks to broaden the mind in order to adjust the tendons, bones, flesh, blood and vessel-pulses for bringing *qi* into flow' (所謂氣者，當調飲食，擇晏日，車步廣志，以適筋骨肉血脈以瀉氣)?[90]

---

[87] The verb *dong* has throughout the Mawangdui vessel texts negative connotations, this is in contrast to its positive connotations in the 'Shiwen' (Ten Questions). See Mawangdui Hanmu boshu zhengli xiaozu (1985).

[88] Correlations of *qi* with the five depositories, wind, and water are characteristic of the 'body ecologic' in Chinese medicine. See Hsu (1999: 78–83). The bladder is in later medical writings classified as the outer aspect of the kidneys, but not in early medicine.

[89] Sivin (1987), 46–7.

[90] *Shiki kaichū kōshō, juan* 105, 55–6. It is odd that five rather than four characters are given in the expression *jingu rouxue mai*. It seems as if *mai* were a concept from a different tradition, here added onto the idiom *jingu rouxue*. If this were so, it would provide further evidence for the argument put forward here that the interrelation between *mai* and *qi* as presented in the 'Canggong zhuan' was innovative for medical practice.

As already stated, *qi* is generally the last constituent of a compound word, a 'categoriser' in terms of lexical semantics. The meaning of a categoriser cannot always be determined by reference to the world outside the linguistic system. Categorisers often have grammatical functions within the linguistic system. It is possible that the meaning of the term *qi*, if used as a categoriser, cannot be determined with reference to objects outside the linguistic system (e.g. to 'vapours' rising from cooking vessels or fermenting foodstuffs), and that *qi* has first and foremost a grammatical function.

Suffixes like '-ity' in 'purity', '-ance' in 'brilliance', or '-ness' in 'brightness' have the grammatical function of making a noun out of an adjective. From a semantic viewpoint, the words composed of adjectives with these suffixes share the meaning of delimiting something like an ideal or an idea. *Qi* as a categoriser in compound words seems to have a grammatical function similar to the above suffixes: *han* 寒 (cold) can be a verb, adjective, or noun while *han qi* 寒氣 (cold *qi*) is always a noun. Compound words with the categoriser *qi* may also share certain semantics: the categoriser *qi* may well indicate a particular aspect of the noun. Thus, if the doctor said that he perceived liver *qi*, liver *qi* might point to an abstraction of liver, say, the Chinese variant of 'liverness'.

If the categoriser *qi* were to designate an abstraction of the things and conditions it modifies, if it were to mark a 'mode of being' particular to a certain worldview, what kind of 'mode of being' would that be? Yi's vocabulary is rather technical, his conceptual framework is relatively sophisticated, and medical explanation takes place within a system of interdependent concepts: the assumption that his concepts were based on as crude a materialism as the translation of *ganqi* as 'vapour of the liver' would suggest is unlikely to be correct. Here, one is best reminded of the previous analogy between *qi* and *dong* (motion, movement, impulsion). The categoriser *qi* may well point to an abstraction of vapour, like its *(upward) movement* or a 'mode of being' that vapour may signify, like a *potential for change*. The Chinese medical doctor's touch goes beyond tactile perceptions, his concepts beyond material entities. Yi may well have been tuned in to a 'mode of being' that modern science does not recognise, and he may have paid particular attention to those states in the body and universe that have a potential for change. The doctor's statement that he got liver *qi* would thus amount to saying that there was a potential for (pathological) change in the liver.

This 'potential for change' would refer to an aspect of a process, regardless of whether change is about to happen or whether it was once in the past about to happen and has now happened.[91] A 'mode of being', like the 'potential for change', which concerns both 'that which has happened' and 'that which may possibly happen' may strike a

---

[91] In linguistics, verbs can be marked by aspect and tempus. Perhaps *qi*, a categoriser in nouns, may have the function of indicating an 'aspect' of the noun.

modern reader as awkward, since we tend to order events chronologically, but it seems to be intrinsic to many notions of the scholarly medical traditions in Asia. When Zimmermann discusses the Sanskrit word *jangala* in 'the Great Triad' of Ayurvedic treatises, he says that *jangala* refers, firstly, to dry lands as opposed to marshy lands (*anupa*). *Jangala* that refers to the dry plains of Brahmin culture is contrasted with the thickets and forests of the *anupa* where the barbarians live. It may refer to cultivated lands but, more importantly, *jangala* refers to the wild, dry space that is uncultivated. This leads, according to Zimmermann, to a paradox of *jangala*'s meaning: 'It is wasteland but also fertile soil.'[92] This paradox is solved if one is interested not in the aspect of what is there (wasteland versus fertile soil), but in the aspect of the 'potential for change' intrinsic to these lands. *Jangala* refers to the lands with the intrinsic potential to be made suitable for Brahmin cultivation. It does not matter whether the dry and fertile area that is open to Brahmin culture was once available for cultivation (and is now cultivated) or whether it promises to be available for cultivation in the future (and is now wasteland). The meaning of the term *jangala* reflects a worldview that is not as interested in the temporal succession of events as in the question of whether or not a thing or quality has a certain inherent 'potential for change'.

Assuming that *qi* is a categoriser signifying 'potential for change', reasoning in terms of compound words with the categoriser *qi* would express adherence to the worldview that a 'potential for change' is immanent in the things or qualities referred to by the first constituent. Naturally, one could use the unmarked form, *bing* (disorder) or *han* (cold), rather than *bingqi* and *hanqi*. But by speaking in terms of *bingqi* or *hanqi* this would stress one's adherence to the worldview that the disorder or the cold intrinsically have a potential for change. In the *Shiji* case histories, *qi* may well indicate such a potential for change. It remains to be seen whether the case of *qi* is like the case of *jangala*, where it did not matter whether the change had already happened in the past or whether it was about to happen in the future.

We observe a fairly close interrelation between the *qi* [coming] from a depository with a potential for pathological change and the same depository in the disease name: in case 5, Yi's examination of *mai* leads to the identification of wind *qi* (*fengqi*) and bladder *qi* (*pangguangqi*) which correlates with the mentioning of wind and bladder in the name of the disorder: a wind heat [due to overexertion] lodged in the bladder (*fengdan ke pao* 風癉客脬). In case 6, the doctor took the pulse and felt lung *qi* (*feiqi*) and the disorder was called a lung consumption (*feixiaodan* 肺消癉). In case 7, the patient suffered from a condition called leaking accumulations and conglomerates (*yijijia* 遺積瘕) which correlates with the doctor's perception of *qi* [coming] from conglomerates

---

[92] Zimmermann (1987), 218.

(*jiaqi*). In case 8, Yi identified, after examining the pulse, an internal wind *qi* (*neifengqi*) and the disorder was called a penetrating wind (*dongfeng*). In case 9, wind *qi* correlated with the mentioning of wind in the name of the disorder, and in case 21 where the lungs were injured, Yi senses *qi* [coming] from the lungs that are *yin*. These examples show that pulse diagnostics allows for the identification of a quality that plays, from the point of view of the naming of the disorder, a category-determining role.[93]

The above examples point to one aspect of Yi's pulse diagnostics, namely that the body parts and other locations from which *qi* comes are often mentioned as one of the constituents in the compound words which make up the name of the disorder. In other words, the quality of *qi* in the *mai* determines *bing*. If the *bing* is curable, Yi treats the patient – always successfully – if not, he predicts death and desists from treatment. Pulse diagnostics is used for determining his treatment strategy and allows him to be infallible.

Xin's condition revisited

Given the above analysis of *qi* as a categoriser in compound words, let us return to the unresolved issues in the case history that concern Xin's condition of a heat disorder *qi* (case 4). If one interprets *qi* to mean 'potential for change', *rebing qi* would designate a 'potential of change in a heat disorder'. Xin's condition was indeed on the verge of changing into another one, namely a coldness and heat (*hanre*). In a similar vein, *shang-piqi* (case 15) would concern a condition with the 'potential for change in a damaged spleen'. In case 15, the condition Yi diagnosed was also on the verge of changing: at the time of Yi's diagnosis, the illness had not yet matured, but he recognised a 'potential for change' (*qi*) in the damaged spleen. It was only in spring that the slave, as anticipated (*guo* 果), fell ill. Yi diagnosed in cases 4 and 15 a disorder on the verge of changing into another one. In those two cases, which differ in this respect from the other twenty-three, the categoriser *qi* probably indicates a 'potential for change'.

The above analysis, that the rubbing of *mai* leads to the identification of certain qualities of *qi* and that those qualities of *qi* determine the name of the disorder, may throw some light on those lines of Xin's condition that could not previously be interpreted. Chunyu Yi states that when he rubbed the *mai* there was a joined *yin* (*bingyin* 并陰; line 26, see also table 2.3). In accordance with the above analysis that the examination of *mai* allows the doctor to identify the quality of *qi* and thereby to determine the name of the disorder, one would expect the joined *yin* to correlate with the name of the disorder.

---

[93] These interrelations between *mai*, *qi*, and *bing* are with few exceptions based on the marked statements in table 2.3.

However, the correlation between the 'potential of change in a heat disorder' (*rebing qi*) and a 'joined *yin*' (*bingyin*) is not immediately evident. Since *bingyin* is not attested in the medical literature, it is difficult to guess to what kind of condition it refers. It seems to refer to *mai* within a new framework of diagnostics that Yi considers necessary to explain. Otherwise why would Yi, in line 30, explain what *bingyin* means: 'In cases of *bingyin*, the *mai* is smooth, clear, and well.' The adjectives smooth (*shun* 順), clear (*qing* 清), and well (*yu* 愈) belong among the technical terms that in the received literature are not attested in the context of pulse diagnostics. Since they are mentioned also in other case histories,[94] they appear to represent a terminology with which Yi was familiar but which has since been lost. These adjectives describe the quality of *mai* in much the same way as the currently standard twenty-eight pulse images (*maixiang* 脈象).[95] While none of these three terms belongs among the currently recognised twenty-eight adjectives for assessing the qualities of *mai*, they are mentioned in other early medical treatises where the quality of *mai* was already described in this fashion (see section III).

Lines 32–36 in case 4 are particularly difficult to interpret because there are hardly any parallels in the attested literature which can explain what Yi means when he says: 'The *qi* of the kidneys was sometimes for a moment murky, the opening of the *taiyin mai*, however, was scarce. This is a case of water *qi*. As long as the kidneys are firm, they control the water. By means of this I knew it.'

The word *zhuo* 濁 (murky) that occurs in the first clause, 'the *qi* of the kidneys was sometimes for a moment murky' (*shenqi youshi jian zhuo* 腎氣有時間濁), modifies *qi* in case 1, 'the *qi* [coming] from the liver was murky but still' (*ganqi zhuo er jing* 肝氣濁而靜); it also modifies *mai* in case 9, 'the *mai* [coming] from the heart was murky' (*xinmai zhuo* 心脈濁). *Zhuo* is in some texts involving correlative thinking opposed to *qing* which indicates, as seen above on line 30, a positive quality.[96] From this, we can deduce that *zhuo* indicates a disturbance of the normal state. The kidneys were evidently murky, but not permanently, since the *qi* [coming] from the kidneys was only sometimes (*youshi* 有時), and then only for a moment (*jian* 間), murky.

The phrase 'the opening of the *taiyin mai*, however, was scarce' (*taiyin maikou er xi* 太陰脈口而希) can either be analysed, following Bridgman,[97] as describing the same

---

[94] These three adjectives all have positive connotations: *shun* (smooth) modifies *mai* in case 15, *ren* 人 (person) in case 15, *bing* in case 20, and *si* 死 (to die) in case 21; *qing* (clear) modifies *mai* in case 15 and *sou* 溲 (urine) in case 10; *yu* (well) modifies *ren* in case 15, *ji* (illness) in case 3, and *bing* (disease) in case 17.
[95] See for instance Deng Tietao et al. (1984), 72.   [96] Graham (1986), 22, 32.
[97] Bridgman (1955), 142.

condition as in the previous clause but within a different framework: the *taiyin mai* would then refer to the kidneys, a correlation well-known in inner alchemy but not emphasised in canonical medical doctrine. The word *xi* would then indicate the same as *you shi jian zhuo*, namely that the *taiyin mai* was only slightly impaired. However, if one takes Yi's line of argumentation seriously, it makes much more sense to interpret the clause 'the opening of the *taiyin mai*, however, was scarce' as referring to a condition that differs from that mentioned in the clause preceding it. In accordance with the Mawangdui vessel texts, *taiyin* may refer to the upper inner parts (*xin* 心),[98] or in consideration of the canonical medical doctrine, it may link up with the lungs (*fei*) which in fact were considered to be located in the epigastrium. If one interprets the joined *yin* to refer to the kidneys which are, according to canonical doctrine, *shaoyin* 少陰,[99] and to the lungs which are *taiyin*,[100] the joined *yin* may well indicate that the two *yin* were affected, namely the kidneys and the lungs.[101]

After describing the above qualities of *mai*, namely that the *qi* of the kidneys was sometimes for a moment murky and that, however, the opening of the *taiyin mai*, which in all likelihood correlated with the lungs, was scarce, Yi explains that this indicated water *qi* (*shuiqi* 水氣). *Shuiqi* occurs fairly frequently in the *Neijing*, often in contexts that have no resemblance to Xin's case at all. *Suwen* 61 is, however, worth noting. Although its contents do not exactly match Xin's case, in its description of various pathological conditions it mentions the kidneys, the lungs, and water, as well as water *qi*. The chapter, entitled 'Shuirexue lun' 水熱穴論 (Treatise on the *loci* [treating] Water and Heat), ends, for no instantly apparent reason, with a discussion of how to treat heat disorders. The parallels are tenuous, but they echo Yi's reasoning that links together the two *yin*, namely the kidneys and the lungs, water *qi*, and heat disorders.[102]

According to the canonical doctrine, Water correlates with the kidneys.[103] In this text, where correlative thinking is mentioned but not elaborated, water also in all likelihood correlates with the kidneys.[104] The analysis of the text would stop short

---

[98] *xin* 心 (heart) is one of the five depositories in canonical medical doctrine, but in early medical texts it generally refers to the entire region of the epigastrium (Catherine Despeux, p.c.).

[99] The kidneys are not always attributed the quality *shaoyin* (lesser *yin*), see for instance below, *Suwen*, *juan* 16, *pian* 61, 164, where they are *zhiyin* 至陰 (extreme *yin*). In case 4, it is possible that the quality of extreme *yin* rather than that of lesser *yin* is attributed to the kidneys.

[100] This interpretation seriously questions Bridgman's (1955), 141–5, hypothesis of the names of *mai* in the *Shiji* case histories being divergent from those of canonical doctrine.

[101] This interpretation has since been modified. See Hsu (2001). For *xi*, see also Ma Jixing (1992), 994.

[102] *Suwen*, *juan* 16, *pian* 61, 164–6.   [103] See for instance *Suwen*, *juan* 2, *pian* 5, 21.

[104] Notice that the accident happened in winter, the season in canonical doctrine explicitly correlated with the kidneys and water, see for instance *Suwen*, *juan* 1, *pian* 2, 10.

here if we had not learnt from the above structural analysis that water *qi* must in some way correlate with the name of the disorder and its concomitant aspects: water *qi* is presumably indicative of the *qi* of the heat disorder or rather of the *qi* of the heat disorder and its concomitant aspect, sweating like in summerheat (*ran shu han* 然暑汗). Considering that the disorder equivalent to *rebing* is in the Mawangdui vessel texts called *re chu han* (heat expels sweat), we can deduce that in early medical reasoning sweating was considered an important aspect of a heat disorder, if not the most important one.

Yi states that the kidneys control the water. He seems to imply that the water that escapes from the kidneys appears as sweat on the body surface. *Suwen* 61 contains a clause in which it is said that the sweat of the kidneys comes out (*shen han chu* 腎汗出). This clause clearly correlates sweating with the kidneys and their function of controlling the water. However, in *Suwen* 61, the sweating is not correlated with a heat disorder but is said to arise from overexertion and physical toil.

This statement, in turn, throws further light on the medical reasoning in the *Shiji* case histories, for it provides a useful explanation of the sweating mentioned as an illness cause that was identified above as indicative of overindulgence in sex. It is well-known in Chinese medical doctrine, past and present, that excessive sex impairs the kidneys. Sweating can therefore be taken as indicative of impaired kidneys. A statement from *Suwen* 33 makes it obvious: 'As for sweat, it is the *qi* of refined essence' (汗者精氣也).[105]

The above findings make it very clear that the condition of the joined *yin*, namely of simultaneously impaired kidneys and lungs, had pulse qualities which indicated water *qi*. According to the analysis given in section II, which interrelates the quality of the *mai* and the disease name, it is water *qi* that correlates with sweating, and sweating was at the time probably such an important aspect of heat disorders that it became their category-determining feature. In this way the quality of *qi* determined the name of Xin's disorder.

This final analysis of Xin's condition nicely shows that the qualities of *qi* that were determined through an examination of the *mai* were category-determining for naming *bing*. It provides evidence that the case histories under discussion contain a systemic account of an early form of pulse diagnostics in Chinese medicine. However, it is still unclear which aspects of Yi's medical skills were innovative. In the third and last section

---

[105] *Suwen*, *juan* 9, *pian* 33, 96. Refined essence (*jing* 精) has been allocated to the kidneys throughout medical history.

of this study, Yi's pulse diagnostics are compared to early medical reasoning in the manuscripts of Mawangdui and Zhangjiashan.

III: *Bing*, *mai*, and *qi* in the early medical manuscripts

The twenty-five case histories in the 'Canggong zhuan' provide a fairly comprehensive account of a medical specialist's notion of *bing* which comprised systematically recorded aspects, namely the name, cause, and 'quality' of the disorder. I showed above that the quality of a disorder, rather than its cause, was the aspect of illness that determined the name of the disorder. It was, *inter alia*, identified after examining *mai* which would inform the doctor about *qi.* This form of pulse diagnostics was for the first time described in the case histories of the 'Canggong zhuan', though it built on specialist knowledge of *bing*, *mai*, and *qi* recorded in other early medical texts.

The notions of *bing* and *mai* in the Mawangdui vessel texts appear to be particularly close to Chunyu Yi's. The vessel texts refer to *mai* that are distinguished from each other by qualities of *yin* and *yang*: namely *taiyin* 太陰, *shaoyin* 少陰, *jueyin* 厥陰 and *yangming* 陽明, *taiyang* 太陽, *shaoyang* 少陽, qualities by which Yi specifies *mai* as well. The *mai* in the vessel texts are further differentiated into two groups, depending on whether the *mai* begins its course at the upper or the lower extremity. This distinction seems to have been known to Yi as well, even though he does not consistently refer to it. In the vessel texts the eleven *mai* are discussed, one by one, in eleven sections. Each section first describes the course of a *mai* and then lists the disorders (*bing*) that are considered characteristic of that *mai*. *Bing* are thus categorised in respect to different *mai*.

Yi seems to engage in the same enterprise of categorising *bing* in respect to *mai*. In case 23, he says he failed to identify the *jingjie* 經解 (explanations according to the ?canons or ?channels) but vaguely knew the location of the illness (*bingsuo* 病所).[106] It is not entirely clear which texts he referred to if he spoke of 'canons', but they may well have been of the same kind as the Mawangdui vessel texts which list a set of symptoms for each *mai*. In order to identify the disorder, Yi appears to have intended to find out where, or more precisely in which *mai*, it resided. Insofar as in the Mawangdui vessel texts *bing* is identified in respect to *mai*, there is nothing new about Yi's diagnostics.

What is new is that Yi examines the *mai* and senses *qi* in order to locate the disorder. The *qi* he senses does not directly inform him about *mai* in terms of *yin* and *yang*, the qualities attributed to *mai* in the vessel texts. As shown above, in the case histories, *qi*

---

[106] Notice that Yi expresses his uncertainty by saying *yiwei* 以為 (I took it for) rather than *yue* (I said).

is mostly a categoriser in compound words which have one of the five depositories (*wuzang* 五藏) as a constituent. Yi's achievement thus consisted in combining medical knowledge which classifies disease with regard to *qi* [coming] from the five depositories with that of the Mawangdui vessel texts, which locates disease in the *mai*. Yi's 'way of doing things' is not recorded elsewhere in the extant early medical literature and his case histories represent the first text that correlates *mai* to the five depositories. Yi established this correlation by interrelating the examination of *mai* with the identification of *qi* which often came from the five depositories. This was innovative.

To be sure, an early form of pulse diagnostics seems to be recorded in the Mawangdui 'Maifa' and in the Zhangjiashan 'Maishu'. It is called *xiang mai* 相脈 (to inspect *mai*; to practise divination with *mai*) rather than *zhen mai* 診脈 (to examine *mai*): 'Place the left hand five *cun* up from the malleolus [i.e. the wrist or ankle] and press on it. Place the right hand at the malleolus and palpate it' (左手上去踝五寸而按之，右手直踝而探之).[107] This procedure enables one to perceive different qualities of *mai*, described with adjectives: 'If other vessels [*mai*] are full and this one alone is empty, it controls the ailment [*bing*]. If other vessels [*mai*] flow evenly and this one alone is blocked, it controls the ailment [*bing*]. If other vessels [*mai*] are still and this one alone is moved, it controls the ailment [*bing*]' (他脈盈，此獨虛，則主病。他脈滑，此獨濇，則主病。他脈靜，此獨動，則主病).[108] Harper translates *mai* as 'vessels' and takes issue with Ma Jixing who translates *mai* as 'pulse images' in the above text passage.

The procedure directed at examining the quality of *mai*, the vessel-pulses, may well refer to a conception of *mai* that comprises simultaneously *mai* as vessel and *mai* as pulse or pulses. It may well describe an early form of pulse diagnostics, since the above text passage has some affinity with Yi's description of the sensations he felt after rubbing the *mai*. At least one of the adjectives, 'still' (*jing*), is identical to those with which Yi describes the qualities of *mai*. These adjectives describe conditions of *mai* which inform the doctor about *bing*, but whereas *bing* remains unspecified in the above text passage of the manuscripts, it is named in the case histories. In the manuscripts not only the quality of *mai*, described with an adjective, but also the quality of one *mai* in relation to others determines whether the *mai* in question governs the disorder or not. In the

---

[107] Mawangdui Han mu boshu zhengli xiaozu (1985), 17, contains many lacunae, but see translation by Harper (1998), 216, and compare with Ma Jixing (1992), 292; *an* 按 (to press) and *tan* 探 (to palpate) may well designate an activity comparable to *qie* 切 (to rub).

[108] See Harper (1998), 216–17, and Ma Jixing (1992), 295.

case histories, this is not usually the case, but there is at least one instance where the condition of the patient is determined on grounds of the interrelation of the three *yin* [*mai*] to each other (case 7). This aspect of Yi's pulse diagnostics strictly speaking is not innovative and has therefore merited only a passing mention.

The 'Maifa' and the 'Maishu' also contain a text passage that interrelates *mai* and *qi*: 'When the vapour [*qi*] ascends and does not descend, discern which *mai* has excess and cauterise it at the ring [i.e. the waist]. If the ailment is severe, go up two *cun* above the ring and perform an additional cauterisation. If vapour [*qi*] emerges, lance the vessels [*mai*] at the poples and elbow with a lancing-stone' (故氣上而不下，則視有過之脈，當還而灸之。病甚而上於還二寸益為一灸。氣一上一下，當邸與肘之脈而砭之). Regardless of how one translates these three sentences,[109] it is clear that they concern therapeutics and not diagnostics. Yi's interrelation of *mai* and *qi* for diagnostic purposes was thus innovative.

The above comparison with early medical texts shows that Yi's pulse diagnostics integrated knowledge previously recorded in a variety of texts. Following the vessel text tradition, Yi investigated *mai* in order to determine *bing*. His innovation was to base on his examination of *mai* the classification of *bing* through the intermediary of *qi*. This innovation did not survive for long because, in the context of pulse diagnostics, the concepts of *mai* and *qi* generally became one, called *mai*. As in many non-medical writings of the Warring States and the Han period, *qi* was used as a categoriser in compound words. Innovative was *qi*'s fairly consistent collocation with the five depositories and other body parts, and Yi's combination of the *qi* [coming] from the five depositories with the *mai* that were categorised, just as in the vessel texts, in terms of *yin* and *yang*. This innovation was fundamental for canonical doctrine. In later texts, as for instance in *Lingshu* 10, the five depositories belong (*shu* 屬) to *mai*. Finally, Yi's case histories stand out for their multifaceted account of illness events. The comprehensiveness with which the doctor accounts for particular occurrences of *bing* is probably the most innovative aspect of medical reasoning in the 'Canggong zhuan'. It comprises a systemic way of interrelating different conditions of *mai* and *qi* for determining *bing*. Chunyu Yi achieved this by recording a series of individual case histories in a formulaic way.

---

[109] See Harper (1998), 214, and Ma Jixing (1992), 282; compare and contrast with translation by Vivienne Lo (this volume), p. 29.

Appendix

Table 2.1. *The name of the disorder* (*yue* 曰: . . . I said: . . .)

1. 此病疽也 this is a case of being ill with a *ju*-abscess
2. 氣鬲病 a disorder of *qi* being separated and blocked off
3. 湧疝也 a gushing amassment
   (other doctors: 蹶入中 a numbness entering and striking the centre)
4. 熱病氣也 the *qi* of a heat disorder (on the verge of becoming a coldness and heat)
5. 風癉客脬 a wind exhaustion-heat, lodged in the bladder
6. 肺消癉也 a lung consumption
7. 遺積瘕也 leaking accumulations and conglomerates
8. 迵風 a penetrating wind
   (other doctors: 寒中 a coldness striking the centre)
9. 風蹶 a wind inversion
10. 病氣疝客於膀胱 she suffers from a *qi* amassment, lodged in the bladder
    (other doctors: 風入中 wind entering and striking the centre)
11. 熱蹶也 a heat inversion
12. 豎傷脾 Shu has damaged the spleen
13. ——
14. ——
15. 此傷脾氣也 this is a case of the *qi* of a damaged spleen
16. 蹶上 an inversion is rising
17. . . . 此所謂腎痹也 . . . this is a case of a so-called obstruction of the kidneys
18. 內寒月事不下也 an internal coldness such that the menses do not descend
    (other doctors: 寒熱 a coldness and warmth)
19. 蟯瘕 a conglomerate of *rao*-worms
    (other doctors: 寒熱篤 a coldness and warmth, considered to be lethal)
20. 當病迵風 if this turns into an illness, it will be a penetrating wind
21. 肺傷 an injury of the lungs
22. 公病中熱 you suffer from a heat striking the centre
23. [以為 replaces 曰] 痹 [I took it for] an obstruction
    (other doctors: 蹶 numbness or inversion)
24. [謂之 replaces 曰] 病苦　沓風 [I said to him] that he was suffering from the wind of sluggishness
25. 牡疝 a male amassment

Table 2.2. *The cause of the disorder* (*bing de zhi* the illness was contracted by/from)

1. drinking alcoholic beverages and having sexual intercourse
2. infantile anxiousness, and frequent rejection of food and drink; being anxious
3. sexual intercourse
4. while bathing in cold water, it is very cold and once this is over, you get hot
5. while profusely sweating she went outside to *xun* (?sunbathe). In the case of *xun*, after one takes off one's clothes, the sweat dries in open sunlight
6. while being in great anger, by taking this emotion into sexual intercourse
7. alcoholic beverages and sexual intercourse
8. alcoholic beverages
9. sweating and lying prostrate on the ground
10. intending to urinate, but not being able to, and having, in this condition, sexual intercourse
11. drinking alcohol and getting extremely drunk
12. profuse sweating
13. wind and sleeping with an open mouth; eating and not rinsing the mouth
14. —
15. sweating and frequently going outside; having roasted by the fire, by being exposed to great winds
16. washing the hair and, while it was not yet dry, going to sleep
17. being fond of picking up heavy [things]
18. while wishing for a son, not being able to conceive one
19. the cold and the damp
20. stuffing onself and thereafter running swiftly
21. falling from a horse and falling supine on a rock
22. —
23. sexual intercourse
24. frequently drinking alcoholic beverages and being exposed to strong wind *qi*
25. sexual intercourse

Table 2.3. *The quality of the disorder* (*suo yi zhi x bing zhe* the means whereby I recognised x's illness were that . . .)[i]

1. when your servant Yi rubbed his *mai*, I got the *qi* [coming] from the liver. The *qi* from the liver was murky but still. (text continues in manner 1: this is . . .)
2. when I examined his *mai*, it was the *qi* [coming] from the heart. It was murky and hurried, yet transient. (text continues in manner 1: this is . . .)
3. at the time when I rubbed his *mai*, at the right opening, the *qi* was taut. The *mai* did not have the *qi* [coming] from the five depositories. At the right opening,[ii] the *mai* were (or was) large and frequent. (text continues in manner 2: in cases where it is frequent . . .)
4. at the time when I rubbed his *mai*, there was a joined *yin*. (text continues in manner 3: the 'Maifa' says . . .)
5. when your servant Yi examined her *mai*, when I rubbed their (or its) opening of the major *yin*, they were (or it was) damp, while there was *qi* [coming] from wind. (text continues in manner 3: the 'Maifa' says . . .)
6. when your servant Yi rubbed his *mai*, the *qi* [coming] from the lungs was hot. (text continues in manner 3: the 'Maifa' says . . .)

Table 2.3. *Cont'd*

7. when your servant Yi rubbed his *mai*, they were (or it was) deep, small, and soft, abruptly they were (or it was) '*qiaqia*'. (text continues in manner 1: this is . . .)

8. when your servant Yi rubbed his *mai*, the coming of the *mai* was slippery (text continues in manner 1: this is . . .)

9. at the time when your servant Yi rubbed his *mai*, it was *qi* [coming] from wind. The *mai* [coming] from the heart was murky. (the text continues in manner 3: the 'Bingfa' (Model of disorders) says . . .)

10. when I rubbed her *mai*, they were (or it was) large and full, their (or its) coming was difficult (text continues in manner 1: this is . . .)

11. —[iii]

12. —

13. —

14. —

15. sentence that concerns the condition of the complexion

16. —

17. sentence that concerns the condition of the complexion

18. at the time when I examined her *mai*, when I rubbed them (or it), it was *mai* [coming] from the kidneys. It was choppy and discontinuous. (text continues in manner 2: in cases where it is choppy and discontinuous . . .)

19. when I rubbed her *mai*, when I stroked their (or its) *chi* area,[iv] their (or its) *chi* area was corded, bristled, and coarse, while the body hair was beautiful x x.[v] (text continues in manner 1: this is . . .)

20. at the time when I examined his *mai*, when I rubbed them (or it), they were (or it was) entirely according to 'the model'.[vi] His illness was placid. (text continues in manner 1: hence . . .)

21. when I rubbed his *mai*, I got *yinqi* [coming] from the lungs. Their coming was dispersed, while arriving by several routes, they were not united. The complexion, moreover, rode on them. (text continues in manner 4: new paragraph beginning with the phrase 'the means whereby I knew x')

22. —

23. at the time when I examined him (no mention of *mai*)[vii]

24. when I examined him, his *mai fa qi ke*.[viii] (text continues in manner 3: the word says . . .)

25. when I rubbed his *mai*, I got the reversed [or spreading] *yang*. (text continues in manner 2: the reversed *yang* . . .)

Manner 1: Yi's perceptions are explained to indicate a certain condition or to refer to certain postulated processes in the body; these clauses are introduced by the character *ci* 此 (this is) or *shi* 是 (this is) or *gu* 故 (hence).

Manner 2: Yi quotes the 'Maifa' or refers to other authorities of medical knowledge; these clauses are introduced by the phrase *maifa yue* 脈法曰 (the model of the pulse says).

Manner 3: by reduplication of the last word in the previous sentence; these clauses are introduced by the standard phrase x *zhe* (in cases where x).

[i] Only those sentences are translated which explicitly mention *mai* in the following phrase.

[ii] Or: 'at the left opening'; text possibly corrupt.

[iii] '—' indicates that the above introductory phrase did not occur in this case.

[iv] *chi* 尺 later takes on the meaning of one of the three locations for taking the pulse at the wrist called *cun* 寸, *guan* 關, *chi* 尺. See 'Difficulty 18' in Unschuld (1986), 243 ff.

[v] *feng fa* 奉髮 (to offer with both hands head hair); text possibly corrupt.

[vi] *bing* is not mentioned in the introductory phrase.

[vii] For parallels see case 24; *zhi* 之 may or may not refer to *mai*.

[viii] *mai fa qi ke* 脈法奇咳; translation uncertain.

References to premodern Chinese and Japanese works

Han Fei zi 韓非子 (Master Han Fei). Zhou, 3rd century BC. References to *Han Fei zi jiaoshi*. Chen Qitian 陳啟天 (ed.). Zhonghua shuju, Shanghai, 1941.

Han shu 漢書 (History of the Former Han). Han, 1st century AD. Ban Gu 班固. Zhonghua shuju, Beijing, 1962.

Huangdi neijing 黃帝內經 (Yellow Emperor's Inner Canon). Zhou to Han, 3rd century BC to 1st century AD. Anon. Reference to Ren Yingqiu 任應秋 (ed.) *Huangdi neijing zhangju suoyin* 黃帝內經章句索引. Renmin weisheng chubanshe, Beijing, 1986.

Huangdi neijing Suwen 黃帝內經素問 (Yellow Emperor's Inner Canon, Basic Questions). Tang, 610. Edited by Wang Bing 王冰. Facsimile of a Ming woodprint of the Song edition of 1067 by Gu Congde 顧從德 et al. Renmin weisheng chubanshe, Beijing, 1956.

Lienü zhuan 列女傳 (Biographies of Outstanding Women). Han, 1st century BC. Liu Xiang 劉向, attributed compiler. References to *Lienüzhuan jiaozhu*, annotated by Liang Duan 梁端. *SBBY*.

Lingshu 靈樞, see *Huangdi neijing* 黃帝內經.

Lunyu 論語. (Analects). Zhou, 3rd to 2nd centuries BC. Anon. References to *Lunyu zhengyi* 論語正義. Qing, 1866. Commentated by Liu Baonan 劉寶楠. Zhonghua shuju, Beijing, 1990.

Maijing 脈經 (Canon of the Vessel-Pulses). Jin, AD 280. Wang Xi 王熙. References to *Maijing jiaozhu*, commentated by Chen Yannan 沈炎南. Renmin weisheng chubanshe, Beijing, 1991.

Mawangdui vessel texts, see Ma Jixing 馬繼興 1992 and Mawangdui Han mu boshu zhengli xiaozu 馬王堆漢墓帛書整理小組 1985.

Shiji 史記. (Records of the Historian). Han, *ca* 90 BC. Sima Qian 司馬遷. Zhonghua shuju, Beijing, 1959. See also: *Shiki kaichū kōshō* 史記會注考證.

Shijing 詩經 (Book of Songs). References to *Shisanjing zhushu* 十三經注疏, vol. II. Qing, 1816. Compiled by Ruan Yuan 阮元. Chūban Shuppansha, Kyoto, 1971.

Shiki kaichū kōshō 史記會注考證 (Examination of the Collected Commentaries to the Records of the Historian). 1932–34. Commentated by Takigawa Kametarō 瀧川龜太郎. Tōyō Bunka Gakuin Tōyō Kenkyūjo, Tokyo.

Shuowen jiezi 説文解字 (Analytic Dictionary of Characters). Han, AD 121. Xu Shen 許慎. References to *Shuowen jiezi zhu* 説文解字注. Qing, 1776–1807. Commentated by Duan Yucai 段玉裁. Shanghai guji chubanshe, Shanghai, 1981.

Suwen 素問, see *Huangdi neijing* 黃帝內經 or *Huangdi neijing Suwen* 黃帝內經素問.

Zhangjiashan manuscripts, see Jiangling Zhangjiashan 江陵張家山 and Gao Dalun 高大倫 1992 in References to modern works.

Zuo zhuan 左傳 (Zuo Tradition). Zhou to Han, 3rd to 1st centuries BC. Anon. References to *Chunqiu Zuo zhuan zhu*, annotated by Yang Bojun 楊伯峻. 4 Vols. Zhonghua shuju, Beijing, 1981.

References to modern works

Bates, Don (ed.) 1995. *Knowledge and the Scholarly Medical Traditions*. Cambridge University Press, Cambridge.

Beasley, W.G. and Pulleyblank, Edwin G. (eds.) 1961. *Historians of China and Japan*. Oxford University Press, London.

Bielenstein, Hans 1980. *The Bureaucracy of Han Times*. Cambridge University Press, Cambridge.

Bodde, Derk 1982. 'Forensic Medicine in Pre-Imperial China'. *Journal of the American Oriental Society* 102 (1), 1–15.

Bridgman, R. F. 1955. 'La médicine dans la Chine antique'. *Mélanges Chinois et Bouddhiques* 10, 1–213.

Brothwell D. and Sandison A. T. (eds.) 1967. *Disease in Antiquity*. Charles Thomas, Springfield.

Chavannes, Edouard 1895. *Les Mémoires Historiques de Se-ma Ts'ien.* 5 vols. Leroux, Paris.

Couvreur S. (repr.) 1951. *Tchouen Tsiou Tso Tchouan: Chronique Lou.* 3 vols. Cathasia, Paris.

Cruse, D. A. 1986. *Lexical Semantics.* Cambridge University Press, Cambridge.

Deng Tietao 鄧鐵濤 (ed.) 1984. *Zhongyi zhenduanxue* 中醫診斷學 (Traditional Chinese Medicine Diagnostics). Shanghai kexue jishu chubanshe, Shanghai.

Epler D. C. 1980. 'Bloodletting in Early Chinese Medicine and its Relation to the Origin of Acupuncture'. *Bulletin of the History of Medicine* 54 (3), 337–67.

Epler, D. C. 1988. 'The Concept of Disease in an Ancient Chinese Medical Text (*Shanghan-lun*)'. *Journal of the History of Medicine and Allied Sciences* 43, 8–35.

Farquhar, Judith 1994. *Knowing Practice: the Clinical Encounter of Chinese Medicine.* Westview, Boulder.
    1995. 'Multiplicity, Point of View, and Responsibility in Traditional Chinese Healing'. In Zito and Barlow, 78–99.

Frake, Charles O. 1961. 'The Diagnosis of Disease among the Subanun of Mindanao'. *American Anthropologist* 63, 113–32.

Gao Dalun 高大倫 (ed.) 1992. *Zhangjiashan Han jian 'Maishu' jiaoshi* 張家山漢簡脈書校釋 (Explanation of the Document of the Mai on Han Dynasty Bamboo Slips from Zhangjiashan). Chengdu chubanshe, Chengdu.

Gernet, Jacques and Kalinowski, Marc (eds.) 1997. *En suivant la voie royale: Mélanges en hommage à Léon Vendermeersch. Etudes thématiques* 7. Ecole Française d'Extrême-Orient, Paris.

Graham, Angus C. 1986. *Yin-yang and the Nature of Correlative Thinking.* Institute of East Asian Philosophies, Singapore.

Granet, Marcel 1934. *La Pensée Chinoise.* La Renaissance du Livre, Paris.

Harper, Donald 1982. 'The Wu Shi Erh Ping Fangi Translation and Prolegomena'. PhD thesis in Oriental Languages, University of California, Berkeley.
    1998. *Early Chinese Medical Literature: the Mawangdui Medical Manuscripts.* Routledge, London.

Hsu, Elisabeth 1987. 'Lexical Semantics and Chinese Medical Terms'. Unpublished MPhil dissertation in General Linguistics, University of Cambridge.
    1999. *The Transmission of Chinese Medicine.* Cambridge University Press, Cambridge.
    2001. 'The Telling Touch: Pulse Diagnostics in Early Chinese Medicine'. Habilitationschrift, Fakultät für Orientalistik und Altertumswissenschaft, Universität Heidelberg.

Hübotter, F. 1927. 'Zwei berühmte chinesische Arzte des Altertums Chouen Yu-I und Hua T'ouo'. *Mitteilungen der deutschen Gesellschaft für Natur- und Völkerkunde Ostasiens* 21A, 3–48.

Hulsewé, A. F. P. 1985. *Remnants of Ch'in Law.* Brill, Leiden.

Jiangling Zhangjiashan Han jian zhengli xiaozu 江陵張家山漢簡整理小組 1989. 'Jiangling Zhangjiashan Han jian "Maishu" shiwen' 江陵張家山漢簡 《脈書》釋文 (Transcript of the 'Maishu' on Bamboo Slips from Jiangling Zhangjiashan). *Wenwu* 7, 72–4.

Johnson, D. 1981. 'Epic and History in Early China: the Matter of Wu Tzu-hsü'. *Journal of Asian Studies* 40 (2), 255–71.

Keegan, David J. 1988. 'The "Huang-ti Nei-Ching": the Structure of the Compilation; the Significance of the Structure'. PhD thesis in History, University of California, Berkeley.

Kuriyama, Shigehisa 1995. 'The Imagination of Winds and the Development of the Chinese Conception of the Body'. In Zito and Barlow, 23–41.
    1999. *The Expressiveness of the Body and the Divergence of Greek and Chinese Medicine.* Zone, New York.

Lau D. C. et al. 1995. *A Concordance to the Chunqiu Zuo zhuan.* Commercial Press, Chinese University of Hong Kong, Institute of Chinese Studies.

Lewis, Mark E. 1990. *Sanctioned Violence in Early China.* State University of New York Press, Albany.

Li Bocong 李伯聰 1990. *Bian Que he Bian Que xuepai yanjiu* 扁鵲和扁鵲學派研究 (Researches on Bian Que and the Bian Que Tradition). Shaanxi kexue jishu chubanshe, Xi'an.

Lloyd, Geoffrey E. R. (1950) 1983. *Hippocratic Writings*. Penguin, Harmondsworth.
  (unpublished). 'Why Case Histories?' 32 pp.

Loewe, Michael A. N. 1997. 'The Physician Chunyu Yi and his Historical Background'. In Gernet and
  Kalinowski, 297–313.

Lu Gwei-Djen and Needham, Joseph 1967. 'Records of Disease in Ancient China'. In Brothwell and
  Sandison, 222–37.

Ma Jixing 馬繼興 (ed.) 1992. *Mawangdui guyishu kaoshi* 馬王堆古醫書考釋 (Explanation of the Ancient
  Medical Documents from Mawangdui). Hunan kexue jishu chubanshe, Changsha.

Mawangdui Hanmu boshu zhengli xiaozu 馬王堆漢墓帛書整理小組 (eds.) 1985. *Mawangdui Hanmu
  boshu* 馬王堆漢墓帛書 (The Silk Documents from a Han Tomb at Mawangdui), vol. IV. Wenwu
  chubanshe, Beijing.

McLeod, Katherina C. D. and Yates, Robin 1981. 'Forms of Ch'in Law: an Annotated Translation of
  Feng-chen shih'. *Harvard Journal of Asiatic Studies* 41, 111–63.

Pfister, Rudolf 1992. 'Tian xia zhi dao tan: Meinungen, wie unter dem Himmel das dao optimal zu erre-
  ichen sei'. Lizentiatsarbeit am Ostasiatischen Seminar der Universität Zürich.

Pulleyblank, Edwin G. 1995. *Outline of Classical Chinese Grammar*. University of British Columbia,
  Vancouver.

Sivin, Nathan 1987. *Traditional Medicine in Contemporary China: a Partial Translation of* Revised
  Outline of Chinese Medicine (1972) *with an Introductory Study on Change in Present-day and Early
  Medicine*. Center for Chinese Studies, University of Michigan, Ann Arbor.

  1995. 'Text and Experience in Classical Chinese Medicine'. In Bates, 177–204.

Tan Qixiang 譚其驤 (ed.) 1982. *Zhongguo lishi ditu ji* 中國歷史地圖集 (Collection of Historical Chinese
  Maps), vol. II. Ditu chubanshe, Beijing.

Twitchett, Denis C. 1961. 'Chinese Biographical Writing'. In Beasley and Pulleyblank, 95–114.

Unschuld, Paul U. 1986. *The Classic of Difficult Issues: with Commentaries by Chinese and Japanese
  Authors from the Third through to the Twentieth Century*. University of California Press, Berkeley.

Watson, Burton 1958. *Ssu-ma Ch'ien: Grand Historian of China*. Columbia University Press, New
  York.

Wilbur, Martin 1943. *Slavery in China during the Former Han Dynasty, 206 BC–AD 25. Anthropological
  Series* 34. Field Museum of Natural History, Chicago.

Yamada Keiji 山田慶兒 1988. 'Hen Shaku densetsu' 扁鵲傳説 (The Legend of Bian Que). *Tōhō gakuhō*
  60, 73–158.

Yin Huihe 印會河 (ed.) 1984. *Zhongyi jichu lilun* 中醫基礎理論 (Fundamental Theory of Traditional
  Chinese Medicine). Shanghai kexue jishu chubanshe, Shanghai.

Yu Yunxiu 余雲岫 1953. *Gudai jibing minghou shuyi* 古代疾病名候疏義 (Explanation of the Nomenclature of Disease in Ancient Times). Renmin weisheng chubanshe, Beijing.

Zimmermann, Francis 1987. *The Jungle and the Aroma of Meats: an Ecological Theme in Hindu
  Medicine*. University of California Press, Berkeley.

Zito, Angela and Barlow, Tani E. (eds.) 1995. *Body, Subject, and Power in China*. University of Chicago
  Press, Chicago.

PART II

Correlative cosmologies

Introduction

By conceiving of the bodily processes in terms of the subtle changes of *mai* and *qi*, imperceptible to the non-initiated, the ground was cleared for the medical authority of the elite to establish itself through medical speculation. The grid for interrelating the subtle changes of *mai* and *qi* with each other in a systemic way was found in so-called 'correlative cosmologies'. This numerological schematism has been singled out as characteristic of the medicine that established itself among the Han elite, which is generally referred to as the 'medicine of systematic correspondences'.[1] The questions are who the proponents were who developed these numerological systems and who the elite physicians were who propagated them in medicine.

Donald Harper's chapter (chapter 3) makes a strong case that the correlative cosmology that dominated Han elite medicine had early precursors in iatromancy (the art of predicting medical events). Harper first provides manuscript evidence documenting a transition from an older divinatory tradition involving propitiations and exorcisms, still dominant in the fourth century BC (documents excavated at Baoshan 包山), to the correlative-cosmology iatromancy of the third century BC (documents excavated at Shuihudi 睡虎地). He then compares the correlative cosmology of iatromancy with that contained in the prognosis in one of Chunyu Yi's 淳于意 case histories, and with that contained in a text passage in the well-known chapter 10 of the *Divine Pivot* (Lingshu 靈樞), the second book of the *Yellow Emperor's Inner Canon*. His article thus discusses two incidences of innovation; one involving modified reasoning within one tradition, that of iatromancy, and the other a transfer of correlative reasoning from one domain of prognostics and diagnostics to another, that is from iatromancy to medicine.

The Baoshan divination manuscript records ten divinations for the years 317 and 316 BC. It refers to a sexagenary cycle of binomials, which were constituted by one of

---

[1] Unschuld, Paul U. (1985), *Medicine in China: a History of Ideas*, University of California Press, Berkeley, 51–100.

the so-called ten stems (*gan* 干) and one of the twelve branches (*zhi* 支) and used for calendrical purposes. This system, which counted days (and later also years) in terms of a sexagenary cycle, is age-old and of uncertain origin. The Baoshan manuscript uses it to predict precisely the day on which respite (*jian* 間) of an illness occurs. Alongside such time-based prognostication, the text also exhorts propitiation of deities through offerings and/or endorsement of exorcistic rites for achieving a cure (*zha* 瘥). Harper points out that the coupling of divinatory with propitiatory and exorcistic acts, which we find in the Baoshan manuscript, reflects a religious pattern already known from the Shang oracle bones of the second millennium BC. The use of the sexagenary cycle undoubtedly had a symbolic significance no longer clear to us now, but Harper stresses that Baoshan iatromancy was not based on a hemerological system, where symptoms and illnesses are considered to follow a clearly set course.

A manuscript from Jiudian 九店 of the late fourth century BC and the Shuihudi manuscripts of the third century BC attest to more elaborate iatromantic systems which are based on hemerological ideas. The iatromantic system of the Jiudian manuscript and one of the Shuihudi manuscripts specifies illness stages with regard to the twelve branches: given the occurrence of a morbid condition (*you ji* 有疾) on a certain day, there are definitive branch days for slight curing (*shaochou* 少廖), great curing (*dachou* 大廖), and for death and life (*sisheng* 死生). Branch iatromancy thus reflects a fairly systematic account of a standard illness course. It also differs from the ailment divination recorded in the Baoshan manuscript in that it does not foresee any medical treatment; recovery is considered to depend solely on the right time.

The Shuihudi manuscripts contain text fragments which record yet another iatromantic system based on hemerological ideas, and those incorporate Five Agent (or Five Phases) correlations. Here the stages of an illness, slightly different from the above, are detailed to occur on a certain stem day: the text distinguishes between a point of origin of a morbid condition (*ji* 疾), a manifest ailment (*bing* 病), respite (*jian* 間), and recovery (*chou* 廖). If there is no recovery, the fault is said to lie with Fever (*fan* 煩) and Year (*sui* 歲), and if Fever and Year both occupy the quarter correlated with the phase that is correlated with the stem day of the illness's point of origin (*ji*), death occurs. These text fragments from Shuihudi on hemerological stem iatromancy are remarkable in that they correlate the ten stem days with the Five Agents.

Harper's argument is that correlative cosmology provided important paradigms for the physicians of the Han dynasty, who by then already reasoned in terms of *mai* and *qi* and were well-versed in what he calls 'vessel theory pathology'. So-called 'Five Agent theory' and the sexagesimal time reckoning system, which were first elaborated in the context of iatromancy, became integrated into medicine when these physicians of 'vessel theory pathology' set about correlating the somatic microcosm with the macrocosm. Harper provides evidence for this in a passage of the *Inner Canon* that correlates the severing of the five different *yin* vessels with the day of death of the five body constituents hair (*mao* 毛), blood (*xue* 血), flesh (*rou* 肉), bone (*gu* 骨), and muscle (*jin* 筋), on the basis of Five Agent correlations.[2] He also gives a striking interpretation for Chunyu Yi's one prognosis that mentions a stem day as the day of death, an explanation not explicitly provided by Chunyu Yi himself, but clearly grounded in the tradition of iatromantic reasoning that Harper discusses in this chapter.

Evidently, astrologers and diviners provided a highly elaborate framework for predicting the course of illness according to a numerological schematism that was later transposed into medical discourse. Harper provides yet another case, in addition to that presented by Lo, where innovation in medical doctrine was achieved by adopting modes of reasoning from a distinct but related tradition into one's own. Vivienne Lo showed that the vocabulary both for landscaping the body and for expressing sensual experience given in manuals on the sexual arts was integrated into medical writings on the body, and Donald Harper explores the numerological schemata developed in iatromancy for predicting the future course of illness and their integration into medical doctrine.

Harper's chapter makes a strong case for the importance of the activities of a group of people called *fangshi* 方士 (recipe gentlemen) and his article suggests that their formulae and calculations laid the foundations for the canonisation of medicine based on the numerological system of 'Five Agent theory'. Two questions arise from this: why was it, once the medical gaze of bodily processes had transcended the static and concrete, and medical language was couched in terms like *mai* and *qi*, that the canonisation of medicine was linked with the acceptance of a certain numerological system for prognostication? And why was it precisely the numerological system of 'Five Agent theory' that became prevalent in the last three centuries BC?

These two questions are radically different in kind, and too far-reaching to be discussed in this volume. While the first is of philosophical import, and ultimately invokes the question of how traditional sciences dealt with problems that the modern sciences phrase in terms of probability, the second is historical in nature. The concept of innovation as arising from the creative tension between conventions in one tradition and their adversaries may provide a guideline for future research. One thing is certain: more needs to be known about these people who were called *fangshi* by others but who did not call themselves so, about their socio-economic background and their intellectual

---

[2] At the end of this text passage the day of death is predicted for the case of a severing of all five *yin* vessels together.

striving, and about the controversies among themselves and with adherents of other traditions of learning.[3]

The second major imposition in Chinese medical history of an elaborate numerological system onto medical doctrine is discussed by Catherine Despeux in chapter 4. The system of the five circulatory phases and the six seasonal influences (*wuyun liuqi* 五運六氣) had existed possibly since the end of the eighth century; Wang Bing, editor of the *Plain Questions* (Suwen 素問) of the *Inner Canon*, is considered one of its chief promotors (though it is uncertain whether he in fact wrote the texts attributed to him). However, the system did not become widely known until the middle of the eleventh century and only took off in the twelfth and thirteenth centuries. This may be due to a discrepancy between what some historians of modern technology have called the 'invention' of a technology and the social process of 'innovation' that leads to its general acceptance. Alternatively, the discrepancy may arise from inexact textual dating. The available detail that Despeux provides on the early texts of this system proves insufficient to solve this question.

The system of the five circulatory phases and the six seasonal influences offers a means to calculate and predict the outcome of medical processes with reference to the basic unit of a cycle of sixty years, where each year is identified by pairing one of the ten celestial stems with one of the twelve terrestial branches. In this system the five circulatory phases (*wuyun* 五運) must not be confused with the Five Phases (*wuxing* 五行), for they differ in their sequential order, and in the pairs that they form with the ten stems. They correspond to five sections in heaven, and in order to make them match the six seasonal influences (*liuqi* 六氣) on earth, fire is divided into a sovereign fire (*junhuo* 君火) and a ministerial fire (*xianghuo* 相火). Despeux points out that this system survived to the present day only in the medical context, though the text passages she cites show that it had been applied also in others.[4]

Already in Song times, there were numerous critiques of the system, and Despeux shows that even its advocates like Shen Gua 沈括 (1031–95), who praised the theory,

[3] For recent discussions of *fangshi*, see Harper, Donald (1998), *Early Chinese Medical Literature: the Mawangdui Medical Manuscripts*, Routledge, London, 42–67, and Sivin, Nathan (1995, VII), 'Taoism and Science', in *Medicine, Philosophy and Religion in Ancient China, Researches and Reflections*, Variorum, Aldershot, 27–30. See also Chen Pan 陳槃 (1948), 'Zhanguo Qin Han jian fangshi kaolun' 戰國秦漢間方士考論 (Examination of the *fangshi* in Warring States, Qin, and Han), *Zhongyang yanjiuyuan lishi yuyan yanjiusuo jikan* 17, 7–57.
[4] The system is outlined by Porkert, Manfred (1974), *The Foundations of Chinese Medicine: Systems of Correspondence*, MIT Press, Cambridge, Mass., 55–106. See also Lu Gwei-djen and Needham, Joseph (1980), *Celestial Lancets: a History and Rationale of Acupuncture and Moxa*, Cambridge University Press, Cambridge, 137–49, and Ren Yingqiu 1960 (1982), *Yunqi xueshuo* 運氣學說 (The Doctrine of the Circulatory Phases and Seasonal Influences), 2nd edn, Shanghai guji chubanshe, Shanghai.

deplored the ignorance of the doctors who employed it in their practice. In her analysis it was the Imperial court which commissioned the production and the dissemination of treatises based on this system, and it was used principally for the prognostication, prevention, and treatment of epidemics. The epidemics of the Song, often seen in relation to advanced innovations in agricultural technology and increased urbanisation, are a commonplace of China's medical history.[5] Given that since antiquity certain seasonal and climatic conditions were correlated with the occurrence of an epidemic, Despeux suggests that the Imperial court promulgated this calendrically based numerological system of the five circulatory phases and the six seasonal influences for very practical reasons. While Daoist priests were busy among the populace, elite doctors of the bureaucratic state issued treatises on epidemics based on this doctrine. Among these the most notable was the *Treatise on Cold Damage Disorders* (Shanghan lun 傷寒論) by Zhang Ji 張機 (*ca* 150–219) which was reconstituted in the Song and had innumerable commentators who were adherents of it.

The doctrine of the five circulatory phases and the six seasonal influences also triggered innovative theories of the body, etiology, pathology, and therapeutics. Fire now corresponded both to the heart and to the kidneys, and as a result the kidneys came to be treated as a double organ comprising fire in the right kidney, called the 'gate of life' (*mingmen* 命門), and water in the left kidney: this was a physiology closely related to the ideas of inner alchemy. Despeux shows that phase energetics contributed significantly to the theories of currently celebrated Song medical scholars, for instance, Chen Yan 陳言 (fl. 1161–74), who put forth the idea of the three disease factors (*sanyin* 三因), or Liu Wansu 劉完素 (1110–1200) and Zhang Congzheng 張從正 (1156–1228), two of the 'four great scholars of the Song and Yuan', and thereby points out that this characteristic of their writings tends to be overlooked nowadays.

In pharmacotherapy the system of five circulatory phases and the six seasonal influences also proved influential where it was used mostly for preventive measures. Notably, it was in this way – by providing a rationale for calculating unknowable future events – that the 'empiricist' tradition of pharmacotherapy came to accept canonical rationale, and thereby became integrated into the realms of medical speculation that had already started to dominate the rationale of acumoxa therapy in the Han dynasty. It is noteworthy, however, that the Song physicians developed for acumoxa a related but different theory, approximated in a literal translation as 'the method that takes account of the flowing and pouring round between noon and midnight' (*ziwu liuzhu fa* 子午流注法).

---

[5] Ma Boying (1994), *Zhongguo yixue wenhua shi* 中國醫學文化史 (A History of Medicine in Chinese Culture), Shanghai renmin weisheng chubanshe, Shanghai, 574, figure 15.3, shows the incidences of epidemics graphically.

This phenomenon is not further explored in Despeux's article, but certainly deserves further investigation: it may well highlight possible controversies between elite doctors practising either acumoxa or pharmacotherapy.

The two articles in this section suggest that numerological schematism was imposed onto medical doctrine in periods of great governmental promotion of and control over medicine, and that the schematism had been developed in related but separate traditions of learning. The techniques and numerological systems of the authors of the iatromantic texts that Harper discusses led, in the course of the canonisation of Chinese medical doctrine, to the integration of 'Five Agent theory' into medical reasoning. Despeux's discussion of the early writers on the system of the five circulatory phases and the six seasonal influences shows that they came from Daoist circles, and that some of them were initiated adherents of a Daoist church. One may question rightly whether it was 'proto-Daoism' that informed the *fangshi* who practised iatromancy, but Despeux's article certainly underlines the importance that Daoist authors had for innovation in Chinese medical doctrine.

3

Iatromancy, diagnosis, and prognosis in Early Chinese medicine

DONALD HARPER

By the second century BC, the vessels (*mai* 脈) carrying blood (*xue* 血) and vapour (*qi* 氣) through the body were seen to constitute the essential physiological structure around which the other constituents of the body were organized. The ascendancy of vessel theory was spurred by a still new, universal model of illness that attributed illness (or nameable ailments) to dysfunctions within the system of vessels. In contrast to older ideas that ailments were the consequence of demonic agents or pathogens occupying the patient's body, the new model considered an ailment to be the manifestation of a deeper physiological dysfunction. The goal of diagnosis and treatment was to determine the nature of the dysfunction and to re-establish somatic harmony. The belief in agents and pathogens represents an ontological view of illness; Chinese vessel theory pathology is the counterpart to humoral pathology and other types of physiological explanation of illness in Western medicine.[1]

The development of vessel theory pathology was stimulated by correlative cosmology. Vessel theory provided a framework for the application of *yinyang* 陰陽 and Five Agent (*wuxing* 五行) theories to the human organism; it allowed physicians to precisely classify the human microcosm and link its operation to phenomenal processes in the macrocosm. Chunyu Yi's 淳于意 (second century BC) account of the invention of the 'model of the vessels' (*maifa* 脈法) testifies to the importance of the new pathology:[2]

> Ailment names are mostly alike and are unknowable. Thus the ancient sages
> created the model of the vessels for them, with which to initiate the measurement
> of dimension and volume, fix the compass and square, suspend the weights and

---

[1] For discussion of ontological and physiological conceptions of illness in Chinese medicine, see Unschuld (1993), 21; Unschuld characterizes vessel theory pathology as a 'functional' view rather than 'physiological'. Hudson (1993) surveys ontological and physiological conceptions of illness in Western medicine.

[2] *Shiji, juan* 105, 21b.

balance, apply the marking-cord ink, and blend *yin* and *yang*.[3] They differentiated the vessels in man and named each one. Matching with heaven and earth,
[the vessels] combine in man to form a trinity. Thus they then differentiated the
hundred ailments, distinguishing between them.

According to Chunyu Yi's medical case histories, vessel diagnosis is the best and most
accurate way to determine the nature of a patient's illness; Chunyu Yi's treatments focus
on ameliorating the morbid condition exhibited by the vessels (except when diagnosis
reveals the condition to be untreatable).[4]

Chunyu Yi's account reveals an intellectual debt to the third-century-BC authors
of the 'Xici zhuan' 繫辭傳 (Tradition on the Appended Texts), the cosmological commentary to the *Yijing* 易經 (Classic of Changes):[5]

> The sages laid out the hexagrams and observed the images. Attaching phrases to
> them, they elucidated the auspicious and the inauspicious. Rigid and pliant fol-
> low one another, giving birth to alteration and transformation . . . [For the] hexa-
> grams, there are lesser and greater [results]; the phrases are devious or candid. As
> for the phrases, each points to the destination. The *Yi* is equivalent to heaven and
> earth. Thus it can wholly envelop the way of heaven and earth. Looking upward
> to observe the design of heaven and downward to examine the pattern of earth;
> for this reason, it knows the cause of dark and bright. It traces back to the begin-
> ning and returns to the end, thus knowing the explanation of death and life.

In the 'Xici zhuan', milfoil divination has become more than an instrument for probing
the unknown, the better to chart an advantageous course of action. The hexagrams
'wholly express the way of heaven and earth'; the system of the *Yijing* is a gauge which
renders life and death knowable.

Chunyu Yi speaks of his success at 'diagnosing ailments and determining death and
life' after completing his three years of medical apprenticeship.[6] Surely this was the
aim of medical training even before vessel theory pathology. However, as correlative
cosmology began to assume greater importance in medicine during the third and second
centuries BC, physicians found themselves in company with other specialists in natural
philosophy who grounded their knowledge in *yinyang* and five agent theories. On
the one hand, this knowledge was superseding old ways of thinking, mostly magico-
religious in nature. On the other hand, correlative cosmology itself was not a new

---

[3] Reference to compass, square, weights, balance, etc., was already a convention by the second century
BC to express the concrete relation between the macrocosm and the microcosm (in this case, the body)
that was established by means of fixed standards. For similar language in the *Huangdi neijing*, see
Suwen, *juan* 2, *pian* 5, 9b; and *Suwen*, *juan* 5, *pian* 17, 3a.
[4] For Chunyu Yi's medical case histories, see Elisabeth Hsu (this volume).   [5] *Yijing*, *juan* 7, 3a–5b.
[6] *Shiji*, *juan* 105, 9a.

rationalism. Despite a kind of rationalistic skepticism that accompanied *yinyang* and Five Agent theories in various fields of knowledge, the theories themselves were not like laws of nature; and there was not a clear break with magico-religious conceptions. A wholly naturalistic explanation of phenomena was a relative interpretation made by the person applying the theories; the theories themselves did not exclude occult interpretation.[7]

The ambivalence felt by thinkers for whom correlative cosmology was the key to naturalistic explanations (including physicians like Chunyu Yi) is concisely expressed in a text included in the Mawangdui 馬王堆 tomb 3 (burial dated 168 BC) manuscript of the *Yijing*. Entitled 'Yao' 要 (Essentials), the text gives Confucius' apology for his attachment to the *Yijing*:[8]

> If men of later generations doubt Qiu [me, Confucius], perhaps it will be because of the *Yi*. I seek the virtue in it, no more. I am one who shares a path with scribes and shamans, but whose final destination is different. How can the virtuous conduct of the gentleman be intended to seek fortune? Thus his performance of sacrificial worship is infrequent. How can his humaneness and sense of duty be intended to seek auspices? Thus his performance of turtle and milfoil divination is rare. Does not the turtle and milfoil divination of the incantors and shamans come after this?

I attribute the sentiments to a third-century-BC mentality. Confucius admits to 'sharing a path' with scribe-astrologers (*shi* 史), shamans (*wu* 巫), and incantors (*zhu* 祝) while rejecting their motives; sacrifices to the spirits intended to gain fortune from them and divination intended to seize the advantage are unworthy of the true gentleman. Yet in the third century BC the *Yijing* remained essentially a divination manual. Confucius' apology occurs as part of his response to a pointed question from the disciple Zigong 子貢: 'Does the Master also believe in its use for milfoil divination?' And Confucius' first words are: 'Of one hundred divinations I have performed, seventy have been on the mark.' The issue in the third century BC was not whether correlative cosmology and divination were incompatible; rather it was where a person chose to take a stand on their relative value.

---

[7] The problem of what labels to apply to theories of nature in early China is important and complicated. I have adopted the expedient of using a pair of terms – 'natural philosophy' and 'occult thought' – to refer to an undivided realm of knowledge in which magico-religious elements were not excluded from naturalistic explanation; see Harper (1998), 8–11. Similarly, Kalinowski (1991), 47, rejects the single label 'natural philosophy', comparing *yinyang* and five agent theories to the hermetic traditions of Greco-Roman times: 'To reduce this to a system of natural philosophy does not take account of the extreme diversity of the elements of which it is composed and of its multiple applications not only in the realm of the investigation of things in general, but also in that of politics, religion, and the arts.'

[8] I follow the transcription in Chen and Liao (1993), 435 (as of this writing a reproduction of the text on the original silk manuscript has not been published).

In the third and second centuries BC, physicians must have been in several minds about the blending of magico-religious and occult beliefs with naturalistic conceptions in correlative cosmology. Socially, they belonged to the same milieu as the *yinyang* specialists and *fangshi* 方士 (recipe gentlemen), who were associated with occult knowledge by the intellectual orthodoxy reflected in virtually all contemporary received sources. If Chunyu Yi as well as the first-century-BC physician-authors of the *Huangdi neijing* (Inner Classic of the Yellow Thearch) appear to have eschewed magico-religious and occult ideas in theory and in practice, we should not conclude that their medicine developed in isolation from such ideas.[9]

I propose to focus on diagnosis and prognosis because of newly discovered bamboo-slip manuscripts from the fourth and third centuries BC that document iatromancy, the practice of medical divination. Manuscripts that treat of hemerology, which concerns the determination of times when people will encounter good or ill fortune, from Jiudian 九店 tomb 56 at Jiangling 江陵, Hubei (burial dated late fourth century BC), and from Shuihudi 睡虎地 tomb 11 at Yunmeng 雲夢, Hubei (burial dated *ca* 217 BC), are particularly significant. In addition to the hemerological content, these manuscripts contain astrological material as well as material related to divination and magic.[10] Han accounts attest to the popularity of this type of literature among the elite. It was one of the vehicles for the dissemination of *yinyang* and five agent theories, whose correlations were at the base of many occult systems. Sections on iatromancy in the Jiudian and Shuihudi manuscripts suggest cross-fertilization between iatromantic prediction of the cause and course of an ailment and the vessel-based diagnosis performed by physicians like Chunyu Yi. Perhaps the iatromantic systems documented in the manuscripts – some of which utilize Five Agent theory – preceded vessel-based diagnosis, which for the first time incorporated *yinyang* and Five Agent ideas into medical diagnosis.[11]

---

[9] For further discussion, see Harper (1990), and Harper (1998), 42–52.

[10] A transcription and photographic reproduction of the Jiudian hemerological manuscript are published in Hubei sheng wenwu kaogu yanjiusuo (1995), 506–11 (transcription) and plates 102–22; a transcription and photographic reproduction of the two Shuihudi hemerological manuscripts are published in Shuihudi Qin mu zhujian zhengli xiaozu (1990), 180–255 (transcription) and 89–141. For a general description of the Shuihudi manuscripts, see Harper (1985), 467–9, and Kalinowski (1986). In addition to the Jiudian and Shuihudi manuscripts, two hemerological manuscripts have been discovered in Fangmatan 放馬灘 tomb 1 at Tianshu 天水, Gansu (burial *ca* 230–220 BC), the second of which includes a section on iatromancy. A transcription of the second manuscript is not yet published. He (1989), 27, refers briefly to the iatromantic content and cites an example.

[11] Yamada (1980) has already demonstrated the influence of wind divination involving the deity Taiyi 太一 (Grand One) in the *Huangdi neijing*; see also Unschuld (1985), 68–71. The occult elements are eliminated or marginalized in the *Huangdi neijing*.

Iatromantic material in the divination manuscript excavated from Baoshan 包山 tomb 2, Hubei (burial dated *ca* 316 BC), represents an iatromantic tradition even older than the iatromancy in the Jiudian and Shuihudi manuscripts. Written in Chu 楚 script in a terse, hieratic style, the manuscript is a personal record of turtle and milfoil divination performed for the benefit of the tomb occupant, Shao Tuo 邵陀, during his lifetime.[12] The last six divination accounts in the manuscript all date to 316 BC and concern the heart ailment that evidently led to Shao Tuo's death. In the typical divination account, diviners present statements regarding the ailment for divination; having arrived at a prediction, a follow-up divination is made concerning precisely what rituals will be performed and what offerings will be sacrificed to which spirits in order to alleviate the ailment; and a prediction concerning these rituals and sacrifices concludes the account.

The world of divination and religion reflected in the Baoshan manuscript belongs to a time preceding the hemerology and nascent correlative cosmology evidenced in the late-fourth and third-century-BC Jiudian and Shuihudi hemerological manuscripts. Significant spiritual and intellectual changes were clearly underway between the fourth and third centuries BC. The changes produced a flowering of specialists in natural philosophy and occult knowledge in the third century BC. Focusing more narrowly on the relation between iatromancy on the one hand and medical diagnosis and prognosis on the other, the manuscript evidence indicates that the second half of the fourth century BC marks the beginning of what I will provisionally call 'correlative cosmology iatromancy' (see the discussion later in this chapter). It is against the background of iatromancy in the third-century-BC Shuihudi manuscripts that I propose to look at diagnosis and prognosis in Chunyu Yi's writings and in the *Huangdi neijing*.

The Baoshan divination manuscript records ten divinations concerning Shao Tuo's heart ailment for the years 317 and 316 BC (four divinations in 317 and six in 316). I translate one divination account from each year to illustrate the general features of fourth century BC iatromancy using turtle and milfoil divination. First, for 317 BC:[13]

---

[12] A transcription and photographic reproduction of the divination manuscript are published in Hubei sheng Jing Sha tielu kaogudui (1991), 32–7 (transcription) and plates 88–109. Several similar divination manuscripts have been discovered in late fourth century BC Chu tombs. See Hubei sheng wenwu kaogu yanjiusuo and Beijing daxue Zhongwenxi (1995), 68–106 (transcription) and 19–50, for the divination manuscript from Wangshan 望山 tomb 1 at Jiangling, Hubei. For an overview of the contents of these divination manuscripts, see Li (1990).

[13] Hubei sheng Jing Sha tielu kaogudui (1991), 34, slip 220. The identification of graphs and their interpretation is often tentative. In addition to the notes accompanying the transcription, I have relied on the invaluable studies of the Baoshan divination manuscript in Li (1990), and Li (1993), 255–75.

In the year that the Guest from Eastern Zhou, Xu Ting, performed sacrifices of allegiance at Ying [317 BC];[14] in the month Cuan [eleventh month]; on the day *jiyou*.[15]

東周之客譽（許）經逵（歸）俊（作）於莪（栽）郢之戠（歲）。奧（爨）月己酉之日。

Ke Guang divines for the Chief Minister of the Left, Shao Tuo, with the Long Rule [turtle]:[16] 'There is illness below the heart, and the vapour is slight.'

苛光以長愲（則）為左尹邵㐌貞（貞）。以其下心而疾少燹（氣）。

[The prediction]:[17] 'The divination is ever auspicious. There will be respite on a *geng* or *xin* [day].[18] The ailment will gradually be cured.[19] Do not perform exorcism[20] at Piyang. Do perform the same elimination rite.'

丞（恆）貞（貞）吉。庚辛又（有）勿（間）。防（病）逮（漸）膚（瘧）。不逗（鬭）於邳易。同禜（奪）。

Ke Guang's 苛光 divination on *jiyou* 己酉 is preceded by the divination of another turtle diviner, Xu Ji 許吉. Whereas Ke Guang predicts 'respite' in the next two days and a gradual cure, Xu Ji predicts a full cure by the day *jiayin* 甲寅, five days after *jiyou* (see table 3.2). The two diviners also differ on the appropriate rituals. In his follow-up divination, Xu Ji stipulates both the Piyang exorcism and the elimination rite; Ke Guang proposes only the elimination rite.[21]

Shao Tuo is suffering from the same general condition in the six ailment-divination accounts for 316 BC. Here is one:[22]

In the year that the Great Director of Horses, Dao Gu, led the army of the Domain of Chu to rescue Fu [316 BC]; in the month Xingyi [fourth month]; on the day *jimao*.[23]

大司馬邵骼䢔（將）楚邦之帀（師）徒以栽（救）郙戠﹦（之歲）。翟（刑）层（夷）育﹦（之月）己卯育﹦（之日）。

[14] The sacrifices indicate Eastern Zhou's status as a vassal state to Chu. Ying is the Chu capital.

[15] 'Cuan' is the eleventh month in the Chu calendar, which corresponds to the eighth month in the Qin calendrical system as explained in the first Shuihudi hemerological manuscript; Shuihudi Qin mu zhujian zhengli xiaozu (1990), 190. *Jiyou* is the forty-sixth day in the sexagenary cycle; see tables 3.1–3.2.

[16] The diviners who perform turtle divination are different from those who perform milfoil divination; and the shell used by each turtle diviner has a proper name.

[17] Usually the words 占之 appear at this point, but they are missing in this divination account.

[18] The two days following *jiyou* in the sexagenary cycle are *gengxu* 庚戌 and *xinhai* 辛亥. 'Respite' (*jian* 間) means that the progress of the ailment is halted.

[19] The reading of 膚 is not certain, but it clearly means 'cure, recover (from an ailment)'; see Li (1990), 82–3, and Li (1993), 268.

[20] I follow Li (1993), 275, in reading *dou* 逗 as 鬭, perhaps referring to exorcism.

[21] The Ke Guang divination account does not include a follow-up divination, no doubt because Ke Guang accepts, with the modification specified, what Xu Ji already proposed in his follow-up divination.

[22] Hubei sheng Jing Sha tielu kaogudui (1991), 36, slips 236–8.

[23] The fourth month in the Chu calendar corresponds to the first month in the Qin calendar. *Jimao* is the sixteenth day in the sexagenary cycle.

Table 3.1. *The ten stems and twelve branches*

Stems	Branches
jia 甲	*zi* 子
yi 乙	*chou* 丑
bing 丙	*yin* 寅
ding 丁	*mao* 卯
wu 戊	*chen* 辰
ji 己	*si* 巳
geng 庚	*wu* 午
xin 辛	*wei* 未
ren 壬	*shen* 申
gui 癸	*you* 酉
	xu 戌
	hai 亥

Table 3.2. *The sexagenary cycle*

1. 甲子	11. 甲戌	21. 甲申	31. 甲午	41. 甲辰	51. 甲寅
2. 乙丑	12. 乙亥	22. 乙酉	32. 乙未	42. 乙巳	52. 乙卯
3. 丙寅	13. 丙子	23. 丙戌	33. 丙申	43. 丙午	53. 丙辰
4. 丁卯	14. 丁丑	24. 丁亥	34. 丁酉	44. 丁未	54. 丁巳
5. 戊辰	15. 戊寅	25. 戊子	35. 戊戌	45. 戊申	55. 戊午
6. 己巳	16. 己卯	26. 己丑	36. 己亥	46. 己酉	56. 己未
7. 庚午	17. 庚辰	27. 庚寅	37. 庚子	47. 庚戌	57. 庚申
8. 辛未	18. 辛巳	28. 辛卯	38. 辛丑	48. 辛亥	58. 辛酉
9. 壬申	19. 壬午	29. 壬辰	39. 壬寅	49. 壬子	59. 壬戌
10. 癸酉	20. 癸未	30. 癸巳	40. 癸卯	50. 癸丑	60. 癸亥

Gu Ji divines for the Chief Minister of the Left, Tuo, with the Precious Home [turtle]: 'There is illness in the abdomen and heart, and rising vapour. [Tuo] finds food unpalatable. For a long time there has been no cure. Would that he gradually be cured, and that there be no trouble.'

盬吉以琛豪（家）為左尹坨自（貞）。既腹心疾以走（上）既（氣）。不甘飤。舊不瘥（瘥）。尚逨（漸）瘥（瘥）。毋又（有）奈（祟）。

The prediction: 'The divination is ever auspicious. The illness is difficult to cure. According to its cause, let there be an elimination rite.'

占之。丞（恒）自（貞）吉。疾難瘥（瘥）。以其古（故）敓（奪）之。

'To be offered in prayer to Taiyi [Grand One],[24] one *fu* sheep;[25] to Lord Earth and to the Director of the Life-mandate, one ewe each. To be offered in prayer to

---

[24] Gu Ji's follow-up divination begins here.
[25] *Fu* 鞴 is not attested in received literature. Li (1993), 273, conjectures that it might denote a black sheep.

Great Water, one *fu* sheep; to the Two Sons of Heaven, one ewe each; to Zuo Mountain, one black sheep. To be offered in prayer to the elders and youths of Chu's forebears, to Zhu Rong, and to Zhu Xiong, two black sheep each for a lavish feast-sacrifice; to High Mound and Low Mound, one whole pig each. May the Chief Minister of the Left, Tuo, walk back to his dwelling place. May Year be attacked and expelled.' Gu Ji's prediction: 'Auspicious.'

舉禱㚇（太一）一𦍩。灰（侯／后）土司命各一牂。舉禱大水一膚。二天子各一牂。侳（坐）山一羖。舉禱楚先老僮祝䨞（融）㜏（鬻）畬（熊）各兩羖亯（享）祭䉈之。高丘（丘）下丘（丘）各一全豢（豢）。由（思）左尹𨚗遜（踐）逡（復）凥（居）。由（思）攻解於𢧢（歲）。盬吉占之曰吉。

The follow-up divination itemising the proposed observances and sacrificial offerings includes the names of three well-known deities in Warring States popular religion: Taiyi 太一 (Grand One, the astrological deity), Lord Earth 后土, and the Director of the Life-mandate 司命; Great Water 大水 may be a Yangzi River deity.[26] Following the list of spirits to be propitiated with sacrificial offerings is the name of one spirit marked for exorcism: Year (*sui* 歲), often associated with the planet Jupiter.[27]

Divination coupled with propitiatory and exorcistic acts continues a religious pattern that is first recorded in the Shang bone and shell inscriptions.[28] It is noteworthy that Xu Ji and Ke Guang make predictions for exact days, and that their predictions differ (cure by the day *jiayin* according to Xu Ji; respite on the *geng* or *xin* day according to Ke Guang). There is undoubtedly symbolic significance in their use of the sexagenary cycle that is no longer clear to us. However, there is no evidence that they are applying hemerological systems such as those in the Jiudian and Shuihudi hemerological manuscripts. The hemerological manuscripts key the occurrence of ailments to the sexagenary cycle and calendar: any ailment occurring on a set day in the cycle, whatever the observable symptoms, follows a set course. Demonic causation remains an element of etiology in the hemerological manuscripts. However, propitiation and exorcism are not employed; the resolution of the ailment lies within the framework of the sexagenary cycle itself.

We should not conclude that old-style divination, propitiation, and exorcism were becoming obsolete in elite medical treatment by the end of the fourth century BC. A *Lüshi chunqiu* 呂氏春秋 essay that treats of medical theories decries the 'current age' (mid-third century BC) that 'elevates turtle and milfoil divination, prayers, and sacrificial offerings' to deal with illness, ensuring that 'illness and ailment come in ever greater numbers'.[29] Yet it is clear that new hemerological ideas and correlative cosmology transformed iatromancy.

[26] See Li (1990), 84–5, and Li (1993), 269–70.

[27] See Kalinowski (1986), 216–19. See below, pp. 112–13, for evidence that *sui* in the Shuihudi hemerological manuscripts is associated with calendrical computations other than the Jupiter cycle.

[28] See Keightley (1978), 212–16. [29] *Lüshi chunqiu*, *juan* 3, 27.

Based on the evidence of the Jiudian hemerological manuscript, the new iatromancy of the late fourth century BC did not yet correlate the ten stems and twelve branches of the sexagenary cycle with *yinyang* or Five Agent theories. The iatromantic material in the manuscript occurs in a section that details lucky and unlucky aspects of each of the twelve branches. A slightly expanded version of this section occurs in the second of the two Shuihudi hemerological manuscripts, which also does not make use of *yinyang* or Five Agent theories. However, both of the Shuihudi manuscripts describe a different iatromantic system that is keyed to the ten stems and is based on Five Agent correlations. Marc Kalinowski's observation that during the third century BC *yinyang* and Five Agent theories gradually incorporated earlier hemerological systems based on the sexagenary cycle fits well with the evidence of iatromancy in the Shuihudi manuscripts.[30] The sections in both manuscripts on stem and Five Agent iatromancy constitute our earliest evidence of correlative-cosmology iatromancy; the section in the second manuscript on branch iatromancy reflects an earlier stage of hemerological iatromancy, as is borne out by the related section in the Jiudian hemerological manuscript.

Branch iatromancy in the Jiudian and Shuihudi manuscripts entails a precise account of the course of an illness. The beginning of an illness is associated with a particular branch and day, and the subsequent stages are also specified by the branch and day on which they occur. However, the branch specifications in the Jiudian and Shuihudi manuscripts are not identical; either the hemerological system changed over time or perhaps there was more than one tradition of branch iatromancy. The Jiudian manuscript is not well preserved. I propose to translate the three passages on branch iatromancy that are complete, for *chen* 辰, *wei* 未, and *hai* 亥; and to translate the corresponding passages in the second Shuihudi manuscript:[31]

Jiudian

When illness occurs [on *chen*], on *you* there is slight curing, on *xu* there is great curing; death and life is situated at *zi*.

吕（以）又（有）疾栖（酉）少翏（瘳）戌大翏（瘳）死生才（在）子。

Shuihudi

When illness occurs [on *chen*], on *you* there is slight curing, on *xu* there is great curing; death and life is situated at *zi*. Dried meat has come from the east quarter; the bearer is azure-coloured. Shaman is the calamity.

以有疾酉少翏（瘳）戌大翏（瘳）死生在子。乾肉從東方來。把者精（青）色。巫為姓（眚）。

---

[30] Kalinowski (1986), 220−4.

[31] See Hubei sheng wenwu kaogu yanjiusuo (1995), 509, slips 64, 67, 71; and Shuihudi Qin mu zhujian zhengli xiaozu (1990), 245−6, slips 165−6, 171−2, 179−80. Only the parts related to iatromancy are translated.

Jiudian

When illness occurs [on *wei*], on *zi* there is slight curing, on *mao* there is great curing; death and life is situated at *yin*.

吕 （以） 又 （有） 疾子少翏 （瘳） 卯大翏 （瘳） 死生才 （在） 寅。

Shuihudi

When illness occurs [on *wei*], on *zi* there is slight curing, on *mao* there is great curing; death and life is situated at *yin*. Red meat has come from the south quarter; the bearer is red-coloured. Mother's brothers and those who have died outside are the calamity.

以有疾子少翏 （瘳） 卯大翏 （瘳） 死生在寅。赤肉從南方來。把者赤色。 母枼 （世） 外死為姓 （眚）。

Jiudian

When illness occurs [on *hai*], on *mao* there is slight curing, on *si* there is great curing; death and life is situated at *shen*.

吕 （以） 又 （有） 疾卯少翏 （瘳） 巳大翏 （瘳） 死生才 （在） 申。

Shuihudi

When illness occurs [on *hai*], on *si* there is slight curing, on *you* there is great curing; death and life is situated at *zi*. Black meat has come from the east quarter. Mother's brothers and shaman[32] are the calamity.

以有疾巳少翏 （瘳） 酉大翏 （瘳） 死生在子。黑肉從東方來。母枼 （世） 見之為姓 （眚）。

The branch specifications for the illness stages match for *chen* and *wei* in the Jiudian and Shuihudi manuscripts; those for *hai* are all different.[33] The Shuihudi passages add three kinds of information regarding the source of the illness: meat, classified by colour and direction, which the sick person presumably consumed; the bearer (*bazhe* 把者), whose precise significance is not clear; and various humans, probably deceased, responsible for causing the calamity (shaman may also designate a category of ghost). Similar information is given for stem iatromancy in the Shuihudi manuscripts; its significance is discussed following translation of stem iatromancy passages below.

---

[32] Reading 見 as *xi* 覡 (male shaman).

[33] Further differences are evident in fragments of the Jiudian manuscript. For example, under the branch *wu* 午, 'slight curing' occurs on a *xu* 戌 day; the Shuihudi manuscript identifies the 'slight curing' day as *chou* 丑. Slips 72–9 in the Jiudian manuscript are extremely fragmentary; they contain phrases that belong together with the passages on branch iatromancy, but it is not possible to determine the correct branch heading.

The stages slight curing (*shaochou* 少瘳), great curing (*dachou* 大瘳), and death and life (*sisheng* 死生) are noteworthy.[34] A late fourth-century-BC divination manuscript from Wangshan 望山 tomb 1, Hubei, which is similar to the Baoshan divination manuscript (unfortunately, the Wangshan manuscript is not as well preserved) includes a fragment with the phrase: 'On *ren* or *gui* there will be great curing' 壬癸大有瘳. A related fragment preserves three graphs 乙丙少, from which we perhaps can restore the phrase: 'On *yi* or *bing* [there will be] slight [curing]'. Another fragment reads: 'On *jiwei* there will be respite; on *xin* or *ren* there will be curing' 己未有閒辛壬戲.[35] Terms such as 'respite', 'slight curing', 'great curing', and 'death and life' were no doubt used by Warring States physicians with or without divinatory or hemerological intent. But the use of these terms in hemerological iatromancy is best seen as a continuation from the formulaic language of the older ailment divination documented in the Baoshan and Wangshan manuscripts.

With regard to the choice of branches assigned to the several stages of an illness, I am unable to determine a regular pattern. For example, 'slight curing' of *chen* and *wei* day illnesses occurs on *you* and *zi* days respectively (following the sequence of branches, five days later); 'slight curing' of a *hai* day illness occurs on a *mao* day in the Jiudian manuscript (four days later) and on a *si* day in the Shuihudi manuscript (six days later). More variations are in evidence with other branches, and differences continue in the stages of 'great curing' and 'death and life'. The similarity between the Jiudian and Shuihudi manuscripts indicates a systematic approach to determining the course of an illness that clearly distinguishes hemerological iatromancy from the ailment-divination of the Baoshan manuscript. However, the hemerological system, whatever its basis may be, bears no relation to *yinyang* or Five Agent correlations.[36]

---

[34] I am uncertain of the exact meaning of 'death and life'. Except for illness associated with the branches *wu* and *wei*, when 'death and life' occurs before the date of 'great curing' in the sequence of branches, the 'death and life' stage occurs after the date of 'great curing'. My guess is that the branch assigned to 'death and life' represents the day on which death can be expected to occur; and that most often this day comes after the period during which a cure can be expected.

[35] Hubei sheng wenwu kaogu yanjiusuo and Beijing daxue zhongwenxi (1995), 74. For the sake of simplicity I give only the modern forms of several graphs as provided by the editors of the transcription. The last statement translated is clearly related to the Baoshan divination account for the day *jiyou* translated above: 'There will be respite on a *geng* or *xin* [day].' And respite (*jian*) has hemerological significance in stem iatromancy in the Shuihudi manuscripts (see below).

[36] There is, for example, no relation between the system of branch iatromancy and the branch/agent correlations given in the second Shuihudi manuscript along with the conquest sequence of the Five Agents. See Shuihudi Qin mu zhujian zhengli xiaozu (1990), 239. There are several lacunae in the text, but it is evident that the branch/agent correlations represent the *sanhe* 三合 system in which wood, fire, metal, and water are associated with three branches each: wood, *mao*, *wei*, *hai*; fire, *yin*, *wu*, *xu*; metal, *chou*, *si*, *you*; water, *zi*, *chen*, *shen* (see Kalinowski (1986), 222–3).

Table 3.3. *Correlation of stems and agents*

wood	*jia* and *yi*	(wood conquers earth)
fire	*bing* and *ding*	(fire conquers metal)
earth	*wu* and *ji*	(earth conquers water)
metal	*geng* and *xin*	(metal conquers wood)
water	*ren* and *gui*	(water conquers fire)

Table 3.4. *Stem iatromancy in the Shuihudi hemerological manuscripts*

	Illness	Ailment	Respite	Recovery
Days	*jia, yi*	*wu, ji*	*geng*	*xin*
	wood	earth	metal	metal
	bing, ding	*geng, xin*	*ren*	*gui*
	fire	metal	water	water
	wu, ji	*ren, gui*	*jia*	*yi*
	earth	water	wood	wood
	geng, xin	*jia, yi*	*bing*	*ding*
	metal	wood	fire	fire
	ren, gui	*bing, ding*	*wu*	*ji*
	water	fire	earth	earth

Stem iatromancy in the Shuihudi manuscripts incorporates Five Agent correlations (see tables 3.3–3.4). The section in the first hemerological manuscript is the better preserved, hence I translate it in full and note additional information contained in the second hemerological manuscript:[37]

> When illness occurs on *jia* or *yi*, father and mother are the calamity. It is obtained from flesh,[38] and comes from the east quarter. Enclose in a lacquer vessel. On *wu* or *ji* the ailment manifests, on *geng* there is respite, and on *xin* recovery. If there is not a recovery, Fever occupies the east quarter. When Year is in the east quarter, azure colour [accompanies] death.[39]

> 甲乙有疾父母為祟。得之於肉。從東方來。裹以桼（漆）器。戊己病庚有
> 閒辛酢（作）。若不酢（作）煩居東。歲在東方青色死。

[37] Shuihudi Qin mu zhujian zhengli xiaozu (1990), 193, slips 68–77; and 246–7, slips 181–7, for the parallel passage in the second hemerological manuscript.

[38] The second manuscript specifies pork.

[39] The parallel in the second manuscript explicitly associates the colours with the complexion of the sick person. The second manuscript also states that death occurs on a day corresponding to the agent associated with the illness; that is, death will be on a *jia* or *yi* day (wood/azure) for illness that began on a *jia* or *yi* day.

When illness occurs on *bing* or *ding*, grandfather is the calamity. It is obtained from red flesh, rooster, and liquor. On *geng* or *xin* the ailment manifests, on *ren* there is respite, and on *gui* recovery. If there is not a recovery, Fever occupies the south quarter. When Year is in the south quarter, red colour [accompanies] death.

丙丁有疾王父為祟。得之赤肉雄雞酉（酒）。庚辛病壬有閒癸酢（作）。若不酢（作）煩居南方。歲在南方赤色死。

When illness occurs on *wu* or *ji*, Shaman Kanhang[40] and grandmother are the calamity. It is obtained from yellow coloured *suo* fish and *jin* liquor.[41] On *ren* or *gui* the ailment manifests, on *jia* there is respite, and on *yi* recovery. If there is not a recovery, Fever occupies the center of the realm. When Year is in the west quarter, yellow colour [accompanies] death.[42]

戊己有疾巫堪行王母為祟。得之於黃色索魚菫酉（酒）。壬癸病甲有閒乙酢（作）。若不酢（作）煩居邦中。歲在西方黃色死。

When illness occurs on *geng* or *xin*, outside demons and the prematurely dead are the calamity. It is obtained from dog flesh and fresh eggs of white colour. On *jia* or *yi* the ailment manifests, on *bing* there is respite, and on *ding* recovery. If there is not a recovery, Fever occupies the west quarter. When Year is in the west quarter, white colour [accompanies] death.

庚辛有疾外鬼傷（殤）死為祟。得之犬肉鮮卵白色。甲乙病丙有閒丁酢（作）。若不酢（作）煩居西方。歲在西方白色死。

When illness occurs on *ren* or *gui* and no person has been encountered, outside demons are the calamity. It is obtained from liquor, dried-meat strips, pounded and spiced dried-meat strips, and meat relish. On *bing* or *ding* the ailment manifests, on *wu* there is respite, and on *ji* recovery. If there is not a recovery, Fever occupies the north quarter. When Year is in the north quarter, black colour [accompanies] death.

壬癸有疾母（毋）逢人外鬼為祟。得之於酉（酒）脯脩節（鱉）肉。丙丁病戊有閒己酢（作）。若不酢（作）煩居北方。歲在北方黑色死。

Before describing the correlative system underlying stem iatromancy, a few general observations are in order. The basic premise in both stem and branch iatromancy is that

---

[40] The identity of Shaman Kanhang is not known; the second manuscript reads Shaman Kan 巫堪.

[41] The meaning of *suo* 索 is uncertain; *suoyu* 索魚 is probably a type of preserved fish. *Jinjiu* 菫酒 is liquor fermented with the herb *jin* (identity uncertain).

[42] The temporal cycles associated with Fever and Year are discussed below. While Fever occupies five positions including the centre at different times, Year occupies only the four cardinal directions. To accommodate the difference between the two cycles, the stem iatromancy described in the Shuihudi manuscripts places Year in the west for illness associated with *wu* and *ji* (the stems assigned to the center); and west is again the position of Year for illness associated with *geng* and *xin* (the stems assigned to the west).

illnesses arising on a particular day share a common etiology and follow a common progression. Having identified day one, a person can anticipate what to expect and in the majority of cases is assured of a cure within a specified period of time – knowing all the while that 'death and life' days or the positions of Fever and Year may prove fatal. The etiologies all identify spirit agents – the source of calamity – as well as foods that serve as the mode of transmission of the illness. Illness is conceived in religious terms as contamination due to angry or malevolent spirits. However, there is no need for prayers or sacrifices to propitiate particular spirits, nor for exorcism; the calamitous activity of the spirit world has been subsumed within the sexagenary cycle and, in the case of stem iatromancy, within correlative cosmology. At the same time, hemerological iatromancy appears to bypass medical treatment; illness follows a set course with or without medical intervention.

Stem iatromancy in the Shuihudi manuscripts is based on the correlation of the stems with the five agents and on the conquest sequence of the five agents. The stem correlations are (see table 3.3): *jia* and *yi*, wood (east, azure); *bing* and *ding*, fire (south, red); *wu* and *ji*, earth (center, yellow); *geng* and *xin*, metal (west, white); *ren* and *gui*, water (north, black).[43] A distinction is made between *ji* 疾 (illness), which is the point of origin of a morbid condition, and *bing* 病 (ailment). Taking *jia* and *yi* as examples, illness on a *jia*/wood or *yi*/wood day becomes an ailment on the following *wu* or *ji* day because *wu* and *ji* are earth, and wood conquers earth; that is, the morbid condition attached to the sign wood becomes a manifest ailment on the days when wood conquers earth. Respite (*jian* 閒) and recovery (*zuo* 作)[44] occur on *geng* and *xin* days because the metal of *geng* and *xin* conquers the wood of *jia* and *yi*. The pattern of initial conquest by an illness followed by its own demise on days when it is conquered remains constant throughout the section (see table 3.4).

In the event that recovery does not occur, the fault lies with Fever (*fan* 煩) and Year (*sui* 歲), whose positions constitute circumstances outside of the five agent correlations. *Fan* (Fever) represents an element of iatromantic pathology to be applied first when an illness is not resolved within the period of time alotted for recovery based on five agent correlations. While *fan* belongs to the early medical vocabulary, it is not attested in received literature in the precise meaning that it has in the Shuihudi manuscripts. Because of its association with Year (*sui*), whose position can be plotted in

---

[43] The stem–agent correlations are given in the second hemerological manuscript along with the conquest sequence of the five agents; see Shuihudi Qin mu zhujian zhengli xiaozu (1990), 239. See also Kalinowski (1986), 222.

[44] *Zuo*, originally written 酢, is not a term attested for recovering from illness in received literature. I concur with the reading of the graph and the meaning given in Shuihudi Qin mu zhujian zhengli xiaozu (1990), 246–7.

a calendrical cycle, I suspect that Fever (*fan*) also follows a cycle. If at the time of illness Fever alone occupies the quarter correlated with the agent of the illness the situation is grave but not necessarily fatal (for example, if Fever is in the east on days *jia* or *yi*, which are correlated with wood and east; or in the south on days *bing* or *ding*, which are correlated with fire and south). If both Fever and Year occupy that quarter, the sick person will die, the complexion having turned the appropriate colour.[45]

Sui (Year) is identified elsewhere in the first Shuihudi manuscript as an astrological entity that occupies the four cardinal directions across the twelve months in the following sequence (branch correlations are in parentheses): first (*yin*), fifth (*wu*), and ninth (*xu*) months, east; second (*mao*), sixth (*wei*), and tenth (*hai*) months, south; third (*chen*), seventh (*shen*), and eleventh (*zi*) months, west; fourth (*si*), eighth (*you*), and twelfth (*chou*) months, north.[46] Although *sui* is often associated with Jupiter, this cycle differs from the usual Jupiter-based cycles known in received literature.[47] It is worth noting that the same cycle occurs in one of the Mawangdui medical manuscripts, in a chart used to determine the proper direction for burial of the afterbirth, where it is identified as the great period (*dashi* 大時).[48]

In the Baoshan ailment-divination account of 316 BC, it is proposed in the follow-up divination statement that Year be exorcised; the ill-omened deity Year is not yet a recurring entity in a calendrical cycle. In the calendrical framework of the Shuihudi hemerological manuscripts, the unlucky months and directions associated with Year can be known. In stem iatromancy, the position of Fever is calculated first. If Fever was positioned in the east on the *jia* or *yi* day when an illness began, this accounts for the sick person's failure to recover (*jia* and *yi* are correlated with wood and east). In addition, if the illness occurred in the first, fifth, or ninth months, the sick person is out of luck, since Year is positioned in the east during these months and death is inevitable.

Before the discovery of the Jiudian and Shuihudi hemerological manuscripts, one might have been inclined to regard such iatromantic practices as derivative of the techniques of diagnosis and prognosis developed by physicians who had already wedded vessel theory pathology and correlative cosmology. The idea that a 'pure' correlative cosmology was adapted in corrupt form to 'superstition' is evident in Wang Chong's

---

[45] Because Year does not occupy the center, west is the fatal location of Year in connection with illness on *wu* and *ji* (earth, center).

[46] Shuihudi Qin mu zhujian zhengli xiaozu (1990), 190. See also Kalinowski (1986), 216–19.

[47] Kalinowski (1986), 216–19.

[48] The manuscript has been assigned the title 'Taichan shu' 胎產書 (Book of the Generation of the Fetus). For the chart, see Mawangdui Hanmu boshu zhengli xiaozu (1985), 134, and Li (1993), 373–4. A Jupiter-based Great Period cycle is known in received literature, but moves counter-clockwise rather than clockwise as in the Mawangdui manuscript; see Harper (1998), 374–5.

王充 critique in the *Lunheng* 論衡 (Weighing of Discourse) of the popular belief in spirits associated with the ten stems:[49]

> When a person is sick and is about to die, the *jiayi* spirits will arrive.[50] If the ail-
> ment occurred on a *jia* or *yi* day, then at death he will see the spirits of *geng* and
> *xin*. What is the principle? In the case of the *jia* and *yi* demons, it is *geng* and *xin*
> that pass judgment on *jia* and *yi*.[51] Thus when the sick person is about to die, the
> killer-demons who arrive are the spirits of *geng* and *xin*.[52] How is this to be
> demonstrated? When an ailment occurs on a *jia* or *yi* day, the time of death and
> life is on *geng* and *xin* days.

For Wang Chong, medical theory 'demonstrates' the 'principle' of Five Agent theory,
according to which the wood of *jia* and *yi* is conquered by the metal of *geng* and *xin*. He
regards the popular belief as a superstition derived from Five Agent theory; that is, the
claim that the spirits of the stems manifest themselves during illness is a false application of the medical concept of crisis days based on the conquest sequence of the agents.

   I will pursue a different line of speculation. Rather than make iatromancy an offshoot
of diagnosis and prognosis in vessel theory pathology, I would argue that the iatromantic ideas recorded in the Jiudian and Shuihudi hemerological manuscripts developed
first as part of the flowering of hemerology and correlative cosmology in the fourth
and third centuries BC. As vessel theory pathology set about correlating the somatic
microcosm with *yinyang* and Five Agent cycles, hemerological iatromancy provided
important correlative paradigms. To be sure, the physician-authors of the *Huangdi
neijing* were skeptical of magico-religious beliefs, and they formulated a new kind
of medicine based on vessel theory. But during the several centuries preceding the
compilation of the *Huangdi neijing* in the first century BC, physicians as a group
belonged to the broader world of technical specialists – including diviners – in which
iatromantic and other 'occult' ideas circulated alongside ideas such as occur in the
Huangdi neijing.

   The treatise on the 'Jingmai' 經脈 (Conduit Vessels) in *Lingshu*, *pian* 10, provides a
convenient illustration of my thesis. I have in mind the passage immediately following
the description of the paths of the twelve vessels and their associated ailments.

---

[49] *Lunheng, juan* 22, 450.
[50] Here Wang Chong uses *jia* and *yi* to refer generically to the ten stems, and he is describing a popular
belief that he subsequently criticizes.
[51] 'Pass judgment' translates *bao* 報, glossed in *Shuowen jiezi*, 10B.13b, as 'to pass judgment on the
guilty person' (*dang zuiren* 當罪人).
[52] Wang Chong's point is that the relation between the two pairs of stems is explained by the conquest
sequence of the Five Agents (the metal of *geng* and *xin* conquers the wood of *jia* and *yi*). According to
Wang Chong, the 'principle' of five agent theory has been misused in the popular belief in spirits associated with the stems.

Beginning with the hand great *yin* vessel, the text lists five *yin* vessels which are linked to five essential body constituents: hand great *yin* vessel, hair (*mao* 毛); hand minor *yin* vessel, blood (*xue* 血); foot great *yin* vessel, flesh (*rou* 肉); foot minor *yin* vessel, bone (*gu* 骨); foot ceasing *yin* vessel, muscle (*jin* 筋).[53]

The passage concerns prognosis. If the vapour of one of the five *yin* vessels is severed (*qijue* 氣絕), the corresponding constituent fails and endangers the body. The symptoms of this failure are described for each vessel, concluding with a prediction of death. Here, for example, is the account of the hand great *yin* vessel:[54]

> When the vapour of the hand great *yin* vessel is severed, the skin and hair shrivel. The great *yin* [vessel] is the one that carries vapour and warmth to the skin and hair. Thus if the vapour is not flourishing, the skin and hair shrivel. If the skin and hair shrivel, the moistening fluids leave the skin and joints. If the moistening fluids leave the skin and joints, the nails dry out and the hair breaks. If the hair breaks, hair has died first. On *bing* it becomes grave; on *ding* death occurs. It is a case of fire conquering metal.

Lingshu 10, does not include a list of body constituent correlations with the Five Agents, but the correlations as given in *Suwen* are: muscle, wood; blood, fire; flesh, earth; hair, metal; bone, water.[55] These correlations match all of the death predictions for the severing of vapour in the five *yin* vessels in *Lingshu* 10. In the above quotation, *bing* and *ding* are fire; hair as a body constituent is correlated with metal; and the days of gravity and death are *bing* and *ding* because fire conquers metal. Severing of vapour of the hand minor *yin* vessel leads to blood (fire) 'dying first'; the days of gravity and death are *ren* and *gui* (water); and water conquers fire. Severing of vapour of the foot great *yin* vessel leads to flesh (earth) 'dying first'; the days of gravity and death are *jia* and *yi* (wood); and wood conquers earth. Severing of vapour of the foot minor *yin* vessel leads to bone (water) 'dying first'; the days of gravity and death are *wu* and *ji* (earth); and earth conquers water. Severing of vapour of the foot ceasing *yin* vessel leads to muscle (wood) 'dying first'; the days of gravity and death are *geng* and *xin* (metal); and metal conquers wood.

The Mawangdui medical manuscripts provide the key to this passage in *Lingshu* 10. The text assigned the title 'Yinyangmai sihou' 陰陽脈死候 (Death Signs of the *yin* and *yang* Vessels) consists of two parts. The first concerns the *yin* and *yang* vessels, and refers to the *yin* vessels as the 'vessels of death'. The second concerns five body constituents, whose failure leads to death:[56]

---

[53] *Lingshu*, *juan* 3, *pian* 10, 7a–b. The hand ceasing *yin* vessel is not included in the list.
[54] *Lingshu*, *juan* 3, *pian* 10, 7a.   [55] *Suwen*, *juan* 2, *pian* 5, 4a–6b.
[56] Mawangdui Han mu boshu zhengli xiaozu (1985), 21. See also Harper (1998), 219–20.

When the lips turn outward and the groove beneath the nose is full, flesh has died first. When the gums become level and the teeth long, bone has died first. When the face is black and the eyes – fixed with fear – gaze obliquely, vapour has died first. When floss-like strands of sweat emerge that stick and do not flow, blood has died first. When the tongue binds and the testicles curl up, muscle has died first. When all five occur, he will not live.

In 'Yinyangmai sihou' the discussion of the *yin* and *yang* vessels is separate from that of the five body constituents; the text dates to a time before a set of five constituents were correlated with particular *yin* vessels. 'Yinyangmai sihou' shows us an early idea of physiology based on body constituents, before vessel theory made the vessels the essential physiological structure subsuming all other body constituents. In *Lingshu* 10, the five constituents are attached to *yin* vessels, and one of the constituents has been changed: vapour in 'Yinyangmai sihou' is replaced by hair in *Lingshu* 10 (evidently vapour is too important a medical concept to remain as one among five body constituents).[57]

'Yinyangmai sihou' provides an early precedent for regarding *yin* vessels as 'vessels of death'; it is *Lingshu* 10, that first integrates *yin* vessels with body constituents. In addition, *Lingshu* 10, incorporates Five Agent correlations, which are the basis for predicting the day of death. Notably, there is no evidence of Five Agent theory in connection with vessel theory in the Mawangdui medical manuscripts.[58] There are generic references to a patient 'dying within three days' and 'dying within ten days' because of *yin* vessel disturbances in the Mawangdui medical manuscripts, but no evidence of calendrically precise death dates based on correlative cosmology.[59]

I submit that the *Lingshu* 10 passage reflects the influence of hemerological iatromancy in the formation of vessel theory pathology. To be sure, the system of stem iatromancy described in the Shuihudi hemerological manuscripts is not directly related to the death prognosis of *Lingshu* 10. The Shuihudi iatromantic system is based on the probability of recovery from illness on a day when the agent of that day conquers the agent of the day on which the illness began; the day of death predicted in *Lingshu* 10, is the day whose agent conquers the agent of the vessel/constituent. However, both the Shuihudi iatromantic system and the *Lingshu* 10, passage share a concern for precise identification of significant days during the course of an illness within the framework of the sexagenary cycle and Five Agent theory.

[57] See Yamada (1979), 77.

[58] The Five Agents are referred to only once, in a description of gestation in 'Taichan shu'; Mawangdui Han mu boshu zhengli xiaozu (1985), 136, and Harper (1998), 379–81.

[59] See the description of the foot ceasing *yin* vessel in the text assigned the title 'Zubi shiyimai jiujing' 足臂十一脈灸經 (Cauterization Canon of the Eleven Vessels of the Foot and Forearm); Mawangdui Han mu boshu zhengli xiaozu (1985), 5, and Harper (1998), 199–200. See also the part of 'Yinyangmai sihou' concerning the *yin* vessels.

The conclusion to the *Lingshu* 10 passage describes a total failure of *yin* and *yang* vessels using the term *zhan* 占 (predict) for the fatal prognosis. In the light of the new iatromantic evidence in the Jiudian and Shuihudi hemerological manuscripts, the use of the vocabulary of divination in a medical context suggests another point of contact between the medicine of the physicians and iatromancy:[60]

> If the vapour of the six *yang* [vessels] is severed, the *yin* [vessels] and *yang* [vessels] separate from one another. Having separated, the skin's webbed pattern [*couli* 腠理] comes apart and a terminal sweat pours out. Thus, at dawn one predicts [*zhan*] death at night; at night one predicts death at dawn.

The cross-fertilization between iatromancy and vessel theory pathology can be attributed, in part, to the nature of vessel theory itself. I have already noted that Chunyu Yi's 'model of the vessels', which serves as the basis for diagnosing all ailments, is a medical counterpart to the *Yijing* and its hexagrams.[61] For Chunyu Yi, vessel theory pathology implicitly linked medicine to the same larger reality crystallized in the cosmo-divinatory system of the hexagrams; it is hardly surprising that the new diagnostic tool – with which, as Chunyu Yi said, the ancient sages 'differentiated the hundred ailments' – would occupy a middle ground between natural philosophy and occult knowledge. This conception of vessel theory is already suggested in the Mawangdui medical text assigned the title 'Maifa' 脈法 (Model of the Vessels), which refers to diagnosing the vessels as *xiangmai* 相脈. *Xiang* is the term for 'occult inspection' of things; in the case of humans, 'physiognomy'.[62]

Looking to Chunyu Yi's medical case histories for evidence of a physician's perspective on diagnosis and prognosis, Chunyu Yi evinces great pride in his skill at knowing the exact condition of a patient upon examining the patient's vessels, including incurable illnesses whose course and final outcome he determines from the initial diagnosis.[63] There is little evidence of iatromantic influence in the case histories as a whole. In one case history, however, Chunyu Yi declares that the patient will die on the day *dinghai* 丁亥. Let me translate the relevant part of the case history, and then examine it for possible iatromantic influence:[64]

---

[60] *Lingshu, juan* 3, *pian* 10, 7b.   [61] See pp. 99–100 above.

[62] The words *xiangmai* are missing on the Mawangdui manuscript, but can be restored based on the second edition of 'Maifa' in the Zhangjiashan 張家山 tomb 247 manuscript *Maishu* 脈書 (Vessel Book); see Jiangling Zhangjiashan Han jian zhengli xiaozu (1989), 74, and Harper (1998), 216.

[63] See Elisabeth Hsu (this volume), p. 79.

[64] *Shiji, juan* 105, 19a. I do not propose to offer a full analysis of the medical terminology used by Chunyu Yi in the passage, the precise meaning of which is not always certain. I would like to thank Elisabeth Hsu for providing me with her own translation of this case history. However, she is not to be held responsible for my translation.

> The Inner Attendant of Qi 齊, Po Shi 破石, was ailing. Your Servant Yi examined the vessels, and declared: 'The lung is injured. Untreatable. Ten days hence on *dinghai* he must die excreting blood.' He in fact died eleven days later excreting blood. Po Shi's ailment was contracted by falling off a horse and landing supine on a rock.[65] As for how I knew Po Shi's ailment, when I pressed the vessels I obtained lung *yin* vapour. Its arrival was dispersed, coming by several paths and not single. Further, the colour overrode it. As for how I knew he had fallen off a horse, when I pressed the vessels I obtained a reverse-*yin* vessel. The reverse-*yin* vessel entered an emptiness and overrode the lung vessel. The lung vessel being dispersed made it certain that the colour would alter.

The case history continues with an explanation of why Po Shi died eleven days later rather than ten, and why he died excreting blood.

Chunyu Yi does not elaborate on why death should be on *dinghai*. Although he does not cite five agent theory, Chunyu Yi's prognosis probably follows the logic of correlative cosmology. *Ding* is a fire day. The correlation of the lung with metal is well attested in the *Huangdi neijing* and other Han sources, along with kidney/water, spleen/earth, heart/fire, and liver/wood. We can be reasonably confident that these correlations were all accepted by Chunyu Yi.[66] Fire conquers metal, hence the injured lung (metal) results in death on a fire day. The logic is the same as in *Lingshu* where fatal damage to the hand great *yin* vessel is manifested in hair/metal, and death occurs on a *ding*/fire day. In addition, I suspect that Po Shi's accident and Chunyu Yi's prognosis occurred on *dingchou* 丁丑, the first day of the *ding* decade preceding the decade of *dinghai*; that is, the processes of fire conquering lung/metal existed from the moment the accident occurred on a fire day.[67] Commentaries also suggest that 'colour overriding' the lung vessel refers to the red of fire overriding the lung's metal.

Rather than confute the prognosis, death on the eleventh day allows Chunyu Yi to introduce a specifically medical rationale for the delay (it concerns the patient's diet, which bolstered the lung). For Chunyu Yi and other physicians, their technical medical knowledge and clinical experience were presumably what distinguished their medical practice from iatromantic systems of the type recorded in the Jiudian and Shuihudi hemerological manuscripts. Yet the main features of Chunyu Yi's prognosis parallel hemerological iatromancy. I suspect that if pressed, Chunyu Yi might have conceded

---

[65] Is it an ironic twist of fate for a man named Po Shi (crushed by rock) to die from landing on a rock?

[66] See the table in Kanō (1987), 178 (only kidney/water and spleen/earth are attested in Chunyu Yi's case histories, but from these two correlations the remaining three ought to be as indicated in the *Huangdi neijing*).

[67] Alternatively, Chunyu Yi's diagnosis took place on the day after *dingchou*, *wuyin* 戊寅. The difference depends on whether the first day of 'ten days later' is counted from the day of the diagnosis (giving *wuyin* as the day of the diagnosis) or from the next day (giving *dingchou*).

(like Confucius) that he 'shared a path' with iatromancers, but would have vehemently insisted that his 'final destination was different'.

In this chapter I have purposely omitted discussion of a physician's natural role as the seer of human mortality, and the sociological and psychological elements of medical diagnosis and prognosis. Nor have I touched on the clinical perspectives that shape a physician's ideas about diagnosis and prognosis. My intention has been to elucidate in formal, textual terms developments of the fourth to second centuries BC that transformed early Chinese medicine: the rise of hemerology and correlative cosmology, for which we now have the testimony of the Jiudian and Shuihudi hemerological manuscripts; and their influence on the formation of vessel theory pathology, particularly the influence of iatromancy on diagnosis and prognosis.

References to premodern Chinese and Japanese works

Lingshu 靈樞 (Divine Pivot). Han, *ca* 1st century BC. Anon. *SBBY*.

Lunheng 論衡 (Weighing of Discourse). Han. Wang Chong 王充 (AD 27–*ca* 100). References to *Lunheng jijie*, edited by Liu Pansui 劉盼遂. Guji chubanshe, Beijing, 1957.

Lüshi chunqiu 呂氏春秋 (Spring and Autumn of Mr. Lü). Warring States. Lü Buwei 呂不韋 (d. 235 BC) and others. References to *Zhuzi jicheng*. Zhonghua shuju, Beijing, 1954.

Shiji 史記 (Records of the Scribe). Han. Sima Qian 司馬遷 (*ca* 145–*ca* 86 BC). Reproduction of 1739 Palace edition. Xinwenfeng chuban gongsi, Taibei.

Shuowen jiezi 說文解字 (Explanation of Primary Signs and Analysis of Graphs). Han. Xu Shen 許慎 (d. AD 146). References are to *Shuowen jiezi zhu* 說文解字注, commentated by Duan Yucai 段玉裁. Facsimile of 1872 woodblock edition. Shanghai guji chubanshe, Shanghai, 1981.

Suwen 素問 (Plain Questions). Han, *ca* 1st century BC. Anon. *SBBY*.

Yijing 易經 (Classic of Changes). Zhou-Han, 7th–1st century BC. Anon. References to *Zhouyi zhushu* 周易注疏 in the *Shisanjing zhushu* 十三經注疏, *SBBY*.

References to modern works

Chen Songchang 陳松長 and Liao Mingchun 廖名春. 1993. 'Boshu "Ersanzi wen," "Yi zhi yi," "Yao" shiwen' 帛書二三子問易之義要釋文 (Transcription of the Silk-texts 'Several Disciples Ask,' 'Properties of the Changes,' and 'Essentials'). *Daojia wenhua yanjiu* 道家文化研究 3, 424–35.

Harper, Donald 1985. 'A Chinese Demonography of the Third Century BC'. *Harvard Journal of Asiatic Studies* 47, 459–98.

 1990. 'The Conception of Illness in Early Chinese Medicine, as Documented in Newly Discovered 3rd and 2nd Century BC Manuscripts'. *Sudhoffs Archiv* 74, 210–35.

 1998. *Early Chinese Medical Literature: the Mawangdui Medical Manuscripts*. Kegan Paul, London.

He Shuangquan 何雙全 1989. 'Tianshui Fangmatan Qin jian zongshu' 天水放馬灘秦簡徐述 (Summary of the Qin Slips from Fangmatan, Tianshui). *Wenwu* 文物 2, 23–31.

Hubei sheng Jing Sha tielu kaogudui 湖北省荊沙鐵路考古隊 1991. *Baoshan Chu jian* 包山楚簡 (Chu Slips from Baoshan). Wenwu chubanshe, Beijing.

Hubei sheng wenwu kaogu yanjiusuo 湖北省文物考古研究所 1995. *Jiangling Jiudian Dong Zhou mu* 江陵九店東周墓 (Eastern Zhou Tombs at Jiudian, Jiangling). Kexue chubanshe, Beijing.

Hubei sheng wenwu kaogu yanjiusuo and Beijing daxue Zhongwenxi 北京大學中文系 1995. *Wangshan Chu jian* 望山楚斷 (Chu Slips fromWangshan). Zhonghua shuju, Beijing.

Hudson, Robert P. 1993. 'Concepts of Disease in the West'. In Kiple, 45–52.

Jiangling Zhangjiashan Han jian zhengli xiaozu 江陵張家山漢簡整理小組 1989. 'Jiangling Zhangjiashan Han jian "Maishu" shiwen' 江陵張家山漢簡《脈書》釋文 (Transcription of the Han Bamboo-Slip 'Vessel Book' from Zhangjiashan, Hubei). *Wenwu* 文物 7, 72–74.

Kalinowski, Marc 1986. 'Les traités de Shuihudi et l'hémérologie Chinoise a la fin des Royaumes-Combattants'. *T'oung Pao* 72, 175–228.

    1991. *Cosmologie et divination dans la Chine ancienne*. Ecole Française d'Extrême-Orient, Paris.

Kanō Yoshimitsu 加納喜光. 1987. *Chūgoku igaku no tanjō* 中國醫學誕生 (Birth of Chinese Medicine). Tōkyō Daigaku Shuppankai, Tokyo.

Keightley, David N. 1978. 'The Religious Commitment: Shang Theology and the Genesis of Chinese Political Culture'. *History of Religions* 17, 211–25.

Kiple, Kenneth F. (ed.) 1993. *Cambridge World History of Human Disease*. Cambridge University Press, Cambridge.

Li Ling 李零 1990. 'Formulaic Structure of Chu Divinatory Bamboo Slips'. *Early China* 15, 71–86.

    1993. *Zhongguo fangshu kao* 中國方術考 (Study of Chinese Technical Arts). Renmin Zhongguo chubanshe, Beijing.

Mawangdui Han mu boshu zhengli xiaozu 馬王堆漢墓帛書整理小組 1985. *Mawangdui Han mu boshu* 馬王堆漢墓帛書 (Silk Manuscripts from the Han Tomb at Mawangdui), vol. IV. Wenwu chubanshe, Beijing.

Shuihudi Qin mu zhujian zhengli xiaozu 睡虎地秦墓竹簡整理小組 1990. *Shuihudi Qin mu zhujian* 睡虎地秦墓竹簡 (Slips from the Qin Tomb at Shuihudi). Wenwu chubanshe, Beijing.

Unschuld, Paul U. 1985. *Medicine in China: a History of Ideas*. University of California Press, Berkeley.

    1993. 'History of Chinese Medicine'. In Kiple, 20–27.

Yamada Keiji 山田慶兒 1979. 'The Formation of the *Huang-ti Nei-ching*'. *Acta Asiatica* 36, 67–89.

    1980. 'Kyū-ku hachi-fu setsu to Shōshiha no tachiba' 九宮八風説ヒ少師 の立場 (The Theory of the Nine Palaces and Eight Winds and the Position of the Followers of Shaoshi). *Tōhōgakuhō* 東方學報 52, 199–242.

4

The system of the five circulatory phases and the six seasonal influences (*wuyun liuqi*), a source of innovation in medicine under the Song (960–1279)

CATHERINE DESPEUX

TRANSLATED BY JANET LLOYD

The Song period is rich in innovations in many domains, including that of medicine, in which one of the most striking is without doubt that of the system of the five circulatory phases and the six influences (*wuyun liuqi* 五運六氣). Under the Song, this system gradually pervaded every field of medicine: prognosis, diagnosis, prevention, pharmacotherapy, and acupuncture. In this period, the Imperial palace recognized the system to be an essential part of scholarly Chinese medicine, and it was included in the examination programme. The series of reforms undertaken from 1071 onward by Wang Anshi 王安石 (1021–86) led to the foundation, in 1076, of an Imperial Bureau of Medicine (*Taiyi ju* 太醫局), to which a school of medicine and a school of pharmacotherapy were attached.[1] This bureau was divided into three sections, consisting in all of nine departments. Each year it received three hundred students, who were divided between three levels of study. It tested the theoretical and clinical knowledge of these students in examinations organised both monthly and annually on the syllabus under the Tang, such

---

[1] On this Bureau, see the *Songshi* 宋史, *juan* 164, 3885. According to the *Yuhai* 玉海, *juan* 63, 25, it was in the fifth month of the ninth year of 1076 that a certain Xu Xiongben 徐熊本 (eleventh century) was appointed Inspector of the Imperial Bureau of Medicine. Then, in the first month of 1136, four Bureaux of Remedies were set up and, in 1151, copies of the Bureau's book of medicinal prescriptions were distributed to the various administrative authorities involved. Each prefecture and each district had schools of medicine, and the practice of the medical art was forbidden to all those who had not passed the examinations or were not registered.

as sphygmology, therapeutic methods, and acupuncture, but also the system of the five circulatory phases and the six influences.[2]

The system of the five circulatory phases and the six influences (*wuyun liuqi*)

The system of the five circulatory phases and the six influences is a cosmological system based upon astro-calendary elements of the sexagesimal cycle; upon a calculation of the development of *yin* and *yang* according to the six modalities taken into consideration by Chinese medicine, namely *taiyin* 太陰 (greater *yin*), *shaoyin* 少陰 (lesser *yin*), *jueyin* 厥陰 (attenuated *yin*), *taiyang* 太陽 (greater *yang*), *yangming* 陽明 (*yang* brightness), and *shaoyang* 少陽 (lesser *yang*); and upon a calculation of the evolution of the Five Phases (wood, fire, earth, metal, water), and the six influences (wind, fire, summer heat, dampness, dryness, and coldness).

In the sexagesimal calendrical system, each year was characterized by a binome formed by combining ten celestial stems and twelve terrestrial branches. The ten celestial stems are divided into five *yang* (*jia* 甲, *yi* 乙, *bing* 丙, *ding* 丁, *wu* 戊) and five *yin* (*ji* 己, *geng* 庚, *xin* 辛, *ren* 壬, *gui* 癸). In similar fashion, the twelve terrestrial branches are divided into six *yang* (*zi* 子, *chou* 丑, *yin* 寅, *mao* 卯, *chen* 辰, *si* 巳) and six *yin* (*wu* 午, *wei* 未, *shen* 申, *you* 酉, *xu* 戌, *hai* 亥). These binomes serve to designate years, but also months, days, and the twelve two-hour periods in a day.

The five circulatory phases (*wuyun* 五運), namely those of the influences of earth (*tu* 土), metal (*jin* 金), water (*shui* 水), wood (*mu* 木), and fire (*huo* 火) are associated with the ten celestial stems in accordance with a correlation that is different from that concerning the Five Phases (see tables 4.1 and 4.2).[3] They follow the cycle of the production relation among the Five Phases, but begin with earth instead of with wood. This association of a *yang* celestial stem with a *yin* celestial stem (eg. *jia* and *ji*) corresponds

---

[2] The monograph on examinations of the *Songshi*, *juan* 157, 3689 runs as follows: 'In the department of sphygmology, the examinations related on the one hand to the three great classics of the *Suwen* 素問, the *Nanjing* 難經 and the *Maijing* 脈經, and on the other to less important classics such as the *Chaoshi bingyuan* 巢氏病源, the *Longshu lun* 龍樹論, and the *Qianjin yifang* 千金翼方. For the departments of acupuncture and ulcers, the *Maijing* was replaced by the *Sanbu zhenjing* 三部針經. In the examinations, the first session consisted of five questions on the general sense of the three classics, and the second session consisted of two questions on sphygmology and the general sense of the system of the five circulatory phases and the six influences. For the two departments of acupuncture and ulcers, the examinations consisted of three questions on the classics of lesser importance and two questions on the meaning of the five circulatory phases and the six influences. The third session consisted of three examples of ailments for which the candidate had to prescribe a treatment.'

[3] Cf. Donald Harper (this volume), table 3.3.

Table 4.1. *Correspondence between the Five Phases and the ten celestial stems*

Five Phases	Ten Celestial Stems	
Wood	*jia* 甲	*yi* 乙
Fire	*bing* 丙	*ding* 丁
Earth	*wu* 戊	*ji* 己
Metal	*geng* 庚	*xin* 辛
Water	*ren* 壬	*gui* 癸

Table 4.2. *Correspondence between the five circulatory phases and the ten celestial stems*

Five Circulatory Phases	Ten Celestial Stems	
Earth	*jia* 甲	*ji* 己
Metal	*yi* 乙	*geng* 庚
Water	*bing* 丙	*xin* 辛
Wood	*ding* 丁	*ren* 壬
Fire	*wu* 戊	*gui* 癸

to the association that results from the distribution of numbers in the *Taixuan jing* 太玄經 (Canon of Supreme Mystery)[4] by Yang Xiong 楊雄 (53 BC–AD 18) of the Han dynasty, which is attested in the almanacs (*rishu* 日書) of the third century BC, discovered in Gansu in 1986.[5]

Whereas the Five Phases (*wuxing*) are related to the five cardinal points (east, south, centre, west, north) (see figure 4.1), the five circulatory phases (*wuyun*) correspond to the five sectors of the sky traversed by the influences of the Five Phases. These five sectors of the sky bear specific names: the cinnabar heaven (*dantian* 丹天), the yellow heaven (*jintian* 黔天), the blue heaven (*cangtian* 蒼天), the pure heaven (*qingtian* 清天), and the dark heaven (*xuantian* 玄天). The beginning and the end of these five sectors are calculated on the basis of the twenty-eight constellations situated in the vicinity of the celestial equator. For example, the influence of fire traverses the cinnabar heaven from the *niu* 牛 (the Ox) and the *nü* 女 (the Girl) constellations, and ends up at the the *bi* 壁 (the Wall) and the *kui* 奎 (the Legs) (see figure 4.2).

The circulatory phases are active, effective, or dominant within certain temporal divisions. First there is a central circulatory phase (*zhongyun* 中運), which is the circulatory phase that is dominant in the course of one year. It is calculated on the basis

---

[4] On the *Taixuan jing* and cosmology, see Nylan and Sivin (1987).
[5] He Shuangquan (1989), 27; see also Kalinowski (1991), 80 and note 262.

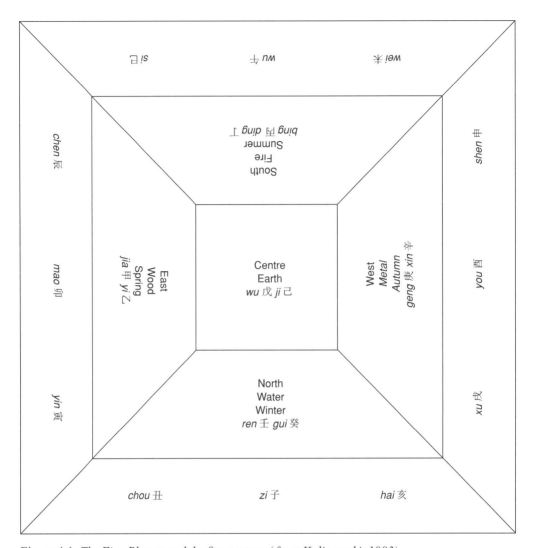

Figure 4.1. *The Five Phases and the five sectors (from Kalinowski, 1983)*

of the celestial stem of that year; if this is *yang*, the circulatory phase of the year is excessive (*taiguo* 太過), if it is *yin*, it is insufficient (*buji* 不及). Next come the domin-ant circulatory phases (*zhuyun* 主運), which reign each year in five consecutive periods, each of seventy-three days. These do not vary from one year to another, and follow each other according to the production cycle of the Five Phases, the first of which is always

圖之天經氣六運五

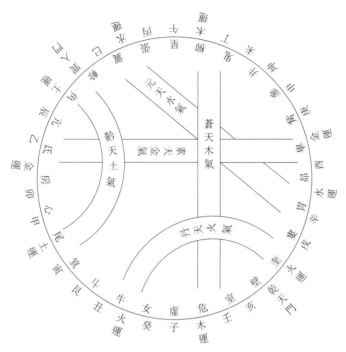

Figure 4.2. *The five circulatory phases in the heavens (from* Jiutian xuannü qingnang haijiao jing 九天玄女青囊海角經 *(Blue Sack Sea Horn Canon of the Mysterious Girl of the Nine Heavens) from the Song, in the* Gujin tushu jicheng 古今圖書集成, Yishu dian 藝術典, juan 651, Kanyu bu 堪輿部 *(geomancy section), 1, 1–10b)*

Inner circle: the five sectors of the sky and the five circulatory phases that traverse them. The cinnabar heaven *dantian* is traversed by the circulatory phase of fire, the yellow heaven *jintian* is traversed by earth, the blue heaven *cangtian* is traversed by wood, the pure heaven *qingtian* is traversed by metal (here rendered as *sutian* 素天), and the dark heaven *xuantian* is traversed by water (here rendered as *yuantian* 元天).

First ring: the distribution of the twenty-eight constellations in four sectors.

Second ring: the twelve celestial branches and the ten celestial stems. At the north-west, north-east, south-east, and south-west corners, the names of the trigrams *qian* 乾, *gen* 根, *xun* 巽, and *kun* 坤 are given in a sequence that is characteristic of the posterior heaven cycle (*houtian* 後天).

Third ring: the four cardinal points, the celestial gate in the north-west, and the human gate in the south-east.

wood. Finally there are the alien circulatory phases (*keyun* 客運), which reign during the same five periods of seventy-three days. The first of these is the same as the central circulatory phase of the year, and the others follow on in the order of the production cycle of the Five Phases.

Table 4.3. *Correspondence between the five circulatory phases and the five notes*

Earth	Metal	Water	Wood	Fire
gong 宮	*shang* 商	*yu* 羽	*jue* 角	*zhi* 徵

Table 4.4. *Correspondences of the six influences*

Seasonal Influence	Circulatory Phase	Modalities of *yin* and *yang*	Binomes		Binomes of the Canonical System[i]	
Wind	Wood	*jueyin*	*si* 巳	*hai* 亥	*yin* 寅	*mao* 卯
Fire	Sovereign Fire	*shaoyin*	*zi* 子	*wu* 午	*wu* 午	*si* 巳
Summer heat	Minister Fire	*shaoyang*	*yin* 寅	*shen* 申	*wu* 午	*si* 巳
Dampness	Earth	*taiyin*	*chou* 丑	*wei* 未	*chou* 丑	*wei* 未
					chen 辰	*xu* 戌
Dryness	Metal	*yangming*	*mao* 卯	*you* 酉	*shen* 申	*you* 酉
Cold	Water	*taiyang*	*chen* 辰	*xu* 戌	*zi* 子	*hai* 亥

[i] 'Canonical system' refers to the medical doctrine in the *Huangdi neijing* and the *Zhenjiu jiayi jing*.

The five circulatory phases are associated with five musical notes (see table 4.3). These sound emblems are major (*taigong* 太宮) or minor (*shaogong* 少宮) depending on whether the circulatory phase is excessive or insufficient, that is to say depending on whether the year is *yang* or *yin*.

The six influences (*liuqi* 六氣) are wind (*feng* 風), fire (*huo* 火), summer heat (*shu* 暑), dampness (*shi* 濕), dryness (*zao* 燥), and the cold (*han* 寒). Each corresponds to two of the twelve terrestrial branches and, so as to get the Five Phases to correspond to each of the six influences, fire is divided into sovereign fire (*junhuo* 君火) and minister fire (*xianghuo* 相火). Finally, these six influences are associated with six modalities of *yin* and *yang* (see table 4.4) and with twelve pitch pipes (*lülü* 呂律). This association between sounds and influences constitutes the system called *nayin* 納音, according to which the years are characterized by a correlation established between the sexagesimal binomes, the five sounds, and the twelve pitch pipes.[6] This system goes back at least as far as the Jin period, since it is mentioned in the *Baopu zi* 抱朴子 (Book of the Master Holding to Simplicity) by Ge Hong 葛洪 (283–341)[7] and also, a little later, in the *Wuxing dayi* 五行大義 (General Significances of the Five Phases) by Xiao Ji 簫吉

---

[6] On the *nayin* system, see the *Mengqi bitan* 夢溪筆談, *juan* 5, 247, and the *Suwen rushi yunqi lun'ao* 素問入式運氣論奧, *juan* 1, 8b – 10a.

[7] *Baopu zi, juan* 11, 190.

(*ca* 530/40−613),[8] which seems to have been partially lost in the days of Shen Gua 沈括 (1031−95).[9]

The six modalities, each of which governs a space, are divided into terrestrial influences or dominant influences (*zhuqi* 主氣) and celestial influences or alien influences (*keqi* 客氣). The six dominant influences, *jueyin, shaoyin, shaoyang, taiyin, yangming, taiyang* succeed one another in the order of the production cycle of the Five Phases in the course of one year, in six steps (*bu* 步) or portions of the year, each of which comprises four of the twenty-four solar periods: these are regular influences that never vary from one year to another. The six alien influences, also divided into six steps, follow one another in the following order: *taiyang, jueyin, shaoyin, taiyin, shaoyang, yangming*. Each of these six modalities corresponds to three kinds of influences: a principal influence (*benqi* 本氣), a secondary influence (*biaoqi* 標氣), and a central influence (*zhongqi* 中氣). For example, for the *taiyang*, the principal influence is cold, the secondary influence is *yang*, and the central influence is *shaoyin*.[10] The six influences are also characterized in the following fashion: they consist of the southern influence or heaven-governing influence (*sitianqi* 氣司天), the northern influence or source influence (*zaiquanqi* 氣在泉), two intermediate influences on the left (*zuo jianqi* 左間氣), and two intermediate influences on the right (*you jianqi* 右間氣). The heaven-governing influence is the superior influence (*shangqi* 上氣), which is calculated according to the branch of the year; it corresponds to the third of the six steps and also to the first half of the year. The source influence is the inferior influence (*xiaqi* 下氣), which is opposed to it and corresponds to the sixth step and also to the second half of the year.

The combination of the circulatory phases and the seasonal influences in the course of a year or a period in the year may be harmonious or unbalanced. When the central circulatory phase is in harmony with the heaven-governing influence, this is called celestial agreement (*tianfu* 天符); when the central circulatory phase is the same as the influence of the yearly branch, this is called year-coincidence (*suihui* 歲會); when the central excessive circulatory phase is in harmony with the source influence, this is called resemblance to the celestial agreement (*tong tianfu* 同天符); finally, when an insufficient central circulatory phase is in harmony with the source influence, this is called resemblance to the year coincidence (*tong suihui* 同歲會).

This complex system of calendrical calculations for the regular and the variable seasonal influences and for the principal and the secondary circulatory phases at any given

---

[8] Kalinowski (1991), 81.

[9] See *Bu bitan* 補筆談, *juan* 2, article 542, 930, on an unexplained correlation between the five sounds and the sixty binomes.

[10] *Suwen, juan* 19, *pian* 68, 352.

moment was used in medicine to forecast the appearance of certain diseases, to explain the pathological processes of some of them, and to choose an appropriate therapy.[11]

The principal sources for the system of the five circulatory phases and the six influences

The various studies so far conducted on this system express divergent opinions as to its origin. As is shown by, among others, a study by Fan Xingzhun 范行準,[12] its earliest origins probably go back to the cosmological and calendrical speculations of the 'gentlemen in possession of techniques' (*fangshi* 方士) of the Han period. However, it turns out that the oldest sources in our possession are seven chapters of the *Suwen* 素問 (Basic Questions) which seem to date, at the earliest, from the mid-eighth century. The system itself was not really developed until the Song period.

The seven chapters of the Suwen

The seven chapters of the *Huangdi neijing Suwen* 黃帝內經素問 (Basic Questions of the Yellow Emperor's Inner Canon) in which the system is described in detail are chapters 66–71 and chapter 74 of the edition with the commentary by Wang Bing 王冰 (*ca* 710–805), which was presented to the Emperor in 762. This is the earliest edition of the *Suwen* to have come down to us and remains the most authoritative.[13] The authenticity of these seven chapters was questioned at a very early date. Already in the eleventh century, when Lin Yi 林億 (eleventh century) and his team began to revise this text (1056–69), they expressed their doubts regarding the antiquity of these seven chapters and suggested that Wang Bing had himself introduced them into the *Suwen*. They pointed out that these chapters did not exist in the commentated editions of the *Suwen* earlier than that of Wang Bing, that is to say the edition produced by Quan Yuanqi 全元起 (sixth century) and the *Huangdi neijing Taisu* 黃帝內經太素 (Grand Basis of the Yellow Emperor's Inner Canon) (666/683), compiled by Yang Shangshan 楊上善 (*ca* 575–670). It is quite true that there are striking differences in length, content, and style between these and the other chapters in the *Suwen*.

---

[11] For more details on this system, see Fan Xingzhun (1951); Liu Jie (1990); Porkert (1974), 55–106; Quan Yijing and Li Minting (1987); de la Robertie and Timon (1984); Ren Yingqiu (1971, 1982a, 1984); Wang Shifu (1958); Zhang Juying (1960).

[12] Fan Xingzhun (1951); see also Lu and Needham (1980), 139–40.

[13] On these chapters, see the work by Fang Yaozhong and Xu Jiasong(1984). Part of chapter 9 also discusses *yunqi*, see Sivin (1993), as do chapters 22 and 29; see Porkert (1974), 56–106, and Ren Yingqiu (1982b), 9–12.

Very little is known of Wang Bing. According to a short biography contained in the *Gujin tushu jicheng* 古今圖書集成 ([Imperially Commissioned] Compendium of Literature and Illustrations, Ancient and Modern),[14] he was a Director of the Imperial Stud (*taipu ling* 太樸令).[15] But one wonders whether that title should not have read *taibu ling* 太卜令, 'Director in Charge of the Bureau of Divination'. If so, it would seem clear that both the commentary on the *Suwen* and the additions to the text, including those seven chapters, were written by Wang Bing, chiefly in order to introduce astrocalendary ideas of the cycle of influences: it is remarkable that the seven chapters on their own constitute one third of the entire work. Wang Bing may well have learned of the cycle of influences from Daoist circles. In the preface to his commentary on the *Suwen*, he declares: 'In my youth, I liked Daoism and the techniques for tending the vital principle . . . From the studio of Master Guo Zizhai (郭子齊), I obtained the secret texts of the previous Master Zhang (張公). The principles set out in those texts were secret and difficult to summarize briefly. That is why I also wrote [apart from this commentary] the "Mysterious Pearl" (Xuanzhu 玄珠), in order to expound this method.'[16]

Wang Bing, who in all likelihood introduced these chapters into the *Suwen*, is in any case considered the advocate of the system of the five circulatory phases and the six influences, for his name is associated with several apocryphal texts on the subject, two of which are described in detail below: the *Qixuan zi yuanhe jiyong jing* 啟玄子元和紀用經 (Master Qixuan's Book on the Use of the Calendar of the Original Harmony) (tenth century), Qixuan zi 啟玄子 being presumed to be a name for Wang Bing; and the *Suwen liuqi Xuanzhu miyu* 素問六氣玄珠密語 (Secret Words of Master Mysterious Pearl on the Six Influences according to the *Suwen*), which calls to mind the reference to the Mysterious Pearl in the preface cited above.

All the same, given that the earliest extant editions of the *Suwen* date from the eleventh century (Northern Song), we cannot dismiss the hypothesis that the seven chapters of the *Suwen* relating to the five circulatory phases and the six influences are later than Wang Bing, especially since the system did not really develop until the time of the Five Dynasties and the Northern Song, and neither the *Ishinpō* 醫心方 (Essential Medical Prescriptions) (984) nor the *Taiping shenghui fang* 太平聖惠方 (Imperial Grace Formulary of the Taiping Period) (992) mention it. It is accordingly prudent to date its development in the field of medicine to no earlier than the eleventh century.

---

[14] *Gujin tushu jicheng*, section 43, *juan* 534, 12b.

[15] The Song editions of the *Suwen* give, following the title, the name of the author of the commentary as either Wang Bing or Qixuan zi 啟玄子. Lin Yi and his team added the following note: 'According to the Tang *Renwu zhi* 人物志 (Monograph on Important Figures), Wang Bing served the dynasty as a *taipu ling*. He died when he was over eighty years old.'

[16] *Suwen*, preface, 1–2.

Qixuan zi yuanhe jiyong jing

The *Qixuan zi yuanhe jiyong jing* 啟玄子元和紀用經 (Master Qixuan's Use of the Calendar of the Original Harmony) (late tenth century) is attributed to Qixuan zi, the 'Master in Harmony with Mysterious [Pearl]', a name that Wang Bing is believed to have adopted after meeting his Daoist master known as Xuanzhu 玄珠, 'Mysterious Pearl'. But this work is believed to have been written in 889, more than a century after Wang Bing's completion of the commentary, by the Daoist Xu Ji 徐寂 (who died in 936). In his youth, Xu Ji was a Daoist on Mount Siming 四明, in the province of Zhejiang. He studied the *Book of Changes* (*Yijing* 易經) with a certain Jin Zhengjun 晉徵君 (tenth century). Then, in 905, he fled with Zhao Kuangming 趙匡明 (tenth century) to the kingdom of Shu, where he served as a minister (*shangshu* 尚書) and, as he was famous for his understanding of calendary calculations, the king of Shu asked him to design a calendar. Later, from 923–6,[17] he was tutor to the heir to the throne, Prince Wang Zongtan 王宗坦 (tenth century), on the recommendation of his friend, the famous Daoist Du Guangting 杜光庭 (850–933), to whom the education of the heir to the throne had been entrusted.[18] It was here, in Daoist circles that the system of the five circulatory phases and the six influences was developed, and was expounded by an expert in the art of calculations, the calendar, and divination, with the aid of the *Book of Changes*.

The *Qixuan zi yuanhe jiyong jing* is divided into three parts. The first concerns the theory of the five circulatory phases and the six influences. For each of the *yin/yang* modalities relating to the principal influence, the secondary influence, and the central influence, it provides a list of remedies chosen on the basis of a correspondence established between their properties, that is to say their flavour (*wei* 味) (sour, bitter, sweet, pungent, or salty), their quality (*qi* 氣) (cold, cool, warm, or hot), and the six *yin/yang* modalities. For example, when the *jueyin* corresponding to the wind reigns at the same time as the circulatory phase of wood, ailments should be treated by remedies with a pungent flavour and a cool quality. The second part lists remedies and prescriptions designed to reinforce the seasonal influences and rebalance them. First, nine procedures are recommended: three alchemical prescriptions (in tune with the sky, the earth, and man), three prescriptions for the kidneys (in tune with the sounds and the pitch pipes), and three prescriptions based on alcohol (in tune with the stars). These are followed by eighty-one prescriptions recommended for treating ailments, the symptoms of which are enumerated, although it is not clear what the link is between these prescriptions and the system of the five circulatory phases and the six influences. The third part consists of

---

[17] *Taiping guangji* 太平廣記, *juan* 196, 1473.   [18] Verellen (1989), 165.

three pages that provide a kind of conclusion. In this work, the system of the five circulatory phases and the six influences is thus applied solely to pharmacotherapy.

Suwen liuqi Xuanzhu miyu

According to the preface of the *Suwen liuqi Xuanzhu miyu* 素問六氣玄珠密語 (Secret Words of Master Mysterious Pearl on the Six Influences according to the *Suwen*) (tenth–eleventh centuries), Xuanzhu was the name of Wang Bing's Daoist master, the presumed author of this work. Xuanzhu is mentioned at least twice in the work discussed above, the *Qixuan zi yuanhe jiyong jing*.[19] He is also cited several times in the edition of the *Suwen* with a commentary by Wang Bing, corrected by Lin Yi.[20] Xuanzhu was thus known as a noteworthy figure, although we do not know whether the text *Suwen liuqi Xuanzhu miyu* already existed. According to Lu Gwei-djen and Needham, it was written by an anonymous author between the tenth and the twelfth centuries.[21] But it is possible to provide a more precise date.

The abbreviated title *Suwen miyu* is cited in the part of the *Huangji jingshi* 皇極經世 (Through the Ages of the August Ultimate) written by a direct disciple of Shao Yong 邵雍 (1012–77), the 'Guanwu waipian' 觀物外篇 (Outer Chapters on the Observation of Things), which contains the following sentence: 'Works such as the *Suwen miyu* have truly reached the peak of the principle of the techniques of calculation.'[22] If the *Huangji jingshi* was completed between 1071 and 1072, as seems likely,[23] these chapters on 'the observation of things' were probably put together from notes taken on Shao Yong's teaching by his disciples. The version included in the *Daoist Canon* (*Daozang* 道藏) (1444), in the Ming period, is probably the closest to the original edition. The edition in the *Siku quanshu* 四庫全書 (Complete Collection of the Works of the Four Storehouses), compiled between about 1711 and 1799, is annotated by Zhang Xingcheng 張行成 (*jinshi* in 1132), who declares in his preface that he has filled in a number of gaps and corrected certain passages. Now, the edition in the *Daoist Canon* contains the following remark: 'Writings such as the *Secret Words of the Suwen* (*Suwen miyu zhi lei* 素問密語之類) constitute the *summum* of the techniques of calculation.'[24] Yet the edition annotated by Zhang Xingcheng states: 'The commentaries on the *Suwen*

[19] *Qixuan zi yuanhe jiyong jing, juan* 1, 2b: 'The many marvellous recipes of Master Mysterious Pearl are dispersed through various works'; and *juan* 3, 50b: 'Several times, I manifested my pure desires to Master Mysterious Pearl.'

[20] *Suwen, juan* 21, *pian* 71, 427, 429, 430, in which Lin Yi cites Xuanzhu in terms that correspond to this text.

[21] Lu and Needham (1980), 140.   [22] *Huangji jingshi, juan* 12, 2, 6b.   [23] Arrault (1995), 59.

[24] *Huangji jingshi, Daozang* 1040, *juan* 12.2, 6b.

such as the "Process of Tablets of Jade of Celestial Origin" (*Tianyuan yuce jiefa* 天元玉策截法) or the "Secret Words of Mysterious Pearl" (*Xuanzhu miyu* 玄珠密語) were written by Wang Bing.'[25] This commentary leaves hardly any doubt that the *Suwen miyu* should be identified as the *Xuanzhu miyu*, which must consequently have existed at the beginning of the twelfth century. Finally, there is also an allusion in chapter 2 of the *Suwen rushi yunqi lun'ao* 素問入式運氣論奧 (Marvellous Introductory Remarks on the Theory of the Circulatory Phases and the Seasonal Influences According to the *Suwen*) (1099) by Liu Wenshu 劉溫舒 (late eleventh century), which simply states, 'Mysterious Pearl also says this.'[26] The *Suwen liuqi Xuanzhu miyu* can thus be dated to before the end of the eleventh century, at the latest. It is clear in any case that the content of the text bearing this title differs greatly from that of the *Suwen* chapters on the system of the five circulatory phases and the six influences, and in all likelihood the text that has come down to us is not the one that Wang Bing is supposed to have written and that he mentions in his preface to the *Suwen*.

The extant *Suwen liuqi Xuanzhu miyu*, in seventeen *juan*, sets out how the system of correlations between the five circulatory phases and the six influences works, including its applications to medicine. The medical data occupy no more than a few chapters. *Juan* 2 presents recommendations of prophylactic acupuncture designed to restore the balance of the six influences. *Juan* 3 and 4 list the symptoms that correspond respectively to the five circulatory phases and the six influences. In contrast to the preceding text, no precise pharmacology is indicated. The only therapeutic references are to acupuncture.

Suwen rushi yunqi lun'ao

The most important work in the history of the system of the five circulatory phases and the six influences is the *Suwen rushi yunqi lun'ao* 素問入式運氣論奧 (Marvellous Introductory Remarks on the Theory of the Circulatory Phases and the Seasonal Influences According to the *Suwen*) by Liu Wenshu, comprising three *juan*, thirty chapters, and seventy-two drawings. It was presented at the court in 1099 and marks the highest point in this system's reputation.[27] Its author was given the title of Vice-Rector of Studies in the Imperial Bureau of Medicine. The illustrations make use of the circle, a frequent feature in Song drawings and one that emphasized the elements' cyclical

[25] *Huangji jingshi Guanwu waipian yanyi, juan* 9, 6b; in *Sikuquanshu* 804-188b.
[26] *Suwen rushi yunqi lun'ao, juan* 2, 8a–10a and *juan* 2, 23a.
[27] *Junzhai dushu houzhi* 郡齊讀書志, *juan* 2, 405.

development in time. The drawings are accompanied by explanations concerning the way to work out the system's various components. There then follows a presentation of the twelve channels, the six types of pathology that are in tune with the six *yin/yang* modalities, the various qualities of the pulse and how these relate to the six influences. The text concludes with therapeutic methods of supplementation (*bu* 補) and discharge (*xie* 泄), using the five flavours in association with the six kinds of seasonal influences at the origin of the ailment. This work thus provides an extensive presentation of the system itself, diagnosis, and pharmacotherapy.

Huangdi neijing Suwen yipian

The *Huangdi neijing Suwen yipian* 黃帝內經素問遺篇 (Recovered Chapters of the Basic Questions in the Yellow Emperor's Inner Canon) (late eleventh century) is claimed to be the text of chapters 72 and 73 of the *Suwen*, which had already disappeared by the time of Wang Bing, who nevertheless passed on their titles: *Cifa lun* 刺法論 (Treatise on the Procedures of Acupuncture) and *Benbing lun* 本病論 (Treatise on Basic Diseases). The *Tongzhi* 通志 *Yiwen lüe* 藝文略 (Brief Bibliography of the Arts and Letters in the Comprehensive Treaty) and the bibliographical catalogue of the *Songshi* 宋史 (History of the Song) both attribute to Liu Wenshu a *Neijing Suwen lun'ao* 內經素問論奧 (Marvellous Remarks [by Way of Introduction to the Theory of Circulatory Phases and Seasonal Influences] According to the Basic Questions of the Inner Canon) in four *juan*.[28] As the text that has come down to us contains only three *juan*, some scholars have thought that the fourth was none other than the *Huangdi neijing Suwen yipian*, which is, in any case, attributed to Liu Wenshu by most bibliographical catalogues.[29] This text contains only therapeutic acupunctural recommendations for epidemic diseases (*yi* 疫) and comas (*jue* 厥). The first chapter expounds the points for acupuncture when influences are not rising or falling correctly and when the displacements of the six influences are out of balance. The points to be punctured are those of the well (*jing* 井), transportation (*shu* 輸), nourishment (*rong* 榮), convergence (*he* 合), and source (*yuan* 原). The second chapter sets out the five forms of comas linked with disorders in the five circulatory phases, and the methods to be applied depending on whether those circulatory phases are excessive or insufficient. The appropriate treatments consist of acupuncture and the recitation of incantations.

Those are the only documents from the periods of the Five Dynasties and the Song specifically devoted to the five circulatory phases and the six influences that have come

---

[28] *Tongzhi, juan* 69, *Yiwen lüe* (7), 810c, and *Songshi, juan* 207, 5319.   [29] Cf. Okanishi (1977), 56–7.

down to us. However, the Song bibliographies have preserved the titles of a dozen or so other works that have been lost.[30]

Applications of the system

To judge from the written sources at our disposal, documents testifying to the social use of the system of the five circulatory phases and the six influences are of later date than the texts themselves. If we accept that Wang Bing was the author of the seven chapters of the *Suwen*, the system itself must have existed at least since the eighth century, but its use in medical practice is not attested before the mid-eleventh century, and did not reach the full height of its popularity until the twelfth and thirteenth centuries. This certainly does not mean that it was not used earlier, only that its use had not been accepted by scholarly medicine and was not yet recognized by the palace doctors. The second half of the eleventh century seems to have been a turning point in this respect. A number of documents from this period testify to the successful use of the system by famous doctors who, thanks to it, managed to cure patients whom the palace doctors had been unable to help: recognition of the efficacy of the system marked its official acceptance.

The development of the system should be set in the context of the cosmological speculations of figures such as Zhou Dunyi 周敦頤 (1017–73) and Shao Yong, around the middle of the eleventh century. There are major resemblances between the history of the development of the five circulatory phases and the six influences and that of the 'Diagram of the Great Ultimate' (*Taiji tu* 太極圖). The famous exposition of the latter by Zhou Dunyi became the cosmological reference *par excellence*. It is recorded that the transmission of this diagram, the origin of which is uncertain, was effected first by Chen Tuan 陳摶, a Daoist of the Five Dynasties period (who died in 989), who was a specialist on the *Book of Changes* and the techniques of divination.[31] It was then passed on by Zhong Fang 種放 (eleventh century) to Mu Xiu 穆休 (eleventh century), and from him to Zhou Dunyi. Now, this eminent philosopher was writing his explanation of the *Taiji* precisely during the period when the system of the five circulatory phases and the six influences was also becoming a cosmogonic system. In both cases, the roots plunged deep into Daoist circles. The development of the *Taiji tushuo* 太極圖説 (Explanations of the Diagram of the Great Ultimate) by Zhou Dunyi and that of the system of the

---

[30] For instance, *Liujia tianyuan yunqi qian* 六甲天元運氣鈐, *Qixuan zi tianyuan yuce* 啟玄子天元玉冊, *Sanjia yunqi jing* 三甲運氣經, *Taishi tianyuan yuce jiefa* 太始天元玉冊截法, *Wuyun liuqi Yusuo zi jing* 五運六氣玉瑣子經, *Wuyun zhizhang futu* 五運指掌賦圖, *Yunqi chao* 運氣鈔, *Tianyuan yuce* 天元玉冊. Cf. Okanishi (1977), 1361–3.
[31] On Chen Tuan, see Knaul (1981).

five circulatory phases and the six influences were also similar in that both presented explanatory models of the mechanisms of the universe. They differed, however, in that the *Taiji tu* presents a model that refers to the *Book of Changes*, whereas the system of the circulatory phases and the seasonal influences proposes a way of calculating disorders in those mechanisms that is based upon the calendar. It is also significant that both in medicine and in the writings of internal alchemy, the 'Diagram of the Great Ultimate' is a model to explain physiological mechanisms, whereas the system of the five circulatory phases and the six influences serves in medicine to foresee disorders and thereby to analyse pathological causes and provide therapeutic answers.

The theories of Shao Yong, the famous cosmologist of the Northern Song period, are also compatible with this.[32] In both cases, a calculation of cosmological cycles is involved, a sort of calendar of the various influences at work in the universe. Furthermore, the doctors famous for their use of the system of the circulatory phases and the seasonal influences tended to gravitate toward circles surrounding Shao Yong. One such was Hao Yun 郝允 (who died in the Huangyou period (1049–54)), details of whose biography were preserved thanks to Shao Yong's grandson, Shao Bo 邵博 (d. 1158).[33] In his youth, Hao Yun travelled with his brother in the Heshuo 河朔 region, where he encountered a Daoist who passed on to him medical techniques relating to the system of the five circulatory phases and the six influences. Thanks to these, he was able to treat a number of officials, sometimes expressing opinions that clashed with those of the court doctors. It is recorded that he knew how to predict the time of death of an individual and could produce infallible prognoses on diseases that tended to be rife in particular regions. The palace doctor Zhao Zonggu 趙宗古 (eleventh century) was presented with his 'Procedures on the Six Origins and the Five Circulatory Phases' (*liuyuan wuyun zhi fa* 六元五運之法); to these he added some drawings, and presented the whole collection to the court (precise date unknown), where these procedures were by and large adopted. Unfortunately, this work has been lost.[34] The son of Hao Yun, Hao Huaizhi 郝懷質 (late eleventh century) apparently inherited the skill of his father, and acquired a reputation as an excellent diagnostician.[35]

---

[32] Cf. his *Huangji jingshi*.

[33] Cf. *Shaoshi wenjian houlu* 邵氏聞見後錄, *juan* 29, 10b–12a. Shao Bo was the second son of Shao Bowen 邵伯溫 (1057–1134), who was a minister at the beginning of the Shaosheng period (1094–95) and was himself the son of Shao Yong; see the biography of Shao Bowen in the *Shongshi*, *juan* 433, 12851–4.

[34] This is probably the work listed in the *Tongzhi*, *juan* 69, *Yiwen lüe* (7), 810b, sphygmology section, under the title *Liujia tianyuan yunqi qian* 六甲天元運氣鈐 in two *juan*, a work also listed in the *Songshi*, *juan* 207, 5313. However, both these bibliographies give the name of the author as not Zhao Zonggu, but Zhao Conggu 趙從古.

[35] This mention of Hao Yun reappears, in abbreviated form, in the *Yishuo* 醫說 *juan* 2, 27b.

Toward the end of the eleventh century, the doctor Yang Zijian 楊子建 (eleventh century) also contributed to the development of the system of the five circulatory phases and the six influences. Reckoning that Wang Bing had not properly understood how to calculate the changes and displacements of the influences, he corrected those errors in a work of 14 *juan* entitled *Tongshen lun* 通神論 (Treatise of Marvellous Comprehension),[36] now unfortunately lost.[37] It was also at about this time that the renowned Pang Anshi 龐安時 (late eleventh century),[38] who was very close to Su Dongpo 蘇東坡 (1037–1101)[39] and Huang Tingjian 黃庭堅 (1045–1105),[40] made use of the system, particularly in his commentary on the *Shanghan lun* 傷寒論 (Treatise on Cold Damage Disorders).

The twelfth century marked the full flowering of the system, which was now applied more widely. First, the medical encyclopaedia produced on the orders of Emperor Huizong 徽宗 (1101–25) and presented to him in 1117, the *Shengji zonglu* 聖濟總錄 (Sagely Benefaction Medical Encyclopaedia), devoted two of its two hundred *juan* to an exposition of the system of the five circulatory phases and the six influences. In the mid-twelfth century, doctors such as Xu Shuwei 許叔微 (1080–*ca* 1154) were influenced by the system.[41] But it was above all toward the end of the twelfth century and the beginning of the thirteenth, with authors such as Chen Yan 陳言 (fl. 1161–74), Liu Wansu 劉完素 (1110–1200), and Zhang Congzheng 張從正 (*ca* 1156–1228), that the innovative function of the system became clearly evident (see the section on innovation in aetiopathogeny).

The titles of works on the system of the five circulatory phases and the six influences preserved in catalogues, along with fragments of the seven chapters of the *Suwen* and the *Suwen liuqi Xuanzhu miyu*, suggest that applications other than medical were found for the system.[42] One detailed document that testifies to this has fortunately survived. It is by Shen Gua, who explains how, thanks to this system, he was able to predict rain:

---

[36] Cf. *Junzhai dushu houzhi* 郡齊讀書後志, *juan* 15, 212a, and the *Wenxian tongkao* 文獻通考, *juan* 222, 1797.

[37] Cf. *Zhongyi renwu cidian* 中醫人物辭典, 198, and Okanishi (1977), 1086.

[38] Style Anchang 安常. He was the author of the *Shanghan zongbing lun* 傷寒總病論, the *Nanjing jieyi* 難經解義, the *Bencao buyi* 本草補遺. His biography appears in the *Songshi*, *juan* 462, 13520–2.

[39] In his *Dongpo zhilin* 東坡志林, Su Dongpo devotes two articles to him, one in *juan* 1, art. 32, 28 and the other in *juan* 3, art. 21, 101.

[40] Huang Tingjian 黃庭堅 in 1100 wrote a preface to his *Shanghan zongbing lun*.

[41] See his *Shanghan fawei lun* 傷寒發微論.

[42] See for instance *Suwen liuqi Xuanzhu miyu*, *juan* 16, 17a: the observation of an excessive cycle of metal and the brilliance of Venus made it possible to predict whether there would be peace or conscription to the army in such or such a sector. In the *Suwen*, *juan* 20, *pian* 69, 366 indicates for each excessive or insufficient cycle not only the corresponding symptoms, but also the corresponding meteorological disorders.

During the Xining period [1068–77], the capital suffered from a prolonged drought. Rites were performed and prayers were said. The weather remained cloudy for several consecutive days and everybody thought it was going to rain. Suddenly [the next day], the sky cleared, the sun came out again, and it became even hotter. As I had been summoned to the palace on that day, the Emperor asked me if it was going to rain. I told him, 'The signs of rain are already visible; it will come tomorrow.' But most people, on the grounds that it had not rained when the sky had remained cloudy for several days and that now the weather was dry and the sky was clear, said to themselves that there was no hope of it raining now. In fact, though, the next day the rain fell. This was a year in which the phase earth reigned along with dampness. The cloudy weather that had lasted several days showed that the influence in conformity [with the season] was present, but that it was dominated by the *jueyin*, and this prevented the rain from falling. The sudden return of the fine weather indicated a manifestation of metal and dryness: the *jueyin* had diminished, allowing the *taiyin* to develop freely so that, the next day, the circulatory phase and the seasonal influence would once again find themselves in conformity. That is how I knew that it was going to rain. My prognosis was made for that particular spot. If I had been elsewhere, the signs would have been different, and so would my prognosis. What is so ingenious about this mechanism is its great accuracy. By reasoning in this way, one inevitably reaches the ultimate principle of things.[43]

Here, Shen Gua certainly presents the system of the five circulatory phases and the six influences as an astrocalendary system that can be used for prognosis. In another passage, on the basis of the fact that Wang Bing cites in his commentary on the *Suwen* a *Dunjia jing* 遁甲經 (Essay on the *dunjia* System),[44] he advances the hypothesis that the origin of certain correspondences in this system should be sought in the *dunjia* system of divinatory calculations.[45] As has been noted above, the system of the five circulatory phases and the six influences makes use of what is known as the *nayin* system. Now, both the *nayin* and the *dunjia* systems, both of which are cited in the *Baopu zi* as techniques of divinatory calculation, had been lost under the Song. Shen Gua also remarks that the correlations given between the five circulatory phases, the cyclical signs, and the twenty-eight constellations were only to be found in the *Suwen*.[46] That fact is crucial. It would certainly appear that ever since antiquity there had existed traditions of

[43] *Mengqi bitan, juan* 7, art.134, 316. See also Hu Daojing and Jin Liangnian (1988), 103.

[44] *Bu bitan*, art. 547, 942. See for instance *Suwen, juan* 19, *pian* 66, 323.

[45] This system is now lost. In divination, use was made of 'tables of divination' (*shi* 式) of which, under the Tang, three types were distinguished: the *Taiyi* 太一 table, the *liuren* 六壬 table, and the Leigong 雷公 table, the last of which was replaced by the *dunjia* table from the Song period onward. The *Baopu zi* records for the first time the fact that the *dunjia* system was used by hermits in their ascetic practices. See Kalinowski (1983), 318–19.

[46] *Bu bitan*, art. 548, 943.

astrocalendary calculations and cosmological speculations relating specifically to medicine. It is certainly noticeable that the six modalities of *yin* and *yang* (*jueyin*, *shaoyin*, *taiyin*, *shaoyang*, *yangming*, and *taiyang*) only appear in medical works, and that the system of the five circulatory phases and the six influences carries on that tradition.

As well as this testimony provided by Shen Gua, other evidence survives to suggest that the system was also used for non-medical purposes. It appears in a text of geomancy believed to have been edited under the Song: the *Jiutian xuannü qingnang hai-jiao jing* 九天玄女青囊海角經 (Blue Sack Sea Horn Canon of the Mysterious Girl of the Nine Heavens).[47] In its first section this describes the evolution of the world ever since the Supreme Non-being (*Taiwu* 太無) down to the deployment in the heavens of the five circulatory phases. We cannot be certain that this text drew upon medical writings, but it seems probable, as the description of the five sectors that correspond to the five circulatory phases repeats, word for word, the description provided in chapter 67 of the *Suwen*.[48] The documentation available is thus insufficient to reconstruct the definitive history of the development of the system of the five circulatory phases and the six influences and its applications. In all likelihood, Wang Bing was responsible for its introduction into the *Suwen*. But we really cannot be certain whether or not it was applied in particular to medicine.

Was the *wuyun liuqi* an innovation that was accepted, or was it rejected?

We know that the palace doctor Zhao Zonggu received a treatise on the system of the five circulatory phases and the six influences, with illustrations, from the doctor Hao Yun, who died in the Huangyou period (1049–54), and that Zhao presented this system to the court. We also know that after the foundation of the Imperial Bureau of Medicine in 1076, the examinations that this body organized related to, among other subjects, the system of the five circulatory phases and the six influences. It must therefore have been between 1054 and 1076 that the system was officially adopted by the court. But even after that official adoption, the system was criticized, either with respect to some of its content, or in its totality. Basically, despite the attempt to establish it as a general theory, individual doctors adopted it only partially and according to their own personal judgement.

The position that Shen Gua adopted *vis-à-vis* the system is extremely interesting. He was appreciative of its precision and harboured no doubts as to the calculations that made it possible to understand the celestial principle (*tianli* 天理) and thereby to accede to the principle of all things (*wuli* 物理). Where he took issue was with the deterministic

---

[47] See *Gujin tushu jicheng, Yishu dian* 藝術典, *juan* 651; *Kanyu bu* 堪輿部, 1, 1–10b.
[48] *Suwen, juan* 19, *pian* 67, 338.

use of those calculations and the insufficient attention paid to variations according to place, as we have seen from his account of weather-forecasting, cited above. Another aspect that he criticised was the manner in which doctors used it. In his preface to the *Su Shen liangfang* 蘇 沈 良 方 (Excellent Prescriptions by Su Dongpo and Shen Gua),[49] he sets out five difficulties that arise in medical practice.[50] In the passage on the second difficulty, which concerns the appropriate ways of remedying a disease, he argues in favour of the system of the five circulatory phases and the six influences. He totally favours the system which, to his mind, belongs to the science of observing the heavenly principles, the changes of nature in accordance with the calendar, and the effects of those changes upon things and men.[51] However, he criticizes his contemporaries for not paying enough attention to the variations of *yin* and *yang* and for being content with the easy way out that consists in applying prescriptions in a mechanical fashion. This is what he says:

> Nowadays, those who tend patients limit themselves to prescribing one or two remedies, and that is all. In antiquity, when a doctor tended patients, he first of all had to detect the changes (*bian* 變)[52] in the development of the *yin* and the *yang*, according to the calendar. He took note of the place where the malady occurred: whether it was a marsh, a plain, a forest, or a mountain. He took into consideration the age of the patient, how corpulent he was, his social situation, where he lived, the hygiene of his life, the qualities and defects of his physique, his worries and

[49] The work written by Shen Gua is the *Shenshi liangfang* 沈 氏 良 方. It has not come down to us in its original form. The work in our possession is the *Su Shen liangfang* 蘇沈良方 (Excellent Prescriptions of Shen Gua and Su Dongpo) in fifteen *juan*. The *Shenshi liangfang* was probably written by Shen Gua when he retired to the Park of the Dream River between 1088 and 1095. Its amalgamation with the prescriptions of Su Dongpo is attested in the *Wenxian tongkao*, *juan* 223, 1797b, and cannot have been earlier than the beginning of the period of the Southern Song (1126). Hu Daojing (1980) has in most cases been able to establish which prescriptions should be attributed to Shen Gua and which to Su Dongpo. On this text and its history, see also Okanishi (1977), 733.

> The *Shenshi liangfang* was one of the first texts, under the Song, to record precise clinical cases, indicating the name of the patient, the place, the date, the symptoms observed, and the treatment given. For example, Shen Gua notes that he treated Ouyang Xiu 歐陽修 (1007–72), who was suffering from diarrhoea and had not been able to be cured by the palace doctors (*guoyi* 國醫) (*Su Shen liangfang*, *juan* 5, 262). The anecdote shows that Shen Gua was successful where other doctors had failed. He stresses the importance of the verification of the value of a method or a prescription. He declares that, in his opinion, an excellent prescription (*liangfang* 良方) is one whose benefits have been seen by one's own eyes.

[50] These are (1) how to make a good diagnosis; (2) how to cure the ailment; (3) how to choose remedies; (4) how to establish prescriptions; (5) how to discern the quality of remedies.

[51] *Su Shen liangfang*, preface, 1. At the fifth point, p. 3, Shen Gua again introduces the *wuyun liuqi*, by citing the *Suwen*: 'When the *yangming* is in the celestial position, flowers and fruits have a vigorous seasonal influence. When the *shaoyang* is at the source, all stones lose their pattern (*li* 理).' I have not been able to trace this quotation in any edition of the *Suwen*.

[52] On this notion of 'change' in medicine, see Hsu (1994).

his joys, whether his environment was peaceful or stressful, and he adapted to the various circumstances . . . His treatment of the patient took account of now the climatic conditions, now human factors. He bore in mind everything to do with the celestial principles (*tianli*): the system of the five circulatory phases and the six influences, the seasons, the climate, intemperate factors such as thunder or hail, the [influence of] demons and supernatural spirits and of poison (*gu* 蠱), flavours, and whether the influences were cold or warm; he watched to see whether these elements were late or early in relation to the calendar, and whether their activity was dominant or impeded.[53]

He also wrote as follows:

In medicine, there is the method of the five circulatory phases and the six influences. In the macrocosm, this procedure consists of rules for foreseeing changes in nature, such as variations in temperature, in temperate conditions, plagues of caterpillars and grasshoppers. In the microcosm, diseases develop in accordance with the circulatory phases and the seasonal in fluences. The people of today use the method without understanding it and stick to fixed rules. That is why their techniques cannot be verified. For example, when the *jueyin* regulates the course of things,[54] that influence is accompanied by much wind, and the people suffer from diarrhoea caused by excessive dampness. Can it really happen that the wind blows throughout the empire at the same time and that the entire population thus suffers from diarrhoea due to the excessive dampness? Even within a single district, there are climatic differences, in that the sun shines in one place while it rains in another. One is bound to make mistakes if one applies the system in that way. Where the principles of things (*wuli*) are concerned, some elements are regular while others vary (*bian* 變). Some are governed by the circulatory phases and the seasonal influences, while others are of an exceptional nature. Phenomena are called 'regular' (*chang* 常) when they are in conformity with the influence peculiar to that period; they are called 'changeable' (*bian* 變) when there are variations that depend on the locality, which in every case lead to changes. That is why, when observing things, the following situations should be distinguished: conformity (*shun* 順), opposition (*ni* 逆), overflow (*yin* 淫), density (*yu* 鬱), domination (*sheng* 勝), reversion (*fu* 復), excess (*taiguo* 太過), insufficiency (*buzu* 不足). Their respective concrete manifestations differ from one another.[55]

---

[53] *Su Shen liangfang*, preface, 1.

[54] The *jueyin* corresponds to the liver, wind, and wood. See *Suwen, juan* 20, *pian* 69, 356: 'In years in which wood is excessive, the spleen is the first to receive the pathogenic agent, and the people suffer from diarrhoea.'

[55] *Mengqi bitan, juan* 7, art. 134, 315–16. These anomalies in the course of seasonal influences are described in various sources on the *yunqi*, such as the *Suwen* and the *Suwen rushi yunqi lun'ao*; e.g. situations involving breathlessness are discussed in the *Suwen, juan* 21, *pian* 71. See also the *Sanyin fang* 三因方, *juan* 5, 64: 'At the time of the five circulatory phases, the latter may be excessive or insufficient. At the time of the rise and the descent of the six influences, there may occur anomalies such as an opposed course, a course in conformity, a dominant course, or an inverted course.'

Another of Shen Gua's criticisms is directly aimed not at the principles underlying the system, but at certain of its components. He thus attacks the way that some people calculate the alien influence (*keqi* 客氣). Noticing that the calculations concerning this are not explained clearly in writings on the five circulatory phases and the six influences and that interpretations differ from one person to another, he gives his own interpretation of what should be understood by the alien influence and how it should be calculated:[56]

> In the annual circulatory phases, there are dominant influences (*zhuqi* 主氣) and alien influences (*keqi* 客氣), which come from outside. [The six influences] from the first, the *jueyin*, down to the last, the *taiyang*, follow the regular progression of the cycle of the seasons, hence their name of dominant influences. Concerning the question of deversant influences, the specialized writings say nothing, and opinions on this point vary widely. For some, the deversant influences designate the cycle of the celestial norm that leads from the first gradation of the clepsydra in years of *jiazi* to the twenty-sixth in years of *yichou* . . . In reality, this is the procedure for calculating the date of the great cold in the calendary system of the four fractions. It bears no relation to the yearly cycle of the seasonal influences.

Other doctors, as well as Shen Gua, criticized an over-deterministic and inflexible application of the system. Chen Yan declares:

> If a doctor does not understand [how to use this system], he falls into a [deterministic] use of the techniques of calculation and divination, and can be compared to blind diviners who use the *Book of Changes*. He allows himself to be trapped by the predictions of good or bad fortune using these techniques. As I see it, this casts a shadow over the path of the sage.[57]

Liu Wansu, for his part, criticizes the lack of education of those who write about this system:

> Many works discuss the five circulatory phases and the six influences, and include songs and formulae, diagrams and seals, but do not fully explain either the theory or the application of the system. They show neither its advantages nor its disadvantages, and this leads people's minds into error, particularly if they are not very intelligent. The authors of these works understand no more than one or two per cent of the classics, and set about writing books simply to show off their learning and to dazzle other people. In this way, the system is never validated.[58]

In the works of the various authors discussed so far, it is now a particular part of the system that is discussed, with each author setting out his own solution, now an aspect of divinatory calculation that is challenged. And, as has been noted above, we ought really to speak of not one, but several systems of the five circulatory phases and the six

---

[56] *Mengqi bitan, juan* 7, art. 135, 316.   [57] *Sanyin fang, juan* 2, 63.
[58] *Suwen xuanji yuanbing shi* 素問玄機原病式 preface, 4.

influences, for in the various sources variants exist in the exposition of the system.[59] It is clear that the scholars and doctors of the Song period were scornful of its divinatory aspect. They certainly used it for the purpose of prognosis, but they regarded it above all as a cosmological system that combined theory and practice and that made it possible to accede to the principle of things, a system at the service of reflection on pathological situations and their analysis. It is an attitude that is comparable with that of the cosmologists of the Song period such as Shao Yong, who drew a distinction between calendary techniques and cosmological speculation.

So the system did not enjoy unanimous approval. Liu Wenshu, who produced the major work on the circulatory phases and the seasonal influences, tells us that in practice only a limited use was made of the system:

> It sometimes happens that, in a given year, one is confronted by a malady that does not correspond to the circulatory phase of the year. It is then necessary to track back to the origin of whatever has affected the patient, for the symptoms, the pulse, and the signs observed are not necessarily all due to the cycle of the seasonal influences. A good doctor understands this and avoids an unrefined comprehension that limits him to the cycle of seasonal influences and leads him into error regarding the way to invigorate or discharge the condition.[60]

However, the most severe critique of the system of the five circulatory phases and the six influences that has come down to us is to be found in the *Chushi yishu* 褚氏遺書 (Books Bequeathed by Master Chu). This is attributed to Chu Cheng 褚澄, a doctor under the Southern Qi, but more probably dates from 1126.[61] Here, it is the very bases of the system, that is to say the calculations, that are questioned. The author roundly refutes the idea that it is possible for man to gain exact knowledge of the periods when climatic changes occur, for those changes do not depend on men, and astrocalendrical calculations are a human invention: such a procedure is therefore untrustworthy and can seldom be verified. He rejects attachment to tradition and adulation of the ancients,[62] opposing all that to clinical experience: a person who is able to surround himself with

---

[59] We have already encountered the problem of the deversant influence, with Shen Gua. For examining the stars, the *Suwen rushi yunqi lun'ao*, *juan* 3, cites a system based on the nine stars and the nine palaces, while the *Suwen liuqi Xuanzhu miyu*, *juan* 16, refers to a system based on the five planets.

[60] *Suwen rushi yunqi lun'ao*, *juan* 3, 17a–b.

[61] This text includes a preface dated 935, by a certain Xiao Yuan 蕭淵 (tenth century). He recounts how, during the rebellion of Huang Chao 黃巢 (875), bandits opened up a family tomb and found in it stones bearing an engraved text in nineteen sections, which somebody passed on to him. According to the *Siku tiyao bianzheng* 四庫題要辯證, *juan* 12, 650, this preface was a forgery. The 1201 postscript by Ding Jie 丁介 (twelfth–thirteenth centuries) states that the stelae of the Xiao family were passed on to the monk Yikan 義堪 at the beginning of the Jingkang period in 1126.

[62] *Chushi yishu*, *pian* 9, 547.

competent masters and to undertake clinical practice acquires true skill and knowledge by dint of feeling pulses, observing symptoms, and making use of the *materia medica*. This is a new attitude, one that stresses the importance of clinical practice.

The system of the five circulatory phases and the six influences: a new tool at the service of epidemics

The relations between the seasons, climatic elements, and certain pathologies, including epidemic diseases, were not a new factor in Chinese medicine. Indeed, they lay at the heart of the system of correspondences between the Five Phases and the system of the six *yin/yang* modalities that had constituted the essential basis of Chinese medicine since the Han period. For the six *yin/yang* modalities, a doctor took into account essentially the cycle of the ten periods in a day, the monthly lunar cycle, and the cycle of the twelve months. In relation to the system of the correlations of the Five Phases, he examined the five periods of the year. However, two chapters – 77 and 79 – of the *Lingshu* 靈樞 (Divine Pivot) present an astrocalendrical system for calculating the climatic elements and their effect upon pathological disorders: the divinatory procedure of the *Taiyi* compass and the eight winds. This served to establish prognoses on various matters of social and individual life, and also on diseases: one determined whether the arrival of each of the eight winds of the eight cardinal points was normal or disordered by calculating the successive circulation of the *Taiji* in each of the nine celestial palaces[63] in the course of one year. Chapter 77 establishes a relation between intermittent fevers (*nüe*) and climatic disorders due to the eight winds and the circulation of the *Taiji* in the nine celestial palaces.[64] This theory did not survive for very long in medicine, but its presence in the *Lingshu* shows that from the time of the Han on, epidemic diseases were associated with the observation of disorders in the weather, by means of astrocalendrical calculations that established correlations other than those of the system of the Five Phases.

The pathologies related more closely to the weather are the categories of cold damage disorders (*shanghan* 傷寒), illnesses caused by seasonal influences (*shiqibing* 時氣病), also known as illnesses brought by the climate (lit. heavenly movements, *tianxingbing* 天行病), warmth factor disorders (*wenbing* 溫病), and epidemic diseases (*yibing* 疫病). In the earliest work to have come down to us that provides an overall view of Chinese pathology, the *Zhubing yuanhou lun* 諸病源候論 (Origins and Symptoms of Medical Disorders), presented to Emperor Yang 楊 (605–18) of the Sui in 610, these

---

[63] On the system of the nine palaces, see Kalinowski (1983).
[64] *Lingshu jing, juan* 11, *pian* 77, 117–19.

pathologies are listed. They are all said to be provoked by a disorder, in relation to the calendar, of climatic elements, and therefore all to belong to the same category. For example, the following pronouncement is made on the subject of epidemic diseases:

> Epidemic diseases belong to the same category as diseases due to an influence contrary to the season, and as diseases due to a hot influence or a warm influence, for they all originate from the fact that, in the course of one year, the influences of the solar periods have not been in harmony, that cold and hot are out of order, that violent wind and heavy rain suddenly occur, or that fog and dew take too long to dissipate. Most of the time this causes epidemic diseases among the people, the manifestations of which are the same for the young and for adults alike and evoke the ferocity of demons. That is why they are also called pestilential diseases (*yilibing* 疫癘病).[65]

The epidemic connotation of these diseases had been well established ever since the Jin, and they were subject to quarantine regulations: 'At the end of the Yonghe period (345–56), epidemic diseases were rife. According to the ancient rules, when the families of court ministers were affected by these diseases and more than three people had been contaminated, those who showed no signs of disease were forbidden to enter the palace for one hundred days.'[66]

Under the Song dynasty, it was to these same pathologies, which stemmed from an astrocalendary disorder, that the system of the five circulatory phases and the six influences was applied, for prognostic, prophylactic, and therapeutic purposes. Most of the sources refer to diseases among the people (*minbing* 民病) and emphasize their collective aspect. 'When epidemic diseases are caused by an excessive warmth (*wenyibing* 溫疫病) or by an influence contrary to the season, the young and adults alike are afflicted, either in a single district or throughout an entire prefecture.'[67] The *Huangdi neijing Suwen yipian*, which in its two chapters deals solely with epidemic diseases (*yi* 疫) and comas (*shijue* 尸厥) due to noxious influences, also remarks upon the collective character of these diseases: 'When there is a disorder in the movement or evolution of the predominant influence in the sky, diseases strike the people. To prevent these diseases and save lives, you need, in the first place, to identify what is the disorder in question.'[68]

The *Shengji zonglu*, which devotes its first two *juan* to the system of the five circulatory phases and the six influences, also describes as epidemic diseases those due to an influence contrary to the season. In the *Sanyin jiyi bingzheng fanglun* 三因極一病證方論 (The Three Causes Epitomized and Unified: the Quintessence of Doctrine on the

---

[65] *Zhubing yuanhou lun, juan* 10, 356.
[66] See the biography of Wang Biaozhi 王彪之 (305–77), *Jin shu, juan* 76, 2009.
[67] *Suwen rushi yunqi lun'ao, juan* 3, 15a.   [68] *Huangdi neijing Suwen yipian, juan* 2, 1a.

Origins of Medical Disorders) (1174) by Chen Yan, the link between the system of the five circulatory phases and the six influences and epidemic diseases is even more marked. The subject is treated essentially in *juan* 5, following the rubric 'cold damage disorders', and also in the passage on epidemic diseases. Two chapters are entitled 'The Care and Symptoms of Diseases of the People Due to Influences Contrary to the Season According to the Five Circulatory Phases' (*Wuyun shiqi minbing zhengzhi* 五運時氣民病證治) and 'The Care and Symptoms of Diseases of the People that are Rife according to the Season's Relations to the Six Influences' (*Liuqi shixing minbing zhengzhi* 六氣時行民病證治).

If the mid-eleventh century marks a decisive turning point in the infiltration of the system of the five circulatory phases and the six influences into the Imperial palace, that is partly because at this time many epidemics were ravaging southern China, and the government was anxious to find a cure for them. A number of documents, such as the *Yuhai* 玉海 (Ocean of Jade) by Wang Yinglin 王應麟 (1223–96), tell us of the concern that the Imperial authorities manifested over the epidemics of the Song period:

> In the eighth year of the Qingli period (1048), as prescriptions and remedies were lacking for the patients afflicted by the poison of the illness (*bingdu* 病毒)[69] in southern China, the Emperor ordered the publication of a work composed of a selection of the best prescriptions from the *Taiping shenghui fang*. This work, entitled *Qingli shanjiu fang* 慶歷善救方 (Prescriptions of the Qingli Period to Save People) was distributed throughout the Empire. The palace doctors were ordered to prepare its prescriptions and distribute them to the people suffering from epidemic diseases.[70]

The reformer Wang Anshi, author of a 1049 postscript to the *Qingli shanjiu fang*, states that he had the text engraved on stelae that were then set up to the left of the district gates, so that passers-by could read them.[71] Two years later, in year 3 of the Huangyou period (1051), the Emperor ordered a new compilation of the most essential prescriptions. The work, in five *juan*, entitled *Jianyao jizhong fang* 簡要濟眾方 (Simple Prescriptions to Save People), became the standard text for the district and prefecture leaders whose job it was to use the prescriptions set out in this work in order to care for people suffering from epidemic diseases.[72] The Emperor is believed to have said to his ministers, 'Outside [the palace] there are no good doctors, and the people suffering from epidemic diseases cannot be cared for properly.'[73]

---

[69] The term probably designates epidemic diseases. Consider *Qianjin yaofang* 千金要方, *juan* 9, 173: 'Epidemic diseases spread in the course of the various seasons are very toxic pathological influences (*dubing zhi qi* 毒病之氣).' *Bingdu* and *dubing* may have been used interchangeably.

[70] *Yuhai*, *juan* 63, pp. 23b–24a.   [71] Cf. *Linchuan xiansheng wenji* 臨川先生文集, *juan* 84, 883.

[72] *Song shi*, *juan* 12, 231.   [73] *Wenxian tongkao*, *juan* 223, 1797a.

Such texts show how very serious epidemics were in the mid-eleventh century and record the Imperial attempts to remedy the situation. Now, it was during this same period that doctors such as Hao Yun and Pang Anshi were becoming famous for their skill at handling the system of the five circulatory phases and the six influences, and that treatises on the circulatory phases and the seasonal influences were applying the system to epidemic diseases. In the past these had been treated chiefly by Daoist masters and shamans using talismans, rituals, and ceremonies, in particular annual ceremonies held to expel the kings of epidemic diseases.[74] Scholarly medicine had, to be sure, been declaring, at least since the *Zhubing yuanhou lun*, that such diseases were caused not by demoniacal influences but by cosmological irregularities. But it had not managed to gain a hearing among the people, who felt a sometimes justifiable scorn for those erudite doctors whose attitudes were similar enough to those of the doctors criticized by Molière in seventeenth-century France. Elaborated therapeutic solutions were in short supply and the necessary conceptual apparatus was lacking, so the appearance of the system of the five circulatory phases and the six influences was certainly timely.

It was against this background of concern about the treatment for epidemic diseases and about the relation between them and seasonal disorders that the *Shanghan lun* became popular during the Song dynasty. Before this time, the work as such had enjoyed no status, and had simply been studied as one pathological rubric among others, inspiring very few commentaries: eight titles at the most can be traced between the Jin and the Tang, whereas under the Song as many as seventy texts linked with the work appeared.[75] Many were commentaries that recommended the use of the system of the five circulatory phases and the six influences, the best known being that by Cheng Wuji 成無己 (after 1126), which has remained the major reference for the *Shanghan lun* right down to the present day. It should be pointed out that the development of the printing press under the Song does not suffice to account for the considerable increase in works associated with the *Shanghan lun*, for there was no equivalent increase in other medical works.

At least three factors predisposed this work to become a basic text for speculation using the system of the five circulatory phases and the six influences. In the first place, it is the only known text that sets out the relations between a constant phenomenon and its variants, that is to say presents first a basic pathological table, then the possible variants and changes to be made in the composition of the basic prescription when taking those variants into account. Secondly 'cold damage disorders' (*shanghan*) is a pathological rubric related to epidemic diseases and, according to Sun Simiao 孫思邈 (581–682), some people considered *shanghan* to be simply the elegant name for epidemic diseases

---

[74] Katz (1995) and Schipper (1985).   [75] Okanishi (1977), 391–502.

(*yibing*), the latter term being more commonly used by country folk.[76] Thirdly, this work classifies diseases according to the six modalities of *yin* and *yang* that are also to be found in the circulatory phases and the seasonal influences. Admittedly, the order of the *Shanghan lun* proceeds from *yang* to *yin*, and corresponds to a progressive movement of the disease from the outside to the inside of the body, whereas the order of the system of the five circulatory phases and the six influences proceeds from *yin* to *yang* and corresponds to a quite different spatial concept of the disease. That difference in the order of the *yin/yang* modalities in the *Shanghan lun* and the system of circulatory phases and seasonal influences forced commentators to make strenuous efforts to get the two to correspond. According to Xu Shuwei, Pang Anshi was the first to explain the order of the *yin/yang* modalities in the *Shanghan lun*, at the same time combining them with the theory of the six dominant seasonal influences that suceeded one another in the course of a year.[77]

The apparently satisfactory use of the system of the circulatory phases and the seasonal influences for epidemics is but one of the many innovations inspired by this system. There is not a single area of medicine, be it physiology, pathology, or therapeutics that is not indebted to it for innovations that have survived right down to the present day. But the very principle of reasoning and establishing new relations between theory and practice prompted new patterns of behaviour for the doctors. The few examples of innovation mentioned below represent only the beginning of a process that was to continue in later periods.

A few innovative uses of the system of the five circulatory phases and the six influences

Innovation and aetiopathogeny

The attention paid to epidemic diseases and the importance of the system of the circulatory phases and the seasonal influences under the Song played a determining role in the clear distinction drawn in this period between external causes and internal causes, a distinction that even prompted such authors as Chen Yan and Zhang Congzheng to restructure one part of pathology.

In his *Sanyin jiyi bingzheng fanglun* 三因及一病證方論 (The Three Causes Epitomized and Unified: the Quintessence of Doctrine on the Origins of Medical Disorders) (1174), Chen Yan[78] distinguishes three sorts of causes: external (*waiyin* 外因), internal (*neiyin* 內因), and neither external nor internal (*bu nei wai yin* 不內外因).

---

[76] *Qianjin yaofang, juan* 29, 2.   [77] *Leizheng puji benshi fang* 類證普濟本事方, *juan* 9, 8b–9a.
[78] His style was Wuze 無擇, his literary name Hexi daoren 鶴溪道人.

However, an attentive reading of this work reveals that the distinction between these three kinds of causes is only made for certain pathological rubrics and does not have a general application. It only makes it possible to refine the analysis of different types of pathological mechanisms for clinical tables that are analogous and that are grouped under the same rubric. The system of the five circulatory phases and the six influences emphasizes the importance of external causes. It provides an alternative interpretation for certain diseases that were previously explained within the system of correlations between the five viscera. It is, incidentally, significant that, under the Song, only three titles were associated with the five viscera: three titles of texts accompanied by illustrations referring to the topography of the body and to drawings made on the basis of vivisections rather than on the way that the five viscera function.[79] In contrast, we know of about sixty titles of works relating to the five viscera for the period stretching from the Han down to the Tang. In the Song period, the system of the five viscera was clearly supplanted, for certain types of pathologies, by the system of the circulatory phases and the seasonal influences.

It was apparently following a discussion with his friends Tang Deyuan 湯德遠 (twelfth century) and Qing Defu 慶德夫 (twelfth century) that Chen Yan came to define three types of causes which, he claimed, clarified the organization of pathology. He wrote as follows:

> When one examines a disease, one should first know its name. Those that are called 'cold damage disorders', 'summer heat disorders', 'wind disorders', 'dampness disorders', 'epidemic diseases' or 'diseases due to an influence contrary to the season' are all due to an external cause. An emptiness or a plenitude of the viscera or other receptacles, the five types of fatigue, and the six types of exhaustion are due to an internal cause. Ailments such as wounds caused by metal, aches, fractures, and harm done by tigers, wolves and venomous creatures stem from causes that are neither external nor internal . . . To treat a malady, one first needs to know its cause. One cannot properly define its origin if one does not know its cause. There are three types of causes: external, internal, and neither external nor internal. The internal causes are the seven emotions (*qiqing* 七情), the external causes are the six excesses (*liuyin* 六淫), the causes that are neither internal nor external are those that stem from an abnormal course of events (*bei jingchang* 背經常). The remarks consigned to the *Jingui yaolüe* 金匱要略 (Essentials in the Golden Casket) set out the essential principles of pathology. The *Treatise on the Origin and Symptoms of Disorders by Master Chao [Yuanfang]* sets out the names of the various disorders in 1,800 articles. But with these three types of causes [that I have defined], I cover all the origins of disorders.[80]

[79] Okanishi (1977), 299–300. The drawings of the five viscera of Ou Xifan 歐希範 (eleventh century) were published by Yang Jie 楊介 (eleventh century) and Zhu Gong 朱肱 (*jinshi* in 1088).
[80] *Sanyin fang, juan* 2, 15.

The system of cosmological speculations thus served as a basis for a partial reordering of the aetiopathogeny. The most representative work in this reordering is without doubt that by Liu Wansu (1110–1200).[81] He considers that, among the external causes, the principle pathogenic agent is fire. To his mind, ailments from wind, cold, dampness, and dryness are all developments of fire-heat; similarly, an excess of the five types of emotions also, according to him, provokes ailments from heat. Consequently, he uses many cooling remedies in his therapy. Elsewhere, he develops a new classification of symptoms according to the five circulatory phases and the six influences – a classification already introduced into the chapters of the *Suwen* devoted to the circulatory phases and the seasonal influences. For example, symptoms due to wind, and also dizziness, are caused by the liver and by wood. The heart and fire are sources of itching, aches, abcesses, and symptoms such as a heated body, shivering, vomiting, distensions, anthrax, swellings, nasal obstructions, nose-bleeds, constipation, urinary problems, verbal delirium, sadness, anxiety, vomitings of blood, cholera, scrofula, etc.[82]

Zhang Congzheng[83] (*ca* 1156–1228) was certainly the man who applied the system of the five circulatory phases and the six influences to aetiopathogeny in the most extensive fashion. For example, he condemns the assertion, in chapter 38 of the *Suwen*, that cold is at the origin of coughing, an assertion that is repeated by the *Zhubing yuanhou lun*.[84] He tries to show that any one of the six climatic influences may induce coughing. Returning to the configurations of the system, Zhang sets up a correspondence between the dominance of each of the celestial influences and particular forms of coughing. He elaborates a number of large clinical tables for which he then indicates the appropriate therapies, at the same time producing a more complex table of the various forms of coughing and their respective treatments.[85] However, like Liu Wansu, he certainly does not make a similar distinction for all the pathological rubrics that he discusses.

We should remember that Liu Wansu and Zhang Congzheng were at the origin of two of the four major currents of medicine in the Jin and the Yuan periods.[86] The founders of

[81] His style was Shouzhen 守真. On him and his disciples, see Wu (1993–94).
[82] *Suwen bingji qiyi baoming ji* 素問病機氣宜保命集 and *Suwen xuanji yuanbing shi* 素問玄機原病式.
[83] His style was Zihe 子和. On him, see Ding Guangdi (1987), Li Congfu and Liu Bingfan (1983).
[84] While *Suwen, juan* 10, *pian* 38, 191, presents the cold as the pathogenic agent of coughing, other passages in this text refer to other external pathogenic agents such as the wind, dampness, and heat as sources of coughing. See Despeux and Obringer (1997), 61–104.
[85] *Rumen shiqin* 儒門事親, *juan* 3, 16–18; see also Despeux and Obringer (1990).
[86] Liu Wansu was the representative of the 'Hejian tradition' (Hejian *pai* 河間派) or the 'tradition that recommends cooling remedies' (*hanliang pai* 寒涼派) and Zhang Congzheng was the representative of the 'tradition recommending the use of laxatives and purgatives' (*gongxia pai* 攻下派). There were also Li Gao 李杲 (1180–1251), whose posthumous name was Dongyuan 東垣, who represented the 'tradition that supplements the earth' (*butu pai* 補土派) and Zhu Zhenheng 朱震亨 (1282–1358), generally known as Zhu Danxi 朱丹溪, who represented 'the tradition that supplements the *yin*' (*ziyin pai* 滋陰派). See Ding Guangdi (1987), Li Congfu and Liu Bingfan (1983), Rall (1970), and Wu (1993–94).

these four currents were responsible for a number of innovations in medical theory and practice, innovations whose roots go back to the system of the five circulatory phases and the six influences.

An innovation in physiology

One major innovation in physiology, on the functional level, was the recognition of two separate kidneys: the left one was associated with water, and the right one, which corresponded to the gate of life (*mingmen* 命門), was associated with minister fire (*xianghuo* 相火). The right kidney's correspondence with the gate of life was not new, for this had already been mentioned in the thirty-sixth and the thirty-ninth difficulty of the *Nanjing* 難經 (Canon of Difficult Issues), which dated from the Eastern Han (second century AD),[87] but until now it had been neglected and had not been used as a basis for speculation on the kidneys' physiological function. Now, the separation of fire into sovereign fire (*junhuo* 君火), associated with the heart, and minister fire, associated with the right kidney (or with the gate of life), which appears in the system of the five circulatory phases and the six influences, makes it possible, without rejecting the traditional correlations between the Five Phases and the five viscera, to connect the kidneys not only with water but also with fire. It should be pointed out that the commentary on difficulty thirty-six in the *Nanjing*, produced by Ding Deyong 丁德用 during the Jiayou era (*ca* 1056–63), introduces these ideas of the cycle of seasonal influences and states: 'The section of the foot (*chi* 尺) where one feels the pulse with the right hand corresponds to the minister fire that carries the orders of the sovereign fire. It is called the gate of life (*mingmen*).'[88]

Several Song works on cosmology integrated the notion of the separation of the kidneys into two entities. For example, this is mentioned in a diagram entitled 'Liuwei sanji tu' 六位三極圖 (Drawing of the Three Poles and the Six Positions),[89] in which the human body is represented by a circle containing the characters and numbers that correspond to the viscera: number one corresponds to the right kidney, two to the lungs, three to the spleen, four to the liver, five to the heart, and six to the left kidney. It also figures in a diagram of the cycle of influences in the *Shangfang dadong zhenyuan miaojing tu* 上方大洞真元妙經圖 (Illustrations of the Marvellous Canon on the True Origin of the Great Cave of the Upper Region),[90] a text that probably dates from the Song period and that contains, in particular, a representation of the *Taiji tu*.

---

[87] Unschuld (1986), 382 and 399.   [88] *Nanjing buzhu* 難經補註, *juan* 1, 3b.

[89] *Zhouyi tu* 周易圖, *juan* 1, 7b. This text dates from the Song period and is later than Shao Yong, who is cited in *juan* 2, 32b.

[90] *Shangfang dadong zhenyuan miaojing tu*, 5b. Although this text, in the *Daozang* edition, contains a preface attributed to Emperor Minghuang 明皇 (712–56) of the Tang dynasty, more likely it dates from the Song period.

This division of fire into sovereign fire and minister fire needs to be restored to the context of the ideas prevalent in Daoist circles, in particular those relating to internal alchemy, concerning the physiological mechanisms of the body and the procedures adopted in order to 'seize upon the mechanism of creations and transformations' (*duo zaohua* 奪造化). In some works on internal alchemy three kinds of fire are associated with various elements in the body. The most ancient known source, the *Taishang jiuyao xinyin miaojing* 太上九要心印妙經 (The Marvellous Canon on the Mind Seal and the Nine Principles of the Most High), which is attributed to Zhang Guo 張果, writing in the mid-eighth century, but which more likely dates from the late Tang or the early Song period, describes the three fires as follows: 'The seminal essence is the fire of the people (*minhuo* 民火), the seasonal influence is minister fire (*chenhuo* 臣火), and the heart is sovereign fire (*junhuo* 君火).'[91] But most texts on internal alchemy from the Song period have sovereign fire correspond to the heart, minister fire to a kidney, and the fire of the people to the bladder.[92] In both alchemical and medical contexts, the relation of sovereign fire to the heart is borrowed from Buddhism, which associates a psychic heat with consciousness (*vijñâna*), which is located in the heart. A text on sovereign fire by Chen Yan, liberally scattered with Buddhist ideas, provides a good example.[93]

In the system of the five circulatory phases and the six influences, in the first place only two fires are retained – and minister fire is called not *chenhuo* 臣火 but *xianghuo* 相火; and secondly, their correlations with elements in the body are rather different, for here fire is associated only with the right kidney. According to alchemical notions, the practitioner had to extract fire from the water of the kidneys and water from the fire of the heart in order to effect the union of opposites and to reverse the course of the process. Similarly, to reverse the cycle of the creation of the Five Phases, he had to extract metal from the water in the kidneys and wood from the fire of the heart.[94] Consequently, when Liu Wenshu declares in the *Suwen rushi yunqi lun'ao* that 'the kidneys do not correspond to metal and water, but the right kidney corresponds to the gate of life and to fire',[95] he is launching a direct attack against the ideas of internal alchemy, and is deliberately distancing himself from them. Thus, in the system of the circulatory phases and the seasonal influences, it is no longer water and *shaoyin* that are associated with the

---

[91] *Taishang jiuyao xinyin miaojing*, 2a.

[92] *Lingbao bifa* 靈寶秘法, *juan* 1, 8a; see Baldrian-Hussein (1981), 106–7. The same goes for the *Daoshu* 道樞, *juan* 7, 13b–14a.

[93] *Sanyin fang*, *juan* 2, 63.

[94] In alchemy this principle is rendered by the metaphorical expression 'extract [the *yang* line] from within the *kan* to complete *li* [which has a central *yin* line] (*qu kan tian li* 取坎添離)'. This is used, for example, in one of the fundamental texts of internal alchemy under the Song, the *Wuzhen pian* 悟真篇 by Zhang Boduan 張伯端 (987–1082). Cf. *Ziyang zhenren Wuzhen pian jiangyi*, *juan* 3, 11a–b (prefaces of 1227 and 1228).

[95] *Suwen rushi yunqi lun'ao*, *juan* 2, 9a.

kidneys, as it was in the traditional system of the Han, but instead two phases, water and minister fire, and two modalities, *taiyang* and *shaoyang*. Shen Gua provides a clear description of this new set of correlations:

> Where the six influences are concerned, doctors who specialize in prescriptions associate them with the six spirits. The blue-green dragon symbolizes the *jueyin* influence from the east; the natural sentiment of this influence is benevolence, its efficient force is transformation, its colour is blue-green, its shape is long, and its animal category is that of scaly animals. The dragon is the animal best adapted to symbolize the qualities of this influence, but that does not necessarily mean that this animal exists. The same applies to the emblems attached to other influences. But the north contains two animals: the dark warrior (tortoise), which designates the influence of *taiyang* water, and the erect snake, which designates the influence of the *shaoyang* minister fire.[96] In the human body, the kidneys are also double. The left one is *taiyang* water, the right one is *shaoyang* minister fire. Fire descends and extinguishes water, water rises and gives rain and dew, which irrigate the five viscera; there is a mutual exchange between above and below: this is the exchange between *kan* 坎 (dark abyss) and *li* 離 (bright flame).[97]

This reflects the predominance of the classification by six based on the system of sexagesimal correspondences (see table 4.4), which is not new: a number of gentlemen in possession of techniques (*fangshi* 方士) and proponents of certain Daoist currents of thought also used a system based on the number six[98] rather than the system of the Five Phases which, when it became established under the Han, over-shadowed the earlier system, of which no more than a few traces remain in the *Suwen*. In truth, when the system of the theoretical bases of medicine became established under the Han, the fusion of the systems of correspondence between the Five Phases and the six *yin/yang* modalities gave prominence to the system of the Five Phases.[99] In the system of the five circulatory phases and the six influences, by contrast, it is the sexagesimal cycle and the sexagesimal system that predominate.

The separation of the kidneys into two is commonly adopted in the medical sources of the Song and later periods. To cite but one example, the *Hua Tuo xuanmen neizhao tu* 華佗玄門內照圖 (Illustrated Text of the Inner Brightness of the Mysterious School

---

[96] This presentation thus returns to the correlations between the six climatic influences and the Five Phases, according to the system of the circulatory phases and the seasonal influences (see table 4.4). These differ from the relations between the phases and the *yin/yang* modalities used in acupuncture, in which the channel of the kidneys is a *shaoyin* channel. There it is the organ coupled with the kidneys, namely the bladder, that corresponds to the *taiyang*. The *shaoyang* modality corresponds to the channel of the triple burner (*sanjiao*).

[97] *Mengqi bitan, juan* 7, art. 136, 317.   [98] Despeux (1994), 110.

[99] Despeux and Obringer (1997), 27–42.

of Hua Tuo)[100] runs as follows on the subject of the gate of life: 'The viscera are single, only the kidneys are double. The left one is the kidney, and corresponds to water; the right one is the gate of life, and corresponds to fire. Similarly [for the cardinal points], the animals that correspond to the north are double: the tortoise and the snake. The tortoise is a *yin* animal, the snake a *yang* animal.'[101]

This innovation prompted lengthy debates on the localization of the gate of life, its role, and its relation to water or to fire.

An innovation in therapeutics

In the eleventh and twelfth centuries, the application of the circulatory phases and the seasonal influences was manifest above all in the domain of pharmacotherapy. It prompted a systematization of correspondences in the *materia medica*, in the principles underlying the interrelations between the drugs and the formulae in which they were used. In the case of certain pathologies at least, the establishment of a prescription for a pathology was based on a more sophisticated theoretical system that combined correspondences with the five circulatory phases and the six influences. The system furthermore made it possible to pick out a selection of prescriptions that could be used equally well for their prophylactic or for their therapeutic effects, depending on the circuit phase of the year. That is precisely what Chen Yan does in his *Sanyin fang*: he lists ten formulae to be prescribed in accordance with the celestial stem of the year on the basis of which the annual circulatory phase is defined, and six formulae that correspond to the six influences. For example:

> In each of the *ren* years, wood is excessive, the influence of wind circulates abundantly and propagates itself, and the earth of the spleen receives the pathogenic agent. People then suffer from diarrhoea, lack of appetite, heaviness in the body, worried and angry spirits, and engorgement of the bronchi and the flanks. In graver cases, the patient is easily enraged, and suffers from dizziness and epileptic fits. There is an inversion of metal, and this provokes aches in the flanks and vomiting. In even graver cases, the pulse in the *chongyang* 重陽 (double *yang*) fails, and death ensues.[102] *Decoction of Magnolia and Atractylodes* (*Lingzhu tang* 苓術湯): this treats symptoms due to wind affecting the spleen and stomach; diarrhoeas, intestinal disorders, rumblings in the bowels, congestion of the abdomen, heaviness and stagnation of energy in the limbs, sudden rushes of anger, vertigo and dizziness, fainting fits, and sometimes unilateral aches in the left flank.[103]

---

[100] Ma Jixing (1990), 137–9.   [101] *Hua Tuo xuanmen neizhao tu, juan* 1, 40.
[102] Apart from a few variants, this text is identical to a passage in the *Suwen, juan* 20, *pian* 69, 366.
[103] *Sanyin fang, juan* 5, 64.

Although Chen Yan returns to the theoretical description of the *Suwen*, he is innovative in so far as he uses that description to introduce a prescription that tallies with the classification of the circulatory phases and the seasonal influences. This reference to prescriptions based on the circulatory phases of the years is also to be found in the *Taiyi ju zhuke chengwen ge* 太醫局諸科成文格 (Composition Models for the Various Departments of the Imperial Bureau of Medicine) of 1212, a work containing dissertation examples for candidates in the Imperial medical examinations. Each of the nine *juan* ends with a section on the five circulatory phases and the six influences, presenting an analysis of how the system works, corresponding symptoms, prescriptions, and an explanation of the composition of the formula. For example, in *jiazi* 甲子 years, one needs to prescribe Aconite decoctions (*Fuzi tang* 附子湯),[104] in *gengwu* 庚午 years, Magnolia decoctions (*Houpu tang* 厚樸湯).[105]

The principles governing the elaboration of formulae became more complex, efforts were made to check their efficacy, and the principles of systematic correspondences were extended to pharmacotherapy.[106] Before the Song, the constitution of formulae had been founded essentially on the principles expounded in the preface to the *Shennong bencao jing* 神農本草經 (Canon of the Divine Husbandman's *Materia Medica*), which outlined combinations between sovereign drugs (*jun* 君), minister drugs (*chen* 臣), and finally assistant drugs (*zuoshi* 佐使). Account was also taken of the principles of compatibility and incompatibility between the drugs (*qing* 情) indicated by Tao Hongjing 陶弘景 (456–536), in accordance with seven kinds of relations between them: the single drug (*danxing* 單行), drugs that help each other (*xiangxu* 相須), that assist each other (*xiangshi* 相使), that fear each other (*xiangwei* 相畏), that detest each other (*xiangwu* 相惡), that oppose each other (*xiangfan* 相反), that annihilate each other (*xiangsha* 相殺).[107] The drugs were chosen on the basis of either symptomatic indications listed in the *materia medica* or their type of action (sudorific, emetic, purgative, regulatory), or their flavour, selected according to the system of correlation between the Five Phases, or the fact that their quality complemented that of the symptoms (e.g. a cold quality for a symptom of heat). The system of the five circulatory phases and the six influences provided new theoretical bases for the choice of drugs, since flavours and qualities were no longer selected on the basis of the system of the Five Phases or a principle of complementarity, but instead on the basis of the relations established between the circulatory phases, the seasonal influences, and the flavours and qualities. Although these methods were defined in chapter 69 of the *Suwen*,[108] no example of their application has survived from any period earlier than the Song, and methods applied after the Song

---

[104] *Taiyi ju zhuke chengwen ge, juan* 1, 29.   [105] *Taiyi ju zhuke chengwen ge, juan* 4, 20.
[106] Unschuld (1985), 167.   [107] This classification is also used in the *Qianjin yaofang, juan* 1, 5a.
[108] *Suwen, juan* 20, *pian* 69.

period are far from unified, for each proceeds according to its own principles, in an inno-vatory fashion.[109]

This system of correspondences reinforcing the relations between ailments and temporal or climatic elements favoured the integration into the pharmacotherapy of ideas and techniques that previously had essentially served acupuncture. Thus the sudorific actions and others mentioned above were now effected by actions of sup-plementing (*bu* 補) or discharging (*xie* 瀉), actions formerly used only in acupuncture. Furthermore, the *materia medica* now noted a new characteristic in its drugs: namely, their clearly defined affinity with a precise channel (*guijing* 歸經). For, given that plants were classified according to their flavour's particular action on one or other of the six influences, it took but a step to attach these drugs to channels corresponding to the six *yin/yang* modalities of the six influences. This affinity with a channel is, it is true, not attested until the Yuan period, in the *Tangye bencao* 湯液本草 (*Materia Medica of Decoctions and Liquors*) by Wang Haogu 王好古 (b. 1200), who was a disciple of Zhang Yuansu 張元素 (twelfth century) and of Li Gao 李杲 (1180–1251),[110] and a contemporary of Liu Wansu. The new rules for the composition of the formulae that he drew up subsequently came to be very influential.

This system of circulatory phases and seasonal influences also lay at the origin of the classification of the formulae into seven categories: major formulae (*dafang* 大方), minor formulae (*xiaofang* 小方), formulae of gentle action (*huanfang* 緩方), formulae of rapid action (*jifang* 急方), odd formulae (*qifang* 奇方), even formulae (*oufang* 偶方), and doubled formulae (*fufang* 復方). The choice between them depended on the nature of the therapeutic action envisaged. All this is expounded in detail in the chapters devoted to the circulatory phases and the seasonal influences in the *Suwen*.[111] The classification is also discussed by Zhang Congzheng in his *Rumen shiqin*.[112]

It is not easy to assess the practical diffusion and application of these new principles. To do so it would be necessary to analyse the prescriptions given in the various works to see how far they conform with the principles. The task is made all the more difficult by the fact that the collections of prescriptions of the Song period do not mention the pro-cedure that resulted in the composition of the formulae, and in their prefaces the system of the circulatory phases and the seasonal influences is referred to only occasionally,[113] even in the rare descriptions of clinical cases. One example is to be found in a work by

---

[109]   *Suwen rushi yunqi lun'ao, juan* 3, 21b.

[110]   In his preface to the *Tangye bencao*, Wang Haogu states that he was a disciple of Li Gao. On that trea-tise, see U. Unschuld (1972).

[111]   *Suwen, juan* 22, *pian* 74, 472.   [112]   *Rumen shiqin, juan* 1, 1–5.

[113]   See *Boji fang* 博濟方, preface of 1047, which begins as follows: 'Between the sky and the earth, the circulatory phases and the cycles occur according to the numbers of birth and growth thanks to the Five Phases.'

Zhang Congzheng who, in a case of leprosy, suspends treatment and waits for the propitious moment in order to benefit from the best conjunction of circulatory phases and seasonal influences.[114]

Curiously enough, the use of the system of the circulatory phases and the seasonal influences is not mentioned in the principal Song works specializing in acupuncture, such as the *Zhenjiu tongren jing* 針灸銅人經 (The Bronze Man Canon of Acupuncture and Moxibustion) (1026) by Wang Weiyi 王惟一 (*ca* 987–1067) or the *Zhen-jiu zishengjing* 針灸資生經(Canon on the Increase of Life by Acupuncture and Moxibustion) (1220) by Wang Zhizhong 王執中[115] (*jinshi* in 1169). The latter simply repeats the prohibitions against needling patients of particular ages and prohibitions against needling on certain days – prohibitions already expounded in the Tang period by Sun Simiao in his *Qianjin yaofang* 千金要方 (Essential Prescriptions Worth a Thousand).[116] Apart from the seven chapters of the *Suwen*, only the works specializing in the circulatory phases and the seasonal influences apply the principles of the system to acupuncture, giving examples of acupunctural instructions and rules governing the choice of the points at which to needle, rules that are based on taking account of the weather and the symptoms to be treated, which are interpreted on the basis of the correlations in the system. The *Suwen rushi yunqi lun'ao* certainly stresses the importance of making a judicious choice of the points to puncture on the basis of the theory of the circulatory phases and the seasonal influences, although it provides no precise examples.[117] And the *Suwen liuqi Xuanzhu miyu*, for its part, describes a prophylactic method of acupuncture designed to counter possible disorders in the cycle depending on the time of year. For example:

> In the twelfth month . . . when wood is in danger of being excessive, it is necessary to disperse [the *qi*] at the source point, that is to say at the *taichong* 太沖 point, the source for the liver. The needle, inserted three-tenths of the way as far as the *yang* position, is left in place for the duration of three exhalations (three is the number for that which is produced by wood). It is then inserted five-tenths of the way (five is the number for the needs of wood). In this way the celestial influence is attracted and the terrestrial influence is obtained. The wood of the liver is thus dispersed so as not to dominate the earth. The drugs used are those of bitter taste and neutral quality . . . In the third month, one disperses [the *qi*] at the source point of the heart . . . that is to say at the *duigu* 兌骨 point . . . In the fifth month, one disperses at the source point of the spleen, at the *taibai* 太白 point . . . In the ninth month one disperses at the source point of the kidneys, at the *taixi* 太溪 point.[118]

---

[114] *Rumen shiqin, juan* 1, case 6, 1–5.   [115] His style was Quanshu 權叔.

[116] *Zhenjiu zisheng jing, juan* 2, 9–10 and 12–13; on the prohibitions of Sun Simiao, see Despeux (1987), 58–62 and 201–10.

[117] *Suwen rushi yunqi lun'ao, juan* 3, 31.   [118] *Suwen liuqi Xuanzhu miyu, juan* 1, 5a.

The *Huangdi neijing Suwen yipian* applies the system of the circulatory phases and the seasonal influences solely to acupuncture, proposing therapeutic acupunctural instructions for epidemic diseases in particular. The choice for needling is made by taking into account the classification of certain points of acupuncture situated at the extremities of the limbs such as the points of the well, of nourishment, of transportation, of regulation, of convergence, and of the source. These categories of points are already mentioned in the *Zhenjiu jiayi jing* 針灸甲乙經 (The ABC of Acupuncture and Moxibustion) (after 256) by Huangfu Mi 皇甫謐 (who died in about 281), where they correspond to the Five Phases. The basic principle is thus readopted, but this time by having the points correspond to the system of the five circulatory phases.

In later sources, acupunctural recommendations connected with the circulatory phases and the seasonal influences become more rare, although some are to be found in Ming works on acupuncture such as the *Zhenjiu juying* 針灸聚英 (Anthology of Acupuncture and Moxibustion) (1527) and the *Zhenjiu dacheng* 針灸大成 (Great Compendium of Acupuncture and Moxibustion) (1601). That rarity is without doubt due to the fact that, in acupuncture, a similar system to that of the five circulatory phases and the six influences supplanted the latter: the new system was 'the procedure consisting of choosing points on the basis of the terrestrial branches' (*ziwu liuzhu fa* 子午流注法). Although the earliest titles relating to this technique appeared in the tenth century, the earliest surviving work is later, dating only from the thirteenth century.[119] It is therefore difficult to evaluate the links between it and the system of the five circulatory phases and the six influences. The technique of the new system consisted in choosing the points of acupuncture on the basis of the five categories of points also used in the system of the circulatory phases and the seasonal influences, and correlations established with cyclical signs, taking into account the hourly, monthly, and annual period. The system is different from the system for calculating the circulatory phases and the seasonal influences, but it stems from a similar procedure of choosing elements on the basis of temporal correlations and speculations on celestial stems and terrestrial branches.

Conclusion

The system of the five circulatory phases and the six influences appears as an innovation under the Northern Song, serving as a basis for medical reflection on aetiopathogeny, physiological processes, and therapeutic applications, even though its beginnings can be traced back to the chapters of the *Suwen* that are attributed to Wang Bing or even further, to techniques of divinatory calculations used in the *nayin* and the *dunjia*

---

[119] On the development of the *ziwu liuzhu* technique, see Lu and Needham (1980), 137–8.

systems, attested as early as the time of Ge Hong. The system nevertheless appears as an innovation under the Northern Song, since it is the basis for reflection on aetiopathogeny, physiological mechanisms, and therapeutic applications.

It is clear that initially the system was used for prognosis rather than for therapy and so was also used in a non-medical context. Thanks to it, Shen Gua was able to predict that it was going to rain; and a work of geomancy also refers to it. In the field of medicine, it is not until the tenth century, with the *Qixuan zi jiyong jing*, that we find detailed prescriptions for every disorder due to the irregularities of the five circulatory phases and the six influences. But despite the close links between this system and astro-calendary calculations, and despite a noticeable Daoist connotation in the earliest texts on the subject, the system came to full blossom in the context of cosmological specula-tion under the Northern Song. The quest for models to explain the mechanisms of the universe was in full swing. The idea that a unity underpinned all phenomena and guided the workings of nature was predominant. It was known variously as the Great Ultimate, the Ultimate Non-Being, and the August Ultimate. In the system of the five circulatory phases and the six influences applied to medicine, people refer to the Mysterious Mechanism (*xuanji* 玄機). In the analysis of the way in which this mechanism worked, a distinction based on calculations was established between regular elements and chang-ing elements. Using calculations as a basis made it possible to apprehend things from outside and to reach greater precision in one's knowledge of the celestial principle, and this in its turn gave access to the ultimate principle of things.

But calculations on their own were not enough. It was also necessary to know how to interpret them and verify the correctness of theories against facts. Here again, it was not a matter of being content to compare theories and facts, for sometimes the facts seemed to contradict the theory, but this did not necessarily mean that the latter was wrong. This is illustrated both by Shen Gua, who shows how theory enables one to pass beyond appearances if, that is, one knows how to reason, and also by an anecdote recorded at the end of the *Suwen rushi yunqi lun'ao*, in which the facts appear to contradict the system for the simple reason that the interlocutor did not make an adequate analysis.

The system of the five circulatory phases and the six influences clearly found a lim-ited application, being chiefly used in the treatment of epidemic diseases, for prophy-lactic and therapeutic purposes. It was in the context of the concern regarding the treatment for epidemic diseases and their relation to seasonal disorders that, in the Song period, the *Shanghan lun* became fashionable: many commentaries on this work now referred to the system of the circulatory phases and the seasonal influences.

Thus the system of the five circulatory phases and the six influences did take over constant elements from traditional medicine, but the complexity of the correlated elements no doubt made it easier to recognize certain clinical realities, and to introduce innovations into various domains of medicine (aetiology, physiology, diagnostics, and therapy) without overturning earlier systems. This provides a good example of the way in which certain innovations, far from breaking with the past, made use of it and reinterpreted it, using new elements. The adoption of this system did not bring about a break with the systems of correspondence between the Five Phases and the six *yin/yang* modalities established under the Han. The example of the doubling of the kidney and of fire itself shows clearly that the new network of correlations did not completely do away with and replace the system of the Five Phases.

References to premodern Chinese and Japanese works

Baopu zi 抱扑子 (The Book of Master Holding to Simplicity). Ge Hong 葛洪. Jin, fourth century, preface of 1049. Cited from the *Baopuzi neipian jiaoshi*, annotated by Wang Ming 王明. Zhonghua shuju 中華書局, Beijing, 1980.

Bencao buyi 本草補遺 (Supplement to *Materia Medica*). Pang Anshi 龐安時. Song, late 11th century. *Siku quanshu* 四庫全書.

Beiji qianjin yaofang 備急千金要方, see *Qianjin yaofang* 千金要方.

Bishu sheng xubiandao siku que shumu 秘書省續編道四庫闕書目 (Catalogue of the Books Missing from the Four Storehouses). Compiled by the Imperial Library as a Continuation of the Comprehensive Catalogue of the [Books held in the Office of the] Exaltation of Literature (*Chongwen zongmu* 崇文總目). Song, 1145. *Siku quanshu* 四庫全書.

Boji fang 博濟方 (Prescriptions to Save the Greatest Number). Wang Gun 王滾. Song, preface of 1047. *Siku quanshu* 四庫全書.

Bu bitan 補筆談 (Supplement to the *Mengqi bitan*), see *Mengqi bitan* 夢溪筆談.

Chaoshi bingyuan 巢氏病源 (The Origins of Diseases According to Master Chao), see *Zhubing yuanhou lun* 諸病源候論.

Chushi yishu 褚氏遺書 (Books bequeathed by Master Chu [Cheng]). Apocrypha attributed to Chu Cheng 褚澄, of the Southern Qi. Song, 1126. *Siku quanshu* 四庫全書.

Daoshu 道樞 (Pivot of the Way). Zeng Zao 曾慥. Song, *ca* 1150. *Daozang* 道藏1017 (fasc. 641–8).

Daozang 道藏 (Daoist Canon). Ming, 1444. Xinwenfeng chubanshe 新文奉出版社, Taibei, 1977. The numbers indicated follow the concordance of Professor Kristofer Schipper.

Dongpo zhilin 東坡志林 (Forest of the Aspirations of Su Dongpo). Su Dongpo 蘇東坡. Song, 1265–74. Huadong shifan daxue chubanshe 華東師範大學出版社, Shanghai, 1983.

Gujin tushu jicheng 古今圖書集成 ([Imperially Commissioned] Compendium of Literature and Illustrations, Ancient and Modern). Chen Menglei 陳夢雷 et al. Qing, 1726. Wenxing shudian 文行書店, Taibei, 1964.

Huangdi neijing Suwen 黃帝內經素問 (Basic Questions of the Yellow Emperor's Inner Canon). Commentary by Wang Bing 王冰. Tang, 762. *Sibu congkan* 四部叢刊. Reproduced by Xuanfeng chubanshe 旋風出版社, Taibei, 1974.

Huangdi neijing Suwen yipian 黃帝內經素問遺篇 (Recovered Chapters of the Basic Questions in the Yellow Emperor's Inner Canon). Liu Wenshu 劉溫舒. Song, late 11th century. *Daozang* 道藏1021 (fasc. 663–4).

Huangdi neijing Taisu 黃帝內經太素 (Grand Basis of the Yellow Emperor's Inner Canon). Yang Shangshan 楊上善. Tang, 666/683. *Siku quanshu* 四庫全書.

Huangji jingshi 皇極經世 (The Governance of the World by the August Ultimate). Shao Yong 邵雍. Song, 1071–77. *Daozang* 道藏1040 (fasc. 705–18) and *Siku quanshu* 四庫全書.

Hua Tuo xuanmen neizhao tu 華佗玄門內照圖 (Illustrated Text of the Inner Brightness of the Mysterious School of Hua Tuo). Attributed to Hua Tuo 華佗. Song, 1095. Reprinted by Sun Huan 孫煥 in 1273 with illustrations by Yang Jie 楊介. Facsimile of *Daozang jinghua* 道藏精華, vol. XIV (2). Ziyou chubanshe 自由出版社, Taibei, 1976.

Ishinpō 醫心方 (Essential Medical Prescriptions). Tambano Yasuyori 丹波康賴. 984, first published 1860. Xinwenfeng chubanshe 新文奉出版社, Taibei, 1976.

Jianyao jizhong fang 簡要濟眾方 (Simple Prescriptions to Save People). Anon. Song, ordered by the Emperor in 1051. *Siku quanshu* 四庫全書.

Jin shu 晉書 (History of the Jin). Fang Xuanling 房玄齡 et al. Tang, 646–48. Zhonghua shuju 中華書局, Beijing, 1974.

Jiutian xuannü qingnang haijiao jing 九天玄女青囊海角經 (Blue Sack Sea Horn Canon of the Mysterious Girl of the Nine Heavens). Anon. Song. *Gujin tushu jicheng* 古今圖書集成, *Yishu dian* 藝術典, *juan* 651, *Kanyu bu* 堪輿部 1, 1–10b.

Junzhai dushu houzhi 郡齋讀書後志 (Monograph on the Books Studied in the Studio of the Commandery). Chao Gongwu 晁公武. Song, 1151. *Siku quanshu* 四庫全書.

Leizheng puji benshi fang 類證普濟本事方 (Classified Prescriptions for Fundamental Events and of Universal Benefit). Xu Shuwei 許叔微. Song, 12th century. *Siku quanshu* 四庫全書.

Linchuan xiansheng wenji 臨川先生文集 (Literary Collection of the Lord of Linchuan). Wang Anshi 王安石. Song, 1140. Based on the 1560 edition. *Sibu congkan* 四部叢刊.

Lingbao bifa 靈寶秘法 (Secret Procedures of the Magic Jewel). Anon. Song. *Daozang* 道藏 1191 (fasc. 874). Full title: *Michuan Zhengyang zhenren Lingbao bifa* 秘傳正陽真人靈寶秘法 (Secret Procedures of the Magic Jewel of the Perfect One of Correct Yang, Secretly Transmitted). Transl. Baldrian-Hussein 1981.

Lingshu jing 靈樞經 (Divine Pivot). Anon. Han. *Sibu congkan* 四部叢刊. Reproduced by Xuanfeng chubanshe 旋風出版社, Taibei, 1974.

Longshu lun 龍樹論 (Treatise of Nāgārjuna), see *Longshu yanlun* 龍樹眼論.

Maijing 脈經 (Classic on the Pulse). Wang Xi 王熙. Jin, late 3rd century. Based on the Yuan edition of 1327. Shiyi shuju 世一書局, Tainan, 1977.

Mengqi bitan 夢溪筆談 (Dream Pool Essay). Shen Gua 沈括. Song, before 1095. Cited from the *Mengqi bitan jiaozheng*, annotated by Hu Daojing 胡道靜. 2 vols. Shanghai guji chubanshe 上海古籍出版社, Shanghai, 1987.

Nanjing 難經 (Canon of Difficult Issues). Anon. Han, 2nd century AD. Cited from the *Nanjing buzhu* 難經補注, commentated by Ding Deyong 丁德用. Song, between 1056 and 1063. *Sibu beiyao* 四部備要, Taibei, 1973. This edition also contains the commentaries by Lü Jiang 呂江 (3rd century), and Yang Xuancao 楊玄操 (7th–8th centuries).

Nanjing jieyi 難經解義 (Commentaries on the Canon of Difficult Issues). Pang Anshi 龐安時. Song, late 11th century. *Siku quanshu* 四庫全書. Transl. Unschuld 1986.

Neijing Suwen lun'ao 內經素問論奧, see *Suwen rushi yunqi lun'ao* 素問入式運氣論奧.

Qianjin yaofang 千金要方 (Prescriptions Worth a Thousand). Sun Simiao 孫思邈. Tang, after 652. Based on a facsimile of a Southern Song edition preserved in Japan. Renmin weisheng chubanshe 人民衛生出版社, Beijing, 1982. Transl. Despeux 1987.

Qianjin yifang 千金翼方 (Appended Prescriptions Worth a Thousand). Sun Simiao 孫思邈. Tang, 681. Based on a facsimile of the Yuan edition of 1307. Renmin weisheng chubanshe 人民衛生出版社, Beijing, 1982.

Rumen shiqin 儒門事親 (A Means for Scholars to Serve their Relatives). Zhang Congzheng 張從正. Song, early 13th century. *Siku quanshu* 四庫全書.

Sanbu zhenjing 三部針經 (Canon of Acupuncture in Three Sections), see *Zhenjiu jiayi jing* 針灸甲乙經.

Sanyin fang 三因方, see *Sanyin jiyi bingzheng fanglun* 三因極一病證方論.

Sanyin jiyi bingzheng fanglun 三因極一病證方論 (The Three Causes Epitomized and Unified: the Quintessence of Doctrine on the Origins of Medical Disorders). Chen Yan 陳言. Song, 1174. Facsimile of the Song edition compiled in the Yuan. Renmin weisheng chubanshe 人民衛生出版社, Beijing, [1957] 1983.

Shangfang dadong zhenyuan miaojing tu 上方大洞真元妙經圖 (Illustrations of the Marvellous Canon of the True Origin of the Great Cave of the Upper Region). Anon. Song. *Daozang* 道藏 437 (fasc. 196).

Shanghan fawei lun 傷寒發微論 (Treatise on Developing the Subtleties of Cold Damage). Song. Xu Shuwei 許叔微. In *Xu Shuwei Shanghan lun zhu san zhong*. Based on Shiwanjuan lou congshu edition of 1881. Renmin weisheng chubanshe 人民衛生出版社, Beijing, 1993.

Shanghan zongbing lun 傷寒總病論 (Treatise on General Cold Damage Disorders). Pang Anshi 龐安時. Song, preface of 1100. *Siku quanshu* 四庫全書.

Shaoshi wenjian houlu 邵氏聞見後錄 (Later Annals on Facts Seen and Heard by Master Shao [Bowen]). Shao Bo 邵博. Song, early 12th century. *Xuejin taoyuan* 學津討原, 18th collection.

Shengji zonglu 聖濟總錄 (Sagely Benefaction Medical Encyclopaedia). Cao Xiaozhong 曹孝忠 et al. Song, 1117. Facsimile of the Yuan edition of 1300, Huagang chuban youxian gongsi 華岡出版有限公司, Taibei, 1978.

Shennong bencao jing 神農本草經 (Canon of the Divine Husbandman's *Materia Medica*). Anon. Han. *Sibu beiyao* 四部備要. Zhonghua shuju 中華書局, Taibei, 1970.

Siku quanshu 四庫全書 (Complete Works of the Four Storehouses). References to *Wenyuan ge Siku quanshu* 文淵閣四庫全書. Qing, 1782. Shangwu yinshuguan 商務印書館, Taibei, 1983.

Siku tiyao bianzheng 四庫提要辯證 (Discussion and Arguments Concerning the Principles of the Catalogue of the Four Storehouses). Yu Jiaxi 余嘉錫. 1937. Zhonghua shuju 中華書局, Hong Kong, 1974.

Song shi 宋史 (History of the Song). Attributed to Tuotuo 脱脱 (1313–55); written by Ouyang Xuan 歐陽玄 (1274/5–1358). Yuan, 1345. Zhonghua shuju 中華書局, Beijing, 1977.

Su Shen liangfang 蘇沈良方 (Excellent Prescriptions by Su Dongpo 蘇東坡 and Shen Gua 沈括). Su Dongpo 蘇東坡 and Shen Gua 沈括. Song, after 1126. *Siku quanshu* 四庫全書.

Suichutang shumu 遂初堂書目 (Catalogue of the Studio of Initial Success). You Mao 尤袤 (1127–93). Song. *Siku quanshu* 四庫全書.

Suwen 素問, see *Huangdi neijing Suwen* 黃帝內經素問.

Suwen bingji qiyi baoming ji 素問病機氣宜保命集 (Collection to Preserve Lives, on the Workings of Diseases and their Relations to the Influences according to the *Suwen*). Liu Wansu 劉完素. Jin, 1186. *Congshu jicheng* 叢書集成.

Suwen liuqi Xuanzhu miyu 素問六氣玄珠密語 (Secret Words of Master Mysterious Pearl on the Six Influences According to the *Suwen*). Attributed to Wang Bing 王冰. Song, 10th–11th centuries. *Daozang* 道藏 1023 (fasc. 665–667).

Suwen rushi yunqi lun'ao 素問入式運氣論奧 (Marvellous Introductory Remarks on the Theory of the Circulatory Phases and the Seasonal Influences According to the *Suwen*). Liu Wenshu 劉溫舒. Song, 1099. *Siku quanshu* 四庫全書.

Suwen xuanji yuanbing shi 素問玄機原病式 (Model on the Origin of Diseases and their Mysterious Workings According to the *Suwen*). Liu Wansu 劉完素. Jin, 1182. *Siku quanshu* 四庫全書.

Taiji tushuo 太極圖説 (Explanations to the Diagram of Ultimate Fate). Zhou Dunyi 周敦頤. Song, 11th century. Cited from *Zhou Dunyi ji* (Collected Works by Zhou Dunyi). Zhonghua shuju 中華書局, Beijing, 1990.

Taiping guangji 太平廣記 (Extended Notes on the Taiping Period). Li Fang 李昉 et al. Song, 978. Facsimile based on three editions, in particular the Ming edition of 1566. Zhonghua shuju 中華書局, Beijing, [1961] 1986.

Taiping shenghui fang 太平聖惠方 (Imperial Grace Formulary of the Taiping Period). Wang Huaiyin 王懷隱 et al. Song, 992. *Siku quanshu* 四庫全書.

Taishang jiuyao xinyin miaojing 太上九要心印妙經 (Marvellous Canon on the Mind Seal and the Nine Principles of the Most High). Attributed to Zhang Guo 張果. Late Tang or early Song. *Daozang* 道藏 225 (fasc. 112).

Taixuan jing 太玄經 (Canon of Supreme Mystery). Yang Xiong 楊雄. Han, 4 BC. Based on *Jizhu taixuan jing* 集注太玄經 (Collection and Commentary on the Canon of Supreme Mystery). Sima Guang 司馬光. Song, preface of 1082. *Daozang* 道藏 1183 (fasc. 860–862).

Taiyi ju zhuke chengwen ge 太醫局諸科成文格 (Composition Models for the Various Departments of the Imperial Bureau of Medicine). Anon. Song, preface by He Daren 何大任, written in 1212. *Siku quanshu* 四庫全書.

Tangye bencao 湯液本草 (Materia Medica of Decoctions and Liquors). Wang Haogu 王好古. Yuan, prefaces of 1298, 1306, 1308. *Siku quanshu* 四庫全書.

Tongren shuxue zhenjiu tujie 銅人輸穴針灸圖解 (Illustrated Explanations of Acupuncture and Moxibustion Pits according to the Bronze Man). Wang Weiyi 王惟一. Song, 1026. Facsimile by Zhonghua shuju 中華書局, Beijing, 1987.

Tongzhi 通志 (Comprehensive Treaty). Zheng Qiao 鄭樵 (1140–62). Song. Based on *Wanyou wenku* 萬有文庫 edition by Wang Yunwu 王雲五, Shangwu yinshu guan 商務印書館, Shanghai, 1936.

Wenxian tongkao 文獻通考 (Examinations of Documents and Writings). Ma Duanlin 馬端臨. Song, late 13th century. Based on Wanyou wenku 萬有文庫 edition by Wang Yunwu 王雲五, Shangwu yinshu guan 商務印書館, Shanghai, 1936.

Xuejin taoyuan 學津討原 (Search for the Origins Based on the Study of Mao jin's 毛晉's *Rarely Accessed Secret Books* 津逮秘書). Qing, 1802–6. Zhang Haipeng 張海鵬. Based on photolithographic reprint of 1831 edition. Shanghai guji chubanshe 上海古籍出版社, Shanghai, no date.

Yishuo 醫説 (Accounts of Medicine). Zhang Gao 張杲. Song, 1189. Based on a facsimile of 1933 of the Song edition that is stored in the library of the Shanghai Medical Institute. Shanghai kexue jishu chubanshe 上海科學技術出版社, Shanghai, 1984.

Yuhai 玉海 (Ocean of Jade). Wang Yingling 王應麟. Yuan, 1371. Facsimile. Huawen shuju 華文書局, Taibei, 1964.

Zhenjiu dacheng 針灸大成 (Great Compendium of Acupuncture and Moxibustion). Yang Jizhou 楊繼洲. Ming, 1601. Renmin weisheng chubanshe 人民衛生出版社, Beijing, 1973.

Zhenjiu jiayi jing 針灸甲乙經 (The ABC of Acupuncture and Moxibustion). Huangfu Mi 皇甫謐. Jin, after 256. Cited from the *Zhenjiu jiayi jing jiaoshi*. Based on Ming edition of 1601 of the *Gujin yitong zhengmai quanshu* 古今醫統正脈全書 (Compendium of the Orthodox Lineage of the Medical System, Ancient and Modern), by Wang Kentang 王肯堂. Renmin weisheng chubanshe 人民衛生出版社, Beijing, 1974.

Zhenjiu juying 針灸聚英 (Anthology of Acupuncture and Moxibustion). Gao Wu 高武. Ming, 1527. Xinya chubanshe 新亞出版社, Taibei, 1967.

Zhenjiu tongren jing 針灸銅人經 (Bronze Man Canon of Acupuncture and Moxibustion). Wang Weiyi 王惟一. Song, 1026. See *Tongren shuxue zhenjiu tujie* 銅人輸穴針灸圖解.

Zhenjiu zisheng jing 針灸資生經 (Canon on the Increase of Life by Acupuncture and Moxibustion). Wang Zhizhong 王執中. Song, 1220. *Siku quanshu* 四庫全書.

Zhouyi tu 周易圖 (The Illustrated Book of Changes of the Zhou). Anon. Song, after 1077. *Daozang* 道藏 157 (fasc. 69).

Zhubing yuanhou lun 諸病源候論 (Treatise on the Origins and Symptoms of Medical Disorders). Chao Yuanfang 巢元方 et al. Sui, 610. Renmin weisheng chubanshe 人民衛生出版社, Beijing, 1978.

Ziyang zhenren wuzhen pian jiangyi 紫陽真人悟真篇講義 (Explanations on the Enlightening Toward the Perfection of Perfected Master Ziyang). Xia Zongyu 夏宗禹; preface by Zhen Dexiu 真德秀 (1227) and Zhang Mizi 張密子 (1228). Song. *Daozang* 道藏 146 (fasc. 66).

References known from citations only

Dunjia jing 遁甲經 (Canon on the *dunjia* System). Anon. Cited in Wang Bing's 王冰 commentary on the *Suwen* 素問, *juan* 19, *pian* 66, 323.

Jingui yaolüe 金匱要略 (Essential Prescriptions in the Golden Casket), cited in the *Sanyin fang* 三因方.

Liujia tianyuan yunqi qian 六甲天元運氣鈐 (Small Bell on the Movements and Influences of Celestial Origin according to the Six *jia* Cyclical Signs). Zhao Conggu 趙從古. Song, 11th century. Cited in the *Tongzhi* 通志, *juan* 69, *Yiwenlüe* 藝文略 (7), 810b; and the *Bishu sheng xubiandao siku que shumu* 秘書省續編道四庫闕書目, *juan* 2, 83a.

Longshu yanlun 龍樹眼論 (Treatise on Ophthalmology from Nāgārjuna). Anon. Sui-Tang. Fragments preserved in the *Yifang leiju* 醫方類聚 and the *Ishinpō* 醫心方. Cited in the *Song shi* 宋史, *juan* 207, 5309.

Qingli shanjiu fang 慶歷善救方 (Prescriptions from the Qingli Period to Save the People). Anon. Song. Cited in the *Yuhai* 玉海, *juan* 63, 23b.

Qixuan zi yuanhe jiyong jing 啟玄子元和記用經 (Book on the Use of the Calendar of the Original Harmony according to Master Qixuan). Xu Ji 許寂. Five Dynasties, 889. Cited from the *Liuli zhai yishu* 六醴齋醫書 edition by Cheng Yongpei 程永培. Qing, 1794.

Qixuan zi tianyuan yuce 啟玄子天元玉冊 (Jade Tablets on the Celestial Origin by Master Qixuan). Anon. Song or earlier. Cited in the *Song shi* 宋史, *juan* 206, 5271.

Sanjia yunqi jing 三甲運氣經 (Book on the Movements and Influences According to the Three *jia* Cyclical Signs). Anon. Song or earlier. Cited in the *Tongzhi* 通志, *juan* 69, *Yiwen lüe* 藝文略 (7), 810b.

Shenshi liangfang 沈氏良方 (Excellent Prescriptions by Master Shen [Gua] 沈括). Lost. See *Su Shen liangfang* 蘇沈良方.

Taishi tianyuan yuce jiefa 太始天元玉冊截法 (Methods on the Jade Calendar on the Celestial Origin and the Supreme Beginning). Anon. Song or earlier. Cited in the *Songshi* 宋史, *juan* 207, 5275.

Tianyuan yuce 天元玉冊 (Jade Tablets on the Celestial Origin). Attributed to Qixuanzi 啟玄子 (the literary name for Wang Bing 王冰). Cited in the commentary on the *Suwen* 素問, *juan* 21, *pian* 71, 429, and in the *Wenxian tongkao* 文獻通考, *juan* 122, 1974.

Tianyuan yuce jiefa 天元玉冊截法 (Methods for the Jade Calendar according to the Celestial Origin). Cited in the *Guanwu waipian* 觀物外篇 edition, annotated by Zhang Xingcheng 張行成. *Siku quanshu* 四庫全書.

Tongshen lun 通神論 (Treatise of Marvellous Comprehension). Yang Kanghou 楊康候. Song, late 11th century. Cited in the *Junzhai dushu zhi* 郡齋讀書志, *juan* 2, 407.

Wuyun liuqi Yusuo zi jing 五運六氣玉瑣子經 (Book on the Five Circulatory Phases and the Six Influences by Master Yusuo). Anon. Song or earlier. Cited in *Tongzhi* 通志, *juan* 69, *Yiwenlüe* 藝文略 (7), 810c.

Wuyun zhizhang fu tu 五運指掌賦圖 (Illustrated Rhapsody to Control the Five Circulatory Phases). Ye Jie 葉玠. Song. Cited in the *Wenxian tongkao* 文獻通考, *juan* 122, 1974.

Yunqi lu 運氣錄 (Manuscript on the Circulatory Phases and the Seasonal Influences). Anon. Song or earlier. Cited in the *Suichutang shumu* 遂初堂書目, 73.

References to modern works

Arrault, Alain 1995. 'Shao Yong (1012–77). Cosmologie, histoire et poésie'. PhD thesis 'nouveau régime', with Kristofer Schipper. Université de Paris VII.

Alleton, Viviane and Volkov, Alexeï (eds.) 1994. *Notions et perceptions du changement en Chine.* Collège de France, Institut des Hautes Études Chinoises, Paris.

Baldrian-Hussein, Farzeen 1981. *Procédés du joyau magique*. Les Deux Océans, Paris.

Despeux, Catherine 1987. *Prescriptions d'acuponcture valant mille onces d'or. Traité d'acuponcture de Sun Simiao (VIIè siècle)*. Guy Trédaniel, Paris.

    1994. *Taoïsme et corps humain: le Xiuzhen tu*. Trédaniel, Paris.

Despeux, Catherine and Obringer, Frédéric 1990. 'Conceptualisation d'un état pathologique dans la médecine chinoise traditionnelle: Exemple de la toux'. *Revue d'Histoire des Sciences* 43 (1), 35–56.

    (eds.) 1997. *La maladie dans la Chine médiévale: la toux*. L'Harmattan, Paris.

Ding Guangdi 丁光迪 1987. *Jin Yuan yixue* 金元醫學 (Medicine of the Jin and Yuan). Jiangsu kexue jishu chubanshe, Nanjing.

Fan Xingzhun 範行準 1951. 'Wuyun liuqi shuo de laiyuan' 五運六氣説的來源 (Origins of the Doctrine of the Five Circulatory Phases and Six Influences). [*Zhonghua*]*Yishi zazhi* [中華]醫史雜志 3 (1), 3–14.

Fang Yaozhong 方藥中 and Xu Jiasong 許家松 1984. *Huangdi neijing Suwen yunqi qipian jiangjie* 黃帝內經素問運氣七篇講解 (Explanations on the Seven Chapters on Circulatory Phases and Seasonal Influences in the *Basic Questions* of the *Yellow Emperor's Inner Canon*). Renmin weisheng chubanshe, Beijing.

Fraser, J. T. et al. (eds.) 1986. *Time, Science and Society in China and the West: the Study of Time*. University of Massachusetts Press, Amherst.

He Shuangquan 何雙權 1989. 'Tianshui Fangmatan Qin jian zongshu' 天水放馬灘秦簡綜述 (Summary of the Qin Dynasty Slips Found at Fangmatan Near Tianshui). *Wenwu* 文物 2, 23–31.

Hsu, Elisabeth 1994. 'Change in Chinese Medicine: *bian* and *hua*; an Anthropologist's Approach'. In Alleton and Volkov, 41–8.

Hu Daojing 胡道靜 1980. '*Sushen neihan liangfang* Chu Shu pan 蘇沈內翰良方楚蜀判' (Distinguishing between the Prescriptions from the Lands of Shu and Chu in the *Excellent Prescriptions by Su Dongpo and Shen Gua*). *Shehui kexue zhanxian* 社會科學戰線 3, 195–209.

Hu Daojing 胡道靜 and Jin Liangnan 金良年 1988. *Mengqi bitan daodu* 夢溪筆談導讀 (Readers' Guide to the Dream Pool Essay). Ba Shu shushe, Chengdu.

Kalinowski, Marc 1983. 'Les instruments astro-calendériques des Han et la méthode Liu Ren', *Bulletin de l'Ecole Française d'Extrême-Orient* 72, 310–416.

    1991. *Cosmologie et divination dans la Chine ancienne: le compendium des cinq agents (Wuxing dayi, VIe siècle)*. Ecole Française d'Extrême-Orient, Paris.

Katz, Paul 1995. *Demon Hordes and Burning Boats: the Cult of Marshal Wen in Late Imperial Chekiang*. State University of New York Press, Albany.

Knaul, Livia 1981. *Leben und Legende des Ch'en T'uan*. Peter Verlag, Frankfurt.

Le Blanc, Charles and Blader, Susan (eds.) 1987. *Chinese Ideas about Nature and Society: Studies in Honour of Derk Bodde*. Hong Kong University Press, Hong Kong.

Li Congfu 李聰甫 and Liu Bingfan 劉炳凡 1983. *Jin Yuan sida yijia xueshu sixiang zhi yanjiu* 金元四大醫家學術思想之研究 (Researches on the Thought of the Four Great Schools of the Jin and Yuan). Renmin weisheng chubanshe, Beijing.

Liu Jie 劉杰 1990. *Zhongguo yunqi xue* 中國運氣學 (China's Doctrine of the Circulatory Phases and Seasonal Influences). Huanghe chubanshe, Jinan.

Loewe, Michael (ed.) 1993. *Early Chinese Texts: a Bibliographical Guide*. The Society for the Study of Early China, Berkeley.

Lu Gwei-djen and Needham, Joseph 1980. *Celestial Lancets: a History and Rationale of Acupuncture and Moxa*. Cambridge University Press, Cambridge.

Ma Jixing 馬繼興 1990. *Zhongyi wenxianxue* 中醫文獻學 (Study of the Chinese Medical Literature). Shanghai kexue jishu chubanshe, Shanghai.

Nylan, Michael and Nathan Sivin 1987. 'The first Neo-Confucianism: an Introduction to Yang Hsiung's *Canon of Supreme Mystery* (*T'ai hsüan ching, ca* 4 BC)'. In Le Blanc and Blader, 41–99. Revised version in Sivin 1995.

Okanishi Tameto 岡西為人 1977. *Song yiqian yiji kao* 宋以前醫籍考 (Researches on the Medical Sources to the Song). Facsimile by Nantian shuju, Taibei.

Porkert, Manfred 1974. *Theoretical Foundations of Chinese Medicine: Systems of Correspondence*. MIT Press, Cambridge, Mass.

Quan Yijing 權依經 and Li Minting 李民聽 1987. *Wuyun liuqi xiangjie yu yunyong* 五運六氣詳解與運用 (Applications of and Detailed Explanations on the Five Circulatory Phases and Six Influences). Gansu kexue jishu chubanshe, Lanzhou.

Rall, Jutta 1970. *Stand und Entwicklung der chinesischen Medizin. Chin und Yuan Zeit. Die vier grossen Medizinschulen der Mongolenzeit*. Franz Steiner, Wiesbaden.

Ren Yingqiu 任應秋 1971. *Wuyun liuqi* 五運六氣 (The Five Circulatory Phases and the Six Influences). Xianggang weisheng chubanshe, Hong Kong.

　　1982a. *Yunqi xueshuo* 運氣學説 (Doctrine of the Circulatory Phases and Seasonal Influences). Shanghai kexue jishu chubanshe, Shanghai.

　　1982b. '*Huangdi neijing* yanjiu shijiang' 《黃帝內經》研究十講 (Ten Lectures on Research on *The Yellow Emperor's Inner Canon*). In Ren Yingqiu and Liu Zhangling, 1–99.

　　1984. *Théorie des mouvements et des énergies: traduction intégrale du Yunqi xueshuo*. Transl. Pierre de la Robertie. Cercle sinologique de l'Ouest, Rennes.

Ren Yingqiu 任應秋 and Liu Zhangling 劉長林 (eds.) 1982. '*Neijing*' yanjiu luncong 《內經》研究論叢 (Collected Essays of Research on the *Inner Canon*). Hubei renmin chubanshe, Wuhan.

De la Robertie, Pierre and Timon, Gérard 1984. *Etude sur les Wu Yun Liu Qi: cinq mouvements et six énergies*. Cercle sinologique de l'Ouest, Rennes.

Schipper, Kristofer 1985. 'Seigneurs royaux, dieux des épidémies'. *Archives des sciences sociales des religions* 59, 31–40.

Sivin, Nathan 1993. 'Huang ti nei ching'. In Loewe, 196–215.

　　1995. *Medicine, Philosophy and Religion in Ancient China: Researches and Reflections.* Variorum, Aldershot.

Unschuld, Paul U. 1985. *Medicine in China: a History of Ideas*. University of California Press, Berkeley.

　　1986. *Nan-ching: the Classic of Difficult Issues*. University of California Press, Berkeley.

Unschuld, Ulrike 1972. 'Das *T'ang-yeh pen-ts'ao* und die Uebertragung der klassischen chinesischen Medizintheorie auf die Praxis der Drogenanwendung'. Dissertation in Sinologie, Ludwig-Maximilians Universität, München.

Verellen, Franciscus 1989. *Du Guangting (850–933): Taoïste de cour à la fin de la Chine médiévale*. Collège de France, Institut des Hautes Etudes Chinoises, Paris.

Wang Shifu 王士福 1958. 'Wuyun liuqi shuo qiyuan de shangtao' 五運六氣説起源的商討 (Discussion on the Origin of the Theory of the Five Circulatory Phases and the Six Influences). [*Zhonghua*]*Yishi zazhi* [中華]醫史雜志 9 (2), 127–131.

Wu Yiyi 1993–94. 'A Medical Line of many Masters: a Prosopographical Study of Liu Wansu and his Disciples from the Jin to the Early Ming'. *Chinese Science* 11, 36–65.

Yao Ruoqin 姚若琴 and Xu Hengzhi 徐衡之 1988. *Song Yuan Ming Qing mingyilei'an* 宋元明清名燦醫案 (Medical Case Records of Famous Physicians of the Song, Yuan, Ming, and Qing). Shanghai shudian, Shanghai.

Zhang Juying 章巨膺 1960. *Song yilai yixue liupai he wuyun liuqi zhi guanxi* 宋以來醫學流派和五運六氣之關係 (Relations between pre-Song Medical Lineages and the Five Circulatory Phases and the Six Influences). *Guangdong zhongyi* 廣東中醫 11, 125 ff.

Zhongyi renwu cidian 中醫人物辞典 1988. *Dictionary of Famous Personages in Chinese Medicine*. Shanghai cishu chubanshe, Shanghai.

PART III

Dietetics and pharmacotherapy

Introduction

Food and medicine have long been the subject of similar traditions of learning in China. Broths, composed of different ingredients, finely chopped and sliced, in order to be blended in carefully regulated amounts, provided, since the Han, a material medium through which people could enact the philosophical principles of systematic correspondence linking the bodily microcosm to the macrocosm at large. Ingredients were added, processed, and mixed according to considerations of season and weather, soil and water, or of the gender, social status, and individual constitution of the consumers; soups formed meals and also medicines.

Drug therapy, in manuscripts from early China, cannot always be clearly distinguished from the preparation of foodstuffs, magic, and demonology.[1] It was, according to Paul Unschuld, 'pragmatic', being grounded in empirical observation of particular instances of treatment rather than in an integrated theory of medical speculation, and existed alongside numerological systematics of canonical medical doctrine for a long time. While the *History of the Former Han* (Han shu 漢書) refers to *bencao* 本草 as a field of knowledge at various instances,[2] it was apparently not until the Liang and Tang that works on drug therapy formed a specialised literary genre which itself was called *bencao*.[3]

The *bencao* genre made the knowledge of drug therapy that had been developed in traditions which took the Divine Husbandman, Shennong 神農, as their patron more

---

[1] See for instance the recipes given in *Wushier bingfang* 五十二病方, translated by Harper, Donald (1998), *Early Chinese Medical Literature: the Mawangdui Medical Manuscripts*, Routledge, London, 221–304.

[2] See *Han shu*, *juan* 25B, 1258, and *juan* 92, 3706, Zhonghua shuju, Beijing, 1962.

[3] The word *ben* is probably best understood as a verb meaning 'to ground' or 'to be based on' and *cao* in this context refers to 'drugs' (*yao*) in general. In translation the *bencao* have been called 'pharmacopeias', a term which is misleading because it is generally used to describe a specialised kind of pharmaceutical literature that has the force of law and subjects drug traders to its rules; the generally accepted translation for *bencao* is now *materia medica*. See Unschuld, Paul U. (1986), *Medicine in China: a History of Pharmaceutics*, University of California Press, Berkeley, 5, 14, and 16.

accessible to Chinese medical doctors, who proclaimed themselves to be followers of the Yellow Emperor, Huangdi 黃帝. This led to the first government sponsored *materia medica*, the *Xinxiu bencao* 新修本草 (Newly Revised *Materia Medica*), which was compiled under the supervision of Su Jing 蘇敬 in the mid-seventh century. The government became even more involved with the publication of *bencao* literature as time progressed, and the Song which 'in various aspects of medicine received the greatest and most effective attention from the state in the entire history of the Chinese Empire' culminated in producing under the supervision of Tang Shenwei 唐慎微 (*ca* 1056–1136) the *Zhenglei bencao* 證類本草(*Materia Medica* Corrected and Arranged in Categories). The article on pharmacotherapy by Frédéric Obringer draws largely on this impressive compendium of state sponsored *bencao* literature.

Bencao works before and after the Song, however, were often the result of an outstanding individual's effort. Tao Hongjing 陶弘景 (456–536) of the Liang,[4] for instance, is renowned, after having spent seven or eight years as a Daoist recluse in the Mao mountains 茅山, for having compiled two different versions of Shennong's *materia medica*, the *Shennong bencao jing* 神農本草經 (*Materia Medica* Canon of the Divine Husbandman) and the *Bencao jingji zhu* 本草經集注 (Notes to the *Materia Medica* Canon), the latter laying the foundations for the above government-commissioned *Xinxiu bencao*. Sun Simiao 孫思邈 (581–682) is a personality of even greater significance, not only for the development of the *materia medica* and *materia dietetica*, as Ute Engelhardt suggests in the first article of this part, but also for innovation and elaboration of Chinese medical practice and doctrine in general.[5]

Engelhardt identifies in her article 'Dietetics in Tang China: Beginnings of a Specialised *Materia Dietetica*' Sun Simiao's chapter on 'Dietary Treatment' (*shizhi* 食治) as the first extant *materia dietetica*. Sun Simiao's student Meng Shen 孟詵 (621–713), author of *Prescriptions to Replenish and Nourish* (*Buyang fang* 補養方), is

---

[4] On Tao Hongjing, the 'virtual founder of Mao Shan Taoism', and his alchemy, see Strickmann, Michel (1979), 'On the Alchemy of T'ao Hung-ching', in Welch, Holmes and Seidel, Anna (eds.), *Facets of Taoism: Essays in Chinese Religion*, Yale University Press, New Haven, 123–92.

[5] Sun Simiao was deified particularly in popular circles as the 'king of drugs' (*yaowang* 藥王). He is also remembered for his concerns with medical ethics, not to speak of his achievements for acumoxa and other therapeutic practices. See Unschuld, Paul U. (1994), 'Der chinesische "Arzneikönig" Sun Simiao; Geschichte–Legende–Ikonographie: zur Plausibilität naturkundlicher und übernatürlicher Erklärungsmodelle', *Monumenta Serica* 42, 211–57; Unschuld, Paul U. (1979), *Medical Ethics in Imperial China: a Study in Historical Anthropology*, University of California Press, Berkeley; Despeux, Catherine (1987), *Prescriptions d'acuponcture valant mille onces d'or: Traité d'acuponcture de Sun Simiao (VIIe siècle)*, Guy Trédaniel, Paris. On his alchemy, see Sivin, Nathan (1968), *Chinese Alchemy: Preliminary Studies*, Harvard University Press, Cambridge, Mass.; for biographical notes, see pp. 81–144.

presented as the first person to write a complete work in the dietetic genre, and Meng Shen's work is known to have been expanded by his student Zhang Ding 張鼎 into the *Materia Medica for Successful Dietary Therapy* (Shiliao bencao 食療本草), the earliest work entirely devoted to 'dietary therapy' (*shiliao* 食療).

Engelhardt indicates that there are obvious affinities between the *materia dietetica* and the 'nurturing life' tradition, although there is a fundamental difference between the Daoist *yangsheng* 養生 ideal of abstaining from cereals and the basic principle of Chinese food systems that a meal should include both cereals and dishes, and she highlights this by citing one small but significant omission in a quotation of Sun Simiao's 'Dietary Treatment' chapter. She also traces how the new genre arose from Sun Simiao's assembling information from earlier works which included interdictions concerning foodstuffs (*shijin* 食禁). About eighty per cent of the foodstuffs discussed were taken from Tao Hongjing's *materia medica*, but Sun Simiao applied in parts a different framework for evaluating them: that of food interdictions found in Zhang Ji's 張機 (150–219) *Essentials and Discussions of Prescriptions of the Golden Casket* (*Jingui yaolüe* 金匱要略). By comparing the text passages on the waterchestnut (*jishi* 芰實) and horse meat (*marou* 馬肉) – one by Sun Simiao and one by Meng Shen – Engelhardt shows that Meng Shen contributed to the formation of the new genre mainly by adding simple prescriptions and drawing attention to cooking techniques.

The reason Sun Simiao himself gives for discussing foodstuffs separately from drugs is that the effects of foodstuffs were less dangerous than those of drugs. A physician should therefore first apply dietary treatment, and only after that is unsuccessful drug therapy. Engelhardt contextualises Sun Simiao's statement by pointing out that state control over medical practice increased during the Tang dynasty; she specifically points to the heightened awareness of the dangers of drug therapy and acupuncture, and considers this one factor that may have facilitated the rise of dietary therapy and moxibustion.

Chinese medical drugs (*yao* 藥) were more potent but also more dangerous. Frédéric Obringer's 'An Innovation of the Song in Pharmacotherapy: some Remarks on the Use of White Arsenic and Flowers of Arsenic' underlines just how dangerous and intoxicating Chinese medical drugs could be. Obringer discusses drugs such as *xionghuang* 雄黃 (As_2S_2), *yushi* 礜石 (various arsenic ores like FeAsS, As_2O_2, etc.), and *cihuang* 雌黃 (As_2S_3), all now identified as arsenical compounds, well known for their therapeutic efficacy since antiquity.

Obringer points out the replacement of the term *yushi* by *pishi* 砒石, a change noticeable in the *materia medica* of the Song, and already discernable in some Tang texts. This change of name is interpreted as reflecting that a change in mining techniques had taken place earlier (AD 973), and Obringer's analysis suggests that the sublimation and crystallisation of *pishi* (i.e. various arsenic ores like crystallised arsenolite, arsenopyrit,

erythrite, smaltite, cabaltite, etc.) allowed one to obtain a new drug called *pishuang* 砒
霜 (arsenious acid). This technological innovation, in turn, permitted an innovation in
medical practice. Arsenious acid (*pishuang*) was used mainly for treating intermittent
fevers (*nüe* 瘧 and *zhang* 瘴), and enjoyed popularity for about two centuries during the
Song. Its dangers had always been known; scholar-physician of the Yuan and Ming like
Zhu Zhenheng 朱震亨 (1281–1358) and Li Shizhen 李時珍 (1518–93) were increasingly critical of it on the grounds of its toxicity.

    Obringer is one of the only authors in this volume to raise the issue of therapeutic
efficacy, and he discusses how we might interpret past evaluations of drug use. But
efficacy alone is not sufficient to explain the disappearance of the arsenical compounds
from the therapeutic repertory. Obringer also identifies economic factors that may have
led to the decline of the technology for producing *pishuang*. Moreover, he raises the
matter of the impact of fashions and trends in the use of particular medical techniques:
Ming doctors, possibly in response to their clientele's demands, were apparently in
favour neither of violent drugs nor of external alchemy,[6] which may partly account for
pishuang's decline in popularity.

    The two articles in this section both discuss aspects of the *bencao* literature, but
they focus on very different facets of innovation. Engelhardt accounts for innovation
primarily by comparing two texts that discuss one and the same subject. Her analysis
highlights in particular the differences between these literary accounts, and these
differences are interpreted to indicate differences between literary genres. Engelhardt
mentions various earlier writings as possible precursors to this literary genre while,
notwithstanding that 'The earliest Chinese work devoted specifically to dietetic therapy
from which at least an extensive fragment has been preserved is the *Shiliao bencao*',[7]
her article emphasises the contribution of Sun Simiao to dietetics.

    The innovation discussed in Frédéric Obringer's article describes a change in a
particular technique of precipitating an arsenical compound, and it explores social and
epidemiological factors which may have led to the wide-spread use of this technique. It
also pertains to the question of 'technological choices' and shows that the 'meaning' or
'social logic' attributed to a technique cannot be neglected.[8] However, while the texts

---

[6] Chao Yuan-ling (1995), 'Medicine and Society in Late Imperial China: a Study of Physicians in
    Suzhou', PhD thesis in History, University of California, Los Angeles, 194–203.

[7] Unschuld (1986), 208.

[8] Lemonnier, Pierre (1993) 'Introduction', in Pierre Lemonnier (ed.), *Technological Choices:*
    Transformation in Material Cultures since the Neolithic, Routledge, London, explains that societies
    make use of certain techniques and technologies not always for technological reasons, but because of
    social and political considerations.

investigated cannot explain whether this technique was developed primarily for solving a technological problem or for specific social or political reasons, the article raises particularly saliently the question of how far a variation in practice seen by an outsider as innovative can be considered so if the insiders themselves do not attribute such a meaning to it. Obringer refers to text excerpts which indicate that this technique was used earlier, but his analysis proposes to consider it as an innovation only when the actors themselves recognised its specific identity and when the product it yielded was given a name. Obringer thereby addresses problems of nomenclatorial definition and the implications they may have for the actors' self-awareness.

5

Dietetics in Tang China and the first extant works of *materia dietetica*

UTE ENGELHARDT

The preoccupation with food and medicine has a long tradition in China. From the time of earliest civilisation in China, there has been a keen awareness of the effects of food on the body and the need for a balanced diet for the well-being of the individual.[1] At the same time, there developed a close relationship between nutrition and medicine which can be traced back at least as far as the third century BC.[2] In these early times no major distinction seems to have been made between the application of drugs and of foodstuffs, as can be testified for example in the 'Wushier bingfang' 五十二病方 (Fifty-two Prescriptions) found in the Han tomb no. 3 at Mawangdui, of which H. T. Huang says: 'The most interesting feature of the "Fifty-two Prescriptions" is that many of the concoctions used to cure ailments could easily pass as dishes eaten at a routine meal and we can learn a good deal about methods of cookery from the recipes used in their preparation.'[3]

In the Tang dynasty, however, one can discern a trend towards a differentiation between various genres of medical and culinary writings. It is from this period that the earliest known texts on dietetics originate. At the time it seems to have come to the first clear distinction between drug therapy and dietary therapy, reflected in the first appearance of the terms dietary treatment (*shizhi* 食治) and dietary therapy (*shiliao* 食療).[4] These Chinese terms refer to a notion of dietetics that is best understood as the knowledge about the effects of foodstuffs on the human organism and the application of this knowledge.

---

[1] As early as 1939 Lu Gwei-djen and Joseph Needham published in *Isis* the first article on Chinese dietetics, mainly focusing on dietary treatment of the beri-beri disease, reissued as Lu and Needham (1977).

[2] Harper (1984), 39–40.

[3] Huang (1990), 140. For the translation of the 'Wushier bing fang', see Harper (1982) and Harper (1998).

[4] As far as is known, both terms appeared for the first time in chapter 26 of Sun Simiao's *Qianjin fang*, in the title of the chapter, as well as in its preface; see below.

The genre of *materia dietetica*[5] clearly has its roots in the *materia medica* (*bencao* 本草) tradition[6] following the same description pattern concerning medicinal effectiveness. The content, however, may be characterised by its predominantly recording individual foodstuffs, regardless of whether they are used in a curative or preventive way.

This article explores the beginnings of dietary literature. First, the various indications of pre-Tang sources are mentioned, and then extant Tang texts that may well mark the beginnings of the ensuing tradition of *materia dietetica* are analysed. Finally, consideration is given to the extent to which these first dietary texts may be considered innovative.

Pre-Tang dietary texts

The bibliographic chapters of the *Han shu* 漢書 (History of the Former Han Dynasty), contain one work, the *Shennong Huangdi shijin* 神農黃帝食禁 (Shennong's and Huangdi's Nutritional Interdictions) in seven *juan*, that can be related to dietetics.[7] In contrast, in the section on medical books in the *Sui shu* 隋書 (History of the Sui Dynasty) the number of titles related to food or nutrition, mostly indicated by the word food (*shi* 食), has increased to between twenty and thirty titles.[8] Among these, titles referring to 'nutritional classics' (*shijing* 食經) are predominant (7), followed by 'nutritional recipes' (*shifang* 食方) (6) and then by 'nutritional interdictions' (*shijin* 食禁) (3). The two first terms, *shijing* (nutritional classics) and *shifang* (nutritional recipes) are common terms for culinary treatises or cookbooks and give no clues as to their dietary application. The term *shijin* (nutritional interdictions), however, seems to point to a possible medical dietary orientation, not least because book titles containing this term are often related to the cultural heroes and medical patrons Huangdi, the Yellow Lord, and Shennong, the Divine Husbandman.

As evidence for the hypothesis that *shijing* (nutritional classics) and *shifang* (nutritional recipes) are common terms for culinary treatises or cookbooks, the example of the quite famous *Cui Hao shijing* 崔浩食經 (Cui Hao's Nutritional Classic) written by Cui Hao 崔浩 (d. 450), which presented his mother's recollections of various foods and

---

[5] The term *materia dietetica* was first used by Buell (1989), 109 ff., although Buell does not define or explain this term explicitly.

[6] I agree with Sivin (1987), 179 ff., in translating the term *bencao* 本草 as *materia medica*, because unlike 'pharmaceutics' (Unschuld (1986), 14, who elsewhere translates *bencao* as *materia medica* too) or 'pharmacopoeia' (Bray (1989), 6) it does not prejudge direct comparison with the West, and includes the descriptions of natural products taken from flora, fauna, and mineralia. For an outline of the *materia dietetica* in English, see Unschuld (1986), 205–28.

[7] *Han shu, juan* 30, 1777.   [8] *Sui shu, juan* 34, 1043 ff.; Okanishi Tameto (1967), 1330 ff.

their preparation methods, may be cited. Only the preface of this book is extant[9] and, owing to its very concise and slightly ambiguous content, the work it represents has frequently been assigned to the category of dietary literature.[10] Since, however, some extracts of this work have been found in the primarily agricultural and gastronomical text *Qimin yaoshu* 齊民要術 (Essential Techniques for the Common People)[11] by Jia Sixie 賈思勰 of the sixth century, it may be assumed that 'Cui Hao's Nutritional Classic' did indeed concern itself mainly with the daily preparation of foods and not with the medical application of foodstuffs.[12]

A number of the above-mentioned titles contain the term *shenxian* 神仙 (immortal), for example *Shenxian fushijing* 神仙服食經 (Nutritional Classic for the Immortal's Intake),[13] which indicates a relation with the tradition of contemporary books on *yang-sheng* (養生 nourishing life), most of which unfortunately have been lost.

One of the most important early handbooks on nourishing life, the *Yangsheng yaoji* 養生要集 (Essential Compendium on Nourishing Life) compiled by Zhang Zhan 張湛 (fl. AD 370–80) seems to have disappeared early on, but was frequently cited in later Chinese and Japanese texts and could be reconstructed to some extent.[14] As far as is known from the reconstructed parts and fragments of this book, it must have included sections dealing with the cultivation of body (*xing* 形), mind (*shen* 神) and *qi* (氣), as well as sections on food, dwelling, behaviour to others, sexual techniques and medical treatment, which were the crucial points in the lifestyle of a would-be sage or immortal. As far as the section on food is concerned, the extant fragments indicate that it mostly included recommendations for the correct way of eating and drinking, along with nutritional prohibitions. It is quite possible that the section on food or the section on medical treatment also involved some descriptions of foodstuffs, for example for rice or sesame, following the description pattern of the *materia medica* (*bencao* 本草) tradition.[15] But these entries seem to have been integrated among many rules which an immortal had to follow in the pursuit of nourishing life. In contrast, the *materiae dieteticae* simply list descriptions of the effects of individual foodstuffs.

---

[9] In the biography of Cui Hao, *Wei shu* 魏書, *juan* 35, 807; Okanishi Tameto (1967), 1332; see translation by Unschuld (1986), 207.

[10] Okanishi Tameto (1967), 1332, and Unschuld (1986), 207–8.

[11] This text has been thoroughly worked on by Françoise Sabban; see Sabban (1993), 81, and Sabban (1990). See also Sabban (1986), 36, and Bray (1984), 55.

[12] Lu Yaodong (1993), 13–18.   [13] *Sui shu*, *juan* 34, 1049.

[14] Despeux (1990), Sakade Yoshinobu (1986), Barrett (1980), Stein (1999).

[15] *Chuxue ji* 初學記, *juan* 27, 660, and *juan* 27, 661; *Taiping yulan* 太平御覽, *juan* 839, 9b, and *juan* 841, 8a. See Despeux (1990), 7 ff.

Nevertheless, it was inevitable that correct diet should become a matter of great importance in an immortal's daily life. For the *yangsheng* (nourishing life) tradition, the most appropriate diet involved abstinence from all cereals, and the strict adherence to this diet became a characteristic mark of the would-be immortal.[16] As will be shown more clearly below, this abstinence from cereal contrasted sharply with the more medically oriented view of dietetics where the proper diet was considered to be mainly based on cereal and, generally, every foodstuff was allowed.

This short glimpse into the biographical chapters of the histories of the Han and Sui dynasties demonstrates that, before the Tang, it is very hard to judge merely from the title of a lost book whether it is a culinary treatise, a cookbook, or a dietary text. If, however, the text fragments are also taken into account, two different currents in the development of nutritional literature between the Northern Wei and the beginning of the Tang may be distinguished: one current emphasised food preparation and technological processing as represented by the *Cuihao shijing* or the *Qimin yaoshu* which can be considered the first extant gastronomic texts. Texts of this type indicate no interest in the therapeutic values of food but provide the reader with instructions as to how to overcome technical problems within food processing.[17] The other current can be related to the above-mentioned nourishing life (*yangsheng*) tradition and thus focuses on the therapeutic value of food and on appropriate diet as part of a religious striving.[18]

The first extant dietary text: Sun Simiao's chapter on dietary treatment

The eminent medical practitioner and author Sun Simiao 孫思邈 (581–682)[19] devoted one whole chapter of his *Beiji qianjin yaofang* 備急千金要方 (Prescriptions Worth a Thousand, for Urgent Need) to dietary treatment. He must have begun his famous compendium of medical knowledge around 650 and completed it by 652.[20] Chapter 26, entitled 'Dietary Treatment' (Shizhi 食治), forms an integrated whole and can be considered as the first small scale extant *materia dietetica*.[21] It can be divided into five parts, comprising a preface, followed by four sections describing the effects of fruits, vegetables, grains, and animals.

[16] See Levi (1983) and Engelhardt (1987), 157 ff.   [17] Sabban (1990), 2.
[18] For further details, see Shinoda Osamu (1987), 116.
[19] For a discussion of Sun's life dates, see Despeux (1987), 22; for Sun Simiao as legendary personage, see Unschuld (1994).
[20] Despeux (1987), 46.
[21] As Watanabe Kōzō (1987), 223–4, has shown, chapter 26 of the *Qianjin fang* 千金方 can be considered quite authentic and has been transmitted fairly directly.

In the preface to chapter 26, Sun explains his intentions in writing this dietary chapter:

> [Zhang] Zhongjing 仲景 said: for the human body to remain in balance and harmony, it is only necessary to ensure its proper nourishment. On no account should drugs be consumed recklessly. The strength of drugs is one-sided and there are occasions when they can be of help. But they lead to an imbalance of the *qi* in a man's *yin* orbs (*zang* 臟), and consequently an external affliction can easily be acquired.
>
> Living beings [lit. the species holding *qi* in their mouths (*hanqi zhi lei* 含氣之類)] all depend on food to maintain their life. But, at the same time, they are unaware of the fact that the consumption of food can bring positive and negative results. [Food is part of] the daily life of all people, but little is known about it. Water and fire are very near, but also difficult to comprehend! I regretted this and have therefore – whenever I had spare time from my other writings – compiled a treatise on dietary treatment [emphasising] the harms and benefits that can result from the five sapors (*wuwei* 五味), in order to pass on this information to our youth. All people should diligently follow [these teachings] and their influence will become more widespread.[22]

Sun describes the advantages of a dietary treatment in contrast to drug therapy, thereby intending to impart his dietary knowledge to all people, especially to the young. It is not yet clear, however, whether his text was aimed at ordinary people, religious adepts, or physicians.

One hint lies in the very first quotation he gives. This passage, beginning 'Zhongjing said', cannot be found in the extant works of Zhang Zhongjing 張仲景 (150–219). But, interestingly, it is quoted in the Japanese *Ishinpō* 醫心方 (Essential Medical Methods) compiled by Tambano Yasuyori (912–95), in a fragment beginning: 'The *Yangsheng yaoji* says: Zhang Zhongjing said: . . .' and closing with the remark: 'Only he who abstains from cereals can continually consume drugs.'[23] This suggests that Sun Simiao might have consciously left out the last sentence in order to eliminate from his own text the *yangsheng* idea of abstinence from cereals and to give the other statements of the text a more medical emphasis.

Sun clarifies his intentions in his preface a few passages later:

> Now, those who practise medicine must first of all recognise the origin of an illness and they must know which violations [have caused it]. Then they must treat it by dietary means. If dietary therapy does not cure the illness, only then can drugs be administered. The nature of drugs is hard and violent, just like that of

---

[22] *Qianjin fang, juan* 26, 464. Based on translation by Unschuld (1986), 209, with author's own amendments.

[23] *Ishinpō* 醫心方, *juan* 1, 15b.

imperial soldiers. Since soldiers are so savage and impetuous, how could any-
body dare to deploy them recklessly? If they are deployed inappropiately, harm
and destruction will result everywhere. Similarly, excessive damage is the consequence if drugs are thrown at illnesses.[24]

One possible reason for separating foodstuffs from all the other sorts of substances
gathered in the *materiae medicae* is given here by Sun himself. He points out that the
effects of foodstuffs are less dangerous than those of drugs. This is the reason why a
physician should first of all apply dietary treatment, and only when that fails should he
turn to the employment of drugs.

Heightened awareness of the dangers of drugs is also reflected in the strict official
regulations governing the use of medicinal drugs under the Tang. It was at this time that
the first official handbook of drugs, the *Xinxiu bencao* 新修本草 (Newly Revised
Materia Medica), was published by a government-sponsored commission and served as
the official basis for treatment by medical practitioners.[25] Moreover, the Tang penal
code, which is the first complete Chinese code extant, required a physician to follow the
fundamental prescriptions (*benfang* 本方) strictly and prescribed two and a half years of
state servitude if a patient died because a prescription was improperly composed; the
penalty was death by hanging if the patient happened to be the Emperor.[26] These laws
are the first known records of any fundamental regulations concerning the misuse of
medicinal drugs and, with slight amendments, they have been adopted in all subsequent
legislative texts.[27]

Similar special caution in the use of relatively dangerous methods of medical treatment capable of serious effects on the human organism is observable with respect to
acupuncture during Tang times. While acupuncture was judged to be too dangerous, the
benefits of moxibustion were emphasised.[28]

All this evidence reflects the tendency during Tang times towards medical methods
which do not represent too severe an intervention. This tendency can also be exemplified in the trend towards a distinction between *materia medica* and *materia dietetica*.

In the passages following the sections of his preface quoted above, Sun emphasises
the necessity of moderation in eating and drinking and gives various rather common
food interdictions. In particular, he quotes lengthy sections from the *Lingshu* 靈樞
(Divine Pivot), mostly chapters 56 and 63, and the *Suwen* 素問 (Basic Questions),

---

[24] My translation follows with slight variations Unschuld (1986), 209; *Qianjin fang, juan* 26, 464.
[25] See Unschuld (1986), 44 ff.
[26] *Tanglü shuyi* 唐律疏議, *juan* 9, 190; *juan* 25, 472; *juan* 26, 483. For translation, see Unschuld (1977),
   363, and Schafer (1963), 177.
[27] Unschuld (1977), 363 ff.   [28] Despeux (1987), 41–6.

Table 5.1. *The four sections of foodstuffs and drugs in Sun Simiao's chapter on dietary treatment*

Fruits (*guoshi* 果實)	29 entries
Vegetables (*caishu* 菜蔬)	58 entries
Cereals/rice (*gumi* 穀米)*	27 entries
Birds/quadrupeds (*niaoshou* 鳥獸)**	40 entries
Total	154 entries

* The section *gumi* includes wine (*jiu* 酒), vinegar (*cu* 酢), and salt (*yan* 鹽).

** The section *niaoshou* has as appendix on worms/insects/fish (虫魚 *chongyu*), including human milk (人乳汁 *ren ruzhi*).

chapters 10 and 22, in order to expound the correspondences between the five sapors, the human organism, the five grains, the *qi*, the orbs, and possible illnesses.[29] With these extracts from the medical classics, Sun seems to provide theoretical foundations enabling the reader to utilise the entries which follow in accordance with classical medical theory.

Moreover, it now becomes clear that Sun's target audience was physicians and young people (see above) desirous of becoming doctors rather than ordinary people interested in the everyday usage of those items. The fact that he quotes from texts like the *Suwen* and *Lingshu* which form the medical classic *Huangdi neijing* 黃帝內經 (Inner Canon of the Yellow Lord), names famous medical writers like Zhang Zhongjing and, in another quotation, Wang Shuhe 王叔和 (3rd century), would suggest that Sun Simiao strives to present his readers knowledge on dietetics in an unambiguously medical context.

The structure of the chapter on dietary treatment

The four sections of the 'Shizhi' chapter following the preface comprise a total of 154 entries on foodstuffs and drugs (see table 5.1).[30]

For a *materia dietetica*, such a grouping, according to origins, is the normal way and the one which most readily suggests itself according to *materia dietetica* tradition. This fourfold division appears in essence in the famous sentence on foodstuffs in the *Suwen* which Sun himself quotes in his preface:

[29] *Lingshu*, *pian* 63, 426 and *pian* 56, 412, *Suwen*, *pian* 10, 34 and *pian* 22, 73.

[30] I follow Lin Yi's edition mentioning the number for each section. There would be more entries, if for instance the jujube fruit, *Zizyphus jujuba* Mill., in its dried and fresh state was counted as two entries.

> The five grains provide nourishment (養 *yang*), the five fruits provide support (助 *zhu*), the [meats of the] five domestic animals provide augmentation (益 *yi*) and the five [sorts of] vegetables provide completion (充 *chong*), thus combining *qi* and sapors in the diet in order to replenish the essence and to augment the *qi*.[31]

Almost eighty per cent of Sun's 154 descriptions of foodstuffs or drugs come from the *Shennong bencao jing jizhu* 神農本草經集注 (Collected Commentaries on the Classic of the Divine Husbandman's *Materia Medica*) compiled by Tao Hongjing 陶弘景 (452–536) around AD 500.[32] Out of Tao Hongjing's total of 730 drug descriptions, Sun seems to have made a special selection of around 110 substances,[33] which can mostly be recognised as foodstuffs.

Within his listing of the entries according to their origins, Sun also followed Tao's division into three classes: upper class (*shangpin* 上品), middle class (*zhongpin* 中品), lower class (*xiapin* 下品), a characteristic of early *materia medica* works since the *Shennong bencaojing* 神農本草經 (Classic of the Divine Husbandman's *Materia Medica*), but he does not mention this division by classes explicitly. For example, Sun begins the section on cereals/rice with grains like Job's tears seeds (*yiyiren* 薏苡仁 Semen Coicis) and Sesame (胡麻 *huma, Sesamum indicum* L.) that appear in the upper class of the older *bencao* works, whereas vinegar (*cu* 酢) and salt (*yan* 鹽), the last entries in this section, are found in the lower class.[34]

In his descriptions of foodstuffs, Sun diverges sometimes from Tao's writings by giving a different corresponding sapor, especially for fruits. For instance, Sun describes grapes (葡萄 *putao*) and jujube fruits (大棗 *dazao*) as having sweet and pungent sapor (甘辛 *gan xin*), and lotus seeds (藕實 *oushi*) as having a bitter sapor (苦 *ku*), differing fundamentally from other known *bencao* works.

Forty-seven descriptions included in Sun Simiao's text mention the additional qualities of lubricating (*hua* 滑) or roughening (*se* 澀), which are lacking in Tao Hongjing's reconstructed text. It is noticeable that the highest proportion of the number of entries that relate to these qualities are to be found in the first section on fruits (16 out of 29); in the second section on vegetables relatively fewer (26 out of 58); in the third section on cereals/rice only four; while in the last section on birds/quadrupeds just one foodstuff, the liver of the rabbit (*tugan* 兔肝), that is described as 'roughening'.

Sun has also omitted some parts of his primary source *Bencao jing jizhu*, such as other names (*yiming* 異名) for the described foodstuff, native location (*chandi* 產地),

---

[31] See *Suwen, pian* 22, 44; *Qianjin fang, juan* 26, 465.
[32] For details of this text, see Unschuld (1986), 41–3.
[33] Watanabe Kōzō (1987), 225, counted 126 quoted descriptions, but I count only 110.
[34] See *Qianjin fang, juan* 26, 460, 461.

and harvesting time (*caiji* 採集). Instead he has added a selection of nutritional inter-dictions at the end of almost every foodstuff description.

Sun's additional information to each entry may help explain the rather unusual sequencing of the four sections. Food interdictions are distributed within the text as fol-lows: in the first section on fruits there are only very few of these interdictions (four out of twenty-nine), the section on vegetables has nineteen (out of fifty-eight), the section on grains has nine (out of twenty-seven), and in the last section on birds/quadrupeds there are twenty-eight of them (out of forty). The increasing number of food interdic-tions in the text might have suggested Sun's arrangement of the sections, beginning with fruits whose application seems to be rather liberal and ending with the meat of various animals, which has to be handled with the greatest of care.

Conversely, the qualities of 'roughening' and 'lubricating' could also have been an indicator for Sun's arrangement of his sections, beginning with fruits and ending with birds/quadrupeds. Most of the later *materia dietetica* begin their monographical sections with grains/rice, according to the principle that the appropiate diet should be based on cereals, as has already been pointed out in the above-quoted passage of the *Suwen*.[35]

Nutritional interdictions

One of the innovative features of many entries in Sun Simiao's chapter on nutritional treatment consists of the inclusion of paragraphs on nutritional interdictions (*shijin* 食禁). Already in the preface, Sun stresses the vital importance of these nutritional interdictions for dietary treatment:

> If the [different] *qi* of foods are incompatible, the essence (*jing* 精) will be damaged. The physical form (*xing* 形) receives the sapors in order to achieve completion. If the [different] sapors of foods are not harmonised, the physical form will be spoiled. This is the reason why the sage first employs nutritional interdictions (*shijin* 食禁) in order to preserve his nature. [Only] after [this has proved unsuccessful], does he resort to the preparation of drugs to sustain life.[36]

In Sun Simiao's concept of dietary treatment, nutritional interdictions, which cannot be found in earlier *bencao* works, seem to have almost the same importance as the adequate knowledge of the effects of food described in the *materia medica* extracts. Nutritional interdictions are also a vital part of dietary therapy in order to prevent and eliminate disorders.

---

[35] See for instance the *Yinshan zhengyao* 飲膳正要, *juan* 3, 117–22.   [36] *Qianjin fang*, *juan* 26, 465.

The great importance accorded to nutritional interdictions in this text is reflected in the sixty-three sections of nutritional interdictions annexed to relevant entries. The following descriptions present typical examples showing the different emphasis accorded to nutritional interdictions and to *bencao* extracts in Sun's text. The first citation derives from the first section on fruits, namely waterchestnut, and the other from the last section on birds/quadrupeds, namely horse meat.

> Waterchestnut (*jishi* 芰實),[37] sapor: sweet, pungent; [*qi*:] neutral, not toxic. Soothes the centre (*anzhong* 安中), refers to splenetic and stomach orb/system), replenishes the *yin* orbs, eliminates the desire to eat and lightens the body. Another name [for *jishi* is] *ling* 菱. The Yellow Lord said: During the seventh month one should not eat raw waterchestnuts, [for] they will cause roundworms.[38]

> 芰實味甘辛平無毒。安中補五藏不飢輕身。一名菱。黃帝云：七月勿食生菱芰作蟯虫。

> Horse (*ma* 馬) . . . meat (*rou* 肉), sapor: pungent, bitter; [*qi*:] neutral, chilling, not toxic; for damage of the centre (*shangzhong* 傷中, refers to the splenetic and stomach orb/system), expels hot heteropathy, brings *qi* down, develops the sinews (*jin* 筋, i.e. muscles, tendons, ligaments, nerve tissues etc.), strengthens waist and spine, makes healthy and fortifies the will, sharpens thought and imagination (*yi* 意), lightens the body and eliminates hunger. The Yellow Lord said: if a white horse has died of natural causes, eating its meat will have harmful effects on a human being. If one eats the brain of a white horse with a dark head, one will have epileptic fits. If a white horse exhibits black colour under the saddle penetrating deep inside the flesh, eating [its meat] will harm the five *yin* orbs of man. If somebody suffering from diarrhoea eats horse meat, this will aggravate his illness. The meat of white horses with green hoofs must not be eaten. All horse sweat and hair should be separated from all food because it is harmful to man. The consumption of horse meat can cause cardiac agitation and [a feeling of] oppression. In such cases one has to drink delicious wine (*meijiu* 美酒) in order to flush out [the toxicity]. If one drinks clear wine (*baijiu* 白酒), [one's state] will get worse. During the fifth month one should not eat horse meat, because this will damage man's spiritual *qi* (*shenqi* 神氣).[39]

> 馬 . . .
> 肉味辛苦平冷無毒。主傷中。除熱下氣。長筋強腰脊。狀健強志。利意輕身不飢。黃帝云：白馬自死。食其肉害人。白馬玄頭。食其腦令人癲。白馬鞍下烏色徹肉裡者。食之傷人五藏。下利者食馬肉必加劇。白馬青蹄。

---

[37] *Trapa bispinosa* Roxb.; see *Zhongyao dacidian* 中藥大辭典, no. 4100.

[38] *Qianjin fang*, juan 26, 466. With the exception of the pungent sapor, Sun quotes exactly an upper class entry of the *Bencao jing jizhu*, juan 7, 465, until the quotation beginning: 'The Yellow Lord said'.

[39] *Qianjin fang*, juan 26, 472. The first part concurs with the description in the *Bencao jing jizhu*, juan 6, 416. The second part beginning with 'The Yellow Lord said' could be found in the *Jingui yaolüe*, juan 24, 14a, with the exception of the sentence: 'White horses with green hoofs must not be eaten.'

肉不可食。一切馬汗氣及毛。不可入食中害人。諸食馬肉心煩悶者。飲以
美酒則解。白酒則劇。五月勿食馬肉。傷人神氣。

Simply from these two descriptions from Sun Simiao's chapter on 'Dietary
Treatment' (Shizhi), it becomes obvious that the nutritional interdictions, always
mentioned in the second part of the description, cover a wide range. We find magico-
religious interdictions including calendrical notions, various effects food can have on
sexuality, as well as interdictions relevant to hygiene like the quite understandable
advice that one should not eat a horse which has died of natural causes.

The sixty-three sections on food interdictions are mostly quotations from sources
that are no longer extant. Forty-eight sections are introduced by 'The Yellow Lord said'.
This might refer to a text mentioned in the *Sui shu*, entitled *Huangdi zayinshi ji*, 黃帝雜
飲食忌 (The Yellow Lord's Various Avoidances Regarding Food and Drink), in two
juan, from the Liang dynasty. Moreover, we find eight sections beginning with 'Bian
Que said' which could tentatively be identified with another text in the *Sui shu*, entitled
Bian Que zhouhou fang 扁鵲肘後方 (Bian Que's Prescriptions [to be Hidden] behind
the Elbows), in three *juan*.[40] Four quotations are introduced by 'Hu Jushi 胡居士 said', a
person who has been identified as Hu Zhao 胡昭 (162–250).[41] And the last three begin
with 'Hua Tuo said' which must refer to the famous Hua Tuo 華佗 (141–203).[42]

Sun's sections on nutritional interdictions, when compared with existing texts, show
a great deal of similarity with the last two chapters of Zhang Zhongjing's *Jingui yaolüe
fang lun* 金匱要略方論 (Essentials and Discussions of Prescriptions in the Golden
Casket) dated around 196–200. Lu Gwei-djen and Needham have already recognised
these two chapters, which comprise various safety regulations concerning nutritional
interdictions and prescriptions against food poisoning, as being very important
evidence for early nutritional hygiene.[43] The similarity between the nutritional interdictions of Sun's 'Shizhi' chapter and Zhang's two chapters is especially true for the
section on fruits and particularly for the parts introduced by 'The Yellow Lord said'.
But neither of Zhang's chapters includes any descriptions of foodstuffs resembling
bencao entries. In addition, Sun's chapter contains similarities to the fragments of the
Yangsheng yaoji quoted in the *Ishinpō*, chapter 29.[44] Although Sun has not quoted the
texts mentioned exactly, it is possible that Sun, Zhang Zhongjing, and the author of

[40] *Sui shu*, *juan* 34, 1046.
[41] For his biography, see *Sanguo zhi* 三國志, *juan* 11, 362. For further details about him, see Despeux
(1990), 25. Two texts, in the *Sui shu*, *juan* 34, 1042, and in the *Jiu Tang shu* 舊唐書, *juan* 47, 2049,
entitled *Hu xia baibing fang* 胡洽百病方 and *Hu Jushi fang* 胡居士方 can be related to him.
[42] Watanabe Kōzō (1987), 225, sees relations between Sun's quotations of Hua Tuo and a text entitled
Hua Tuo shilun 華佗食論 mentioned in the *Taiping yulan* 太平御覽, *juan* 867, 3a.
[43] Needham and Lu (1962), 453.   [44] *Ishinpō*, *juan* 29, 270.

the *Yangsheng yaoji*, Zhan Zhan, employed roughly the same sources for nutritional interdictions that must have been very popular during the period between the Han and Tang dynasties.

Sun's combination of nutritional interdictions with the description of individual foodstuffs following the same pattern as in the *materia medica* tradition can be considered as innovative and characteristic of the newly evolved literary genre of *materia dietetica*. Although, as the next work of this genre to be described would suggest, not all texts of the *materia dietetica* tradition put as much weight on food interdictions as Sun did, nevertheless they became an integral and important part of dietary literature as a whole.[45]

The earliest complete dietary work: the *Shiliao bencao*

The earliest Chinese work specifically devoted to dietetic therapy from which at least an extensive fragment has been preserved is the *Shiliao bencao* 食療本草 (*Materia Medica* for Successful Dietary Therapy). A forerunner to the *Shiliao bencao* was a work entitled *Buyang fang* 補養方 (Prescriptions to Replenish and Nourish), that is no longer extant, written by Meng Shen 孟詵 (621–713) around 701–704. Another otherwise unknown author, Zhang Ding 張鼎 (eighth century), expanded the *Buyang fang* of Meng Shen some time between 721 and 739. His version expanded the original by eighty-nine descriptions to a total of 227 entries arranged in three chapters.[46] He entitled this new work *Shiliao bencao*.[47]

Meng Shen held various official posts, especially under the Empress Wu, and appears to have been associated with the Daoist circles of his time. In his youth he studied alchemy and followed Sun Simiao as his teacher. After retirement, he withdrew to the mountains and devoted himself to the study of drugs and food (*yao'er* 藥餌).[48]

Both versions, the original *Buyang fang* and the *Shiliao bencao*, appear to have been preserved until the eleventh century.[49] During the years that followed, the *Shiliao bencao* must have shared the same fate as many *bencao* works of its time: although the most important passages were incorporated into later works, the rest fell into oblivion and, sooner or later, were lost.

---

[45] See for example the *Yinshan zhengyao*, which begins with many nutritional interdictions in *juan* 1, 2–7, before giving dietary prescriptions and finally ending with *materia dietetica* descriptions in *juan* 3, 117–77.

[46] See Nakao Manzō (1930), 71 ff., Xie Haizhou et al. (1986), 160.   [47] See Nakao Manzō (1930), 26.

[48] For further details on Meng Shen's life, see Unschuld (1986), 209, and Schafer (1963), 177.

[49] For further details, see Unschuld (1986), 210.

Until the beginning of this century, the most important sources for quotations from the *Shiliao bencao* were the Japanese *Ishinpō* and several Chinese *bencao* works such as the *Zhenglei bencao* 證類本草 (*Materia Medica* Corrected and Arranged in Classes).[50] Fortunately, a fragment of the *Shiliao bencao* was found among the materials discovered in the Dunhuang caves by Sir Aurel Stein in 1907. This fragment comprises twenty-five entries, mostly common foodstuffs such as various kinds of gourds, grapes, and walnuts. Their order seems to follow neither the scheme based on three classes nor one based on origins.[51] In each case, the name of the foodstuff is followed by the typical *bencao* descriptive pattern (which gives the *qi*, sapor, and main indications), food interdictions, preparation methods, and simple recipes. The main text of the fragment, which today is located in the British Museum, is written in black ink. The names of the foodstuffs and the symbols separating sentences are emphasised by the use of red ink.[52]

Nakao Manzo published a detailed analysis of the reconstructable parts of the *Shiliao bencao*, comparing these twenty-five entries of the Dunhuang fragment with quotations mainly from the *Zhenglei bencao* and the *Ishinpō*. He was thus able to reconstruct more than two hundred entries, which appear in the same order as in the chapters of the *Zhenglei bencao*.[53] They begin with precious stones/minerals (with salt as first entry), turning to herbs, trees, quadrupeds, fowl, worms/insects/fish, fruits, rice/ grains, and finally to vegetables.[54] This grouping of entries in the reconstructed fragments is not necessarily identical to that of the original text. In the opinion of Nakao Manzo, who compared the Dunhuang fragments with the later quotations, the later sources give a significantly shortened or changed form.[55] Moreover, he compared Sun Simiao's chapter on dietetics with the contents of the *Shiliao bencao* and came to the conclusion that Meng Shen was strongly influenced by the knowledge of his teacher Sun Simiao.[56]

The two examples quoted above from Sun Simiao's *Qianjin fang* may be compared with the following corresponding entries of the fragments of the *Shiliao bencao*:

> Waterchestnut (*jishi* 芰 實), [*qi*] neutral. For treating and soothing the middle *jiao* (*zhongjiao* 中焦 refers to splenetic and stomach orb/system), replenishes *qi* in the orbs, eliminates hunger. [According to] 'The Immortal's Prescriptions' (Xianfang 仙方) [waterchestnuts] have to be cooked by steaming, then dried in the sun, pulverised, mixed with honey and eaten as a substitute for cereals. All

---

[50] For further details on the *Zhenglei bencao*, see Unschuld (1986), 70 ff.
[51] Nakao Manzō (1930), 73 ff.   [52] Unschuld (1986), 211.
[53] Nakao Manzō (1930), 73 ff.   [54] Unschuld (1986), 75 ff.
[55] Nakao Manzō (1930), 6–9. See also Unschuld (1986), 211, and Xie Haizhou et al. (1986), 163.
[56] Nakao Manzō (1930), 58–71.

fruits which grow in water develop an extremely chilling *qi*. [For this reason] one may not [employ them] for treating illnesses, [otherwise] the *yin* will suffer and the penis will become weak. For those whose [abundant intake of waterchestnuts] has caused distentions in the abdomen, they should drink one *qian* of ginger wine (*jiangjiu* 薑酒), and then [the disorder] will subside.[57]

芰實：平。右主治安中焦，補藏腑氣，令人不饑。仙方亦蒸熟，曝乾，作末，和蜜，食之休糧：凡水中之果，此物㝡發冷氣。不能治眾疾，損陰，令玉莖消衰，令人或腹脹者以薑酒一盞飲即消。

Horse (*ma* 馬) . . . meat (*rou* 肉), chilling, slightly toxic; for heat heteropathies in the intestine; expels and lowers *qi*, helps the growth of sinews and bones. Not to be eaten together with granary rice (*cangmi* 倉米), [otherwise] this will suddenly cause various evil [disorders] from which nine out of ten people will die. Not to be eaten together with ginger, [otherwise] this will bring on coughing. If while being cooked horse meat is often soaked and washed, it becomes tender and thoroughly cooked and equally all blood is removed, then one can begin to cook and eat[58] it. The same applies if [the meat is] fat. If one does not proceed in this way, the toxicity will not be eradicated.

肉冷有小毒，主腸中熱，除下氣，長筋骨。不與倉米同食，必卒得惡(病)，十有九死。不與薑同食，生氣嗽。其肉多著浸洗，方煮得爛熟兼去血盡，始可煮食。肥者亦然。不邇毒不出。

If [the meat] of a white horse with a dark head is eaten, it will cause epileptic fits. Eating a white horse that has died of natural causes will have harmful effects on [the health of] a human being . . .

白馬黑頭，食令人癲。白馬自死，食之害人。

When the consumption of any kind of horse meat leads to [a feeling of] pressure on the chest, one has to drink clear wine in order to flush out [the toxicity], whereas with cloudy wine (濁酒) [the disorder] will be aggravated.[59]

食諸馬肉心悶，飲清酒，既條揶，濁酒即加。

---

[57] The translation follows the Dunhuang fragment. See Nakao Manzō (1930), 156; Xie Haizhou et al. (1986), 36; Zheng Jinsheng et al. (1993), 42.

[58] Nakao Manzō (1930), 107, gives, in consideration of the *Chongxiu Zhenghe bencao* 重修政和本草, the character 灸 instead of 食, but I follow Xie Haizhou et al. (1986), 63, and Zheng Jinsheng et al. (1993), 67.

[59] The entry on horse meat has not been preserved in the Dunhuang manuscript, but there are several quotations of the *Shiliao bencao* in the *Zhenglei bencao* and the *Jiayou bencao* 嘉佑本草 (Expanded and Annotated *Materia Medica* of the Jiayou Period). The first part of the above citation is based on Xie Haizhou et al. (1986), 63; the following parts on Nakao Manzō (1930), 107. See also Zheng Jinsheng et al. (1993), 42. The fragments have been sequenced so as to accord with Sun Simiao's.

When one compares the two sections from Sun's chapter on dietetics with those from the *Shiliao bencao*, a partial resemblance is obvious: the heading under the descriptive pattern according to the *materiae medicae* or *materiae dieteticae*, the description of the medicinal effects of this particular foodstuff, and also the food interdictions. Nevertheless, as far as can be judged from the preserved fragments, Meng Shen does not appear to have attached so much importance to the nutritional interdictions as Sun did. Instead, he introduced some daily preparation methods and simple prescriptions. Thus, he drew more attention to the practical handling of foodstuffs and their preparation. Yet in contrast to the culinary treatises mentioned above, which predominantly provide the reader with techniques of food processing, Meng Shen always keeps in mind the therapeutic value of foodstuffs and how it can be changed by different preparation methods.

Conclusion

Nathan Sivin's observations about Sun Simiao's works can generally be said to be true also of Meng Shen's works: 'It is precisely in their eclecticism, the ease with which they incorporate elements from the folk traditions as well as from the medical traditions of other cultures into a close rational structure, that Sun's books are most representative of the major trends in Chinese medicine.'[60]

This rational structure is obvious in Sun's chapter on dietetics: on the one hand it comprises extracts about foodstuffs taken directly from Tao Hongjing's *materia medica*, the *Bencao jing jizhu*, on the other hand it gives nutritional interdictions which can be related to different earlier sources. Thus, in combining the basic pattern of the *bencao* monographs with interdictions concerning foodstuffs, Sun Simiao appears to have written the first extant *materia dietetica* and with this, he has contributed to the establishment of an ensuing genre of *materia dietetica*.

Sun's student, Meng Shen, was stimulated by his master's impetus and seems to have expanded the *materia dietetica*, especially by adding simple preparation methods and prescriptions. Thus, it may be said that Sun, in his chapter on dietetics, gives the theoretical framework, whereas Meng Shen's *Shiliao bencao*, the first extant complete work, which is based upon the theories of Sun's work and emphasises the practical application of dietary knowledge. With these two outstanding texts, the genre of *materia dietetica* took a distinct shape during the Tang, on the basis of which it developed during the following centuries.

---

[60] Sivin (1967), 270.

References to premodern Chinese and Japanese works

Beiji qianjin yaofang 備急千金要方 (Prescriptions Worth a Thousand, for Urgent Need). Tang, 652. Sun Simiao 孫思邈. Facsimile of a Ming print of Lin Yi's 林億 edition of 1066. Zhonghua shuju 中華書局, Beijing 1955. Reprint 1992.

Chongxiu Zhenghe bencao 重修政和本草, see *Zhenglei bencao* 證類本草.

Han shu 漢書 (History of the Former Han). Han, 1st century AD. Ban Gu 班固. Zhonghua shuju 中華書局, Beijing, 1962.

Huangdi neijing 黃帝內經 (Yellow Emperor's Inner Canon). Han, 1st century BC. Anon. References to Ren Yingqiu 任應秋 (ed.) *Huangdi neijing zhangju suoyin* 黃帝內經章句索引. Renmin weisheng chubanshe 人民衛生出版社, Beijing, 1986.

Ishinpō 醫心方 (Essential Medical Methods). Tambano Yasuyori 丹波康賴 (comp.). 982, first published 1860. Xinwenfeng chubanshe 新文奉出版社, Taibei, 1955.

Jingui yaolüe fanglun 金匱要略方論 (Essentials and Discussions of Prescriptions in the Golden Casket). Han, 196–200. Zhang Zhongjing 張仲景. *Sibu beiyao* 四部備要, Zhonghua shuju 中華書局, Beijing, 1955.

Jiu Tang shu 舊唐書 (Old History of the Tang Dynasty). Later Jin, 945. Liu Xu 劉昫 et al. Zhonghua shuju 中華書局, Beijing, 1963.

Lingshu 靈樞 (Divine Pivot), see *Huangdi Neijing* 黃帝內經.

Qimin yaoshu 齊民要術 (Essential Techniques for the Common People). Wei, *ca* 535. Jia Sixie 賈思勰. Cited from *Qimin yaoshu jiaoshi*, annotated by Miao Qiyu 繆啟愉. Nongye chubanshe 農業出版社, Beijing, 1982.

Sanguo zhi 三國志 (History of the Three Kingdoms). Western Jin. Chen Shou 陳壽 (d. 297) et al. Zhonghua shuju 中華書局, Beijing, 1959.

Shennong bencaojing jizhu 神農本草經集注 (Notes to the Divine Husbandman's Canon of *Materia Medica*). Liang, ?492. Tao Hongjing 陶弘景. Annotated by Shang Zhijun 尚志鈞 and Shang Yuansheng 尚元勝. Renmin weisheng chubanshe 人民衛生出版社, Beijing, 1994.

Sui shu 隋書 (History of the Sui Dynasty). Tang, 636. Wei Zheng et al. 魏徵. Zhonghua shuju 中華書局, Beijing, 1973.

Suwen 素問 (Basic Questions), see *Huangdi neijing* 黃帝內經.

Taiping yulan 太平御覽 (Encyclopedia of the Great Peace and Prosperous State Era for Imperial Scrutiny). Tang, 983. Li Fang 李昉 et al. Zhonghua shuju 中華書局, Beijing, 1985.

Tanglü shuyi 唐律疏議 (Official Commentaries to the Tang Law). Tang. Zhangsun Wuji 張孫無忌 (comp.). Zhonghua shuju 中華書局, Beijing, 1983.

Wei shu 魏書 (History of the Wei Dynasty). Northern Qi, 551. Wei Shou 威收 et al. Zhonghua shuju 中華書局, Beijing, 1974.

Xinxiu bencao 新修本草 (Newly Revised *Materia Medica*). Tang, *ca* 660. Su Jing 蘇敬. Shanghai guji chubanshe 上海古籍出版社, Shanghai, 1985.

Yinshan zhengyao 飲膳正要 (Correct and Essential Principles for Drink and Food). Yuan, 1456. Hu Sihui 忽思慧. Reprint of the Yuan edition. Beijingshi zhongguo shudian 北京市中國書店, Beijing, 1985.

Zhenglei bencao 證類本草 (*Materia Medica* Corrected and Arranged in Classes). Song, *ca* 1082. Tang Shenwei 唐慎微. Short title of *Chongxiu Zhenghe jingshi zhenglei beiyong bencao* 重修正和經史證類備用本草. Based on the Song edition of 1249. Nantian shuju 南天書局, Taipei, 1976.

References known from citations only

Bian Que zhouhou fang 扁鵲肘後方 (Bian Que's Prescriptions [to be Hidden] behind the Elbows). Anon. Cited in *Sui shu, juan* 34, 1046.

Buyang fang 補養方 (Prescriptions to Replenish and Nourish). Tang, 701–4. Meng Shen 孟詵. Basis of *Shiliao bencao* 食療本草 (*Materia Medica* for Successful Dietary Therapy).

Cui Hao shijing 崔浩食經 (Cui Hao's Nutritional Classic). Wei. Cui Hao 崔浩 (d. 450). Preface cited in *Wei shu* 魏書, *juan* 35, 807.

Hu Ju shi fang 胡居士方 (Recipes by Master Hu Ju). Attributed to Hu Zhao 胡昭. Cited in *Sui shu, juan* 34, 1042 and in the *Jiu Tang shu, juan* 47, 2049.

Hu xia baibing fang 胡洽百病方 (Recipes by Master Hu to Treat the Hundred Illnesses). Attributed to Hu Zhao 胡昭. Cited in *Sui shu, juan* 34, 1042 and in *Jiu Tang shu, juan* 47, 2049.

Hua Tuo shilun 華佗食論. Attributed to Hua Tuo 華佗. Cited in *Taiping yulan, juan* 867, 3a.

Huangdi zayinshi ji 黃帝雜飲食忌 (The Yellow Lord's Various Avoidances Regarding Food and Drink). Liang. Anon.

Jiayou bencao 嘉佑本草, short title of *Jiayou buzhu Shennong bencao* 嘉佑補注神農本草 (Expanded and Annotated *Materia Medica* [commissioned] in the Jiayou Period). Song, 1061. Zhang Yuxi 掌禹錫 et al. Cited in *Zhenglei bencao* 證類本草.

Shennong bencao jing 神農本草經 (*Materia Medica* Classic of the Divine Husbandman). Anon. Han, 1st century AD. Lost. References to *Shennong bencaojing jiaozheng*, revised by Wang Yunmo 王筠默 et al. Jilin kexue jishu chubanshe 吉林科學技術出版社, Changchun, 1988.

Shennong Huangdi shijin 神農黃帝食禁 (Shennong's and Huangdi's Nutritional Interdictions). Anon. Cited in *Han shu, juan* 30, 1777.

Shenxian fushi jing 神仙服食經 (Nutritional Classic for the Immortal's Consumption). Anon. Cited in *Sui shu, juan* 34, 1049.

Shiliao bencao 食療本草 (*Materia Medica* for Successful Dietary Therapy). Tang, 721–39. Based on the *Buyang fang* 補養方 by Meng Shen 孟詵. Expanded and renamed in 1886 by Zhang Ding 張鼎. Lost. For reconstructions, see Nakao Manzo 1930, Xie Haizhou 謝海洲 et al. (comp.) and Zheng Jinsheng 鄭金生 et al. (comp.) 1993, in 'References to modern works'.

Yangsheng yaoji 養生要集 (Essential Compendium on Nourishing Life). Eastern Jin, 4th century. Zhang Zhan 張湛. Cited in *Ishinpō* 醫心方, *passim*.

References to modern works

Aymard, Maurice, Grignon, Claude and Sabban, Françoise (eds.) 1993. *Le temps du manger Alimentation, emploi du temps et rythmes sociaux*. Editions de la Maison des Sciences de l'Homme, Paris.

Barrett, Timothy H. 1980. 'On the Transmission of the *Shen tzu* and of the *Yang-sheng yao-chi*'. *Journal of the Royal Asiatic Society* 2, 168–76.

Bray, Francesca 1984. *Agriculture*. In Joseph Needham, *Science and Civilization in China*, vol. VI: *Biology and Biological Technology*, part 2. Cambridge University Press, Cambridge.

1989. 'Essence and Utility: the Classification of Cultivated Plants in China'. *Chinese Science* 9, 1–13.

Buell, Paul 1989. 'The *Yin-shan cheng-yao*, a Sino-Uighur Dietary: Synopsis, Problems, Prospects'. In Unschuld, 109–27.

Despeux, Catherine 1987. *Préscriptions d'acuponcture valant mille onces d'or*. Guy Trédaniel, Paris.

1990. 'Le *Yangsheng yaoji*'. Unpublished manuscript, 44 pp.

Engelhardt, Ute 1987. *Die klassische Tradition der Qi-Übungen: Eine Darstellung anhand des Tang-zeitlichen Textes Fuqi jingyi lun von Sima Chengzhen*. Franz Steiner, Wiesbaden.

Harper, Donald 1982. 'Wu Shih Erh Ping Fang, Translation and Prolegomena'. PhD thesis in Oriental Languages, University of California, Berkeley.

Harper, Donald 1984. 'Gastronomy in Ancient China'. *Parabola* 9, 39–47.

1998. *Early Chinese Medical Literature: the Mawangdui Medical Manuscripts*. Routledge, London.

Huang, H. T. 1990. 'Han Gastronomy: Chinese Cuisine in *statu nascendi*'. *Interdisciplinary Science Reviews* 15 (2), 139–52.

Levi, Jean 1983. 'L'abstinence des céreales chez les taoïstes'. *Etudes Chinoises* 1, 3–47.

Lu Gwei-djen and Needham, Joseph 1977. 'A Contribution to the History of Chinese Dietetics.' In Nathan Sivin (ed.), *Science and Technology in East Asia: Articles from* Isis *1913–1975*, 85–92. Science History Publications, New York.

Lu Yaodong 1993. 'Bei Wei *Cui shi shijing* de lishi yu wenhua yiyi' 北魏崔氏食經的歷史與文化意義 (The Historical and Cultural Significance of Master Tsui's Recipes). *Diyi ceng Zhongguo yinshi wenhua xueshu yantao hui lunwenji* 第一層中國飲食文化學術研討會論文集 (The First Symposium on Chinese Dietary Culture). Zhongguo yinshi jijinhui, Taibei, 13–38.

Nakao Manzō 中尾万三 1930. 'Shokuryō honzō no kōsatsu' 食療本草の考察 (Studies on the *Shiliao bencao*). *Shanghai ziran kexue yanjiusuo huibao* 上海自然科學研究匯報 1, 5–216.

Needham, Joseph and Lu Gwei-djen 1962. 'Hygiene and Preventive Medicine in Ancient China'. *Journal of the History of Medicine and Allied Sciences* 17, 429–78.

Okanishi Tameto 岡西為人 1967. *Songyiqian yiji kao* 宋以前醫籍考 (Studies of Medical Books through the Song Period). Jinxue shuju, Taibei.

Sabban, Francoise 1986. 'Un savoir-faire oublié: le travail du lait en Chine ancienne'. *Zinbun Memoirs of the Research Institute for Humanistic Studies, Kyoto University* 21, 31–65.

1990. 'Food Provisioning, the Treatment of Foodstuffs and other Culinary Aspects of the *Qimin yaoshu*'. Paper read during the 6th Conference on the History of Science in China, Cambridge, 12 pp.

1993. 'Suivre les temps du ciel: économie ménagère et gestion du temps dans la Chine du VIe siècle'. In Aymard, Grignon and Sabban, 81–108.

Sakade Yoshinobu 阪出祥伸 1986. 'Cho Tan no "Yōsei yōsū" itsubun to sono shisō' 張湛の《養生要集》件文とその思想 (Zhang Zhan's *Yangsheng yaoji* and its Thinking). *Tōhō shūkyō* 東方宗教 68, 1–25.

Schafer, Edward 1963. *The Golden Peaches of Samarkand: a Study of T'ang Exotics*. University of California Press, Berkeley.

Shinoda Osamu 筱田統 1987. *Zhongguo shiwushi yanjiu* 中國食物史研究 (Research on the History of Chinese Food). Gao Guilin 高桂林 et al. (transl.). Shangye chubanshe, Beijing.

Shinoda Osamu 筱田統 and Tanaka Seiichi 田中靜一 (eds.) 1972. *Chūoku shokukei sōsho* 中國食經叢書 (Collection of Chinese Food Classics). Shoseki Bunbutsu Ryūtsūkui, Tokyo.

Sivin, Nathan 1967. 'A Seventh-Century Chinese Medical Case History'. *Bulletin of the History of Medicine* 41 (3), 267–73.

1987. *Traditional Medicine in Contemporary China: a Partial Translation of* Revised Outline of Chinese Medicine (1972) *with an Introductory Study on Change in Present-day and Early Medicine*. Center for Chinese Studies, University of Michigan, Ann Arbor.

(ed.) 1989. *Science and Technology in East Asia*. Science History Publications, New York.

Steih S. 1999. *Zwischen Heil und Heilung: Zur frühen Tradition des Yangsheng in China*. Medizinische literarische Verlagsgesellschaft, Uelzen.

Unschuld, Paul U. 1977. 'Arzneimittelmißbrauch und heterodoxe Heiltätigkeit im kaiserlichen China: Ausgewählte Materialien zu Gesetzgebung und Rechtsprechung'. *Sudhoffs Archiv* 61, 353–86.

1986. *Medicine in China: a History of Pharmaceutics*. University of California Press, Berkeley.

1994. 'Der chinesische "Arzneikönig" Sun Simiao: Geschichte – Legende – Ikonographie'. *Monumenta Serica* 42, 217–57.

(ed.) 1989. *Approaches to Traditional Chinese Medical Literature*. Kluwer, Dordrecht.

Watanabe Kōzō 渡邊幸三 1987. 'Son Shibō senkin-yohō shokujihen bunkengaku no kenkyū' 孫思邈千金要方食治篇文獻學の研究 (Research on the Chapter on Dietetics of Sun Simiao's Prescriptions Worth a Thousand). Repr. of 1955 in *Honzo sho no kenkyu* 本草書研究, Tokyo.

Xie Haizhou 謝海洲 et al. (comp.) 1986. *Shiliao bencao* 食療本草 (*Materia Medica* for Successful Dietary Therapy). Renmin weisheng chubanshe, Beijing.

Zheng Jinsheng 鄭金生 et al. (comp.) 1993. *Shiliao bencao yizhu* 食療本草譯注 (Annotated *Materia Medica* for Successful Dietary Therapy). Shanghai guji chubanshe, Shanghai.

Zhongyao dacidian 中藥大辭典 (Dictionary of Chinese *Materia Medica*) 1977. Jiangsu xinyi xueyuan 江蘇新醫學院 (eds.). Shanghai kexue jishu chubanshe, Shanghai.

6

A Song innovation in pharmacotherapy: some remarks on the use of white arsenic and flowers of arsenic

FRÉDÉRIC OBRINGER
TRANSLATED BY JANET LLOYD

When applying the notion of innovation directly to the history of China, with all that notion's recently formulated implications, particularly in the economic domain, considerable prudence is undoubtedly called for. Nevertheless, to seek to draw too rigid an opposition between on the one hand an industrial world – for example, that of the West from the end of the eighteenth century down to the present day – intoxicated by innovation and 'scientific and technical revolutions', and, on the other, the cold world of tradition – for example, pre-modern China – immobilised in stagnation, is of course an untenable position, particularly following the work of Joseph Needham and Lu Gwei-djen.

My aim is to single out a case of innovation – in the widest sense of the word – in the domain of pharmacotherapy and to explore its various facets: its origin, its birth, its progress, and its success or failure. If we adopt the distinction proposed by François Sigaut[1] between radical and non-radical innovations, this case seems on the face of it to belong to the latter category, in that it developed, without any noticeable break, within a tradition of skills and practices: it was thus a 'modest' innovation, which came about at a pivotal point in Chinese history, the Song dynasty; and its main interest lies in the fact that its nature is such that it enables us to pick out a number of circumstances that are necessary for such a phenomenon to occur. Very often, in the field of the history of medical matters and ethno-pharmacology, it is tempting to attribute the use of drugs to a rather vague kind of empiricism, in a context that is, generally speaking, hard to pin down, given the lack of sufficiently precise information. In such conditions, any

---

[1] See Sigaut (1994) who draws a distinction between radical and non-radical innovations.

192

enquiry into the criteria underlying the use of such and such a remedy usually turns out to be incomplete.[2] In some cases, however, we possess a certain amount of extra information, as in the case of drugs from foreign parts, whose introduction into China it is possible to date, or in that of others that were the product of a preparation the earliest description of which is known to us. It is more or less such a situation that, while recognising that some arsenical substances had been used by doctors ever since antiquity, I propose to examine here: namely, the appearance in the therapeutic arsenal of arsenic anhydride, a derivative of arsenic.

Arsenic derivatives in China: an ancient history

First, it is important to point out that, if we are to consider the history of arsenic derivatives in China, we need, *a posteriori*, to introduce as it were the whole community of products covered by the notion of the chemical element 'arsenic'. However, there are no grounds for thinking that at any particular moment in the period in which we are interested, the doctors (*yi* 醫), the 'masters of prescriptions' (*fangshi* 方士), and the alchemists did actually conceptualise this notion of a chemical element. So what we shall here retrospectively classify as a group are substances that were not then thought to be linked by any such common element.[3]

As Nathan Sivin and Zhao Kuanghua have shown,[4] very probably Chinese alchemists, in the course of their manipulations and depending on the somewhat elusive nature of the material, did sometimes obtain metallic arsenic (As). Thus, a passage in the *Baopuzi* 抱朴子 (Book of Master Holding-to-Simplicity) by Ge Hong 葛洪 (281–341),[5] describes obtaining a product that must be this metal from a mixture of realgar, pig's intestines, pine resin, and salt. However, what was obtained was not referred to by a specific name, and substances that we link chemically with arsenic, such as its sulphides – realgar or orpiment – were not conceived to be derivatives from that body of ingredients.

However that may be, even in antiquity, there are many references to the use of three mineral substances that we now identify as arsenical compounds. They are already

---

[2] On the history of drugs in the West, see for example Dagognet (1964), Riddle (1992), and Touwaide (1995).

[3] On the history of arsenic in China, see Schafer (1955); Needham (1974), 282 f.; Zhao Kuanghua (1985), 14–79; in particular Wang Kuike et al. (1985); Needham (1987), 114 f.; Zhang Hongzhao ((1927) 1993), 218.

[4] See Sivin (1968), 180–3; Zheng Tong and Yuan Shuyu (1985); and Zhao Kuanghua and Luo Meng (1985).

[5] *Baopuzi* 抱朴子, *juan* 11, 203.

distinguished clearly in the *Shennong bencao jing* 神農本草經 (The Canon of the Husbandman's *Materia Medica*), which dates from the first century AD, in which they are studied separately.

Xionghuang 雄黃 (lit. 'male yellow') is realgar, that is to say red sulphide of arsenic: As_2S_2.[6] In connection with this identification, it should be remembered on the one hand that realgar (As_2S_2) and orpiment (As_2S_3) are often found together in seams and, on the other, that realgar gradually becomes discoloured in the open air and in the light, producing pulverulent orpiment (As_2S_3) and arsenolite (As_2O_3). It is therefore unlikely that all the mining products designated by the term *xionghuang* were invariably realgar. However, the texts do specify that the authentic drug was the colour of a cock's comb:[7] so what was being sought was certainly realgar. *Xionghuang* is already mentioned several times in the *Shanhaijing* 山海經 (Classic of the Mountains and Lakes),[8] compiled under the Han, and is cited twice in the 'Wushier bing fang' 五十二病方 (Prescriptions for Fifty-two Ailments), excavated at Mawangdui 馬王堆 (from a tomb closed in 168 BC)[9] and once in the prescriptions written on bamboo slips from Wuwei 武威 (from a tomb closed between AD 55 and 68).[10] This drug had a bitter (*ku* 苦) taste and was of a neutral (*ping* 平) nature, according to the *Shennong bencao jing*, which classified it in the second of its three categories.[11] As a therapy, realgar was recommended, as early as in the 'Wushier bing fang', against cutaneous and external parasitical complaints, as it also was in the first-century *Shennong bencao jing* and the fifth-century *Mingyi bielu* 名醫別錄 (Informal Records of Famous Physicians).[12] According to the *Shennong bencao jing*, it was also capable of killing ghosts, harmful demons, and perverse *qi* (*jingwu egui xieqi* 精物惡鬼邪氣), and according to the *Mingyi bielu*, it could cure possession by demons (*guizhu* 鬼疰), so clearly the product was highly prized for its magical powers.

---

[6] See *Zhongyao dacidian* (1979), no. 4853; in general, throughout this article, I depend largely upon this fundamental work for the identification of substances, although I sometimes suggest complements or modifications. On *xionghuang*, see also *Zhenglei bencao* 證類本草, *juan* 4, 3a–6a. The *Wu Pu bencao* 吳普本草 (third century), 8, stated that the name *xionghuang* came from the fact that this ore was found at the level of the sunny (*yang* 陽) slopes of mountains, equivalents of the male (*xiong* 雄) category.

[7] See for example *Baopuzi*, *juan* 11, 203, and *Bencao tujing* 本草圖經, in *Zhenglei bencao*, *juan* 4, 4a. This text also indicated that certain forms, called *chouhuang* 臭黃 , with a disagreeable smell (lit. 'yellow with a bad smell'), had to be reserved for external use. The smell was probably the alliaceous odour of arsenic anhydride, a substance to which we shall be returning in this chapter.

[8] *Shanhaijing* 山海經, *juan* 2, 34, 63 and *juan* 5, 156.

[9] 'Wushier bing fang', 63 (prescription 210) and 70 (prescription 250).

[10] *Wuwei Han dai yijian* 武威漢代醫簡, 16b (slat 85b); realgar is here designated solely by the *xiong* 雄 character.

[11] For an outline of these three categories in the *Shennong bencao jing*, see Georges Métailié (chapter 7, this volume), p. 224.

[12] *Shennong bencao jing*, *juan* 3, 281, and *Mingyi bielu*, *juan* 2, 99.

It also enjoyed a great reputation (particularly in the form of amulets to be worn on one's person) for its power to put dangerous animals to flight[13] and to destroy the venom of poisonous snakes.[14] Finally, a hierarchy was established between the various qualities of the drug: according to Ge Hong,[15] the drugs that were collected on their own, not mixed together, and those that were shiny and the colour of cocks' combs were suitable for the preparation of elixirs of immortality, whereas those of lower quality were reserved for the treatment of ailments.

Cihuang 雌黃 (lit. 'female yellow') is orpiment, a yellow sulphide of arsenic, As_2S_3,[16] which, as we have noted above, is frequently present in seams, along with realgar. On the basis of its pungent (*xin* 辛) flavour and its neutral (*ping*) nature, the *Shennong bencao jing*[17] classified it in the intermediary category of drugs. It was also recommended against cutaneous conditions but, under the Song, the *Bencao yanyi* 本草衍義 (Dilations upon *Materia Medica*), published in 1116 by Kou Zongshi 寇宗奭 (eleventh–twelfth centuries) noted that it was very seldom used as a medicament.[18] In a very different field, as early as the *Qimin yaoshu* 齊民要術 (Essential Techniques for the Peasantry),[19] published in about 535, it was noted that orpiment was used to correct mistakenly written characters in texts, as it was the same colour as the paper. The *Mingyi bielu* noted that it was often to be found mixed with realgar, in the mountains.[20]

Yushi 礜石 (lit. '*yu* stone') designated arsenic ores:[21] for instance, arsenopyrite (also known as mispickel), FeAsS, of a silvery white or grey colour, with metallic reflections; and arsenolite or claudetite: arsenolite, in the cubic system, is the crystalline translucent variety of arsenic anhydride (As_2O_3 or As_4O_6), also known as 'flowers of arsenic' and claudetite is the monoclinical form of this anhydride. In all likelihood, the term *yushi* also applied to native arsenic (As), although this was rarely found. All these bodies are light grey or white in colour – with variations depending on how long they are exposed to the open air – and this is borne out by certain synonyms of *yushi* noted in the *Mingyi*

---

[13] See *Yaoxinglun* 藥性論 (Treatise on the Nature of Drugs) (Tang), in *Zhenglei bencao*, *juan* 4, 4a; see also Obringer (1997), 78.

[14] *Mingyi bielu*, *juan* 2, 99. [15] *Baopuzi*, *juan* 11, 203.

[16] See *Zhongyao dacidian* (1979), no. 5324, and *Zhenglei bencao*, *juan* 4, 8b–9b.

[17] *Shennong bencao jing*, *juan* 3, 282. [18] *Bencao yanyi*, *juan* 5, 30.

[19] *Qimin yaoshu*, *juan* 3, 164; this work gives a method of preparing the product for use. On this subject, see also Shen Gua 沈括 (1031–95), who, in his *Mengqi bitan* 夢溪筆談, *juan* 1, 67, stresses that orpiment is the best means of correcting errors in books.

[20] *Mingyi bielu*, *juan* 2, 100.

[21] See *Zhongyao dacidian* (1979), no. 2728, and *Zhenglei bencao*, *juan* 5, 5b. Other entries in the *bencao* also correspond to particular forms of *yushi*: *tesheng yushi* 特生礜石 (lit. '*yu* stone formed in a special way'), *Zhenglei bencao*, *juan* 5, 26b, and *cangshi* 蒼石 (lit. 'blue-green stone'), *Zhenglei bencao*, *juan* 5, 30a.

bielu, such as *baiyushi* 白礜石 (lit. 'white *yu* stone'), or *taibaishi* 太白石 (lit. 'very white stone').[22] The latter had already been mentioned in the *Shanhaijing* as a rat-poison.[23] It was classified by the *Shennong bencao jing* among the drugs of the lowest – and therefore toxic – category, was said to have a sharp taste and a very hot nature (*da re* 大熱), and was recommended by that same work against cold or hot flushes (*hanre* 寒熱), certain cutaneous conditions (*shulou shichuang* 鼠瘻蝕瘡), obstructions caused by wind (*fengbi* 風痺), hard lumps in the abdomen (*fu zhong jian* 腹中堅), heteropathic *qi* (*xieqi* 邪氣), and to expel heat (*chu re* 除熱).[24] Elsewhere, Tao Hongjing 陶弘景[25] noted that the substance was frequently used in formulae for elixirs for long life and in alchemical techniques.

It should immediately be emphasised that the toxicity of these compounds was well known. The *Mingyi bielu*, for example, mentioned that prolonged consumption of *yushi* provoked convulsions, which calls to mind the polyneuritis characteristic of chronic intoxication resulting from arsenic. The damage could take an even more dramatic turn if care was not taken to treat the mineral with heat (*lian* 煉), for then it was considered to be lethal.[26] Throughout the history of Chinese pharmacy and alchemy, one of the recurrent procedures for detoxification was treatment using heat. In the case of *yushi*, Tao Hongjing noted, for example, that the drug needed to be heated for a day and a night, after being enclosed in yellow mud.[27] Then after being pulverised, it could be used. From the point of view of modern chemistry, if arsenopyrite is subjected to heat, a toxic iron arsenate ($FeAsO_4$) is produced, then, at higher temperatures, an arsenic oxide (AsO_3) and a gaseous sulphur dioxide (SO_2). What is left is a non-toxic ferric oxide (Fe_2O_3), but also small quantities of toxic arsenopyrite and neo-formed iron arsenate.[28]

The terms *xionghuang*, *cihuang* and *yushi* continued to be used in the medical documents of the Tang, the Song, and the Ming. But – and here we come to the nub of

[22] *Mingyi bielu, juan* 3, 210.   [23] *Shanhaijing, juan* 2, 30.
[24] *Shennong bencao jing, juan* 4, 436. The *Tang bencao* 唐本草, also known as *Xinxiu bencao* 新修本草, published in 659, includes a passage that is very remarkable in that it implies a procedure that could be described as experimental. In this passage, *yushi* is claimed to be excellent for attacking ailments due to accumulations (*jiju* 積聚) or to chronic cold (*guleng* 固冷), and states that 'if the drug is replaced by another substance, the treatment becomes ineffective'; cited in *Zhenglei bencao, juan* 5, 6b, see *Xinxiu bencao, juan* 5, 128. It is worth noting that *yushi* was probably an element in the composition of the famous powder known as 'for eating cold' (*hanshi san* 寒食散), which was so fashionable among the gentry, the scholars, and circles of power from the third century AD until at least the Tang dynasty; on this subject see Obringer (1997), 145–223.
[25] Cited in *Zhenglei bencao, juan* 5, 6b.   [26] *Mingyi bielu, juan* 3, 210.
[27] Cited in *Zhenglei bencao, juan* 5, 6b.   [28] Wang Kuike et al. (1985), 21.

the matter – a new entry made its appearance in the pharmaceutical works of the Song period, classified immediately after *yushi*. This 'new drug', introduced into the *materia medica* by the *Kaibao bencao* 開寶本草 (*Materia Medica* of the Kaibao Period),[29] completed in 973, was known as *pishuang* 砒霜 (lit. '*pi* frost').[30] The same *Kaibao bencao* also cited under the name *pihuang* 砒黃 (lit. 'yellow *pi*') a substance that could produce *pishuang* when treated by fire and sublimation (*feilian* 飛煉).[31] However, the *Bencao tujing* 本草圖經 (*Materia Medica* with Illustrations),[32] published in 1062 by Su Song 蘇頌 (1019–1101), declared that the *pishuang* drug was not mentioned in ancient works, and that the type with the best reputation came from Xinzhou 信州, in what is now Jiangxi province, which suggests that *pishuang* itself originated from mines. By contrast, in 1116, the *Bencao yanyi* noted that *pihuang* was the name for *pi* in the raw state (*shengpi* 生砒).[33] Several centuries later, under the Ming, Li Shizhen 李時珍 (1518–93), in his *Bencao gangmu* 本草綱目 (Systematic *Materia Medica*),[34] edited for the first time in 1596, drew the following distinction at the *pishi* 砒石 (lit. '*pi* stone') entry: in its raw state, the substance was called *pihuang*, and that which had been submitted to heat was known as *pishuang*. It seems likely that the *Bencao tujing* did not yet – for the innovation recorded in the *Kaibao bencao* was a recent one – distinguish between the product from the mine and that which resulted from some kind of preparation, and that the classification only gradually became more precise.

To sum up, the new organisation of the names of arsenic derivatives, which began under the Song and became established under the Ming, was as follows:

- *xionghuang*, *cihuang*, and *yushi* continued to designate respectively realgar (As_2S_2), orpiment (As_2S_3), and arsenic ores (arsenopyrite (FeAsS) and arsenolite (As_2O_3));
- the character *pi* 砒 entered into the composition of the names of several substances: the generic *pishi* became an entry in the *Bencao gangmu* in its own right, while

---

[29] The *Kaibao bencao* attributes a bitter, acid (*suan* 酸) flavour to *pishuang*, and considers it to be toxic (*you du* 有毒). Cited in *Zhenglei bencao*, *juan* 5, 7a–8b.

[30] *pi* could be written using two characters: 砒 and 貔; Li Shizhen 李時珍 (1518–93) notes in his *Bencao gangmu* 本草綱目, *juan* 10, 606, that the name of the drug, *pi*, comes from its nature, which is as fierce as the animal *pi* 貔. This creature was likened to the bear, the leopard, and the tiger, and is impossible to identify precisely. On this subject, see the *Shuowen jiezi* 説文解字, 198, which notes that one of the most famous references to this animal name occurs in the *Shijing* 詩經, Daya 大雅, Hanyi 韓奕, *juan* 18.4, 572, and the *Shujing* 書經, Mushi 牧誓, *juan* 11, 183. Li Shizhen also mentions two synonyms for *pishi*: *Xin shi* 信石 (lit. 'the stone from Xin[zhou]', Xinzhou being the principal source for it), and *renyan* 人言 (lit. 'human word'), a graphic decomposition of the character *xin*: 信.

[31] Cited in *Zhenglei bencao*, *juan* 5, 7b; *pihuang* is also cited by the *Rihuazi bencao* 日華子本草, *ibid.*

[32] Cited in *Zhenglei bencao*, *juan* 5, 7b.   [33] *Bencao yanyi*, *juan* 6, 43.

[34] *Bencao gangmu*, *juan* 10, 606.

pishuang, which had been an entry in the *Zhenglei bencao* (*Materia Medica* Corrected and Arranged in Classes) (*ca* 1082) by Tang Shenwei 唐慎微 (*ca* 1056–1136), disappeared as such, to be treated along with *pihuang* under the *pishi* entry. In this context, the term *pihuang* designated ores which, when heated, produced *pishuang*. Some of the substances named *pihuang* were arsenic ores also designated by the term *yushi*,[35] such as arsenopyrite and arsenolite: in this connection, the *Bencao tujing* noted that products from Xinzhou, which fetched very high prices on the market, took the form of very large chunks, the colour of the pale yolks of goose-eggs;[36] this description could also apply to certain varieties of arsenolite (of a more or less white, grey, or yellowish colour). But other ores, which were not to be classified under the rubric *yushi*, as their colour was neither white nor grey, were also included under the name *pihuang*. In his *Bencao yanyi*,[37] Kou Zongshi states that the native drug is either the colour of beef or else it is whitish.[38] Another Song treatise, the *Bieshuo bencao* 別説本草 (More Sayings on *Materia Medica*), by Chen Cheng 陳承 (eleventh century), for its part declares that the most renowned substances from the Xinzhou mine, which was heavily guarded, were of a red colour close to that of *xionghuang*, or realgar.[39] So it seems probable that *pishi* also referred to arsenic ores that were red or purplish, such as erythrite ($As_2O_5.3CoO.8H_2O$), cobaltine (CoAsS), and smaltine ($CoAs_2$), and possibly also, in some cases, to realgar itself. In truth, the coherence of the naming was determined by a technical process: the term *pishi* designated substances used to prepare *pishuang*, the central subject of our study, by means of sublimation and condensation.

A technical innovation

The *Bencao yanyi* describes the method for preparing *pishuang*.[40] The ore in its raw state (*shengpi*) was placed on a fire and grilled; it was then subjected to sublimation (*fei* 飛) and condensation (*ning* 凝), which was carried out in a crucible turned upside

---

[35] This partial synonym is not mentioned in the texts but is implicit if, *a posteriori*, one draws up a table of the various products concerned. It is also worth noting that in works containing medical prescriptions written in the Ming and the Qing periods, the term *yushi* tends to be used more rarely, and is usually replaced by the term *pishi*.

[36] Cited in *Zhenglei bencao, juan* 5, 7b.   [37] *Bencao yanyi, juan* 6, 43.

[38] See Wang Kuike et al. (1985), 17–18.

[39] Cited in *Zhenglei bencao, juan* 5, 8a. Li Shizhen, for his part, notes that the drug *pihuang*, in its raw state, should be red if it is of good quality, whereas *pishuang* should be white; see *Bencao gangmu, juan* 10, 607.

[40] *Bencao yanyi, juan* 6, 43.

down. The substance obtained, which hung from the surface of the crucible in an amorphous mass, had a nipple-like appearance: the longest of the 'nipples' were the most prized as a drug.

By this method, through the oxidation of the arsenic ore, white arsenic (As_2O_3) was obtained, or vitreous arsenolite, which is a kind of arsenic anhydride that takes the form of an opaque vitreous mass. It is worth pointing out that this vitreous arsenolite (that is to say *pishuang*) in time develops spontaneously into crystalline arsenolite, with an identical chemical formula, which is the more stable form of arsenic anhydride. As will be remembered, crystalline arsenolite, 'flowers of arsenic', appears in nature in earthy masses and encrustations. As we have seen, it is one of the acceptable identifications of *yushi* and *pihuang* (or *shengpi*).

What seems fundamental in the case that we are studying is thus not so much the actual nature of the 'new' drug, from a chemical point of view; for Chinese doctors and alchemists had already for a long time been manipulating a product known as *yushi* that was very similar to *pishuang*, even if its outward appearance was different. Rather, what is remarkable is that the product now integrated into the *materia medica* was a synthetic product that benefited from the improvement believed to be effected by transforming it by means of fire.

We thus find ourselves in the presence of a new product, the fruit of a codified manipulation that made it possible for the procedure to be repeated. The product also received a new name. In other words, this was a technical *innovation*.

At this point we must take a leap of several centuries backward in time, and recall an explanation given by Zheng Xuan 鄭玄, the author of a commentary on the *Zhouli* 周禮 (Records of the Rites of the Zhou Dynasty), who lived in the second century AD. On the subject of the passage in this treatise[41] that mentions the treatment of various cutaneous infections or wounds by means of five poisons (*wudu* 五毒), Zheng Xuan reports that these five substances were minerals: chalcanthite (*shidan* 石膽), cinnabar (*dansha* 丹砂), realgar (*xionghuang* 雄黃), an arsenic ore (*yushi* 礜石), and magnetite (*cishi* 磁石). He also declares that the doctors of his time (the end of the Han period) placed all five ingredients in an earthenware crucible with a lid, which was then heated for three days and three nights; the drug thus obtained (on the crucible) was then collected by means of a hen's feather, and was applied to the infected parts. This drug was probably arsenic anhydride in the form of a vitreous arsenolite. Today, we know that subjecting arsenic derivatives and mercury (and likewise cinnabar and red sulphide of

---

[41] *Zhouli*, 'Tianguan zhongzai' 天官冢宰, 47–8.

mercury) to heat, in the presence of oxidising agents, in an enclosed space, leads to the formation of this compound of mercuric oxide.[42]

On the evidence of this procedure that led – fortuitously – to what would, several centuries later, be called *pishuang*, we might say that, even then, this represented a technical innovation. However, the fact that the product obtained was not given a particular name of its own (according, at least, to the little documentation at our disposal) and that it was not recorded in written medical records prevents us from considering the product obtained as a true innovation, since at the time it was not really, or at least not sufficiently, 'conceptualised'. The glorious therapeutic destiny of *pishuang* under the Song shows that the integration of any particular drug into the *materia medica* depended upon a number of factors, among which – at the very least – was its acquisition of an individual identity thanks to being given a particular name, and also that it should offer a number of advantages over the drugs that were previously used.

A therapeutic innovation

As has been mentioned above, *pishuang* was used as a remedy under the Song. The *Rihuazi bencao* 日華子本草 (*Materia Medica* by Master Sun-Rays), of the tenth century, for example, recommended it as treatment for a number of women's complaints.[43] The *Kaibao bencao*, for its part, gave the following therapeutic directions: 'For all intermittent fevers (*nüe* 瘧), mucus resulting from wind in the chest and diaphragm; can be used as an emetic. Not to be taken over long periods, can be harmful.'[44] The first

---

[42] A text preserved in the *Daozang* 道藏 also cites another preparation designed to obtain the product under consideration, arsenic anhydride. The *Taiqing shibi ji* 太清石壁記, the compilation of which is attributed to a certain Chu Ze xiansheng 楚澤先生 (late eighth century?), appears originally to have been the work of Su Yuanlang 蘇元朗 [that last character *lang* was replaced by *ming* 明, as a result of either an error in copying or a taboo against the character, in a number of bibliographical catalogues such as the bibliographical monograph *Yiwen lüe* 藝文略 of the *Tongzhi* 通志, *juan* 5, 638]; the text may date from the sixth century, between the Liang and the Sui: see Ren Jiyu 任繼愈 (1991), 644. This text (in Lu Guoqiang 陸國強 et al.'s edition of the *Daozang* 道藏, vol. 18, 754, cites a method of obtaining the product called *shuangxue* 霜雪 (lit. 'frost-snow') from the following seven substances: *cengqing* 曾青 (azurite), *yushi* 礜石 (arsenic ore), *shiliuhuang* 石硫黃 (sulphur), *rongyan* 戎鹽 (rock salt), *ningshuishi* 凝水石 (various sulphates, epsomite, glauberite . . .), *daizhe* 代赭 (hematite), and *shuiyin* 水銀 (mercury). In my own view, what was obtained was certainly arsenic anhydride. But the product under consideration, *shuangxue*, was not integrated into any work on *materia medica*, nor was it used for therapeutic purposes, and its mode of preparation was different from that used under the Song to obtain *pishuang*.

[43] The *Rihuazi bencao* recommends boiling the drug in vinegar in order to destroy its poison. Cited in *Zhenglei bencao, juan* 5, 7b.

[44] Cited in *Zhenglei bencao, juan* 5, 7b.

recommendation in this treatise was certainly a major therapeutic application of *pishuang* as treatment for this category of complaints associated together as a particularly important nosological entity, namely intermittent fevers (*nüe* and *zhang* 瘴). It included malaria, but also other conditions in which fevers recurred at regular intervals.[45]

The nosological classification of intermittent fevers continued to evolve throughout the history of Chinese medicine. The *Zhubing yuanhou lun* 諸病源候論 (Origins and Symptoms of Medical Disorders), presented to the Emperor in 610,[46] considered that intermittent fevers were due to heat-stroke suffered in the summer, and that they manifested themselves in the autumn, when the weather was cold and windy. But the text explores several forms of these fevers, and some passages attribute all *nüe* to the action of wind. It also contains references to the fevers characteristic of the mountains of Lingnan 嶺南 (by and large the present-day provinces of Guangdong and Guangxi), which were believed to be caused by miasmas (*zhang* 瘴).[47]

As for malaria, in all likelihood the extension of irrigated rice cultivation under the Song contributed to its becoming endemic in territories that were previously hardly touched by it or, at any rate, had been less highly populated. The increase in the population itself probably contributed towards the development of marsh fevers, for it swelled the reservoir of individuals who could fall victim to parasites.[48] These fevers must thus have constituted a serious public health problem, as had already been suggested by Shen

---

[45] On the subject of malaria, see the article by Miyasita Saburō (1979); it should be remembered that the term *yao* (*nüe*) 瘧 can certainly not be assimilated solely to malaria (see Chapter 2, this volume). On the history of malaria in Europe, see Bruce-Chatt and de Zulueta (1980) and Grmek (1983), 397. The haematozoan responsible for malaria (*Plasmodium*) was identified by Laveran in 1880, and the vector role played by the female mosquitoes of the *Anopheles* species was recognised by Grassi in 1899. Nowadays human beings are invaded by parasites in four kinds of *Plasmodium*: *P. vivax* (benign tertian fever in temperate countries); *P. malariae* (quartan fever); *P. ovale* (benign tertian fever in Africa); and *P. falciparum* (daily or malignant tertian fever), the most pathogenic type.

[46] *Zhubing yuanhou lun*, *juan* 11, 362. On the concept of disease in general in this work, see Despeux and Obringer (1997), 69–89.

[47] This question of southern fevers was to be tackled in the very interesting *Lingnan weisheng fang* 嶺南衛生方 (Prescriptions for Hygiene from Lingnan), a work by Li Qiu 李璆 (*jinshi* in *ca* 1114) and Zhang Zhiyuan 張致遠 (*jinshi* in 1121), composed in the Song and published in the Yuan (preface of 1283).

[48] On the subject of the Song 'agricultural revolution', see Song Xi ((1962) 1979), 82; Elvin (1973), 113–30; Golas (1980); Bray (1984), 55; Cheng Minsheng 程民生 (1992), 71. One of the main sources on these various points is the *Wang Zhen nongshu* 王禎農書 (1313), in particular chapters 13 and 14, on hydraulic techniques.

Gua 沈括 (1031–95),[49] and the innovation introduced into their treatment may well have been a response to a pressing need.[50]

The drug *pishuang*, arsenic anhydride, appeared in prescriptions designed to fight fevers at the same time as it was introduced into treatises on *materia medica*, that is to say at the end of the tenth century. The *Taiping shenghui fang* 太平聖惠方 (Imperial Grace Formulary of the Taiping Period), a large formulary compiled by order of the government in 992, in its section devoted to intermittent fevers,[51] proposes 139 formulae, 36 of which (about 26 per cent) contain *pishuang*. Considering that the *Kaibao bencao*, which was the first to include *pishuang* in a *bencao* 本草, dated from 973, the drug was integrated into the arsenal of medications at about the same time as it first appeared in treatises on *materia medica*.

A number of prescriptions for treating intermittent fevers contained in another large formulary of the Song period, the *Shengji zonglu* 聖濟總錄 (Sagely Benefaction Medical Encyclopaedia), compiled by order of the Emperor Huizong 徽宗 in 1118, also use *pishuang*, particularly in the following two nosological categories:

- intermittent fevers of demoniacal origin (*guinüe* 鬼瘧), against which eight formulae out of fourteen (57 per cent) resort to *pishuang*.[52] According to the text, the treatment consisted mainly of sacrifices (*rang* 禳), but drugs could be useful for chasing out the demoniacal element and to calm the spirit.
- the condition known as *nüemu* 瘧母 (lit. 'mother of intermittent fevers'), which corresponds to recalcitrant intermittent fevers that would not respond to treatment. Medication had to be administered to fight against the hard abdominal lumps (*zhengjia* 癥瘕) that characterised this illness:[53] four out of six formulae (66 per cent) contained *pishuang*.

In the above two cases, the use of a toxic drug such as arsenic anhydride was altogether in line with the therapeutic tradition that went back at least as far as the *Shennong*

---

[49] *Mengqi bitan, juan* 24, 777.

[50] A number of different drugs were used, throughout the history of Chinese medicine, against intermittent fevers. The *Zhenglei bencao, juan* 2, 6b–7a, for example, lists many remedies to be used against these disorders. They include: the effective *changshan* 常山 (the root of *Dichroa febrifuga*) which, however, was difficult to administer in an appropriate way; *shuqi* 蜀漆 (the leafy twigs of *D. febrifuga*); *muli* 牡蠣 (oyster); *fangji* 防己 (*Stephania tetranda*); *mahuang* 麻黃 (*Ephedra sinica*); and a whole variety of artemisias, among them the famous *Artemisia annua* (*qinghao* 青蒿), which has again become famous in the late twentieth century, thanks to the active principles that it contains and its marked anti-malarial qualities.

[51] *Taiping shenghui fang, juan* 52, 1592–622.   [52] *Shengji zonglu, juan* 35, 718.

[53] *Shengji zonglu, juan* 35, 720.

bencao jing, which recommended treating demoniacal possessions (*guizhu* 鬼疰) and accumulations (*jiju* 積聚) with toxic remedies.[54]

In any event, the striking eruption of *pishuang* into the curative arsenal proposed against intermittent fevers by the *Taiping shenghui fang* and the *Shengji zonglu*, two works of an encyclopaedic nature lucky enough to enjoy Imperial approval, corresponds to a veritable *therapeutic method* that was commonly found between the end of the tenth century and the beginning of the twelfth.

The life and survival of a toxic therapeutic method

How did this method fare? An examination of the medical texts of the Southern Song, the Jin and the Yuan reveals that *pishuang* continued to be quite regularly prescribed. The drug is mentioned, for example, in the *Jifeng puji fang* 雞峰普濟方 (Prescriptions for All from the Hen's Peak), compiled in 1133 by Zhang Rui 張銳 (twelfth century), which included arsenic anhydride in nine out of forty-two prescriptions suggested for the treatment of intermittent fevers.[55] It also features in the *Weisheng baojian* 衛生寶鑒 (Precious Examination of Hygiene), compiled under the Yuan by Luo Tianyi 羅天益 (thirteenth century), a pupil of Li Gao 李杲 (1180–1251). In the latter work, the 'elixir of arsenic and cinnabar' (*chensha dan* 辰砂丹), for example, which the author claims to have used with success, contains cinnabar, arsenic anhydride, and realgar.[56] During this same period, authors also tried to justify the use of *pishuang* on 'theoretical' grounds. Zhang Congzheng 張從正 (1156–1228) declared in his *Rumen shiqin* 儒門事親 (A Means for Scholars to Serve their Relatives) published in 1228, that, in such a case, heat attacked heat (*yi re gong re* 以熱攻熱), that is to say the heat of the drug attacked the heat felt by those suffering from intermittent fevers.[57]

Although *pishuang* continued to be used under the Southern Song, the Jin, and the Yuan, the tendency seems to have been for its prestige to diminish, and a number of treatises from this period use it only seldom, as has been pointed out by Miyasita Saburō.[58] For example, the *Sanyin jiyi bingzheng fanglun* 三因極一病證方論 (The Three Causes Epitomized and Unified: the Quintessence of Doctrine on Medical Disorders) (1174), by Chen Yan 陳言 (late twelfth century),[59] resorts only twice to the use of *pishuang*. Similarly, Zhu Zhenheng 朱震亨 (1281–1358) in his works draws attention to the danger of the drug, which can lead to the aggravation of complaints

---

[54] *Shennong bencao jing, juan* 1, 36, and 84. See also Obringer (1997), 28–9.
[55] *Jifeng puji fang, juan* 14, 177–83.   [56] *Weisheng baojian, juan* 16, 260.
[57] *Rumen shiqin, juan* 1, 846, cited from *Zhongguo yixue dacheng* 中國醫學大成.
[58] Miyasita (1979), 97 f.   [59] *Sanyin jiyi bingzheng fanglun, juan* 6, 77 f.

rather than to their hoped-for alleviation, particularly in the treatment of chronic intermittent fevers.[60]

This tendency was to be largely confirmed during the Ming and Qing dynasties,
when the prescription of *pishuang* (or *pishi*), without entirely disappearing, at least
became secondary compared to the use of other drugs. Under the Ming, important
works such as the *Yixue gangmu* 醫學綱目 (Principles of Medicine), by Lou Ying 樓英
(1320–89), published posthumously in 1565,[61] the *Yifang kao* 醫方考 (Examination
of Medical Prescriptions) (1584), by Wu Kun 吳崑 (1551–1620),[62] the *Renshu bianlan* 仁術便覽 (A Vade-mecum of Human Techniques) (1585), by Zhang Hao 張浩
(sixteenth century),[63] and the *Shoushi baoyuan* 壽世保元 (Preserving the Original
Principle in Order to Obtain Longevity) (author's own preface 1615), by Gong Tingxian
龔廷賢 (fl. 1615)[64] all make either very little use of arsenic anhydride or none at all.
Under the Qing, in the section devoted to intermittent fevers in the medical part of the
Gujin tushu jicheng 古今圖書集成 ([Imperially Commissioned] Compendium of
Literature and Illustrations, Ancient and Modern) (1726),[65] only 7 of the 179 formulae
mentioned – apart from the 'simple formulae' (*danfang* 單方) – against such ailments
contain *pishuang* (or *pishi*), that is to say about 4 per cent. These figures should be com-
pared to those that reflect the prescription of other drugs: for instance, *chaihu* 柴胡
(*Bupleurum chinense* D.C.),[66] which features in the composition of forty-three formulae (24 per cent); *chenpi* 陳皮 (the rind of the fruit of *Citrus tangerina* Hort. and
Tanaka),[67] in thirty-eight formulae (21 per cent); *huangqin* 黃芩 (*Scutellaria baicalensis*
Georgi),[68] in twenty-eight formulae (16 per cent); *changshan* 常山 (*Dichroa febrifuga*
Lour.),[69] in twenty-seven formulae (15 per cent); and *baizhu* 白朮 (*Atractylodes macro-
cephala* Koidz.),[70] in twenty-six formulae (14 per cent).

It would, however, be exaggerated to say that from the time of the Ming onward
the use of arsenic anhydride against intermittent fevers was rejected. That dynasty's
treatises on *materia madica* do retain *pishuang* among their entries. The *Bencao pinhui
jingyao* 本草品匯精要 (Essentials of *Materia Medica*, Classified by Degrees) (1505)
by Liu Wentai 劉文泰 (fl. 1488–1505), for example, lists the drug mainly as the treatment
for all intermittent fevers.[71] The *Bencao gangmu*, by Li Shizhen also contains refer-

[60] See *Danxi zhifa xinyao* 丹溪治法心要, *juan* 1, 17, and *Gezhi yulun* 格致餘論, 21.
[61] *Yixue gangmu*, *juan* 6, 182 f. [62] *Yifang kao*, *juan* 2, 99 f. [63] *Renshu bianlan*, *juan* 2, 136 f.
[64] *Shoushi baoyuan*, *juan* 3, 170 f. [65] *Gujin tushu jicheng*, *Yibu quanlu*, *juan* 290, 1503 f.
[66] *Zhongyao dacidian* (1979), no. 3763. [67] *Zhongyao dacidian* (1979), no. 5535.
[68] *Zhongyao dacidian* (1979), no. 4147. [69] *Zhongyao dacidian* (1979), no. 4321.
[70] *Zhongyao dacidian* (1979), no. 1376. [71] *Bencao pinhui jingyao*, *juan* 5, 181.

ences of a kind to the drug.[72] Not only does it integrate into the text the therapeutic indications mentioned in earlier treatises, but it also introduces others such as that the remedy 'gnaws away the rotten flesh of boils (*yongju* 癰疽)'. Furthermore, it recognises
that the drug can be very effective against certain ailments, in particular intermittent
fevers with catarrh (*tannüe* 痰瘧) and respiratory difficulties with very loud breathing
(*houchuan* 齁喘).[73] But at the same time it points out the extreme toxicity of *pishuang*,
underlines how difficult it is to use, and criticises the Song authors for not having
sufficiently drawn attention to this point:

> *Pi* is a very hot and very toxic drug, and the poison of *pishuang* is extremely vio-
> lent. Mice and sparrows die immediately after having absorbed a small quantity
> of it; the cats and dogs that eat those mice and sparrows also die. The consump-
> tion of one *qian* 錢 of the drug [about 3.7 g] provokes death in a human being. The
> power of the poison of *gouwen* 鉤吻 (*Gelsemium elegans* Benth.) or of *shewang*
> 射罔 (lit. 'net for hunting', a hunting poison prepared from aconite)[74] is less
> strong than that of *pishuang*, yet the *materia medica* of the Song have very little
> to say about the toxicity of the latter. Why is that?[75]

In truth, when Li Shizhen accuses the Song authors of having neglected the dangers
of the drug, he is wrong, as is proved by certain passages in the *bencao* of the Song
period. The *Bieshuo bencao*, for example, observed:

> Recently *pi* 砒 has been much in use as a treatment for intermittent fevers. The
> basic idea is that with the raw (*sheng* 生) drug one can neutralise the hot poison.
> Now, intermittent fevers result, basically, from heat-stroke, hence its use.
> Nowadays, doctors of the common people have not thoroughly studied that prin-
> ciple, and they use the frost obtained after heating (*yi suo shao shuang* 以所燒
> 霜), that is to say arsenic anhydride, *pishuang*, which is bound to provoke vomit-
> ing and diarrhoea. If, with good luck, this calms down, they persevere in applying
> the method, causing damage of many kinds. One must be vigilant: at the beginning
> of the preparation of *pishuang* by grilling and sublimation, men stand more
> than ten *zhang* 丈 away, up-wind; all the trees and grasses that are close by and

---

[72] *Bencao gangmu, juan* 10, 606 f. Elsewhere, the same author considers that *pishi* is the origin (the
expression used is 'young sprout' (*miao* 苗)) of tin, *xi* 錫. This explained why wine contained in new
receptacles made of tin could become poisonous. In this connection, it is worth noting that the presence
of arsenic in bronzes confers upon alloys a fine golden colour (with a 2 per cent proportion of arsenic),
or a silvery colour (4–6 per cent). An analysis of certain copper or bronze pots of the Shang-Yin
dynasty has revealed percentages of arsenic as high as 4.72 per cent; see Needham (1974), 223, and
Zhao Kuanghua (1985), 15.

[73] *Bencao gangmu, juan* 10, 608.   [74] On aconite, see Obringer (1997), 91–143.

[75] *Bencao gangmu, juan* 10, 608.

that are down-wind die. Similarly, we often see the drug mixed with food to poison rats. If cats or dogs eat it, they too die. This poison is far stronger than *shewang*.[76]

As can be seen, a certain inconsistency surrounds the subject of *pishuang*, which is accused of being more dangerous than the drug before it has been heated. Such denunciations became frequent, under the Song, on the subject of a number of minerals which, according to the precepts and practices of external alchemy, had to be subjected to the action of fire before being used.[77] In a similar vein the *Bencao yanyi*, after setting out the method for preparing *pishuang*, notes that people suffering from intermittent fevers who use excessive doses of this drug are afflicted by vomiting and diarrhoea.[78]

Plenty of troubles thus seem to have plagued cures based on *pishuang*.[79] In an attempt to seize upon the 'technical' and 'clinical' reality of such treatment, I have studied the posology proposed by prescriptions in the *Shengji zonglu* that are intended to counter intermittent fevers and that contain arsenic anhydride among their ingredients.

My first example is the Cinnabar Pill (*dansha wan* 丹砂丸),[80] recommended against intermittent fevers of a demoniacal origin. The pill was composed as follows:

- *dansha* 丹砂 (cinnabar): $\frac{1}{2}$ *qian*
- *awei* 阿魏 (*Ferula* sp.): $\frac{1}{2}$ *qian*
- *pishuang* 砒霜 (arsenic anhydride): 1 *qian*
- *chi* 豉豆 (fermented soya beans): 49 beans

---

[76] Cited in *Zhenglei bencao*, juan 5, 8a.

[77] Consider, for example, the anecdote recorded by Shen Gua, under the Song, in his *Mengqi bitan*, juan 24, 761, about his cousin Li Shansheng 李善勝 (eleventh century), one of whose disciples died after taking an elixir made from cinnabar that had been treated by fire. See Ho and Needham (1959) and Obringer (1997), 42.

[78] *Bencao yanyi*, juan 6, 43.

[79] In a completely different historical and cultural context, Trousseau (1873), vol. III, 487, notes that J. Ch. M. Boudin, in his *Traité des fièvres intermittentes et continués des pays chauds et des contrées marécageuses, et de leur traitement par les préparations arsenicales*, published in Paris in 1842, restored the reputation of the use of arsenic acid as a remedy for bouts of intermittent fevers. Elsewhere, the twelfth edition of the *Dictionnaire de médecine* (1865), known as the Nysten dictionary (after Nysten, one of its earliest authors), ran as follows (see Littré and Robin (1865), 108):

> The arsenicals act efficaciously as anti-periodicals on intermittent fevers and other malarial conditions both recent and longstanding, even when the sulphate of quinine has no effect. It is above all arsenic acid that is used in a daily dose of 5 centigrammes in a solution. It is administered in fractional doses, which are increased or decreased according to the patient's tolerance.

[80] *Shengji zonglu*, juan 35, 719.

The four ingredients had to be reduced to a powder and 49 pills were then made by adding water, drop by drop. The posology was one pill for each dose. If we adopt the equivalence commonly accepted for the Song period of 1 *qian* = about 4 g,[81] and if we assume the powder to have been homogeneously mixed – which is rather unlikely – with each dose one absorbed a quantity of arsenic anhydride approximately equivalent to: $^1/_{49}$ *qian* = $^1/_{49} \times 4 = 0.082$ g, or 82 mg.

A similar procedure enabled me to determine the quantity of *pishuang* absorbed where two other prescriptions were followed:

- the Powder with *Euonymus alatus* (*guijianyu san* 鬼箭羽散球),[82] for which the daily dose of arsenic anhydride was about 100 mg.
- the Pill of Marvellous Application (*miaoying wan* 妙應丸),[83] which involved taking a dose of about 100 mg of arsenic anhydride.

From these calculations – subject, it will be remembered, to the imprecise measuring techniques of the period – we find that the doses of *pishuang* prescribed under the Song (around 80–100 mg), if strictly adhered to in the cure, were strong, even positively dangerous. According to certain authors,[84] a lethal dose would be 120 mg. However, it should be pointed out that this would vary considerably from one individual to another, and also depending on how fine a powder the product was reduced to.[85]

To be sure, the Song doctors did take precautions, as can be seen from the formulation of prescriptions containing *pishuang*: they were frequently forbidden for pregnant women (as in the case of *miaoying wan*, studied above), they sometimes contained an

---

[81] See Guo Zhengzhong (1993), 203–23. This quantity is, of course, approximative, on account of the variability of the calibration and the complexity of the system of weights and measures. For the Song, equivalences were on average as follows: 1 *jin* 斤 = 633 g; 1 *liang* 兩 = 40 g; 1 *qian* 錢 = 4 g; 1 *fen* 分 = 0.4 g.

[82] *Shengji zonglu, juan* 35, 719; the dose given is the same as for the preceding formula; the composition of this powder was as follows: *guijianyu* 鬼箭羽 (*Euonymus alatus* (Thunb.) Sieb.), 1 *fen*; *pishuang* 1 *qian*; *wulingzhi* 五靈脂 (the faeces of various kinds of flying squirrels, including *Trogopterus xanthipes*, Milne-Edwards), 1 *liang*; in total, *pishuang* thus represented 10 per cent, in weight, of the prescription (assuming that 1 *liang* = 10 *qian*, and 1 *qian* = 10 *fen*). The daily dose was equal to one half-*qian* spoonful (*banqian bi* 半錢匕), considered to be the equivalent of about 1 g (or slightly more). See *Zhongyi dacidian: fangji fence* (1983), 606.

[83] *Shengji zonglu, juan* 36, 733. The pill was recommended against intermittent fevers characterised by thirst and a feeling of nausea. The composition of this pill was as follows: *lüdou* 綠豆 (*Phaesolus radiatus* L.), 40 beans; *heidou* 黑豆 (Glycine max (L.) Merr.), 30 beans; *pishuang*, $^1/_2$ *qian*; *dansha* 丹砂 (cinnabar), a quantity as large as two soya seeds; *qiandan* 鉛丹 (minium Pb_3O_4), 1 *qian*. This made twenty pills, the posology being one pill.

[84] Buchanan (1962), 43.

[85] The nineteenth-century Western doctors mentioned in note 79 recommended a dose of 50 mg.

antidote to the drug (for example, *lüdou* 綠豆, *Phaseolus radiatus* L.),[86] and *pishuang* was never used in a decoction. All the same, the general tendency to prescribe overdoses – or at least very strong doses – must have resulted in a number of accidents, and given the methods of preparation then followed and the relatively imprecise weighing techniques, the difficulties involved in controlling the regularity of the doses administered certainly considerably handicapped the therapeutic use of the drug. It was one of the dangerous remedies that were banned from sale in 1268, under the Yuan, at the same time as aconites and *badou* 巴豆 (*Croton tiglium* L.).[87] The reactions of distrust, if not rejection, evinced by the doctors of the Yuan, the Ming, and the Qing periods were thus to a certain extent justified and go at least some way towards explaining the relative failure and difficult survival of a practice that was a real technical innovation, even if it did not represent a true break in pharmacotherapy.

Quite apart from the undeniable toxicity of arsenic anhydride (*pishuang*), another hypothesis, of an economic order, might be advanced in an attempt to explain the situation. It concerns the problem of obtaining supplies of the *pishi* ore used to prepare *pishuang*. I have already mentioned the fact that, under the Song, there existed only one mine, in Xinzhou, which was expected to supply the entire Empire. Now, a local monograph dated 1873, the *Guangxinfu zhi* 廣信府志 indicates that, under the Qing, it was no longer known what some of the mining products cited in the Song text were.[88] However, under the Ming, the *Tiangong kaiwu* 天工開物 (Exploitation of the Works of Nature), dating from 1637, by Song Yingxing 宋應星 (1587–1666), mentions several places where arsenic ores (*pishi* 砒石) were produced: [Guang]xin [廣]信 (Jiangxi), Xinyang 信陽 (Henan), and Hengyang 衡陽 (Hunan), which was the most important source at that time.[89] So it would seem that the decline in the use of *pishuang* cannot, after all, be explained by problems relating to the supply of the raw material.

All in all, it seems to me that the technical and therapeutic innovation represented by the preparation of arsenic anhydride (*pishuang*) from arsenic ores, and its use as a remedy for intermittent fevers encountered too many difficulties for it to last: the definition and classification of the various substances necessary for the technical procedure frequently suffered from a lack of precision. The very nature of arsenic

---

[86] *lüdou* 綠豆 ('green bean'): as early as the Song period, this leguminosa, of which the seed (a small bean) was used, was recognised to be an antidote to mineral poisons (*Kaibao bencao*, in *Zhenglei bencao*, *juan* 25, 18a), and even nowadays is recommended, for example, in cases of intoxications from pesticides. Its ability to counter the hot nature of the poisons was attributed to its own cold nature. The drug contains many phospholipides and a roughly 22 per cent proportion of proteins. The presence of some of the latter might explain its general action against the poisons, as they render toxic minerals insoluble.
[87] *Yuan shi* 元史, *juan* 105, 2687.   [88] *Guangxinfu zhi*, *juan* 1, 116.
[89] *Tiangong kaiwu*, *juan* 11, 301, and Sun and Sun (1966).

anhydride, from a chemical point of view, and its instability must sometimes have disoriented the Chinese doctors. And finally, the danger represented both by the preparation, which involved heating the ores, and by the extreme toxicity of the drug when it was used as a therapeutic treatment probably outweighed any possible curative benefit that the innovation provided.

References to premodern Chinese and Japanese works

Baopuzi 抱朴子 (Book of Master Holding-to-Simplicity). Jin, *ca* 320. Ge Hong 葛洪. Cited from *Baopuzi neipian jiaoshi* 抱朴子內篇校釋, annotated by Wang Ming 王明. Zhonghua shuju, Beijing, 1985.

Bencao gangmu 本草綱目 (Systematic *Materia Medica*). Ming, 1596. Li Shizhen 李時珍. 4 vols. Renmin weisheng chubanshe, Beijing, 1975–81.

Bencao pinhui jingyao 本草品匯精要 (Essentials of *Materia Medica*, Classified by Degrees). Ming, 1505. Liu Wentai 劉文泰. Renmin weisheng chubanshe, Beijing, 1982.

Danxi zhifa xinyao 丹溪治法心要 (Essentials of the Therapeutics of [Zhu] Danxi). Yuan, 14th century. Zhu Zhenheng 朱震亨. Renmin weisheng chubanshe, Beijing, 1983.

Daozang 道藏 (Taoist Canon). Lu Guoqiang 陸國強 et al. (eds.). 36 vols. Wenwu chubanshe / Shanghai shudian / Tianjin guji chubanshe, Beijing/Shanghai, 1988.

Gezhi yulun 格致餘論 (Supplementary Comments on a Deep Understanding of Things). Yuan, 14th century. Zhu Zhenheng 朱震亨. Jiangsu kexue jishu chubanshe, Nanjing, 1985.

Gujin tushu jicheng 古今圖書集成 ([Imperially Commissioned] Compendium of Literature and Illustrations, Ancient and Modern). *Yibu quanlu* 醫部全錄 (Comprehensive Record of the Section on Medicine). Qing, 1726. Chen Menglei 陳夢雷 et al. 12 vols. Renmin weisheng chubanshe, Beijing (1959–62) 1982–83.

Guangxinfu zhi 廣信府志 (Gazetteer of the Prefecture of Guangxin). Qing, 1873. Jiang Jizhu 蔣繼洙 et al. Cited from *Zhongguo fangzhi congshu* 中國方志叢書, *Huazhong difang* 華中地方 no. 106. Chengwen chubanshe, Taibei, 1970.

Jifeng puji fang 雞峰普濟方 (Prescriptions for All from the Hen's Peak). Song, 1133. Zhang Rui 張銳. Shanghai kexue jishu chubanshe, Shanghai, 1987.

Lingnan weisheng fang 嶺南衛生方 (Prescriptions for Hygiene from Lingnan). Song manuscript published in Yuan, preface of 1283. Li Qiu 李璆 and Zhang Zhiyuan 張致遠. Annotated by Ji Hong 繼洪. Zhongyi guji chubanshe, Beijing, 1983.

Mengqi bitan 夢溪筆談 (Dream Pool Essays). Song, *ca* 1086. Shen Gua 沈括. Cited from *Mengqi bitan jiaozheng* 夢溪筆談校證, annotated by Hu Daojing 胡道靜. 2 vols. Shanghai guji chubanshe, Shanghai, 1987.

Qimin yaoshu 齊民要術 (Essential Techniques for the Peasantry). Wei, *ca* 535. Jia Sixie 賈思勰. Cited from *Qimin yaoshu jiaoshi* 齊民要術校釋, annotated by Miao Qiyu 繆啟愉. Nongye chubanshe, Beijing, 1982.

Renshu bianlan 仁術便覽 (A Vade-mecum of Human Techniques). Ming, 1585. Zhang Hao 張浩. Renmin weisheng chubanshe, Beijing, 1985.

Rumen shiqin 儒門事親 (A Means for Scholars to Serve their Relatives). Jin, 1228. Zhang Congzheng 張從正. Cited from *Zhongguo yixue dacheng* 中國醫學大成, edited by Cao Bingzhang 曹炳章, vol. II, 839–956. See also *Gujin tushu jicheng* 古今圖書集成, *Yibu quanlu* 醫部全錄, vol. VII, 1465–7.

Sanyin jiyi bingzheng fanglun 三因極一病證方論 (The Three Causes Epitomised and Unified: the Quintessence of Doctrine on Medical Disorders). Song, 1174. Chen Yan 陳言. Renmin weisheng chubanshe, Beijing, 1983.

Shanhaijing 山海經 (Classic of the Mountains and Lakes). Warring States – Han, *ca* 3rd – 1st centuries BC. Anon. Cited from *Shanhaijing jiaozhu* 山海經校注, annotated by Yuan Ke 袁珂. Shanghai guji chubanshe, Shanghai, 1980.

Shengji zonglu 聖濟總錄 (Sagely Benefaction Medical Encyclopaedia). Song, 1118. Zhao Ji 趙佶 et al. 2 vols. Renmin weisheng chubanshe, Beijing, (1962) 1987.

Shijing 詩經 (Book of Songs). Zhou, 1000–600 BC. Anon. Cited from *Maoshi zhengyi* 毛詩正義. In *Shisanjing zhushu* 十三經注疏.

Shisanjing zhushu 十三經注疏 (Commentary to the Thirteen Canons). Qing, 1816. Ruan Yuan 阮元. Reprint in 2 vols. by Zhonghua shuju, Beijing, 1980.

Shoushi baoyuan 壽世保元 (Preserving the Original Principle in Order to Obtain Longevity). Ming, author's preface of 1615. Gong Tingxian 龔廷賢. Annotated by Lu Taolin 魯兆麟. Renmin weisheng chubanshe, Beijing, 1993.

Shujing 書經. *ca* 1000 BC–AD 400. Anon. Cited from *Shangshu zhengyi* 尚書正義. In *Shisanjing zhushu* 十三經注疏.

Shuowen jiezi 説文解字 (Analytical Dictionary of Characters). Han, 121. Xu Shen 許慎. Zonghua shuju, Beijing, (1963) 1979.

Taiping shenghui fang 太平聖惠方 (Imperial Grace Formulary of the Taiping Period). Song, 978–92. Wang Huaiyin 王懷隱 et al. 2 vols. Renmin weisheng chubanshe, Beijing, (1958) 1982.

Taiqing shibi ji 太清石壁記 (Records from the Stone Wall of the Great Purity). Tang, 758–60. Based on an earlier version of the Jin, 3rd century. Earlier version by Su Yuanlang 蘇元朗, Tang compilation attributed to Chu Ze xiansheng 楚澤先生. In *Daozang*, vol. XVIII, 763–76.

Tiangong kaiwu 天工開物 (Exploitation of the Works of Nature). Ming, 1637. Song Yingxing 宋應星. Annotated by Zhong Guangyan 鍾廣言. Zhonghua shuju, Hong Kong, 1978. Transl. Sun and Sun, 1966.

Tongzhi lüe 通志略 (Collection of Monographs). Song, 1161. Zheng Qiao 鄭樵. Shanghai guji chubanshe, Shanghai, 1990.

Wang Zhen nongshu 王禎農書 (Agricultural Treatise of Wang Zhen). Yuan, 1313. Wang Zhen 王禎. Nongshu chubanshe, Beijing, 1981.

Weisheng baojian 衛生寶鑒 (Precious Examination of Hygiene). Yuan, 13th century. Luo Tianyi 羅天益. Renmin weisheng chubanshe, Beijing, 1987.

Xinxiu bencao 新修本草 (Newly Revised *Materia Medica*). Tang, *ca* 660. Su Jing 蘇敬. Annotated by Shang Zhijun 尚志鈞. Anhui kexue chubanshe, Hefei, 1981.

Yifang kao 醫方考 (Examination of Medical Prescriptions). Ming, 1584. Wu Kun 吳崑. Renmin weisheng chubanshe, Beijing, 1990.

Yixue gangmu 醫學綱目 (Principles of Medicine). Ming, 1565 (posthumous). Lou Ying 樓英. Annotated by Gao Dengying 高登瀛 and Lu Zhaolin 魯兆麟. 2 vols. Renmin weisheng chubanshe, Beijing, 1987.

Yuan shi 元史 (History of the Yuan). Ming, 1370. Song Lian 宋濂 et al. Zhonghua shuju, Beijing, 1976.

Zhenglei bencao 證類本草 (*Materia Medica* Corrected and Arranged in Classes). Song, *ca* 1082. Tang Shenwei 唐慎微. Cited from the *Chongxiu Zhenghe jingshi zhenglei beiyong bencao* 重修正和經史證類備用本草. Facsimile of 1249 edition. Renmin weisheng chubanshe, Beijing, 1957.

Zhouli 周禮 (Records of the Rites of the Zhou Dynasty). Pre-Han or Han. Anon. Cited from *Zhouli jinzhu jinyi* 周禮今注今譯. Song, 11th century. Annotated by Lin Yin 林尹. Taiwan shangyin yinshuguan, Taibei, 1972.

Zhubing yuanhou lun 諸病源候論 (Origins and Symptoms of Medical Disorders). Chao Yuanfang 巢元方 et al., 610. Cited from *Zhubing yuanhou lun jiaoshi* 諸病源候論校釋. Edited by Nanjing zhongyixue yuan 南京中醫學院. 2 vols. Renmin weisheng chubanshe, Beijing, 1980. See also *Tōyō igaku zenpon sōsho* 東洋醫學善本叢書, volume 6, Tōyō igaku kenkyūkai, Osaka, 1981.

References known from citations only

Bencao tujing 本草圖經 (*Materia Medica* with Illustrations). Song, 1062. Su Song 蘇頌. Cited in *Zhenglei bencao*.

Bencao yanyi 本草衍義 (Dilations upon *Materia Medica*). Song, 1116. Kou Zongshi 寇宗奭. Reconstituted from citations. Renmin weisheng chubanshe, Beijing, 1990.

Bieshuo bencao 別説本草 (More Sayings on *Materia Medica*). Song, 11th century. Chen Cheng 陳承. Introduced into the *Zhenglei bencao* in 1108 by Ai Sheng 艾晟.

Kaibao bencao 開寶本草 (*Materia Medica* of the Kaibao Period). Song, 973. Liu Han 劉翰, Ma Zhi 馬志 et al. Cited in *Zhenglei bencao*.

Mingyi bielu 名醫別錄 (Informal Records of Famous Physicians). ?Wei–Jin, 3rd century. Attributed to Tao Hongjing 陶弘景. Reconstituted from citations and annotated by Shang Zhijun 尚志鈞. Renmin weisheng chubanshe, Beijing, 1986.

Rihuazi bencao 日華子本草 (*Materia Medica* by Master Sun-Rays). Song, 10th century. Da Ming 大明. Cited in *Zhenglei bencao*.

Shennong bencao jing 神農本草經 (The Divine Husbandman's Canon of *Materia Medica*). Late Han, 1st century AD. Cited from *Shennong bencao jing jiaozheng* 神農本草經校證. Reconstituted from citations and revised by Wang Yunmo 王筠默. Jilin kexue jishu chubanshe, Changchun, 1988.

Wu Pu bencao 吳普本草 (*Materia Medica* by Wu Pu). Wei, 3rd century. Attributed to Wu Pu (*ca* 149–250). Reconstituted from citations by Shang Zhijun 尚志鈞 et. al. Renmin weisheng chubanshe, Beijing 1987.

Wuwei Han dai yijian 武威漢代醫簡 (Slips on Medicine from the Han Period, Found in Wuwei). Gansu sheng bowuguan 甘肅省博物館 (eds.). 1975 Wenwu chubanshe, Beijing.

Yaoxing lun 藥性論 (Discourse on the Nature of Drugs). Tang. Attributed to Zhen Liyan 甄立言 and Zhen Quan 甄權. Cited in *Zhenglei bencao*.

References to modern works

Boudin, J. Ch. M. 1842. *Traité des fièvres intermittentes, rémittentes et continues des pays chauds et des contrées marécageuses, et de leur traitement par les préparations arsenicales*. Baillière, Paris.

Bray, Francesca 1984. *Agriculture*. In Joseph Needham. *Science and Civilisation in China*, vol. VI, *Biology and Biological Technology*, part 2. Cambridge University Press, Cambridge.

Bruce-Chwatt, L. J. and de Zulueta, J. 1980. *The Rise and Fall of Malaria in Europe*. Oxford University Press, Oxford.

Buchanan, W. D. 1962. *Toxicity of Arsenical Compounds*. Elsevier, Amsterdam/London/New York.

Cheng Minsheng 程民生 1992. *Songdai diyu jingji* 宋代地域經濟 (Regional Economy under the Song). Henan daxue chubanshe, Kaifeng.

Dagognet, François 1964. *La raison et les remèdes*. Presses Universitaires de France, Paris.

Despeux, Catherine and Obringer, Frédéric (eds.) 1997. *La maladie dans la Chine médiévale: la toux*. L'Harmattan, Paris.

Elvin, Mark 1973. *The Pattern of the Chinese Past*. Stanford University Press, Stanford.

Gansu sheng bowuguan 甘肅省博物館 1975. *Wuwei Han dai yijian* 武威漢代醫簡 (Slips on Medicine from the Han Period, Found in Wuwei). Wenwu chubanshe, Beijing.

Golas, Peter J. 1980. 'Rural China in the Song'. *Journal of Asian Studies* 39 (2), 291–325.

Grmek, Mirko D. 1983. *Les maladies à l'aube de la civilisation occidentale.* Payot, Paris.
  (ed.) 1995. *Histoire de la pensée médicale en Occident.* Editions du Seuil, Paris.
Guo Zhengzhong 郭正忠 1993. *San zhi shisi shiji Zhongguo de quanheng duliang* 三至十四世紀中國的
  權衡度量 (Units of Measure in China from the Third to the Fourteenth Century). Zhongguo shehui
  kexue chubanshe, Beijing.
Ho Pingyü and Needham, Joseph 1959. 'Elixir Poisoning in Medieval China'. *Janus* 48, 221–51.
Littré, Émile and Robin, Charles 1865. *Dictionnaire de médecine, de chirurgie, de pharmacie, des sci-
  ences accessoires et de l'art vétérinaire*, 12th edition. J.-B. Baillière et Fils, Paris.
Mawangdui Han mu boshu zhengli xiaozu 馬王堆漢墓帛書整理小組 (eds.) 1985. *Mawangdui Han mu
  boshu* 馬王堆漢墓帛書 (Manuscripts on Silk Excavated from a Han Tomb in Mawangdui). Wenwu
  chubanshe, Beijing.
Miyasita Saburō. 1979. 'Malaria (*yao*) in Chinese Medicine during the Chin and Yuan Periods'. *Acta
  Asiatica* 36, 90–112.
Needham, Joseph 1974. *Spagyrical Discovery and Invention: Magisteries of Gold and Immortality.* In
  Joseph Needham, *Science and Civilisation in China*, vol. V: *Chemistry and Chemical Technology*
  part 2. Cambridge University Press, Cambridge.
  1987. *Military Technology: the Gunpowder Epic.* In Joseph Needham, *Science and Civilisation
  in China*, vol. V: *Chemistry and Chemical Technology*, part 7. Cambridge University Press,
  Cambridge.
Obringer, Frédéric 1997. *L'aconit et l'orpiment: drogues et poisons en Chine ancienne et médiévale.*
  Fayard, Paris.
Ren Jiyu 任繼愈 1991. *Daozang tiyao* 道藏提要 (A Summary of the Daoist Canon). Zhongguo shehui
  kexue chubanshe, Beijing.
Riddle, John M. 1992. *Quid pro quo: studies in the History of Drugs.* Variorum, Hampshire/Brookfield.
Schafer, Edward H. 1955. 'Orpiment and Realgar in Chinese Technology and Tradition'. *Journal of the
  American Oriental Society* 75, 73–89.
Sigaut, François 1994. 'Compte-rendu de Daumas M. 1991. *Le cheval de César, ou le mythe des révolu-
  tions techniques*'. Editions des Archives contemporaines, Paris. *Annales (Histoire, Sciences
  Sociales)* 49 (4), 903–5.
Sivin, Nathan 1968. *Chinese Alchemy: Preliminary Studies.* Harvard University Press, Cambridge, Mass.
Song Xi 宋晞 (1962) 1979. *Song shi yanjiu luncong* 宋史研究論叢 (A Collection of Articles on the
  History of the Song). Zhongguo wenhua yanjiusuo, Taibei.
Sun Zen E-tu and Sun Shiou-chuan (transl.) 1966. *T'ien-kung k'ai-wu. Chinese Technology in the
  Seventeenth Century, by Sung Ying-Hsing.* Pennsylvania State University Press, University Park/
  London.
Touwaide, Alain 1995. 'Stratégies thérapeutiques: les médicaments'. In Grmek, vol. I, 227–37.
Trousseau, Armand 1873. *Clinique médicale de l'Hôtel-Dieu de Paris.* J. B. Baillière et Fils, Paris.
Wang Kuike 王奎克, Zhu Sheng 朱晟, Zheng Tong 鄭同 and Yuan Shuyu 袁書玉 1985. 'Shen de lishi zai
  Zhongguo' 砷的歷史在中國 (A History of Arsenic in China). In Zhao Kuanghua, 14–38.
Yang Yuan 楊遠 1982. *Tangdai de kuangchan* 唐代的礦產 (Mineral Ores under the Tang). Taiwan
  xuesheng shuju, Taibei.
Zhang Hongzhao 章鴻釗 (1927) 1993. *Shiya* 石雅 (*Lapidarium Sinicum*). Shanghai guji chubanshe,
  Shanghai.
Zhao Kuanghua 趙匡華 (ed.) 1985. *Zhongguo gudai huaxue shi yanjiu* 中國古代化學史研究 (Research
  into the History of Chemistry in Ancient Times in China). Beijing daxue chubanshe, Beijing.
Zhao Kuanghua 趙匡華 and Luo Meng 駱萌 1985. 'Guanyu woguo gudai qude danzhi shen de jin yi bu
  quezheng he shiyan yanjiu' 關於我國古代取得單質砷的進一步確證和實驗研究 (Experimental
  Research and New Proofs concerning the Obtainment of Metallic Arsenic in Ancient China). In Zhao
  Kuanghua 45–62.

Zheng Tong 鄭同 and Yuan Shuyu 袁書玉 1985. 'Danzhi shen lianzhi shi de shiyan yanjiu' 單質砷煉制史的實驗研究 (Experimental Research into the History of the Preparation of Metallic Arsenic). In Kuanghua, 39–44.

Zhongyao dacidian 中藥大辭典 (Great Dictionary of Chinese *Materia Medica*) 1979. Jiangsu xinyi xueyuan 江蘇新醫學院 (ed.). Shanghai kexue jishu chubanshe, Shanghai.

Zhongyi dacidian: fangji fence 中醫大辭典方劑分冊 (Great Dictionary of Chinese Medicine: Prescriptions) 1983. 'Zhongyi dacidian' bianji weiyuanhui《中醫大辭》典編輯委員會 (eds.). Renmin weisheng chubanshe, Beijing.

Zhongguo yixue dacheng 中國醫學大成 (Compendium of Chinese Medicine). (1936) 1990. Cao Bingzhang 曹炳章 (ed.). 6 vols. Yuelu shushe, Changsha.

PART IV

The canons revisited in Late Imperial China

Introduction

Innovation in the Song is often opposed to the consolidation of Neo-Confucian doctrine in the Ming and Qing, the implication being that Late Imperial China had little to offer by way of medical innovation. This view is clearly outdated. The sheer wealth and diversity of records which have survived from this period is overwhelming, and it has enabled researchers to explore a wide range of medical practices – from reproductive technologies to the treatment of smallpox – in social domains as varied as those of household-based health care or urban venues of medical patronage.[1] These studies have highlighted important changes to which medical doctors, their clientele, and their learning were subject, changes that in part have had a lasting impact on present-day practices.

This section is limited to the discussion of works, currently celebrated as canonical, that were then recompiled and reinterpreted. Among the doctrinal texts (*jing* 經) the *Yellow Emperor's Inner Canon* (*Huangdi neijing* 黃帝內經) is an example *par excellence* of late Ming revision. Over time this work was repeatedly reworked and now contains vocabulary with a layer of meaning dating to the Zhou, grammatical constructions characteristic of the Han, and sections and chapters that were probably composed in the Tang, while the two books that it comprises were edited into their extant form no

---

[1] Among recent works in the West belong, for instance, Bray, Francesca (1997), *Technology and Gender: Fabrics of Power in Late Imperial China*, University of California Press, Berkeley, 275–368; Chang Chiafeng (1996), 'Aspects of Smallpox and its Significance in Chinese History', PhD thesis in History, School of Oriental and African Studies, University of London; Wu Yi-li (1998), 'Transmitted Secrets: the Doctors of the Lower Yangzi Region and Popular Gynecology in Late Imperial China', PhD thesis in History, Yale University; Hanson, Marta (1997), 'Inventing a Tradition in Chinese Medicine: from Universal Canon to Local Medical Knowledge in South China, the Seventeenth to the Nineteenth Century', PhD thesis in History and Sociology of Science, University of Pennsylvania. See also works mentioned in the part V introduction.

earlier than in the Song.[2] Yet those parts of this work that are currently taught to medical students and constitute the core of the canonical doctrine practitioners are familiar with, are basically those considered as relevant in the late Ming. At that time, Zhang Jiebin 張介賓 (1563–1640) pointed out that related medical topics were dealt with in entirely different chapters of the two books that constituted the *Neijing*. He therefore compiled the *Leijing* 類經 (Canon of Categories) (1624) which conflated the *Suwen* 素問 (Basic Questions) and *Lingshu* 靈樞 (Divine Pivot) into one book, and regrouped their contents thematically into twelve categories (*lei* 類). In contemporary China it is his work which provides the basis for medical theory.[3]

   The two chapters in this part are concerned, not with the medical canons (*jing*), but with two other important genres, the *materia medica* (*bencao* 本草) and the formularies (*fang* 方): the *Bencao gangmu* 本草綱目 (Hierarchically Classified *Materia Medica*) (1596) by Li Shizhen 李時珍 (*ca* 1518–93) is generally considered the apex of the *bencao* tradition and the *Shanghan lun* 傷寒論 (Treatise of Cold Damage Disorders) from the second century AD by Zhang Ji 張機 (150–219) is the canonical formulary book. The articles explore the interests of the compiler Li Shizhen, in the first case, and the claims of Zhang Ji's critics, in the second case.

   In chapter 7 Georges Métailié examines the structure of this monumental compendium and shows that Li Shizhen's concerns were not only those of a medical doctor but also those of a scholar interested in the 'investigation of things' (*gewu* 格物). In an introductory chapter, Li Shizhen declared the need to reorganise the existing knowledge on drug products, and he did it by hierarchically ordering the material into sixteen sections (*bu* 部), sixty categories (*lei* 類), and about 1,895 kinds (*zhong* 種).

   While the now lost canonical *Shennong bencao jing* 神農本草經 (Divine Husbandman's *Materia Medica* Canon) had grouped all drugs into three classes (*sanpin* 三品) in respect of their therapeutic qualities, Tao Hongjing 陶弘景 (456–536), in his *Bencao jing jizhu* 本草經集注 (Notes to the *Materia Medica* Canon), had proposed to categorise them into sections (*bu*) that took account of more naturalistic criteria. Li Shizhen not only created new sections but also changed their sequencing. For instance, rather than grouping the two sections of wild plants and the three sections of cultivated plants together, he ordered the five plant sections, as he said, 'from the smallest to the biggest', i.e. from herbs (*cao* 草) to trees (*mu* 木), an ordering which has been likened to

---

[2] These two books each with eighty-one chapters had a very different textual history, see Sivin, Nathan (1993), 'Huang ti nei ching', in Loewe, Michael (1993), *Early Chinese Texts: a Bibliographical Guide*, Society for the Study of Early China and the Institute of East Asian Studies, University of California, Berkeley, 196–215.

[3] Hsu, Elisabeth (1999), *The Transmission of Chinese Medicine*, Cambridge University Press, Cambridge, 186–206.

the *scala naturae*[4] although it certainly reflects primarily a Chinese philosophical concern with degrees of consciousness and perhaps also with cosmological studies on 'outward appearance'.[5]

Categories (*lei*) constituted a level of classification subordinate to sections (*bu*) and superordinate to kinds (*zhong*). Their use as an independent structuring device was innovative, but the criteria which determined whether or not a kind was included in a category are rather diverse and difficult to identify retrospectively. The article shows that in many cases 'ecological' criteria seemed important, which would corroborate Lu Gwei-djen's observation that Li Shizhen paid great attention to the ecology of the living beings from which the drugs of the *materia medica* were derived.[6]

Zhong (kind) is the same word as currently used for designating Linnaean species, but Métailié stresses that none of the three classificatory entities that Li Shizhen used has any affinity with modern taxonomic categories. Rather, the rationale for many aspects of Li Shizhen's classifications is best understood in respect of recent researches in ethnobiology and the cognitive psychology of living kinds. The sections (*bu*) and kinds (*zhong*), in particular, reflect ethnobiological considerations found cross-culturally, while the categories (*lei*) seem to have traits of a characteristically Chinese (folk-) scientific approach to living kinds and their habitat.

The monographs on the kinds were structured in a new way that again underlined Li Shizhen's concern with 'the investigation of things': he clearly distinguished between systematically provided entries with information on the natural history of the animals, plants, and minerals, and other entries which informed the physician on the medicinal properties of the products derived from them. His description of living kinds, such as that of the well-known *tong* 桐 trees, testifies to his incorporation of knowledge from agricultural and horticultural treatises into the *bencao* literature, to which he added his own observations. Such detailed accounts of living kinds were certainly innovative for the *bencao* genre. But in other instances Li Shizhen collated information from different sources without having seen a specimen. Clearly, he was not a modern botanist but motivated by philologial concerns and primarily guided by the Confucian concern with the 'investigation of things'.

---

[4] Needham, Joseph (with Lu Gwei-djen) (1986), *Science and Civilisation in China*, vol VI: *Biology and Biological Technology*, part 1: *Botany*. Cambridge University Press, Cambridge, 315.

[5] Unschuld, Paul U. (1986), *Medicine in China: a History of Pharmaceutics*, University of California Press, Berkeley, 135–8, points out that the compilers of the *Bencao pinhui jingyao* categories systematised the sections in light of Shao Yong's (1011–77) cosmological studies on 'outward appearances'. It is possible that such considerations were applied also by Li Shizhen.

[6] Lu Gwei-djen (1966). 'China's Greatest Naturalist: a Brief Biography of Li Shih-Chen', *Physis* 8 (4), 383–92.

The *Treatise on Cold-Damage Disorders* (*Shanghan lun* 傷寒論) from the second century AD, which has remained *the* canonical work on formulae (*fangji*), forms the core of Marta Hanson's chapter insofar as the polemic of late Ming and Qing medical authors centred on it. In chapter 8 Hanson examines the importance of ideas about space and geographically specific ecologies in the formation of this new medical tradition formed in contradistinction to the universality of the *Shanghan lun*. China was seen as divided into major geographic regions: the dry highlands of the north and west were opposed to the damp lowlands of the east and south. To each region corresponded dominant types of bodily constitution, language, food preference, tastes, desires, and diseases. Hanson suggests that this ecological contrast, expressed in a theory of 'local *qi* (*diqi* 地氣)', parallels the contrast between wet and dry regions in Ayurvedic classifications of therapeutic substances and of cosmic processes.[7]

The *Shanghan lun* was long presumed to be applicable throughout China. However, although it had apparently been composed in response to an outbreak of epidemics in Hunan during the later Han, by Qing times certain physicians in the Jiangnan region viewed it as a northern teaching. By emphasising that its prescriptions were limited not only in time (i.e. it was outdated) but also in space (i.e. it only applied to the north), they were able to promote *wenbing* 溫病 (warm factor disorders) as a southern tradition of medical theory and practice. The rationale of *wenbing* was predicated on a denial of the universal validity of the *Shanghan lun*.

Hanson examines two texts of what she identifies as a trajectory towards the new tradition of *wenbing*. They were published within a century of one another in Suzhou and she considers them indicative of the situation before and after *wenbing* was defined as a southern medical tradition. The *Discriminating Examination of Southern Diseases* 南病別鑑 (*Nanbing biejian*), first published in 1878 by Song Zhaoqi 宋兆其, includes essays by Ye Gui 葉桂 (1667–1746), Xue Xue 薛雪 (1661–1750), and Xue Chengji 薛承基 (*ca* 1800), whom Song Zhaoqi portrays as the most influential physicians of the new *wenbing* tradition. Writings by all three had also been included in Tang Dalie's 唐大烈 *Compilation of Lectures by Suzhou Physicians* 吳醫彙講 (*Wuyi huijiang*) of 1792, but there, as Hanson points out, the three did not figure as representatives of the same tradition but merely as writers from the same area. They did not refer to each other in their essays nor did they cover similar topics. She shows that in the later work shared geographic space was used to legitimate grouping these three practitioners together as the originators of the *wenbing* doctrine: it was argued that *wenbing* medical theory and

---

[7] Zimmermann, Francis ((1982) 1987), *The Jungle and the Aroma of Meats: an Ecological Theme in Hindu Medicine*, University of California Press, Berkeley.

therapy were developed in response to the conditions and diseases characteristic of the local soil.

In order to highlight the new trends of the *wenbing* tradition, Hanson begins her article by discussing at length two of the four extant essays of an eighteenth-century representative of the cold-damage tradition, Guan Ding 管鼎. In the first essay Guan refutes the claims made by critics of the cold-damage tradition, namely that the natural endowment of primordial *qi* (*yuanqi* 元氣) had decreased over time and that the formulae in the *Shanghan lun* were therefore too strong. In the second essay, he counters the idea that these formulae were effective only for disorders arising due to cold *qi* in winter by arguing that cold damage is ultimately the underlying cause for other disorders too, such as the febrile illnesses arising in spring or summer, and that these need not be treated according to a different rationale. Notably, the editor of *Suzhou physicians*, Tang Dalie, disagreed with Guan Ding's viewpoint, as becomes obvious in his own essay on the 'Eight Masters', but he nevertheless had included Guan's writings in his compilation.

By contrast, Song Zhaoqi's compilation on the *Southern Diseases* republished the writings of the above-mentioned three physicians, who in his view laid the ground for the *wenbing* tradition, because 'their methods are best suited for the diseases of Jiangnan people'. Hanson, rather than discussing the contents of these authors' medical writings, examines the six prefaces to Song Zhaoqi's volume. These prefaces not only reveal the social relations that made its publication possible, they are shown to give cohesion and meaning to the new medical tradition and were, according to Hanson, the site of its invention. Clinical inadequacies of the *shanghan* methods are mentioned here, alongside the claim of reviving a tradition of ancient orthodoxy and the idea of local *qi* to legitimate an ideal of local medical knowledge. Hanson concludes that the epistemological shift from attributing universal validity to the *Shanghan lun* to the localist *wenbing* tradition paralleled the political transition from a court-dominated central authority in the eighteenth century to the rise of regionalism in the late nineteenth century. The revision of canonical works in Late Imperial China, motivated by various scholarly and political interests, was clearly coupled with an innovative reinterpretation of the canonical past.

7

The *Bencao gangmu* of Li Shizhen: an innovation in natural history?

GEORGES MÉTAILIÉ
IN COLLABORATION WITH ELISABETH HSU

Li Shizhen 李時珍 (1518–93), author of several books on medicine and of the famous *Bencao gangmu* 本草綱目 (Classified *Materia Medica*) (1596), was evaluated by Lu Gwei-djen as 'the greatest naturalist in Chinese history, and worthy of comparison with the best of the scientific men of the Renaissance period in Western countries'.[1] Since the time of this appreciation, an important corpus of literature has been devoted to his life and work,[2] and in the People's Republic of China he is celebrated – often in a hagiographic tone – as a great empiricist and innovator.[3] The number of recent editions of his *Bencao gangmu* is proof of the great interest that the book still commands not only among historians of science and medicine,[4] but also among practitioners.[5] Besides its unquestionable value as a rich source for research in the history of pharmacology and medicine, mineralogy, botany, and zoology in China, Li Shizhen's writings have even

---

[1] Lu (1966), 383.
[2] See for instance Cai Jingfeng (1964), Lu (1966), Sivin (1973), Qian Yuanming (1984), Chen Xinqian et al. (1985), Needham and Lu (1986), 308–21, Unschuld (1986), 145–68; for a comparison with a European Renaissance author, see Métailié (1989).
[3] See for instance Liu Hongyao (1994).
[4] 'His scholarly attitude towards the wealth of previous literature makes him also the greatest Chinese historian of science before modern times, and his work an unparalleled source of information on the development of scientific knowledge in East-Asia' (Lu (1966), 383).
[5] The standard edition in four volumes between 1977 and 1981 had the main purpose of restoring the original text and illustrations. In 1992 another editing committee headed by Chen Guiting published the *Bencao gangmu tongshi* in which the original text is followed by (a) explanations; (b) information about modern researches, if available; (c) examples of clinical usage; and (d) a bibliography of modern references. This edition also provides a scientific identification of the plants and animals.

proved to be interesting for linguistic studies.[6] With all these very laudative apprecia-
tions in mind, we explore aspects of the *Bencao gangmu* perceived as innovative within
the *bencao* 本草 (*materia medica*) tradition. Through an analysis of Li Shizhen's scientific approach we wish to present what we consider his main innovative achievement:
this was, alongside his main purpose of curing people effectively the re-classification
of the entire *materia medica* according to a new logic which was to a certain extent
motivated by the 'investigation of things' (*gewu* 格物).[7]

The textual sources for the *Bencao gangmu*

Li Shizhen begins the work by quoting his various bibliographic sources, so it is worth
considering what they are.[8] The way in which they were used is discussed below. His
first list introduces and briefly describes forty books, called *bencao* from 'all the authors
in history' (*lidai zhujia* 歷代諸家), which, in fact, represents only those works of
importance to which Li Shizhen had access. As the final item, this list includes the
Bencao gangmu itself and the short note that Li Shizhen devotes to his own book
contains details about the compilation of the work. It took him some twenty-six years,
from 1552 to 1578. He obtained data from many people, and 'visited and collected
everywhere' (*fangcai sifang* 訪采四方).[9] A second list quotes the titles of books written
by ancient and contemporary physicians (*gujin yijia shu* 古今醫家書). It is divided
into two parts: the first is a list of eighty-four books that were already cited by the
authors of previous *bencao* (since the sixth century), the second part introduces 277
authors quoted for the first time by Li Shizhen. A third list mentions ancient and
contemporary non-medical works like canonical, historical, technical, and philosophical texts, travel diaries, scholars' notes, dictionaries, encyclopaedias, and poems (*gujin
jingshi baijia shu* 古今經史百家書). It is divided into two parts in the same way as the
previous list: 151 texts were already used by Li Shizhen's predecessors and 440 are
quoted for the first time. Altogether the bibliography includes 932 titles. Among them,
following Li Shizhen's own differentiation, 36 per cent are medicinal and pharmacological works and 76 per cent, if we trust Li Shizhen, are quoted for the first time in the
bencao literature. This alone indicates a first innovative aspect of the *Bencao gangmu*,

---

[6] See for instance Shi Guanfen and Wang Lingmin (1991). The authors analyse the phenomenon of
trisyllabic terms with a duplication of the first syllable which frequently occurs in Li Shizhen's
writings.

[7] We would like to thank John Moffett for his kind bibliographical cooperation and Clare Cleret and
Penny Herbert who combed the English of a previous draft.

[8] *Bencao gangmu, juan* 1, 1–40.   [9] *Bencao gangmu, juan* 1, 11.

namely the introduction of a considerable amount of data, known but new to the *bencao* literature.

The Confucian legacy

Li Shizhen explains in the preliminary chapter, 'Fanli' 凡列 (Directions), why and how he decided to undertake this tremendous work. He insists on the complexity of the problem of nomenclature:

> Drugs possess many names, different today and formerly. However, I indicate (*biao* 表) the correct name (*zhengming* 正名) as the main entry (*gang* 綱), all the other ones being annexed in the rubric for 'explaining the names' (*shiming* 釋名). The correct name is given at the beginning; then I comment on the names and subordinates from the different *bencao*, recording their origin.[10]

This stress on accurate nomenclature which can be taken as evidence for Li Shizhen's basic Confucian attitude – linked to the concern with *zhengming*[11] – is crucial for him as a physician, considering that any error in the identification of the *materia medica* can have very dangerous consequences for patients' health, but Li Shizhen's interests are not limited to those of a medical practitioner. In the context of writing about the products that he has added to the Chinese *materia medica*, Li Shizhen explicitly declares that his undertaking is also of a scholarly nature:

> The 319 kinds (*zhong* 種) which the Tang and Song works do not have, but the many doctors of the Jin, Yuan, and our present Ming dynasty have used, have additionally been incorporated. I, Shizhen, carried on supplementing 374 kinds. Although they are considered drugs for physicians, by doing researches and explaining their nature and principle (*xingli* 性理), I have actually practised what we Confucian scholars call the 'investigation of things'[12] (*gewu zhi xue* 格物之學). This can fill the hiatus in the commentaries on the *Erya* 爾雅 (Approaching what is Correct) and the *Shijing* 詩經 (Book of Songs).[13]

We realise here that Li Shizhen's revision of the *materia medica* and the subsequent compilation of his book is for the author not merely the production of a work in the field of medicine but explicitly belongs to the long tradition of *gewu* (the investigation of things). This 'investigation of things' can be defined as a method of observation of the

---

[10] *Bencao gangmu*, 'Fanli', 33.

[11] On *zhengming*, see Cheng (1991), 221–32; Fung ((1952) 1973), *passim*; and Mei (1951).

[12] In this context *ru* means Confucian as well as scholarly.   [13] *Bencao gangmu*, 'Fanli', 34.

natural world from a moral perspective.[14] Li Shizhen's interest in *gewu* may well provide the main key to understanding his approach to the Chinese *materia medica*.

Li Shizhen uses various categories for ordering the knowledge compiled in this monumental work. First, he stresses the need to distinguish between *gang* 綱 and *mu* 目 (main and secondary levels), then he uses notions like *bu* 部 (sections), *lei* 類 (categories), and *zhong* 種 (kinds) for taxonomically ordering items that were often the 'living kinds' from which were derived products used as drugs in the Chinese *materia medica*. Most of these notions already figured in earlier works of the *bencao* tradition, but they are in part used in a different way by Li Shizhen. As will become more evident in the course of this study, interests not only of a physician but also of a *gewu* scholar gave the book its structure. Hence we raise the question as to whether the largest *materia medica* of Chinese medical history is in fact primarily innovative for natural history.

The structure of previous *bencao* works

In the *Shennong bencao jing* 神農本草經 (Divine Husbandman's Canon on *Materia Medica*), the canonical text for *materia medica* compiled around the second and first centuries BC,[15] drugs (*yao* 药) were classified from a pharmacodynamic point of view into three grades (*sanpin* 三品). The 120 drugs of the upper grade (*shangpin* 上品) were considered to act as princes (*jun* 君); non-toxic, they could not cause harm even when taken in large quantities and for a long time. They provided the basis for longevity. The 120 drugs of the intermediate grade (*zhongpin* 中品) acted as ministers (chen 臣); since they could be toxic depending on the dose, their use had to be well balanced. They were used to treat illness and recover from weakness. The 125 kinds of drugs of the lower grade (*xiapin* 下品) acted as government assistants (*zuoshi* 佐使); they were very toxic and could not be taken over a long period. They were used to expel noxious influences, balance coldness and heat, dissolve engorgements, and cure illness. Within this system reflecting the social order, the use and action of drugs were also linked to a conception of the cosmos, revealed above all by the number of drugs quoted in this book: they numbered 365, that is one for every day of the year. Moreover, drugs of the upper grade

---

[14] Through this formulation Li Shizhen alludes to a long tradition in China. In the first part of *The Great Learning (Da Xue* 大學), one of the canonical texts attributed to Confucius, reference is made to the ancient rulers who, in order to let natural virtues brighten the hearts of the people, began to become better themselves and, for this purpose, broadened their knowledge as much as possible through the investigation of things. This behaviour became one of the leitmotives of the Neo-Confucians after the eleventh century. During the nineteenth century, the term *gewuxue* came to be used to translate 'science' from Western languages. On *gewu*, see Chan (1957), Lau (1967), and Ching (1976), 75–103.

[15] Needham and Lu (1986), 244.

were mainly concerned with the nourishing of life in its essence (*yangming* 養命) and depended on Heaven (*tian* 天), those of the intermediate grade were mainly concerned with the nourishing of life as part of human nature (*yangxing* 養性) and depended on Man (*ren* 人), while those of the lower grade were mainly concerned with curing illness and depended on Earth (*di* 地). We acknowledge here a direct relationship with another concept of Chinese antiquity, namely that of the three powers (*sancai* 三才) Heaven, Earth, and Man, which resulted in the *sanpin* system of classification that organised the book into three parts. There was yet another classificatory system in the *Shennong bencao jing*, namely that of the Five Phases (*wuxing* 五行) which was used for assessing the flavour (*wei* 味), and what later became known as the nature or quality (*xing* 性 or *qi* 氣), of each drug. But this division into Five Phases never appeared as a structuring scheme for the book as a whole.

Tao Hongjing 陶弘景 (456–536) introduced a second partition in the *materia medica* when revising and completing the first canonical text in his *[Shennong] Bencao jing jizhu* [神農]本草經集注 (Notes to the [Divine Husbandman's] Canon of *Materia Medica*) in possibly AD 492. He took into account natural categories and made a first distinction between minerals, plants, and animals, then subdivided each of the categories following the *sanpin* system. After a first section on jades and stones (*yushi* 玉石), he sorted plants into five groups: herbs (*cao* 草), trees (*mu* 木), fruits (*guo* 果), vegetables (*cai* 菜), and staples (*mishi* 米食). The herbs and trees formed one part, the fruits, vegetables, and grains another, and inserted between them was the part on animals (*chongshou* 蟲獸). This system of different sections (*bu*) each of which were subdivided into three grades became the model for subsequent *bencao*.

The *Bencao jiyao* 本草集要 (Essentials of the *Materia Medica*) published in 1496 by Wang Lun 王綸 (mid fifteenth – early sixteenth centuries), however, distinguished between ten different sections: herbs, trees, vegetables, fruits, grains, minerals, quadrupeds, birds, 'insects'/fishes, and man.[16] Chen Jiamo 陳嘉謨 (1496–1600), in his *Bencao mengquan* 本草蒙荃 (Enlightenment on the *Materia Medica*) which was published in 1565, in Li Shizhen's time, adopted this new model, though with a few modifications: the plants came first (herbs, trees, grains, vegetables, and fruits), the minerals second, and then the animals and man last.

Gang and *mu*, and emphasis on a hierarchical order

In the opening sentence of the 'Fanli' chapter, Li Shizhen recapitulates the above information on earlier works, in an abbreviated form:

[16] See Okanishi (1977), 236–7.

The *Divine Husbandman's Materia Medica* in three chapters, with three hundred
and sixty kinds, is divided into three grades: upper, intermediate, and lower. Tao
Hongjing of the Liang dynasty added drugs so that their number was doubled,
adding them following their grade. During the Tang and Song dynasties, there
were duplications and revisions, each author made additions, including some,
omitting others; doing so, the levels of grading (*pinmu* 品目) still existed but the
ancient headings were all mixed up and the true meaning was lost. Now I have
ordered all under sixteen sections (*bu*) which represent the higher level *gang* 綱
and sixty categories (*lei*) which represent their subordinates *mu* 目, each according to its own category.

In this opening statement, *gang* and *mu* are newly introduced as a structuring device
for the compilation to follow. The *gang–mu* interrelation appears to be central to Li
Shizhen's reorganisation of the *materia medica* because he even mentions it in the title
of his work. As separate morphemes, *gang* and *mu* refer to the main rope and the meshes
of a net. It is in this way that they were probably explained to the Jesuit missionaries
since du Halde in his *Description . . .* (1735) gives a metaphoric interpretation: 'Like a
net with its main line [*gang*] and meshes [*mu*], this Herbal has main titles under which
are arranged the subjects dealt with, in the same way as meshes are arranged and
linked with the main line.'[17] As a disyllabic term, *gangmu* has the meaning of an organised whole. In this way it may refer to an administrative organisation or to the structure
of a book. Perhaps Li Shizhen in coining this title intended to make reference to the
Tongjian gangmu 通鑑綱目 (Summary of the Comprehensive Mirror) published in
1189 by Zhu Xi 朱熹 (1130–1200), which presented the main points of the famous book
on history, the *Zizhi tongjian* 資治通鑑 (Comprehensive Mirror to Aid in Government),
written between 1072 and 1084 by Sima Guang 司馬光 (1019–86). Li Shizhen may
thereby have intended to indicate his ambition to produce an encyclopaedic piece of
work.

A closer look at the *gang–mu* interrelation shows that it stands for a hierarchical relation, regardless of the level at which different structuring categories are related to each
other: in the opening paragraph of the 'Fanli' chapter, cited above, Li Shizhen presents
the sections (*bu*) as *gang*, the categories (*lei*) as *mu*. In the third paragraph of the same
chapter, cited at the very beginning of this chapter (p. 223), he attaches great importance
to the names of drugs, and expresses awareness that they have changed over time. He
distinguishes between the correct name (*zhengming*) of an entry on a kind (*zhong*) –
which is *gang* – and other names known from more recent *materia medica* that are presented in a subordinate rubric – which are *mu*. In the fourth paragraph, after accusing
his predecessors of dealing with the inclusion or omission of drugs into the *materia*

---

[17] Du Halde (1735), 586 (our transl.).

medica in a confused and undifferentiated manner, he claims not only to have engaged in evidential research (*kaozheng* 考正), analytic procedures (*fenbie* 分別), and synthesising operations (*guibing* 歸并), but also to have highlighted the *gang* and subordinated the *mu*. Thus, the dragon is *gang*, and its teeth, horns, bones, brain, afterbirth, and saliva are *mu*; or, millet is *gang*, and the red and yellow millet grains are *mu*. The *gang–mu* interrelation thus indicates a hierarchical order, regardless of whether it concerns the hierarchy between the higher order sections (*bu*) and the categories (*lei*) or the hierarchical organisation of information within a monograph on a kind (*zhong*).

The *gang–mu* interrelation evidently expresses the author's concern with ordering knowledge hierarchically which, in the 'Fanli' chapter, he himself puts forward as innovative. The notions *gang* and *mu* are thus best understood as expressing a *motto* according to which Li Shizhen structured his compilation; they do not designate taxa of any kind. However, the three notions which hierarchically structured his compilation of the Chinese *materia medica* – *bu*, *lei*, and *zhong* – appear to reflect an increased interest in a taxonomy of living kinds.

The sections (*bu*), and the grading of the myriad things

If Li Shizhen was not the first to introduce a new order in relation to Tao Hongjing's presentation of the *materia medica*, he was as far as we know innovative in ordering the sections (*bu*) according to a new 'logic' against the previous disorder he claimed to have found in the old books. He writes in the second paragraph of the 'Fanli' chapter:[18]

> The old books treat in an undifferentiated manner jades, minerals, waters, and earths, they do not distinguish between 'insects', scaly creatures, and creatures with shells; some 'insects' have an entry in the tree section and some trees in the herb section . . . I have now ordered (*lie* 列) everything into sections (*bu* 部) beginning with waters and fires, followed by earths, [because] Water and Fire precede the myriad things (*wanwu* 萬物) and the Earth is the mother of the myriad things. Then [follow] the metals and minerals, [because] they come from the Earth; then the herbs, grains, vegetables, fruits, and trees, from the smallest to the biggest; then the clothes and utensils, [made] from herbs and trees; then the 'insects',[19] the scaly creatures, the shelled creatures, the birds, the four-legged animals, to finish with man: from the vile to the precious.[20]

---

[18] *Bencao gangmu*, 'Fanli', 33.
[19] The *chong* 蟲 category includes, besides 'insects', spiders, snails and slugs, worms, myriapods, frogs, and toads.
[20] This is a literal translation. For another more elegant translation, see Needham and Lu (1986), 315.

Table 7.1. *The sixteen sections in the* Bencao gangmu

Waters	(*juan* 5)	*shui bu* 水部
Fires	(*juan* 6)	*huo bu* 火部
Earths	(*juan* 7)	*tu bu* 土部
Metals and Minerals	(*juan* 8–11)	*jinshi bu* 金石部
Herbs	(*juan* 12–21)	*cao bu* 草部
Grains	(*juan* 22–25)	*gu bu* 穀部
Vegetables	(*juan* 26–28)	*cai bu* 菜部
Fruits	(*juan* 29–33)	*guo bu* 果部
Trees	(*juan* 34–37)	*mu bu* 木部
Clothes–Utensils	(*juan* 38)	*fuqi bu* 服器部
'Insects'	(*juan* 39–42)	*chong bu* 蟲部
Scaly Creatures	(*juan* 43–44)	*lin bu* 鱗部
Shelled Creatures	(*juan* 45–46)	*jie bu* 介部
Birds	(*juan* 47–49)	*qin bu* 禽部
Quadrupeds	(*juan* 50–51)	*shou bu* 獸部
Man	(*juan* 52)	*ren bu* 人部

From this we can see that Li Shizhen explicitly wished to introduce innovations into the way in which knowledge in the *materia medica* was organised (see table 7.1). He not only created new sections by, for instance, differentiating between 'insects', scaly creatures, and shelled creatures, but also changed the usual sequencing of the sections. Compared to previous *bencao* books, the first three sections of the *Bencao gangmu* are innovative, for the waters, fires, and earths are newly treated as classified objects of a *materia medica*. Within the plant kingdom, Li Shizhen keeps to the old five sections, but he breaks with the former rationale based on the opposition of wild plants (trees and herbs) and crops (grains, vegetables, and fruit trees). This opposition was underlined by the way in which, in most of the former *bencao* books, the two sections on trees and herbs were separated from the three sections on crops by several sections concerning animals. By presenting the herbs, grains, vegetables, fruits, and trees in a sequence, Li Shizhen, as he himself explicitly states, takes account of a progression from the smallest to the biggest, from herbs to trees.

The section on clothes and utensils may be taken to reflect the concern to distinguish between drugs obtained from artefacts made of plant material and those obtained from plants directly, now clearly conceived of as living kinds.

The following five sections on the animals featured in part in other *materia medica*, though they would not always total five. Again it may be observed that the sequencing from 'insects' to scaly creatures to shelled creatures to birds and quadrupeds follows a new order: it goes, in Li Shizhen's own words, 'from the vile to the precious', ending with 'man as a medicine'.[21]

We notice that in doing so Li Shizen proposed a real *scala naturae*, as Lu Gwei-djen and Joseph Needham have already pointed out.[22] This grading of the myriad things from the lowest to the highest, an innovation for the *Bencao* tradition, actually expressed an ancient conception already found in *Xunzi* 荀子 of the third century BC,[23] which referred to degrees of consciousness. As Zhu Xi said: 'The consciousness of plants is inferior to that of animals, which in turn is inferior to that of human beings.'[24]

The categories (*lei*), and the ecology of living kinds

The categories (*lei*) constitute a level of classification subordinate to that of the sections (*bu*). The concept *lei* 類 already features widely in the Han and pre-Han literature and its increasing importance in the context of the *bencao* tradition is reflected in its occurrence in the title of the Song compilation *Zhenglei bencao* 證類本草 (*Materia Medica Corrected and Arranged in Classes*) (*ca* 1082). Despite its title, however, the compiler Tang Shenwei 唐慎微 (*ca* 1056–1136) made no use of *lei* as an independent structuring device. Li Shizhen is one of the first, if not the first, to use *lei* as a classificatory scheme for ordering his *materia medica* without, however, being explicit about his understanding of *lei*. In light of this, the meaning of *lei* can only indirectly be deduced from the way in which Li Shizhen uses it as a classificatory category.

The compilation begins with the section on waters (*shui bu*) – medicinal ones only – which is divided into two *lei*: sky waters (*tianshui* 天水) with thirteen kinds (*zhong*) and earth waters (*tushui* 土水) with thirty kinds.[25] The sky waters include rain and dew, the earth waters natural waters from seas, rivers, springs, and wells or byproducts of man's activities, such as knife sharpening, baby washing, hand and foot washing.

The section on fires (*huo bu*) does not distinguish between different *lei*, but directly subsumes eleven kinds (*zhong*) of which the first comprises *yang* 陽 fires as well as *yin* 陰 fires. Li Shizhen explains that this first kind, called *yanghuo yinhuo* 陽火 陰火, can be divided into three *gang* and twelve *mu*: fires from the sky (with four *mu*), fires from

---

[21] On 'Man as a Medicine', see Cooper and Sivin (1973).
[22] Lu (1966), 385; and Needham and Lu (1986), 315.
[23] *Xunzi, pian* 9, 84–5.   [24] Bodde (1991), 327.
[25] The author speaks of *zhong*, which we translate as 'kind'. More precisely, *zhong* designates a separate entry with a monograph that usually describes a 'kind', but several entries also provide lists of different types of living kinds such as, for instance, the poisonous fish, birds, or meats (at the end of chapters 44, 49, and 50) or different types of peoples (at the end of chapter 52). Notice also that the *zhong* in the section on man (chapter 52) mostly concern human body parts and not living kinds.

the earth (with five *mu*), and fires from man (with three *mu*).[26] He draws a distinction similar to that between the sky and earth waters, but it is made on a different level. Notably, in this case he uses the classificatory terms *gang* and *mu*.

The section on earths (*tu bu*) is formed by sixty-one kinds (*zhong*) of which more than half (thirty-nine kinds) used to be listed within the section on jades and minerals (*yushi* 玉石) in previous *materia medica*.[27]

The section on metals and minerals (*jinshi bu*) quotes four *lei* with altogether 161 kinds (*zhong*): metals (*jinlei* 金類) with twenty-eight kinds, jades (*yulei* 玉類) with fourteen kinds, minerals (*shilei* 石類) with seventy-two kinds and salted minerals (*lushilei* 鹵石類) with twenty kinds, followed by an appendix of twenty-seven kinds that 'have a name but are not (yet) used' (*youming weiyong* 有名未用). The *jinlei* begins with an entry on gold and silver and includes iron rust and all kinds of iron tools; the *yulei* discusses, besides jades, many precious stones, corals, and glass; the *shilei* is by far the longest and describes among other items cinnabar (*dansha* 丹砂), magnetic stones (*cishi* 磁石), arsenic compounds (*pishi* 砒石),[28] as well as including an entry on stone needles (*bianshi* 砭石); the *lushilei* which begins with table salt (*shiyan* 食鹽) comprises many kinds with a salty (*xian* 咸) or bitter (*ku* 苦) flavour, but also others. The criteria for distinguishing between these four *lei* are sometimes the same as those a lay-person currently makes in daily life between metals, precious stones, minerals, and salts, on the grounds partly of their appearance, partly of their use, and partly of the value society attributes to them, but it seems difficult, if not impossible, to find generally valid criteria.

The first three sections on waters, fires, and earths, as well as the section on *jinshi* (metals and minerals) – which in previous *bencao* carried the label of *yushi* (metals and minerals) and formed the first section – obviously seem to be linked to the desire of Li Shizhen to stress the significance of Five Phase doctrine. Water (*shui* 水), Fire (*huo* 火), and Earth (*tu* 土) are three of the Five Phases, and Li Shizhen's choice of *jinshi* rather than *yushi* seems to allude to the fourth of the Five Phases, Metal (*jin* 金). The fifth Phase, Wood (*mu* 木) is not specified, but if it were, one surmises, it would probably refer to the entire plant kingdom and not only to the trees which form one of the work's sections (*mu bu*). The polysemy of the term *mu* comprises both the meaning of tree and wood, so in recognition of there being 'herb in wood' (see p. 235) would allow Li Shizhen to incorporate all plants in the cosmological order of Five Phase doctrine.

For the plant kingdom, keeping to the five traditional sections, Li Shizhen distinguishes between thirty-one *lei*. The herb section (*cao bu*) is divided into the following ten *lei*: mountain herbs (*shancao lei* 山草類) with 70 kinds (*juan* 12–13), fragrant herbs

---

[26] *Bencao gangmu, juan* 6, 415.   [27] *Bencao gangmu, juan* 8, 455.
[28] Discussed by Obringer (this volume).

(*fangcao lei* 芳草類) with 56 kinds (*juan* 14), marshland herbs (*xicao lei* 隰草類) with 126 kinds (*juan* 15–16), poisonous herbs (*ducao lei* 毒草類) with 47 kinds (*juan* 17), creepers (*mancao lei* 蔓草類) with 73 kinds followed by an appendix with 19 kinds (*juan* 18), water herbs (*shuicao lei* 水草類) with 23 kinds (*juan* 19), stone herbs (*shicao lei* 石草) with 19 kinds (*juan* 20), and the 'mosses and his kindes'[29] (*tailei* 苔類) with 16 kinds (*juan* 21). This last chapter on the herbs also includes a listing of the names of 9 kinds of sundry herbs (*zacao* 雜草) and 153 kinds of plants which 'have a name but are not (yet) used' (*youming weiyong* 有名未用, *juan* 21), both of which, when listed, are not labelled as *lei*.[30]

The grains section (*gu bu*) comprises four *lei*: hemp–wheat–rice (*mamaidao lei* 麻麥稻類) with 12 kinds (*juan* 22), millets (*jishu lei* 稷黍類) with 18 kinds (*juan* 33), soja and legumes (*shudou lei* 菽豆類) with 14 kinds (*juan* 24), and fermented products (*zaoniang lei* 造釀類) with 29 kinds (*juan* 25). Evidently, three of the Five Grains (*wugu* 五穀) have been grouped into one *lei*, two of the Five Grains are presented as two separate *lei*, and one *lei* comprises products derived from some of the living kinds listed in the other three *lei*.

The vegetables section (*cai bu*) includes five *lei* defined as such on much more diverse grounds: those for seasoning (*hunxin lei* 葷辛類) with 32 kinds (*juan* 26), the soft and slippery (*rouhua lei* 柔滑類) with 41 kinds (*juan* 27), the gourd-like vegetables (*luocai lei* 蓏菜類) with 11 kinds (*juan* 28), the aquatic vegetables (*shuicai lei* 水菜類) with 6 kinds (*juan* 28), and the fungi (*zhi'er lei* 芝栭類) with 15 kinds (*juan* 28).

The fruit section (*guo bu*) is divided into six *lei*, again by taking account of many different criteria: the Five Fruits[31] (*wuguo lei* 五果類) with 11 kinds (*juan* 29), mountain fruits (*shanguo lei* 山果類) with 34 kinds (*juan* 30), exotic fruits (*yiguo lei* 夷果類) with 31 kinds (*juan* 31), spices (*weilei* 味類) with 13 kinds (*juan* 32), gourd-like fruits (*luolei* 蓏類) with 9 kinds (*juan* 33), and aquatic fruits (*shuiguo lei* 水果類) with 6 kinds (*juan* 33). The appendix lists the names of 21 kinds about which no further information was found.

---

[29] Following the terms in 'The Tables of English Names' of *The Herbal* by John Gerard ((1633) 1975); for Li Shizhen, *tai* – which in modern Chinese means specifically 'moss' – also had a broader meaning, including other plants like lichens.

[30] However, in the introductory text of the section, Li Shizhen explicitly says that he divides the herbs (*cao*) for therapeutic usage into ten *lei*, namely the above eight and the last two called *za* and *youming weiyong*. See *Bencao gangmu, juan* 12, 687.

[31] Under this heading are quoted the main fruits cultivated in Northern China, the 'classical fruits'. See Sivin (1973).

The tree section (*mu bu*) has six different *lei*: fragrant trees (*xiangmu lei* 香木類) with 35 kinds (*juan* 34), tall trees (*qiaomu lei* 喬木類) with 52 kinds (*juan* 35), lesser trees (*guanmu lei* 灌木類) with 51 kinds (*juan* 36), parasitic trees (*yumu lei* 寓木類) with 12 kinds (*juan* 37), trees in clusters (*baomu lei* 苞木類) with 4 kinds (*juan* 37), and miscellaneous woods (*zamu lei* 雜木類) with 7 kinds (*juan* 37), followed by an appendix listing the names of 19 kinds.

From the above, it becomes obvious that categories (*lei*) are the result of sorting based on very different criteria. They are sometimes determined by 'ecological' criteria that concern the habitat of the plants (mountains, marshlands, water, and stones) and possibly also by the attributes of being exotic (fruits) or parasitic (trees); the 'morphological' aspect (creepers, mosses, fungi, gourd-like, tall trees, lesser trees, trees in clusters); the aspect of whether a plant is wild or cultivated (the Five Fruits were cultivated); pharmacodynamic aspects such as toxicity (poisonous herbs); culinary and medicinal aspects of flavour and consistency (fragrant herbs, fragrant trees, fermented grains, vegetables for seasoning, soft and slippery vegetables, spices); and the traditional agricultural categories for the grains (hemp–wheat–rice, millets, soja and legumes); very diverse criteria indeed.

The section on clothes and utensils (*fuqi bu* 服器部) differentiates between two *lei*: clothes (*fubo lei* 服帛類) with 25 kinds (*juan* 38) and utensils (*qiwu lei* 器物類) with 54 kinds (*juan* 38).

The animals, like the plants, comprise five different sections, but are subdivided into only eighteen *lei*. These are determined by similar criteria of ecology and morphology as well as animal husbandry and life-cycle physiology.

Thus, the section on 'insects' (*chong bu*) is divided into three *lei*, all three being identified on the basis of their physiology in respect to the life cycle, i.e. their way of coming into being: the oviparous (*luansheng lei* 卵生類) with 45 kinds (*juan* 39–40), those produced by metamorphosis (*huasheng lei* 化生類) with 31 kinds (*juan* 41), and those produced by moisture (*shisheng lei* 濕生類) with 23 kinds (*juan* 42), followed by an appendix listing the names of 7 kinds.

The section on the scaly ones (*lin bu*) includes four *lei*, one of which is actually designated 'without scales': dragons (*longlei* 龍類) with 9 kinds (*juan* 43), snakes (*shelei* 蛇類) with 17 kinds (*juan* 43), fishes (*yulei* 魚類) with 31 kinds (*juan* 44), and fishes without scales (*wulinyu lei* 無鱗魚類) with 28 kinds to which the full description of another 9 kinds is added (*juan* 44).

The section on those with shells (*jie bu*) comprises two *lei*: turtles and tortoises (*guibie lei* 龜鱉類) with 17 kinds (*juan* 45), and scallops (*bangha lei* 蚌蛤類) with 29 kinds (*juan* 46).

The section on birds (*qin bu*) is divided into four *lei*, all of which are determined by the ecological factor of habitat: aquatic birds (*shuiqin lei* 水禽類) with 23 kinds (*juan* 47), grassland birds (*yuanqin lei* 原禽類) with 23 kinds (*juan* 48), forest birds (*linqin lei* 林禽類) with 17 kinds (*juan* 49), and mountain birds (*shanqin lei* 山禽類) with 13 kinds, followed by one additional kind (*juan* 49).

The section on quadrupeds (*shou bu*) differentiates between five *lei*, partly taking account of whether they are domesticated or not: domestic animals (*xulei* 畜類) with 28 kinds (*juan* 50), wild animals (*shoulei* 獸類) with 38 kinds (*juan* 51), rodents (*shulei* 鼠類) with 12 kinds (*juan* 51) as well as the wanderers (*yulei* 寓類) and monsters (*guailei* 怪類) which together comprise 8 kinds (*juan* 51).

The last section on man (*ren bu*), without being subdivided into categories, comprises 37 'kinds' (*juan* 52).

Li Shizhen's compilation aims at comprehensiveness which is reflected in the numerology in that it comprises, as stated in the 'Fanli' chapter, sixty different categories (*lei*). The above list shows that he explicitly refers only to fifty-seven. Evidently he adds to them those three sections (*bu*) – on fires, earths, and man – which have not been subdivided into categories.[32] Plants clearly form the most important part with 1,094 out of approximately 1,895 different kinds or, more precisely, entries (*zhong*).[33] Animals, which include dragons and monsters side by side with the well-known domestic animals, comprise only 409 different kinds.[34] Waters, fires, earths, metals, and minerals comprise 276 different kinds,[35] clothes and utensils 79 kinds.

From the above, it becomes very clear that Li Shizhen's categorisation of knowledge based on *lei* in no way represents a system as understood by modern taxonomists,[36] since Li Shizhen's criteria are largely based on subjective judgement and are not mutually exclusive. His classification of plants can be compared to the one created by his European contemporary Jacques Dalechamp (1513–88).[37] But it cannot be considered of the same nature as that of Andrea Cesalpino[38] who, in *De Plantis libri*, dated 1583, was the first botanist to attempt a systematic approach to botany[39] and whom Linnaeus

---

[32] Lu (1966), 386, counts sixty-two instead of sixty categories, for reasons that are not entirely transparent to us.

[33] This investigation does not purport to calculate how many entries describe living kinds. The calculation of the sum of living kinds mentioned in this compilation is complicated by the fact that the main text and the appendices (*fulu*) to some monographs on a kind list additional kinds.

[34] When Lu (1966), 386, speaks of 444 kinds belonging to the 'zoological domain', she obviously includes the entries (*zhong*) listed in the section on man which mostly concern body parts of man; they are in the present edition 37 but could arguably be considered 35.

[35] Lu (1966) counts 275 different kinds. The discrepancy may have arisen from a contradictory statement in the opening paragraph of chapter 6. See *Bencao gangmu, juan* 6, 413.

[36] A system, according to Germain de Saint-Pierre (1870), 1257, consists of the 'classification of plants following some principles'.

[37] Métailié (1989).   [38] As suggested by Chen Jiarui (1978), 106.   [39] Atran (1987), 195.

classified as a 'fructist' among the 'universal orthodox systematics' because he established his classification on the basis of fructification.[40] Notably, Linnaeus did not quote
Li Shizhen in his *Philosophia botanica*. According to Linnaeus' criteria, Li Shizhen
probably would not have been considered a 'true botanist' 'who knows botany by its
own principles and must know how to give an easily comprehensible name to any of the
plants'.[41] It is more likely that he would have thought of Li Shizhen as the 'physician'
('who has researched the virtues of plants and their action on the human body') among
the 'botanophilous' ('who have left some observations on plants though their works had
no direct link with the botanical science').[42] Since Li Shizhen was 'worthy of commen-
dation by some book on botany', he certainly was a 'phytologous'.[43]

   We have sought to give convincing reasons for considering Li Shizhen's sorting of the
materia medica in no way to constitute a modern taxonomy of natural kinds. Indices for
what guided his classification are embedded in his writings, more or less hidden, over-
shadowed by the table of contents (*zongmu* 總目),[44] which has wrongly been considered
the outline of a taxonomy of modern biology.[45]

The sections (*bu*) and categories (*lei*) in the light of modern taxonomy

In what follows, Li Shizhen's notions of *bu* 部 and *lei* 類 are explored by comparing
them with modern taxa in a preliminary study that focuses on the plant kingdom. As
already stated, the five sections (*bu*) on herbs, trees, grains, vegetables, and fruits were
well known in the *bencao* literature, but the notion of category (*lei*) is in the *Bencao
gangmu* applied for the first time as a structuring scheme of knowledge. Our attempt is
directed at teasing out the innovative aspect of Li Shizhen's classification of the *materia
medica* by, on the one hand, having recourse to an already given term (*bu*) and, on the
other hand, introducing a new classificatory term (*lei*). We will see that his classification reflects an interest in living kinds which is folk taxonomic rather than modern
taxonomic.

   Among the five sections (*bu*) of the plant kingdom, two refer, from an ethnobiological
viewpoint, to 'life forms',[46] namely the herbs (*cao* 草) and trees (*mu* 木). The distinction

---

[40] Linaeus (1751).   [41] Linaeus (1751), 4.   [42] Linaeus (1751).

[43] Linaeus (1751).   [44] *Bencao gangmu*, 25–32.

[45] For instance in the *Zhongyi dacidian yishi wenxian fence* 1981, 100, one reads that 'in biological
    classification, he possessed evolutionist ideas, relatively advanced'. Pei (1984), 9, states that the
    Bencao gangmu 'is one of the earliest works on plant systematics in ancient China'. Chen (1978), 110,
    considers that Li Shizhen's 'Body of principles for scientific naming, based on simple materialism, is
    still applicable today'.

[46] 'A salient characteristic of folk biological life-forms is that they partition the plant and animal cat-
    egories into contrastive lexical fields' (Atran 1990, 17).

between these two life forms, which can be traced in the Chinese context to the *Erya*,[47] is well known cross-culturally and parallels the Aristotelian distinction between the woody and the non-woody.[48] The singling out of vegetables (*cai* 菜) is probably derived from culinary practice. Fruits (*guo* 果) were consumed after the meal but they were not actually considered part of the meal.[49] Though found as foodstuffs in Han archaeological sites like Mawangdui,[50] they do not figure as a culinary category in the Mawangdui medical texts.[51] But in the *Liji* 禮記 (Book of Rites),[52] fruits (*guoshi* 果實) are a generic category, mentioned in a phrase parallel to one on the Five Grains (*wugu* 五穀) and in the *Guanzi* 管子,[53] the idiom of the Five Grains and Hundred Fruits (*wugu baiguo* 五穀 百果) expresses one idea: *gu* 穀 (grains) and *guo* 果 (fruits) are crops, emblems of seasonal regularity resulting in rich harvests.

The above five sections, which structured the knowledge of the plant kingdom in the *materia medica* since the Liang, reflect a categorisation that, apart from the well-known aspects of utility, also takes account of criteria derived from observation of the phenomenal world, even before Li Shizhen's time (e.g. the division into the life forms herbs and trees). Notably, their usage for therapeutic purposes was not primary among these criteria. Rather, habits of culinary practice and important social events in the agricultural cycle, like harvesting, seem to have coined the meaning of these terms.

Li Shizhen's somewhat modified understanding of these terms is revealed in the short introductory texts to each section. Thus the herbs section (*caobu*) opens by recording the origin of the plants: 'Heaven creates, Earth transforms, and so the plants are born' (*tian zao di hua er caomu sheng yan* 天造地化而草木生焉). Roots and bulbs (*gengai* 根荄) are the result of the action of the hard principle (*gang* 剛) on the soft (*rou* 柔), and branches and trunks (*zhigan* 枝干) result from the reverse. Leaves and sepals (*ye'e* 葉 萼) belong to *yang*, flowers and fruits (*huashi* 花實) to *yin*. In 'herb' there is wood/tree and in wood there is 'herb' (*cao zhong you mu, mu zhong you cao* 草中有木，木中有 草).[54] In this context Li Shizhen says: 'Setting aside grains and vegetables, the herbs that can be used as medicine comprise 611 kinds.' For him, grains and vegetables are herbs although they are not listed as subsections to the 'herb section'. This is confirmed by his statement at the beginning of the grains section (*gu bu*): 'I have regrouped the fruits of herbs (*caoshi* 草實) which can be eaten as grains in the grains section.'[55]

---

[47] *Erya, juan* 8, 1–24, and *juan* 9, 1–22.
[48] It need, however, not be universal, for size rather than woodiness and position (above or below) can also belong among the necessary criteria for determining basic life forms.
[49] Yu (1977), 69–70. [50] Yu (1977), 56.
[51] The one text passage in which *guo* occurs invokes its shape to which that of the embryo is likened. See Ma Jixing (1992), 786.
[52] *Liji*, 'Wang zhi' 王制. *Liji zhengyi* 禮記正義, *juan* 13, 1069. [53] *Guanzi, juan* 14, *pian* 40, 6a.
[54] *Bencao gangmu, juan* 12, 687. [55] *Bencao gangmu, juan* 22, 1433.

As for vegetables (*cai bu*), Li Shizhen writes: 'All the plants (*caomu* 草木) that can be eaten are called vegetables (*cai* 菜) . . . So, I select the herbs that one can eat, altogether 105 kinds, to make the vegetables section.'[56] Evidently vegetables and grains are herbs. By subordinating the vegetables and grains to the life form of herbs, Li Shizhen emphasises their complementarity. In the introductory texts to the grains and vegetables sections, he quotes only the phrases referring to the Five Grains (*wugu* 五穀) and Five Vegetables (*wucai* 五菜) from the *Suwen* 素問 (Basic Questions), and omits mention of the Five Fruits (*wuguo* 五果) and the Five Domestic Animals (*wuchu* 五畜) given in the original.[57]

The fruits section (*guo bu*) begins with: 'The fructification (*shi* 實) of trees is called *guo* 果,[58] the fructification of herbs is called *luo* 蓏[59] . . . So I have regrouped the fructifications of plants which are called *guo* and *luo* into the fruits section, altogether 127 kinds.'[60] That 'fruits are the fructification of trees' (*guo mu shi ye* 果木實也) is already given in the *Shuowen jiezi* 説文解字 (Explanation of Graphs and Analysis of Characters).[61] Li Shizhen's distinction between *luo* and *guo* as fruits of herbs and trees echoes that of Kong Yingda 孔穎達 (574–648), commentator to the *Yijing* 易經 (Book of Changes).[62] It fits the pattern that primarily distinguishes between *cao* and *mu*, but modifies the parallelism between the tree-fruits and the grains given in the above *Liji* and *Guanzi* quotations. The parallelism between *guo* and *gu* relies on their seasonal significance for a cultural activity, harvesting, while that of *guo* and *luo* seems to be based on the observation of living kinds, their appearance and ecological proclivity.

The trees section (*mu bu*) states:[63] '*mu* 木 (tree/wood) is a plant (*zhiwu* 植物), [it] is [also] one of the Five Phases. Its nature (*xing* 性) is linked to the soil: the mountains, valleys, plains, and marshes. At the beginning it is through the transformation of the material force (*qi* 氣) that it receives shape and quality (*xingzhi* 性質): standing up, with drooping branches, in clusters and in thickets.[64] Roots, leaves, flowers, and fruits; firmness, softness, beauty, and the ugly; all depend on the Supreme Pole (*Taiji* 太極).'

From the above text excerpts it is possible to deduce that plants, referred to as *caomu* (lit. 'herbs-trees') or *zhiwu* (planted things), represent the uppermost rank of Li Shizhen's classification which is called 'unique beginner' in ethnobiology.[65] In this rank, Li Shizhen distinguishes two 'life forms', herbs (*cao*) and trees (*mu*). He contin-

---

[56] *Bencao gangmu*, *juan* 26, 1571.   [57] Cf. *Suwen*, *juan* 7, *pian* 22, 73.
[58] Note that the character *guo* 果 has a tree radical (no. 75).
[59] Note that the character *luo* 蓏 is composed of two gourds and a grass radical (no. 140).
[60] *Bencao gangmu*, *juan* 29, 1725.   [61] *Shuowen jiezi*, *pian* 6, *shang*, 249.
[62] *Yijing* 'Shuo gua' 説卦 *Zhouyi zhengyi* 周易正義, *juan* 9, 83b.
[63] *Bencao gangmu*, *juan* 34, 1911.   [64] These four terms are borrowed from the *Erya*, *juan* 9, 11–12.

ues to use the five traditional categories of Tao Hongjing, but he in fact ranks the plant kingdom primarily into herbs and trees. The herbs form a section just like the grains and vegetables, but they are conceived of as superordinate. The fruit section comprises fruits from herbs as well as trees but differentiates between fruits of trees (*guo*) and fruits of herbs (*luo*).

The categories (*lei*) are subordinate to the sections (*bu*) and superordinate to kinds (*zhong*). The criteria according to which Li Shizhen distinguishes between them are outlined in the introductory commentary to the tree/wood section:[66] '[With] colour and fragrance, quality and flavour, one distinguishes grades and categories' (*se, xiang, qi, wei, qubian pinlei* 色香氣味區辨品類). Here Li Shizhen explicitly states that his categorisation accounts for the appearance of trees, their colour, and fragrance. Additionally, he says, categories (*lei*) are also determined by criteria linked to pharma-codynamic properties for therapeutic use; *qi* refers to the qualities cold (*han* 寒), hot (*re* 熱), cool (*liang* 涼), warm (*wen* 溫), and also neuter (*ping* 平) and *wei* to the Five Flavours sour (*suan* 酸), bitter (*ku* 苦), sweet (*gan* 甘), pungent (*xin* 辛), and salty (*xian* 咸).

To a modern botanist's eye, it is striking that within a category (*lei*), the names of various plants, today considered as belonging to the same botanical family, are quite often listed in a sequence. Joseph Needham has already observed this: 'The Chinese perceived very clearly relationships between plant genera, even though they were often "submerged" within their oecological and physiological classification.'[67] Li Shizhen groups together different kinds belonging to 'natural' families that were among the earliest ones to be recognised in the West, as reflected through the unorthodox structure of their names in modern taxonomy: they include the *Cruciferae* (versus the orthodox *Brassicaceae*), the *Labiatae* (versus *Lamiaceae*), the *Umbelliferae* (versus *Apiaceae*), the *Gramineae* (versus *Poaceae*), and several others. For instance, seven *Cruciferae* are quoted in a row within the seasoning category (*hunxin lei*)[68] and ten *Labiatae* are given at the end of the fragrant herbs category (*fangcao lei*).[69] The most salient example, however, concerns plants of the carrot family (*Umbelliferae*). Admittedly, the twenty-seven botanical species of the *Umbelliferae* identified by Read[70] occur in ten differ-

[65]   See Atran (1990), 5; also called 'kingdom' (Berlin 1992) or 'folk kingdom' (Atran et al. 1997).
[66]   *Bencao gangmu, juan* 34, 1911.   [67]   Needham and Lu (1986), 177.
[68]   *Wuxincai* 五辛菜, *yuntai* 芸薹, *song* 菘, *jie* 芥, *baijie* 白芥, *wuqing* 蕪菁, *laifu* 萊菔. See *Bencao gangmu, juan* 26, 1602–20.
[69]   *Xiangru* 香薷, *shixiangmao* 石香茅, *juechuang* 爵床, (*chicheshizhe* 赤車使者 which is an *Urticaceae*, a family with species in habitus similar to those of the *Labiatae*), *jiasu* 假蘇, *bohe* 薄荷, *jixuecao* 積雪草, *su* 蘇, *ren* 荏, *shuisu* 水蘇 *jining* 薺薴. See *Bencao gangmu, juan* 14, 909–26.
[70]   Read (1936), 54–61.

ent categories in the *Bencao gangmu* and seven categories name only one kind of *Umbelliferae*, but in three categories, entries on plants from this family are listed consecutively. In the seasoning category (*hunxin lei*) of the vegetables section, six species are mentioned in a row;[71] in the fragrant herbs category (*fangcao lei*) and the mountain herbs category (*shancao lei*) of the herbs section, two rows of seven are given.[72] In the case of botanical taxa with homogenous chemical properties, and also rather particular morphological features, like plants from the mint or carrot families, it is not entirely surprising to observe some convergence between Li Shizhen's 'folk classification' and modern scientific taxonomy. Other examples of partial overlapping of 'submerged families' may be found in the *Bencao gangmu* and botanical families, such as species of the *Rosaceae*, the *Compositae*, the *Euphorbiaceae*, or the *Araceae*, are listed consecutively within a category.[73] But this is not the rule and the grouping of taxa in a way that may look very unfamiliar to a modern taxonomist should not provoke surprise.

Needham and Lu's observation corroborates the relevance of 'covert categories' that ethnobiological research has detected on grounds of their operational significance in folk taxonomies. Typically, these covert categories have no name but psychological tests have revealed that they represent tacit knowledge of native speakers and the above-presented sequencing of kinds from modern botanical families is best interpreted in light of this research. Ordinarily Li Shizhen would not give a name to categor-

---

[71] *Bencao gangmu, juan* 26, 1632–40; *huluobo* 胡蘿卜: *Daucus carota* L.; *shuiqin* 水芹: *Oenanthe javanica* (Bl.) DC.; *jin* 堇 with synonym *hanqin* 旱芹: *Apium graveolens* L.; *zijin* 紫堇 *Corydalis edulis* Maxim. which is a *Fumariaceae* but has the name *jin* 堇; *maqi* 馬蘄: *Angelica yabeana* Mak. (according to Read 1936, 55); *huaixiang* 懷香 with synonym *huixiang* 茴香: *Foeniculum vulgare* Mill.; *shiluo* 蒔蘿: *Anethum graveolens* L. The Chinese names and synonyms sometimes refer to a range of different species, of which only one is given here. Plant identification is based on *Zhongyao dacidian* (1977) which often differs from Read (1936).

[72] One reads as follows: *chaihu* 茈胡: *Bupleurum chinense* D.C.; *qianhu* 前胡: *Peucedanum praeruptorum* Dunn; *fang feng* 防風: *Saposhnikovia divaricata* (Turcz.) Schischk.; *duhuo* 獨活: *Angelica pubescens* Maxim.; *tudanggui* 土當歸: *Aralia cordata* Thunb.; *duguancao* 都管草: *Angelica kiusiana* Maxim. (according to Read 1936, 54); *shengma* 升麻: *Cimifuga foetida* L. or *Cimifuga dahurica* (Turcz.) Maxim. See *Bencao gangmu, juan* 13, 785–98. The other comprises: *danggui* 當歸: *Angelica sinensis* (Oliv.) Diels; *xiongqiong* 芎藭 with synonym *chuanxiong* 川芎: *Ligusticum chuanxiong* Hort.; *miwu* 蘼蕪: sprouts of *chuanxiong*, here identified as *Ligusticum wallachii* Franch.; *shechuang* 蛇床: *Cnidium monnieri* (L.) Cusson; *gaobe* 藁本: *Ligusticum sinense* Oliv.; *zhizhuxiang* 蜘蛛香: *Pimpinella candolleana* Wight et Arn.; *baizhi* 白芷: *Angelica dahurica* (Fisch ex Hoffm.) Benth. et Hook. See *Bencao gangmu, juan* 14, 833–49.

   Note on *tudanggui*: possibly, Li Shizhen considered it a kind of *danggui* 當歸: *Angelica sinensis* (Oliv.) Diels; it is in modern Jilin province identified as *Angelica gigas* Nakai. On the other hand, the above given *Aralia* sp. would for obvious morphological reasons have been mentioned among the *Umbelliferae* (Métailié 1988).

[73] Needham (1971), Chen (1978).

ies of this kind, but in encyclopaedic texts, they are often named by the juxtaposition of two generic names like *tao-li* 桃李 (peach-prune) or *song-bai* 松柏 (pine-cypress).[74]

The above discussion shows that Li Shizhen was guided by interests that liken him to a botanist-naturalist and not merely a pharmacist-doctor, but he was not a modern taxonomist. The example given below, listing all the different kinds (*zhong*) within a particular category (*lei*), corroborates this. The category in mind is the first of the four in the grains section, called hemp–wheat–rice category (*mamaidao lei*), a name that is somewhat unusual insofar as it is trisyllabic with the three morphemes having a generic meaning.[75] Hemp, wheat, and rice were considered to constitute the Five Grains, together with beans (*shudou*) and millet (*jishu*), which the *Bencao gangmu* discusses in two separate categories (*lei*).[76] The *mamaidao lei* comprises twelve *zhong*: three entries on *ma* 麻 (hemp), six on *mai* 麥 (wheat), and three on *dao* 稻 (paddy rice, all written with the rice radical). The entries on hemp comprise *huma* 胡麻 (sesame), *yama* 亞麻 (wax), and *dama* 大麻 (hemp), identified with species from different families, namely *Sesamum indicum* L. from the family *Pedaliaceae*, *Linum usitatissimum* L. from the family *Linaceae*, and *Cannabis sativa* L. from the family *Cannabinaceae* respectively. The six wheat kinds have been equated with three species from the same family and two from the same genus: *xiaomai* 小麥 (wheat) with *Triticum aestivum* L., *damai* 大麥 (barley) and *kuangmai* 穬麥 (barley) with *Hordeum vulgare* L., and *quemai* 雀麥 which has the synonym *yanmai* 燕麥 (oat) with *Avena fatua* L., all three of which belong to the family of the *Graminaceae*; *qiaomai* 蕎麥 and *kuqiaomai* 苦蕎麥 are considered to be two *Fagopyrum* (buckwheat) species of the *Polygonaceae* family, namely *Fagopyrum esculentum* Moench. and *Fagopyrum tataricum* Gaertn. The three kinds of paddy rice called *dao* 稻, *jing* 粳, and *xian* 秈 or 籼, by contrast, refer to one and the same species, *Oryza sativa* L. This example shows not only the incongruence between Li Shizhen's notion of *zhong* and the modern species concept but further highlights how difficult, if not impossible it is to identify retrospectively the criteria that motivated Li Shizhen to group different *zhong* into a *lei*. The grains of the six *mai* and three *dao* were used as staple food while hemp, wax, and sesame seeds were used for making oils, all being essential in domestic economy. But Li Shizhen was certainly motivated by other considerations too.

In this particular case, where the polysyllabic names end in *ma*, *mai*, and *dao*, it is tempting to take the names of the various kinds as a lead to Li Shizhen's ordering of knowledge in his compilation. As will be shown below, this is indeed an important key

---

[74] Métailié (1997), 314.

[75] Following Atran et al. (1997), each of these morphemes would be a 'generic species'.

[76] *Bencao gangmu, juan* 22, 1435–70.

to understanding Li Shizhen's rationale, but names need not necessarily provide further guidance. While Li Shizhen must have taken account of the name when he listed the three *ma* (sesame, wax, and hemp) in a sequence, it is noticeable that he did not group all polysyllabic names ending with *ma* into a category (*lei*). Joseph Needham and Lu Gwei-djen discuss plants belonging to the *ma* group at length.[77] 'More than twenty plants and trees have this character in their names, though belonging in terms of modern botany to more than a dozen families.' They add: 'The resemblances were perfectly real, whether in fibres fit for textiles, in oil extractable from the seeds, or in the shapes of leaves, the polygonal character of the stem cross-section, the position of the seeds in the capsules, etc.'[78] These criteria make apparent why these plants were all called *ma*, the type evidently being hemp *Cannabis sativa* L. However, textile fibres, oil-seeds, and the like have no botanical significance, and the different plants called *ma* appear to be of a different order from Li Shizhen's folk taxa.

Needham and Lu's explorations thus suggest that there are different kinds of folk-taxonomic classification. One form of classification is reflected in the ending of polysyllabic names, the other one, discussed here, concerns criteria for grouping kinds into categories. To account for the differences between these two folk taxonomic classifications, it seems necessary to remind ourselves of the distinction between taxonomies of natural kinds and artefacts. This difference is now well established in cognitive psychology.[79] It appears Li Shizhen was primarily interested in natural kinds, that is 'basic-level categories of naturally occurring objects',[80] which 'scientific disciplines evolve to study'.[81] The different kinds of *ma*, by contrast, may have acquired their name from certain parts of the plant, like the fibres or seeds, which, like flowers and fruits, are not living natural kinds.[82] The use and function of these parts of the plant in social life probably determined their name. In other words, the polysyllabic names ending in *ma* are indicative of a folk-taxonomic classification, but not one of living kinds, while Li Shizhen's folk taxonomy is marked by an interest in the living kinds themselves.

Kinds (*zhong*), and the investigation of things

Folk taxonomies of living kinds, according to Atran, are 'universally and primarily composed of three absolutely distinct hierarchical levels, or ranks: the levels of *unique beginner*, *generic-specieme* and *life-form*'.[83] The ethnobiological viewpoint suggests

[77] Needham and Lu (1986), 170–6.   [78] Needham and Lu (1986), 170.   [79] For instance Keil (1986).
[80] Gelman (1988), 69.   [81] Carey (1985), 171.   [82] Atran (1990), 72.   [83] Atran (1990), 5.

that these three ranks characteristic of folk taxonomies can be found in Li Shizhen's
work but not within the explicitly given hierarchical orders *bu*, *lei*, and *zhong*. It has
been shown above that Li Shizhen differentiates between the ontological categories of
plants and those of animals (excluding humans), which is what the 'unique beginner'
does.[84] He is also well aware of the 'life-form' level, at least as we have seen, with regard
to the life forms herbs (*cao*) and wood/trees (*mu*), and this is so although he continues
to use the traditional categorisation of plants into five sections (*bu*). The 'generic-
specieme' level, though logically subordinate, is generally considered psychologically
prior to the life-form level. In the *Bencao gangmu*, it coincides with the notion of *zhong*
種 (kind).

The term *zhong* means 'species' in modern taxonomy, and modern authors often
wrongly translate it in this way when referring to ancient *bencao* literature. However, as
seen above the *zhong* entry does not always correspond to a botanic or zoologic species
and so must be considered as a generic-specieme.[85] Needless to say, within a certain
culture approaches to the classification of natural kinds differ. In the course of history,
foundations laid by predecessors are likely to be taken up again, but they may also be
transformed in the process. Li Shizhen elaborates on the entries that are kinds (*zhong*) in
earlier *materia medica*. The information he adds is written in a style that is innovative
in several ways, as will be examined in more detail in this section. The way in which
he structures the monographs on each entry of a kind will be explored in the following
section. But firstly his research methods will be examined.

As Li Shizhen himself professes, his first step is always a concern with names. This
stress on accurate nomenclature, repeatedly mentioned above, reflects Li Shizhen's
basically Confucian attitude. It is primarily as cultural objects that plants interest Li
Shizhen and other Chinese *literati*. New introductions as entries in the *Bencao gangmu*
are not newly discovered plants or animals that Li Shizhen would describe and name for
the first time – as would a modern botanist or zoologist. Firstly, this is not the purpose of
the compilation and, secondly, it is unlikely that this would at all be conceivable for a
Chinese scholar of the Ming time. His work represents a reorganisation of knowledge; it is
not a report on new discoveries after a botanical investigation into an unknown vegetation.

Li Shizhen's field work is of an anthropological rather than a field-botanical kind. He
goes to the countryside or to a mountain area in order to question people living there and

---

[84] Since Li Shizhen includes a section on man in his work, in this respect he can be considered to tran-
scend the folk-taxonomic domain, like Linné, who subordinated man into the natural world by creating
the species *homo sapiens*.

[85] See Atran (1990), 5; also called folk generic (Berlin (1992), 52–101), or generic species (Atran et al.
(1997)). In the *Bencao gangmu*, *zhong* need not always refer to a living kind, see above, note 25.

to try to find the plants corresponding to the names he has found in the huge corpus of texts already investigated. He is a naturalist for whom the first tool is philology.

This philological concern, closely linked with the *zhengming* tradition, is for us the fundamental aspect of Chinese natural history. One is reminded of the injunction of Confucius to his pupils to study the *Book of Songs* where one becomes 'largely acquainted with the names of birds, beasts, and plants'.[86] It is also what is advocated by Zheng Qiao 鄭樵 (1103–62) in his famous *Essay on Animals and Plants* (Kunchong caomu lue 昆蟲草木略)[87] written between 1149 and 1161. Without cooperation between Confucian scholars who ignore things of nature, on the one hand, and peasants and gardeners 'who do not know the taste of *Book of Songs*', on the other hand, it is impossible to study plants and animals.[88] The rectification of names is still at the basis – and even in the title – of the book by Wu Qijun 吳其濬 (1789–1847), published several centuries later, in 1848, called *Zhiwu mingshi tukao* 植物名實圖考 (Researches on Illustrations and the Authenticity of the Names of Plants).

When comparing Li Shizhen with his contemporaries in Europe, his philological concern must be kept in mind. Some European naturalists, particularly during the fifteenth and sixteenth centuries, had a similar attitude. They were interested in the first place in plants and animals named in books by the great authors of Latin and Greek antiquity. In fact, modern natural science began to appear only when this attitude changed, that is when people began to consider that what they saw around them might have been unknown to the Roman and Greek masters. Chinese scholars never changed their attitude to the same extent as their European contemporaries, with the exception of the above-mentioned Wu Qijun who was unusual insofar as he included the description of previously unknown plants in his work (without giving them a name).[89] Scholars like Cheng Yaotian 程瑤田 (1725–1814), for instance, did manifest an obvious sense of acute naturalistic observation, but they did so in order to solve a philological problem.[90]

The concern with *zhengming* which appears to have motivated the physician Li Shizhen to engage in prolonged researches made him into a natural historian, observant and interested in the phenomenal appearance of living kinds. Sometimes, however, the author of this compilation had no opportunity to investigate specimens of the kinds (*zhong*) described in earlier *materia medica* that he included in his compilation. Two examples which reflect his writing about plants follow. In one case, he must have studied the specimen, in the other, it is very unlikely that he did so.

---

[86] *Lunyu* 論語, *pian* 17, *zhang* 9. See Legge (1861), 187.   [87] *Tongzhi* 通志 1, *juan* 75–6, 865–85.
[88] Métailié (1992), 171.   [89] Métailié (1993).
[90] See *'Shicao' xiaoji* 《釋草》小記. An example of Cheng Yaotian's mode of argumentation is discussed in Métailié (1992), 176.

The *tong* trees

Lu Gwei-djen has already drawn attention to Li Shizhen's treatment of the kind (*zhong*) called *tong* (桐).[91] Formerly scattered among various sections of the *bencao* literature, the various plants whose names end with the morpheme *tong* are grouped together by Li Shizhen within the tree/wood section (*mu bu*), with the exception of one, *hutong* 胡桐, which, under the heading 'tears of *hutong*' (*hutonglei* 胡桐淚), is put into the fragrant trees category (*xiangmu lei*), in all likelihood because of its fragrant exudation.[92] All the others, i.e. *tong*, *wutong* 梧桐, *yingzitong* 罌子桐, with *yingtong* 櫻桐 in the appendix, and *haitong* 海桐, with *jitong* 雞桐 in the appendix, belong to the next category of tall trees (*qiaomu lei*).[93]

Li Shizhen proceeds in the same way for every entry on *tong* trees. First, he quotes famous authors of former *bencao*, mainly Tao Hongjing (456–536), author of the above-mentioned *Bencao jing jizhu* and the *Mingyi bielu* 名醫別祿 (Informal Records of Famous Physicians) (510); Su Song 蘇頌 (1019–1101) author of the *Bencao tujing* 圖經本草 (Illustrated Canon of *Materia Medica*) (1061); and Kou Zongshi 寇宗奭, author of the *Bencao yanyi* 本草衍義 (Dilations upon *Materia Medica*) (1116). Then he gives his own opinion, drawing on non-pharmacological books like the agricultural treatise *Qimin yaoshu* 齊民要術 (Essential Techniques for the Peasantry) (535) by Jia Sixie 賈思勰 (sixth century)[94] or the monograph devoted to *tong* trees, titled *Tongpu* 桐譜 (Treatise on the *Tong*) (preface of 1049) by Chen Zhu 陳翥 (1009–?56/63).

For example, under the *tong* heading, in the rubric 'explaining the names' (*shiming*), he begins by indicating the various synonymous terms and their sources: '*Baitong* 白桐 (white *tong*) < [Tao] Hongjing, *huangtong* 黃桐 (yellow *tong*) < *[Bencao] tujing, paotong* 泡桐 (bullate *tong*) < *[Bencao] gangmu, yitong* 椅桐 (meaning unclear) < [Tao] Hongjing, *rongtong* 榮桐 < (flowering *tong*)'. Then he writes:

> [Li] Shizhen says: the *tong* leaves in the *Canon of the Divine Husbandman's Materia Medica* refer to *baitong*. The *tong* flower is tubular (*tong* 筒), the name comes from that. The wood is light and hollow, its appearance white and veined. Hence it is called *baitong* (white *tong*) and *paotong* (bullate *tong*). Formerly called *yitong*.[95] The flowers come before the leaves; it is the reason why the *Erya* calls it flowering *rongtong* (flowering *tong*).[96] Some say that it flowers but

[91] Lu (1966), 385.   [92] *Bencao gangmu, juan* 34, 1972.

[93] *Bencao gangmu, juan* 35, 1997–2002.   [94] See Bray (1984), 55–9.

[95] See for instance *Shijing*, 'Xiaoya' 小雅, 'Zhanlu' 湛路. See *Maoshi zhengyi* 毛詩正義, *juan* 10.1, 421b.

[96] *Erya, juan* 9, 9b.

does not give fruit. I have not analysed this in detail. Lu Ji 陸璣[97] considers that *yi* is *wutong*, Guo Pu 郭 璞 [98] considers that *rong* is *wutong*, they are both wrong.[99]

〔時珍曰〕本經桐葉，即白桐也。桐華成筒，故謂之桐。其材輕虛，色白而有綺文，故俗謂之白桐，泡桐，古謂之椅桐也。先花後葉，故而雅謂之榮桐。或言其花而不實者，未之察也。陸璣以椅為梧桐，郭璞以榮為梧桐，并誤。

In the following rubric on 'grouped explanations' (*jijie* 集解), Li Shizhen first quotes what the *Mingyi bielu*, Tao Hongjing, Su Song, and Kou Zongshi say about morphology, ecology, various kinds, common use, and the like of the *tong*:

> The *Informal Records* say: *tong* leaves are produced in the mountains and valleys with *tong* and *bai* (cypress) trees.[100]
>
> [Tao] Hongjing says: there are four kinds of *tong* trees: [1] the *qingtong* 青桐 (bluegreen *tong*): the leaves and bark are bluegreen, it resembles the *wutong* but does not have seeds. [2] The *wutong*: the bark is white, the leaves resemble those of the *qingtong*, but it has seeds, the seeds are fatty and edible. [3] The *baitong* (white tong), also *yitong*: often cultivated, no different from the *gangtong* 岡桐 (ridge *tong*), but with flowers and seeds; it flowers in the second lunar month [February–March], yellowish purple colours. It is the one of which the *Rites* says: 'In the third month the *tong* begins to blossom.'[101] It can be used for making cithars. [4] The *gangtong* has no seeds; this one is the one for making cithars. When the *materia medica* refers to the flowers of *tong* trees, it means those of the *baitong*.[102]
>
> [Su] Song says: *tong* are ubiquitous. Lu Ji's *Commentary on Herbs and Trees*[103] says: 'The *baitong* is appropriate for cithars.' The people of Zangge in Yunnan take the fine white hairs from the middle of the flower, soak them, and spin them into thread in order to make cloth; it resembles woollen fabric, one calls it flowery cloth. *Yi* is the *wutong*. What the people of Jiangnan nowadays use to make oils is the *gangtong*. It has larger seeds than those of the *wutong*. In Jiangnan there are *chengtong* 檉桐 (red *tong*), they flower in autumn, no fruits. There are *zitong* 紫桐 (purple *tong*), the blossoms are like those of lilies (*baihe* 百 合),[104] their

[97] Lu Ji (third century AD) wrote a commentary on the names of plants and animals quoted in the *Shijing*. See *Lu Ji Maoshi caomu niaoshou chongyu shu* 陸璣毛詩草木鳥獸蟲魚疏, *juan* 1, 23.
[98] Guo Pu (276–324) was a commentator of the *Erya*. See *Erya, juan* 9, 9b.
[99] *Bencao gangmu, juan* 35, 1997.
[100] *Mingyi bielu, juan* 3, 240. Rather than giving *verbatim* quotes, Li Shizhen paraphrases and summarises the works he refers to, in this and all the following cases.
[101] *Liji* 禮記, 'Yueling' 月令. See *Liji zhengyi* 禮記正義, *juan* 15, 1363a.
[102] Cf. *Bencao jing jizhu, juan* 5, 352. Li Shizhen, however, follows in some places the wording given in the *Zhenglei bencao* more closely. Cf. *Zhenglei bencao, juan* 14, 53.
[103] *Lu Ji Maoshi caomu niaoshou chongyu shu, juan* 1, 23.
[104] *Lilium brownii* F. E. Brown, *Lilium pumilum* D. C., or *Lilium longiflorum* Thunb. and many other species.

fruits can be simmered into sweets for chewing. In Lingnan there are *citong* 刺桐 (thorny *tong*), the colour of their flowers is deep red.[105]

[Kou] Zongshi says: the *tong* leaves mentioned in the *Canon of the Divine Husbandman's Materia Medica* do not indicate for certain which kind of *tong* they are, and so it is difficult to apply them. However, the four kinds each have a therapeutic effect. The *baitong*: leaves are three-forked, with white flowers, does not form seeds. Those without flowers are *gangtong*, [the wood that is] not in the centre makes cithars, its body is heavy. The *rentong* 荏桐 (soft *tong*): the seeds can be used for making *tong* oil. The *wutong*: it forms seeds that are edible.[106]

〔別錄曰〕桐葉生桐柏山谷。

〔弘景曰〕桐樹有四種　青桐，葉　皮青，似梧而無籽，梧桐，皮白，葉似青桐而有籽，籽肥可食，白桐，一名椅桐，人家多植之，與岡桐無異，但有花籽，二月開花，黃紫色，禮云：三月桐始華者也，堪作琴瑟，岡桐無籽，是作琴瑟者。本草用桐華，應是白桐。

〔頌曰〕桐處處有之。陸璣草木疏言白桐宜為琴瑟。雲南牂牁人，取花中白氎淹漬，績以為布，似毛布，謂之華布。椅，即梧桐也。今江南人作油者，即岡桐也，有籽大於梧籽。江南有䪷桐，秋開紅花，無實。有紫桐，花如百合，實堪糖煮以啖。嶺南有刺桐，花色深紅。

〔宗奭曰〕本經桐葉不指定是何桐，致難執用。但四種各有治療。白桐，葉三杈，開白花，不結籽。無花者為岡桐，不中作琴，體重。荏桐，籽可作桐油。梧桐，結籽可食。

Then, Li Shizhen gives his own opinion again:

[Li] Shizhen says: Tao [Hongjing] notices that there are four kinds of *tong*. The seedless ones are *qingtong* and *gangtong*, those with seeds are *wutong* and *baitong*. Kou [Zongshi] says that *baitong* and *gangtong* are both seedless. Su [Song] identifies *gangtong* with *youtong* 油桐 (*tong* for making oils), though in the *Qimin yaoshu* by Jia Sixie it is said: 'What fructifies and has a bluegreen bark is *wutong*, what flowers but does not fructify is *baitong*.'[107] What appear in winter on the *baitong* and look like seeds are the buds of next year's flowers and not seeds. In this way, to say that *gangtong* is *youtong* 油桐 (*tong* for making oils), that its seeds are big and possess oil, to say so is in contradiction with Mr Tao [Hongjing's statement]. When we make inquiries today, there are contradictions. Certainly *baitong* is *paotong*: its leaves are big, one foot in diameter; it grows very quickly, the colour of its bark is whitish, its wood is light and hollow, it does not grow 'insects', excellent to make objects or building posts. In the second lunar month it flowers like morning glory[108] but is white. It forms fruits as large as jujubes,[109] more than one inch long, inside the skin there are seeds on strips, very

---

[105] Cf. *Zhenglei bencao, juan* 14, 53.

[106] Cf. *Zhenglei bencao, juan* 14, 54, and *Bencao yanyi, juan* 15, 97.

[107] Cf. *Qimin yaoshu, juan* 5, 254–5.   [108] *Pharbitis nil* (L.) Choisy.   [109] *Zizyphus jujuba* Mill.

light, like elm-pods or mallow fruits;[110] when they are old the shells open, and [the seeds] drift with the wind. The one with a purple flower is called *gangtong*. *Rentong* is a synonym for *youtong*. *Qingtong* is the seedless kind of *wutong*. According to the *Treatise on the tong* by Chen Zhu, the distinction between *baitong* and *gangtong* is very clear. It says: '*Baihuatong* (white flowered *tong*): wood structure coarse, trunk texture loose, likes to grow in sunny places. Coming from seeds, in one year it can grow to three or four feet; coming from a root, it may reach five to seven feet. Its leaves are big and circular but stretching out to make a point, they are glossy with very fine hairs. The flowers come before the leaves. The flowers are white, in the centre slightly red. Its fruits are big, two to three inches; inside are two segments, inside the segments there is flesh, on this flesh are thin strips, they are its seeds. *Zihuatong* 紫花桐 (purple flowered *tong*): wood structure thin, trunk texture dense, it also grows in sunny places but does not grow as easily as the *baitong*. Its leaves are triangular but rounded, as big as those of *baitong*, bluegreen in colour with many hairs and not glossy, tough and slightly red. The flowers also come before the leaves, the colour of the flowers is purple. The fruits are similar to those of *baitong* but thinner, looking like fruits of myrobalans,[111] but sticky; the flesh inside the segments is yellow. The colour of the bark of the two *tong* is identical but flowers and leaves are slightly different, wood textures completely different; one dense, one loose. There are also some which in winter have a second flowering'.[112]

〔時珍曰〕陶注桐有四種，以無籽者為青桐，岡桐，有籽者為梧桐白桐。寇注言白桐　岡桐皆無籽。蘇注以岡桐為油桐。而賈思勰齊民要術言　實而皮青者為梧桐，華而不實者為白桐。白桐冬結似籽者，乃是明年之華房，非籽也。岡桐即油桐也，籽大有油。其説與陶氏相反。以今咨訪，互有是否。蓋白桐即泡桐也。葉大徑尺，最易生長。皮色粗白，其木輕虛，不生虫蛀，作器物　屋柱甚良。二月開花，如牽牛花而色白。結實大如巨棗，長寸余，殼內有籽片，輕虛如榆莢　葵實之狀，老則殼裂，隨風飄揚。其花紫色者名岡桐。荏桐即油桐也。青桐即梧桐之無實者。按陳翥桐譜，分別白桐岡桐甚明。雲：白花桐，文理粗而體性慢，喜生朝陽之地。因籽而出者，一年可起三四尺，由根而出者，可五七尺。其葉圓大而尖長有角，光華而毳，先花後葉。花白色，花芯微紅。其實大二三寸，內為兩房，房內有肉，肉上有薄片，即其籽也。紫花桐，文理細而體性堅，亦生朝陽之地，不如白桐易長。其葉三角而圓，大如白桐，色青多毛而不光且硬，微赤。亦先花後葉，花色紫。其實亦同白桐而微尖，狀如訶籽而粘，房中肉黃色。二桐皮色皆一，但花　葉小異，體性堅，慢不同爾。亦有冬月复花者。

   If we compare the description of the *tong* trees in the *materia medica* that Li Shizhen cites with the descriptions quoted under his name, we find continuity in some respects

---

[110] *Ulmus parviflora* Jacq. which produces samaras and *Malva verticillata* L. which produces samara-like achenes.

[111] *Terminalia chebula* Retz.   [112] *Bencao gangmu, juan* 35, 1998. Cf. *Tongpu, juan* 2, 17–18.

and innovative features in others. Tao Hongjing, whom Li Shizhen takes as the most distinguished authority, accounts for a kind of *tong* by comparing and contrasting it with another rather than by providing a focused description of each in its own right. For instance, the leaves are compared with those of other kinds without being described in more detail. He pays attention to the leaves, bark, and whether the plant forms fruit or not. He does mention the use of *tong* wood, but he does not describe its quality. In the case of *baitong*, he mentions, apart from the colour of its flowers which gives it its name, the flowering time as recorded in the canonical literature. Su Song's account is primarily oriented towards reporting on the use of *tong* tree products. It is noteworthy that Li Shizhen attacks Su Song first, accusing him not of inaccurate observation, but of contradicting the authority, Tao Hongjing. Kou Zongshi's description of *baitong*, the shape of the leaves, the colour of the blossoms, and whether or not the *baitong* bears fruits comes already quite close to the quotations Li Shizhen gives under his own name, but Kou Zongshi describes in each case a different aspect of the plant. The text passage which expresses Li Shizhen's viewpoint is not only more elaborate, it is systematic in its comparison of several aspects of one variety with the same aspects of another. Li Shizhen is careful to point out structures that can be confused one with the other, for instance, flower buds that can be mistaken for fruits. He emphasises the habitats in which the trees grow, whether sunny or shady.[113] He quotes descriptions of the leaves, fruits, and the entire plant which relate absolute measurements. Some of them must have been derived from direct observation of their appearance (for instance the degree of hairiness) or of the developmental cycle (the observation that the shell of a fruit can open, with the effect that the seeds drift in the wind). Li Shizhen's main innovation thus consists of incorporating descriptions given in texts on agriculture and arboriculture into the *bencao* literature. These detailed observations on living kinds are given within the same framework as that found in the *materia medica* where a kind is not so much described in its own right, but in comparison with another; the descriptions of the white flowered *tong* and the purple flowered *tong* are, for instance, complementary. This comparative style of description is common to both writings on arboriculture and *materia medica*, though the newly included descriptions are more elaborate and more systematic.

This example is intended to give an idea of Li Shizhen as a naturalist. Details on other *tong* trees are omitted here.[114] Thanks to Li Shizhen's minute philological and botanical research, we have been able to find a possible solution to big problems of synonymies

---

[113] Li Shizhen mentions this ecological aspect at the beginning of the partly restructured quote from the *Tongpu.*

[114] The whole saga of the *tong* trees is in the second part of the botanical section of *Science and Civilisation in China*, vol. VI, part 4 (not yet in press).

Table 7.2. *Tentative identification of various* tong *trees*

Category of Fragrant Trees		
• *hutong*	胡桐	*Populus diversifolia* Schrenk.
Category of Tall Trees		
• *tong*	桐	*Paulownia fortunei* (Seem.) Hemsl. with the synonyms: *baitong* 白桐, *baihuatong* 白花桐, *huangtong* 黃桐, *paotong* 泡桐, *yitong* 椅桐, *rongtong* 榮桐
• *gangtong*	岡桐	? *Paulownia tomentosa* (Thunb.) Stend. synonym: *zihuatong* 紫花桐
• *wutong*	梧桐	*Firmiana simplex* Wight. synonym: *chengtong* 赬桐 aspermous variety: *qingtong* 青桐
• *yingzitong*	罂子桐	*Aleurites fordii* Hemsl. synonyms: *huzitong* 虎子桐, *rentong* 荏桐, *youtong* 油桐
• *yingtong*	罃桐	unidentified
• *haitong*	海桐	*Erythrina indica* Lam. synonym: *citong* 刺桐, *jitong* 雞桐

among the *tong* trees and have proposed the following identifications for the various plants involved (table 7.2).[115]

This example of the *tong* trees points out the qualities of Li Shizhen as a naturalist, and gives a clear insight into his approach to the investigation of plants. His main criteria of classification appear to be, firstly, the quality and structure of the wood and, secondly, the size of the leaves. Even though his researches were primarily motivated by a philological concern, he showed great interest in, familiarity with, and detailed observation of the natural world.

The almond tree (*Prunus amygdalus* Batsch.)

In the category of the Five Fruits (*wuguo lei*) in the fruit section (*guo bu*), Li Shizhen introduces a new fruit under the name *badanxing* 巴旦杏 (apricot *badan*).[116] He gives as synonym *badanxing* 八擔杏 from the *Yinshan zhengyao* 飲膳正要 (Principles of Correct Diet) (1330), compiled by the Mongol doctor Hu Sihui 忽思慧 (fourteenth

[115] Métailié (1988), 35. [116] *Bencao gangmu, juan* 29, 1735.

century),[117] and another name, *huluma* 忽鹿麻,[118] without indicating from where the name comes. *Badan* is a transcription of a Persian term *badam* which is the name of the sweet almond, *Prunus amygdalus* Batsch.[119] Li Shizhen expresses awareness that it comes from the West, for he firstly refers to its geographical distribution: 'It comes from the home lands of the Hui people and is now also in all the lands of the west.' He then comments on the morphology of this plant and its usage: 'The tree is like the apricot but its leaves are smaller; the fruit is pointed and small, the flesh thin. Its kernel is like a plumstone, the skin is thin and the almond is sweet and nice. It is eaten for tea, its taste is similar to that of a hazelnut. The people in the west consider it a local speciality.'

The entry on *badanxing* includes two brief rubrics quoting the *Yinshan zhengyao*, with only minor amendments.

The peach (*tao* 桃) is discussed within the same category (*lei*).[120] Li Shizhen begins with saying that there are many varieties of peaches (*tao pin shen duo* 桃品甚多). Some take their name from their colour, others from the shape (of the fruit), and still others from the season (of fructification). Among those which take their name from the shape of the fruit, we find the horizontal board peach (*biantao* 匾桃) and the peach with a flat stone (*pianhetao* 偏核桃). Li Shizhen writes, without acknowledging that he is quoting Duan Chengshi's 段成式 (?–863) *Youyang zazu* 酉陽雜俎 (Miscellanea from [Mount] You Yang) (no date):[121] 'The *biantao* (horizontal board peach) comes from the southern Fan, it looks like a horizontal board (*bian* 匾), its flesh is astringent (*se* 澀), the shape of its stone looks like a box, its almond is sweet and nice. The foreigners highly value it, they call it *botan* 波淡 (*badam*) tree, the tree is very high.'[122] Immediately thereafter he describes *pianhetao* (the peach with a flat stone): '[It] comes from Persia, its form is thin and slender, the crown is bent over [to the effect that] its shape is like a half-moon; its almond has a good taste like the seeds of Korean pines, it is edible, its nature is hot.'

In these three cases, Li Shizhen is describing the same plant three times over. That he never had the opportunity to see either the almond tree or its fruits seems probable since the study of the case of the *tong* trees has just proved him able to be a good observer. In

---

[117] The current editions give *badanren* 八桓仁. See *Yinshan zhengyao* (1986), *juan* 3, 138, and (1935), *juan* 3, 159.

[118] This is a transcription from the Persian *xurma (khurma)*, a word which refers to the date (*Phoenix dactylifera* L.). See Laufer (1919), 406, note 4.

[119] Laufer (1919), 406.   [120] *Bencao gangmu, juan* 29, 1741.   [121] Laufer (1919), 407.

[122] Cf. *Youyang zazu*, 178, no. 792. Actually, Li Shizhen seems to have used little of the description given by Duan Chengshi, leaving aside the details about the tree itself: 'Tree five to six *zhang* 丈 [fifty to sixty feet] high, circumference four to five feet, leaves looking like those of the peach tree but bigger. Flowers during the third month, white flowers, the flowers fall and it gives fruits, the shape of a peach but flat, hence its name.'

Table 7.3. *The structure of the entries on* zhong *(as outlined in the 'Fanli' chapter)*

shiming	釋名	'explaining the names': gives the correct name
jijie	集解	'grouped explanations': explains the place of origin and production, form and appearance, and collection [time]
bianyi	辨疑	'explanation of the doubtful': evaluates that which is doubtful
zhengwu	正誤	'correction of mistakes': corrects the erroneous
xiuzhi	修治	'preparing the therapy': details (preparatory) roasting processes and cauterisation
qiwei	氣味	'quality and flavour': explains the nature
zhuzhi	主治	'main therapeutic indications': records indication and therapeutic effect
faming	發明	'bringing light': comments on meaning and significance
fufang	附方	'appended recipes': lists all applications
fulu	附錄	'appendix': records all those objects that are of a complementary category (*xianglei* 相類) and without having a (known) effect and application are conducive to consultation or those which have (therapeutic) use, but are not yet widely known

this case, it is obvious that the names determined his choice. He considered the plant called '*badan* apricot' a kind of apricot tree, and discussed it in a separate entry. In the other case, he listed the plants known by the name *bian*-peach and *pianhe*-peach as two distinct varieties/species of the peach tree.[123]

The structure of the entries on *zhong*

The entries on each kind (*zhong*) have a common structure which is outlined in the fifth paragraph of the 'Fanli' chapter of the *Bencao gangmu* (table 7.3).[124] Such systematic presentation of information within each entry, however, was not strictly speaking an innovation within the *bencao* literature because it was already used in the *Bencao pinhui jingyao* 本草品匯精要 (Classified Essential *Materia Medica*), compiled by 1505 under the supervision of Liu Wentai 劉文泰 (fl. 1488–1505). The *Bencao pinhui jingyao* remained a manuscript in the Imperial Library, and was apparently never seen by Li Shizhen; it is therefore not surprising that his structure differs greatly from it.[125]

Only rarely are all the above rubrics included for describing one single kind, the most frequent ones being *shiming* and *jijie, qiwei* and *zhuzhi*. The *shiming* and *jijie* rubrics are often very well documented and generally describe the natural object or living kind

[123] All these names are now considered synonyms. See *Zhongyao dacidian* (1977), no. 1035.
[124] Cf. summaries of these rubrics in Lu (1966), 386; Sivin (1973), 392; and Unschuld (1986), 152. Unschuld (1986), 153–8, translates an entire monograph on a *zhong* entry, that on the Ba bean (*badou* 巴豆).
[125] Cf. Sivin (1973), 394.

from which drugs for medicinal usage are made. These two rubrics are primarily responsible for the reputation of the *Bencao gangmu* as an important text on natural history. In the *shiming* rubric come the synonyms, each with its source indicated. Sometimes philological and etymological remarks are added. The *jijie* rubric concerns information about geographical distribution and sometimes the ecological niche of the kind, its place of production, morphology, behaviour (for animals), and the like. Li Shizhen usually quotes various authors and then gives his own opinion in reference to these various sources.

The *zhengwu* and *bianyi* rubrics, which are only occasionally included, express doubts of previous authors about the name and identity of the kind that Li Shizhen discusses. Some entries also have a *jiaozheng* rubric, a rubric not mentioned in the 'Fanli' chapter which indicates from where an entry has been dislocated (*yi ru ci* 移入此) or where else it has been incorporated (*bing ru* 并入). Li Shizhen often reallocates kinds into different sections (*bu*), as for instance in the case of the *tong* trees, where the *hutonglei*, as the *jiaozheng* indicates, has been moved from the herbs section (*cao bu*) into the trees section (*mu bu*).

The knowledge presented in each monograph on a kind (*zhong*) can thus be partitioned into two parts: the first part records information derived from *gewu* scholarship, mostly in the *shiming* and *jijie* rubrics; the second part contains information on medicinal issues.

So far, the innovative aspects of Li Shizhen's compilation derived from *gewu* scholarship have been emphasised. Our account would, however, be incomplete if we were to leave unmentioned innovations relevant to the medical practitioner. Nathan Sivin has already drawn attention to the preliminary chapters in which Li Shizhen presents a classification of drugs according to the disorders they were deemed to cure.[126] Previous works contained such a listing too, but 'Li's carefully appended notes on the physiological functions of each drug with respect to each disease (phrased in the abstract terminology of rational medicine) were his own innovation.'[127] The monographs on each *zhong* contain a wealth of information that is similar in kind, particularly in the *zhuzhi* and *fufang* rubrics, both of which list complaints and symptoms alongside nosological entities.

While the *zhuzhi* rubric which records the main therapeutic indications follows largely the tradition, the *fufang* rubric has been newly created. It gives the conditions for which there are recipes which include the drug discussed, the textual source often, but not always, being indicated. The information on these conditions is quite varied in kind: it may include information on how to administer the drug, on the cause and course of the illness it is to be used for, and on the effectiveness of the drug. It indicates the number of old (*jiu* 久) and newly incorporated (*xin* 新) recipes, though in the list itself they are not

---

[126] *Bencao gangmu, juan* 3–4, 131–386.   [127] Sivin (1973), 392.

differentiated one from the other. The compilation of these recipes should not be under-estimated, for it makes the *Bencao gangmu* a precious reservoir of practical medical knowledge accessible to physicians in the late Ming. As Li Shizhen himself states in the 'Fanli' chapter, previous *bencao* had recorded only 2,935 recipes, while he introduced 8,161 for the first time, making the respectable sum of 11,096.[128]

The *fulu* is just like the *fufang* a rubric that has been created for accommodating newly acquired knowledge. Li Shizhen explicitly states this in the 'Fanli' chapter: 'There is that which was hidden from the ancients and is clear to contemporaries.'[129] Within this rubric, he mentions the names of kinds related to the kind discussed in the monograph and also provides *gewu* scholarship-derived and medicinal information. In the context of the *tong* trees, for instance, he mentions the *rentong* and the *jitong* in the *fulu*, once quoting from another work, once referring to himself.

The *faming* rubric is also new. It contains notes, from Li Shizhen and other authors, on flavour, therapeutic nature, and many other properties of the drug, and it sometimes gives anecdotes and relates *curiosita*. The *xiuzhi* rubric, newly named as such, provides information on the preservation and processing of drugs that can also be found in earlier *bencao*.[130]

There remains the *qiwei* rubric, by which most *bencao* commenced the description of a drug, indicating its flavour and quality (*qiwei* 氣味), and whether it was potent and toxic (*you du* 有毒) or non-toxic (*wu du* 無毒). This rubric, together with the *zhuzhi* rubric, is not only the most common in the *bencao* literature, but also most frequently mentioned in Li Shizhen's monographs on *zhong*.

All rubrics compile information from different textual sources. Yet Li Shizhen claims that he introduced certain kinds for the first time into the *bencao* literature, altogether totalling 374 kinds.[131] The content of these new entries will therefore now be compared with what he says about items already mentioned in previous *bencao* books.

'Old entries'

'Old entries' consist of a patchwork of quotations. For instance, under bear (*xiong* 熊),[132] thirty-one different texts are used with fifty-two quotations. The monograph on the bear begins with a *shiming* rubric where Li Shizhen quotes himself and a *jijie* rubric where he quotes other *bencao*, followed by a long text passage with his own comments.

---

[128] *Bencao gangmu*, 'Fanli', 33. See also Lu (1966), 386.   [129] *Bencao gangmu*, 'Fanli', 33.
[130] In the *Bencao pinhui jingyao*, for instance, it can be found in the rubric called *shi* 時.
[131] *Bencao gangmu*, 'Fanli', 33.
[132] *Bencao gangmu*, *juan* 51, 2837–41; *xiong* 熊 is *Ursus arctos* L. or *Selenaretos thibetanus* G. Cuvier, see Chen Guiting (1992), 2158. Cf. *Zhongyao dacidian* (1977), 5412.

It ends with the *fulu* rubric on the *pi* 羆 and the *tui* 魋 bears, which consists entirely of a quotation by Li Shizhen himself.[133] The limbs (*zhi* 脂), flesh (*rou* 肉), paws (*zhang* 掌), gall bladder (*dan* 膽), brain and marrow (*naosui* 腦髓), blood (*xue* 血), and bones (*gu* 骨) are separately discussed with regard to their main therapeutic properties (*zhuzhi*) in all cases and their pharmacodynamic properties (*qiwei*) in most cases. In some cases, discussion also includes *shiming, xiuzhi, faming,* and *fufang* rubrics. The information on the bear's gall bladder is by far the longest. This is particularly interesting since the source indicated for the monograph on the bear, the *Benjing* [*Shennong bencao jing*], contains in its reconstructed form[134] only an entry on the bear's limbs with information that Li Shizhen largely reproduces in the *qiwei* and *zhuzhi* rubrics.[135] He adds to it information from other sources, in these two as well as in three new rubrics (*shiming, xiuzhi,* and *fufang* rubrics). Evidently, the patchwork of quotations represents an unprecedented richness in information, but Li Shizhen's additive cumulation of information is not innovative in itself.

Keeping in mind the three categories of his bibliographic sources, it may be noted that the *bencao* literature is quoted almost exclusively in the *shiming, qiwei,* and *zhuzhi* rubrics.[136] Books by physicians are used as sources for the recipes (*fufang*),[137] and reference to these texts clearly represents an innovative aspect for the *bencao* genre. Excerpts from other texts are often cited in the *shiming* and *jijie* rubrics,[138] and anthropologically elucidated 'folk' knowledge, often concerned with local names, tends to be recorded in the *shiming* rubric.

In this monograph on the bear, Li Shizhen quotes himself eight times: in five cases he backs his argument with quotations from other authors (eight in all); in three cases he reports on information from folk sources. Obviously, it is not the case that wherever Li Shizhen quotes himself, he provides information that he himself claims to have dis-

---

[133] *Xiong* 熊, *pi* 羆, and *tui* 魋 are three different kinds of bears that all belong into the same category (*san zhong yi lei ye* 三種一類也). See *Bencao gangmu, juan* 51, 2841.

[134] *Shennong bencaojing jizhu, Shennong bencaojing juan* 2, 176–7.

[135] Cf. *Zhenglei bencao, juan* 16, 16.

[136] They include among others: the *Benjing* 本經: *Shennong bencao jing* 神農本草經, *Bencao tujing* 本草圖經, *Mingyi bielu* 名醫別錄, *Leigong baojiu lun* 雷公炮灸論, *Rihua zhujia bencao* 日華諸家本草, *Yaoxing bencao* 藥性本草, the titles of which are given in the list on the *bencao* literature.

[137] They include among others: *Song Taizong Taiping shenghui fang* 宋太宗　太平聖惠方, *Sun zhenren Qianjin yifang* 孫真人　千金翼方, *Yangshi Chanru jiyan fang* 楊氏　產乳集驗方, *Zan Yin Shiyi xinjing* 昝殷　食醫心鏡, *Wang Tao Waitai biyao fang* 王燾外台密要方, *Doumen fang* 斗門方 which are listed among the medicinal works.

[138] They include among others: *Ren Fang Shuyi ji* 任昉　述異記, *Taoshi Dusou shenji* 陶氏　讀搜神記 *Lu Ji Maoshi caomu niaoshou chongyu shu* 陸璣　毛詩草木鳥獸蟲魚疏, *Huainanzi* 淮南子, *Zhuangzi* 莊子.

covered. This aspect of Li Shizhen's work requires systematic analysis for we have
found that, in some cases, he may quote an author without any mention of his name.
The case of the winter-sweet (*lamei* 臘梅), *Chimonanthus praecox* (L.) Link., is a good
example.[139] On reading the entry, the only reference is to Li Shizhen; but actually the
two texts in the *shiming* and *jijie* rubric are just an adaptation of parts of the 'Meipu'
梅譜 (Treatise on Japanese Apricot) (1186) by Fan Chengda 范成大 (1126–93).[140]

New entries

Let us now turn to some examples of the *materia medica* that Li Shizhen introduced into
the *bencao* literature. They are recognisable as such if the textual source of a name is
given as [*Bencao*] *gangmu*. With regard to the *tong* trees discussed above, the entry on
the *wutong* tree was always discussed within the monograph on the *tong* tree in previous
materia medica.[141] Li Shizhen separates *wutong* from *tong* and introduces *wutong* as
an autonomous kind (*zhong*). In the *shiming* rubric of the *wutong* monograph, he
quotes the *Erya* and *Zuo zhuan* 左傳 (Zuo Tradition) and in the *jijie* rubric, he cites Tao
Hongjing, Su Song, and Kou Zongshi, followed by his own description of the tree. From
this it is obvious that the fact that a plant or animal is a 'new' entry in the *Bencao
gangmu* does not mean that it has been discovered by Li Shizhen but simply that he has
introduced this item for the first time as an autonomous *zhong* entry.

An example of a new entry that concerns a new drug is *afurong* 阿芙蓉[142] with the
synonym *apian* 阿片 and the popular form *yapian* 鴉片,[143] which is mentioned just
after the entry for the opium poppy (*yingzisu* 罌子粟), *Papaver somniferum* L., that is
recorded in the grains section (*gu bu*), probably because of its many edible seeds.
Afurong, Li Shizhen says, was seldom heard of in previous times,[144] and only began to
be used in contemporary recipes, defined as the 'liquid of the flower of the opium
poppy' (*yingsuhua zhi jinye* 罌粟花之津液). He does not refer to a previous textual
source in the *shiming* rubric and only to one in the *jijie* rubric; these two rubrics contain
information that seems to have been found by Li Shizhen himself. The first relates
speculations on the meaning of its name *afurong*, the second reports on techniques to

[139] *Bencao gangmu, juan* 36, 2132.
[140] 'Meipu', 1. Métailié (1995) systematically compares the two texts.
[141] See for instance *Zhenglei bencao, juan* 14, 53.
[142] *Bencao gangmu, juan* 23, 1495. Cf. Unschuld's (1986), 158–60, translation into English.
[143] According to Edkins (1898), 18, Li Shizhen actually borrowed these different terms from the *Yilin jiyao* 醫林集要 by Wang Xi 王璽 who died in 1488.
[144] This in contrast to *yingzisu* the first mention of which Li Shizhen traces to the *Kaibao bencao* (*Materia Medica* of the Kaibao Period) (947).

obtain opium. In the *faming* rubric, Li Shizhen notes that the populace uses opium for the art of the bedroom (*fangzhongshu* 房中術) and that it is sold in the capital as a theriac, called *yilijindan* 一粒金丹 (one-grain-gold-cinnabar), but he dismisses these usages as tricks of charlatans (*fangjijia* 方伎家).

In the *qiwei* rubric, *afurong* is ascribed a sour flavour and astringent qualities which are the same as those of the hard capsule of the poppy. However, unlike the hard capsule which is described as slightly cooling and not toxic, *afurong* has warming qualities and is slightly toxic (*weidu* 微毒).

The *zhuzhi* rubric mentions long-term diarrhoea resulting in a prolapse of the anus (*xieli tuogang buzhi* 瀉痢脫肛不止) and maintains that *afurong* can halt men's essential *qi* (*neng se zhangfu jingqi* 能澀丈夫精氣), which seems to imply that it can cure loss of semen. Li Shizhen refers to himself as the source for these two indications. The recipes listed in the *fufang* rubric are primarily against long-term diarrhoea (*jiuli* 久痢), red- and white-coloured diarrhoea (*chibailixia* 赤白痢下), and they include also the one-grain-gold-cinnabar which is added to other decoctions for treating a vast variety of ailments, from different kinds of headaches to incessant blood loss. All four recipes are said to be new, but Li Shizhen indicates for two of them a textual source.

In summary, we cannot detect a clear difference between old and new entries. Old and new entries both compile information from the literature. In old and new entries there are quotations by Li Shizhen himself, which in both cases need not necessarily be based on his anthropological field researches, but may refer to Li Shizhen quoting from another textual source.

For the monographs on *zhong*, Li Shizhen no longer follows the canonical model of the *Shennong bencao jing*, where the flavour, nature or quality, and main therapeutic properties were given at the beginning of each entry. His main innovation consists of drawing a clear distinction between information on the natural history of animals, plants, and minerals (names, morphology, ecology, common use) and information on the medicinal properties of the products derived from them (pharmacodynamic aspects, main indications, recipes). This new ordering of the different rubrics within a *zhong* monograph is probably also related to Li Shizhen's concern with *gewu*.

Conclusion

Considering what has been said about the scientific botanical milieu in Renaissance Europe, we would be inclined to agree with Joseph Needham[145] that 'the classification adopted by Li Shizhen has close similarities to that of his French contemporary

---

[145] Needham (1971), 131.

d'Alechamps [Dalechamp]'.[146] The *Bencao gangmu* may be considered 'China's greatest herbal' but this in no way makes it 'the greatest pre-modern botanical work in any language';[147] its conception is based on concerns alien to modern taxonomy and it deals also with animals and minerals. In any case, before assertion of this kind, one should proceed to a close comparison of its botanical content with the many books on plants written by European contemporaries of Li Shizhen.[148]

This article has attempted to explore those notions which seem to have been of major concern to Li Shizhen himself insofar as he used them for hierarchically ordering knowledge – the sixteen sections (*bu*), the sixty categories (*lei*), and the approximately 1,895 entries on different kinds (*zhong*).

The rationale of the categories (*lei*), newly introduced as a structuring device into the *bencao* literature, remains the most difficult to assess. From an ethnobiological viewpoint, the categories (*lei*) do not correspond to any of the more or less universally found three ranks of folk taxonomies. As Lu Gwei-djen noted long ago, many categories (*lei*) take account of the ecological aspects of living kinds. Our researches corroborated this while simultaneously highlighting that the criteria for forming a category were not exclusively naturalistic; it was not possible to find generally valid characteristics for all categories (*lei*).

Sections (*bu*) and kinds (*zhong*), notions according to which the *materia medica* was already previously ordered, continued to be used for organising the knowledge accumulated by Li Shizhen. The modified way in which they are presented nicely reveals the interests of the compilation's author, otherwise not immediately evident. With regard to the sections (*bu*) of the plant kingdom, for instance, we showed that Li Shizhen was primarily interested in the basic life forms of plants, as either herbs (*cao*) or trees (*mu*), although he continued to present plants in terms of the traditional five sections. These concerns, characteristic of a 'folk taxonomist', would suggest that Li Shizhen was not merely a medical doctor but also a natural historian.

From the way in which information on kinds (*zhong*) is presented, Li Shizhen's concerns as a *gewu* scholar become even more evident. While previous *materia medica* often began by providing information on the flavour and quality of a drug (*qiwei*), and its main indications (*zhuzhi*), Li Shizhen provides far more information on each kind. In particular, his descriptions are contained in newly created rubrics which deal with problems linked to naming and to information concerned with living kinds.

[146] Métailié (1989). [147] Anderson (1997), 147.
[148] For a non-exhaustive list of some fifty-six titles of the 'principal herbals and related botanical works' published during the sixteenth century, see for instance Arber (1938), 273–82. For a good insight into pre-modern botanical works, see also Greene (1983).

Since the sheer wealth of information in this compilaton has often been considered innovative and Li Shizhen himself claimed to have newly integrated many more kinds and recipes into the *bencao* literature, we decided to compare old with newly established entries. No great difference was found between new and old entries. We conclude from our explorations that Li Shizhen's main innovation consisted of the structure according to which he reallocated knowledge from previous textual sources. This structure reveals, within the *bencao* tradition often primarily of pharmacological and medical significance, interests of a philologically motivated, but acutely observant, natural historian.

References to premodern Chinese and Japanese works

Bencao gangmu 本草綱目 (Classified *Materia Medica*). Ming, 1596. Li Shizhen 李時珍. 4 vols. Renmin weisheng chubanshe, Beijing, 1977–81.

Bencao jiyao 本草集要 (Essentials of the *Materia Medica*). Ming, 1496. Wang Lun 王綸. See Okanishi Tameto 1977, 236–7. See also *Quanguo zhongyi tushu lianhe mulu* 1991, no. 02252.

Bencao mengquan 本草蒙筌 (Enlightenment on the *Materia Medica*). Ming, 1565. Chen Jiamo 陳嘉謨. Punctuated and annotated by Wang Shumin 王淑民 et al. Renmin weisheng chubanshe, Beijing, 1988.

Bencao pinhui jingyao 本草品匯精要 (Classified Essential *Materia Medica*). Ming, 1505. Liu Wentai 劉文泰. Renmin weisheng chubanshe, Beijing, 1982.

Bencao tujing 本草圖經 (Illustrated Canon of *Materia Medica*). Song, 1061. Su Song 蘇頌. Cited in *Bencao gangmu*, passim.

Bencao yanyi 本草衍義 (Dilations upon *Materia Medica*). Song, 1116. Kou Zongshi 寇宗奭. Renmin weisheng chubanshe, Beijing, 1990.

Congshu jicheng 叢書集成 (Compilation of *Collectanea*). Wang Yunwu 王雲五 (ed.). Shangwu yinshuguan, Shanghai, 1935–37.

Erya 爾雅 (Approaching what is Correct). 3rd century BC. Anon. *SBBY*.

Guanzi 管子 (Master Guan [Zhong]). Han, 26 BC. Liu Xiang 劉向. *SBBY*.

Kaibao bencao 開寶本草 (*Materia Medica* of the Kaibao Period). Five Dynasties, 973. Cited in *Bencao gangmu*, passim.

Liji 禮記 (Book of Rites). Han, 1st century AD. Anon. Cited from *Liji zhengyi*. In *Shisanjing zhushu* 十三經注疏.

Maoshi caomu niaoshou chongyu shu 毛詩草木鳥獸蟲魚疏 (Commentary to the Plants, Animals and 'Insects' mentioned in the *Book of Songs*). Wu, 3rd century AD. Lu Ji 陸璣. *Congshu jicheng* 叢書集成.

'Meipu' 梅譜 (Treatise on Japanese Apricot). Song, 1186. Fan Chengda 范成大. In *Shenghuo yu bowu congshu*, vol. I, 1–2. Shanghai guji chubanshe, Shanghai, 1993.

Mingyi bielu 名醫別錄 (Informal Records of Famous Physicians). Liang, 510. Attributed to Tao Hongjing 陶弘景. Reconstituted and annotated by Shang Zhijun 尚志鈞. Renmin weisheng chubanshe, Beijing, 1986.

Qimin yaoshu 齊民要術 (Essential Techniques for the Peasantry). Northern Wei, 535. Jia Sixie 賈思勰. Cited from *Qimin yaoshu jiaoshi*, annotated by Miao Qiyu 繆啟愉. Nongye chubanshe, Beijing, 1982. See also *Qimin yaoshu jinshi*, annotated by Shi Shenghan 石聲漢. 4 vols. Beijing kexue chubanshe, Beijing, 1957.

Shennong bencao jing 神農本草經(Divine Husbandman's Canon on *Materia Medica*). Han. Anon. Cited from *Shennong bencaojing jizhu*. Edited and annotated by Ma Jixing 馬繼興. Renmin weisheng chubanshe, Beijing, 1995.

[Shennong] Bencao jing jizhu 神農本草經集注 (Notes to the Divine Husbandman's Canon of *Materia Medica*). Liang, ?492. Tao Hongjing 陶弘景. Annotated by Shang Zhijun 尚志鈞 and Shang Yuansheng 尚元勝. Renmin weisheng chubanshe, Beijing, 1994.

'Shicao' xiaoji 《釋草》小記 (Remarks on the 'Explanation of Herbs'). Qing, Preface of 1803. Cheng Yaotian 程瑤田. In *Tongyilu* 通藝錄 11. Chengshi kanben, Shexian.

Shijing 詩經 (Book of Songs). Zhou, 1000–600 BC. Anon. Cited from *Maoshi zhengyi*. In *Shisanjing zhushu* 十三經注疏.

Shisanjing zhushu 十三經注疏 (Commentary to the Thirteen Canons). Qing, 1816. Ruan Yuan 阮元. Reprint in 2 vols. by Zhonghua shuju, Beijing, 1980.

Shuowen jiezi 説文解字 (Explanation of Graphs and Analysis of Characters). Han, 121. Xu Shen 許慎. Cited from *Shuowen jiezi zhu*. Qing, 1807. Annotated by Duan Yucai 段玉裁. Facsimile by Shanghai guji chubanshe, Shanghai, 1981.

Siku quanshu 四庫全書 (Collection of the Works from the Four Storehouses). Cited from *Wenyuan ge Siku quanshu* 文淵閣 四庫全書 (Wenyuan Pavilion Edition of the Complete Collection of the Works from the Four Storehouses). Shangwu yinshuguan, Taibei, 1983.

Suwen 素問 (Basic Questions). Han. Anon. Tang, 762. Edited by Wang Bing 王冰. Cited from *Huangdi neijing zhangju suoyin* 黃帝內經章句索引, edited by Ren Yingqiu 任應秋. Renmin weisheng chubanshe, Beijing, 1986.

Tang bencao 唐本草, see *Xinxiu bencao*.

Tongjian gangmu 通鑒綱目 (Summary of the Comprehensive Mirror). Song, 1189. Zhu Xi 朱熹. *Siku quanshu.*

Tongpu 桐譜 (Treatise on the *Tong*). Song, preface of 1049. Chen Zhu 陳翥. Cited from *Tongpu xiaozhu.* Annotated by Fan Falian 藩法連. Nongye chubanshe, Beijing, 1981.

Tongzhi 通志 (Comprehensive Treatise). Song. Zheng Qiao 鄭樵 (1104–62). Cited from Wang Yunwu 王雲五 (ed.), *Wanyou wenku* 萬有文庫. 3 vols. Shangwu yinshuguan, Shanghai, 1935.

Xinxiu bencao 新修本草 (Newly Revised *Materia Medica*). Tang, *ca* 660. Su Jing 蘇敬. Shanghai guji chubanshe, Shanghai, 1985.

Xunzi 荀子. Warring States, 3rd century BC. Xun Qing 荀卿. Cited from *Xunzi jianzhu.* Annotated by Zhang Shitong 章詩同. Shanghai renmin chubanshe, Shanghai, 1974.

Yijing 易經(Book of Changes). Zhou–Han. Anon. Cited from *Zhouyi zhengyi.* In *Shisanjing zhushu* 十三經注疏, 5–108.

Yilin jiyao 醫林集要 (The Essentials of Medicine) by Wang Xi 王璽 (?–1488). For same title attributed to another author see Yan Shiyun 嚴世芸 (ed.) 1990–94. *Zhongguo yiji tongkao* 中國醫籍通考 2, 2776.

Yinshan zhengyao 飲膳正要 (Principles of Correct Diet). Yuan, 1330. Hu Sihui 忽思慧. Shangwu yinshuguan, Shanghai, 1935. See also edition punctuated and annotated by Liu Yushu 劉玉書. Renmin weisheng chubanshe, Beijing, 1986.

Youyang zazu 酉陽雜俎 (Miscellanea from [Mount] You Yang). Tang. Duan Chengshi 段成式 (?–863). Punctuated and annotated by Fang Nansheng 方南生. Zhonghua shuju, Beijing, 1981. See also *Siku quanshu* 1047–637 – 1047–658.

Zhenglei bencao 證類本草 (*Materia Medica* Corrected and Arranged in Classes). Song, *ca* 1082. Tang Shenwei 唐慎微. Annotations by Cao Xiaozhong 曹孝忠. *Siku yixue yeshu* 四庫醫學業書. Shanghai, Shanghai guji chubanshe, 1991.

Zhiwu mingshi tukao 植物名實圖考 (Researches on Illustrations and the Authenticity of the Names of Plants). Qing, 1848. Wu Qijun 吳其濬. Facsimile of the 1880 edition. Shanxisheng gu jianzhu baohu yanjiusuo (eds.). Wenwu chubanshe, Beijing, 1993.

Zizhi tongjian 資治通鑒 (Comprehensive Mirror to Aid in Government). Song, 1072–84. Sima Guang 司馬光. Punctuated and annotated by Hu Sanxing 胡三省. Guji chubanshe, Beijing, 1956.

References to modern works

Anderson, Eugene N. 1997. 'Vegetables, Roots, and Wisdom in Old China', *Journal of Ethnobiology* 17 (1), 147–8.

Anon. (ed.) 1971. *Histoire des Sciences Naturelles et de la Biologie*. (Tome 7, Actes du 12ième Congres International des Sciences. Paris, 1968.) Abel Blanchard, Paris.

Arber, Agnes (1912) 1938. *Herbals: their Origin and Evolution. A Chapter in the History of Botany.* Cambridge University Press, Cambridge.

Atran, Scott 1987. 'Origin of the Species and Genus Concepts: an Anthropological Perspective'. *Journal of the History of Biology* 20 (2), 195–279.

 1990. *Cognitive Foundation of Natural History: towards an Anthropology of Science.* Cambridge University Press, Cambridge.

Atran, Scott, Estin, Paul, Medin, John C. D. 1997. 'Generic Species and Basic Levels: Essence and Appearance in Folk Biology'. *Journal of Ethnobiology* 17 (1), 17–43.

Berlin, Brent et al. 1968. 'Covert Categories and Folk Taxonomies'. *American Anthropologist* 70, 290–9.

Berlin, Brent 1992. *Ethnobiological Classification.* Princeton University Press, Princeton.

Bodde, Derk 1991. *Chinese Thought, Science and Society.* University of Hawaii Press, Honolulu.

Bowers, John Z. et al. (eds.) 1988. *Science and Medicine in Twentieth-Century China: Research and Education.* Center for Chinese Studies, University of Michigan, Ann Arbor.

Bray, Francesca. 1984. *Agriculture.* In Joseph Needham, *Science and Civilisation in China*, vol. VI: *Biology and Biological Technology*, part 2. Cambridge University Press, Cambridge.

Cai Jingfeng 蔡景峰 1964. 'Shilun Li Shizhen ji qi zai kexueshang de chengjiu' 釋論李時珍及其在科學上的成就 (Appreciation of Li Shizhen and his Scientific Achievements). *Kexueshi jikan* 科學史集刊 7, 63–80.

Carey, Susan 1985. *Conceptual Change in Childhood.* MIT Press, Cambridge, Mass.

Chan, Wing-tsit 1957. 'Neo-Confucianism and Chinese Scientific Thought'. *Philosophy East and West* 6 (4), 309–32.

Chang, K. C. 1977a. 'Ancient China'. In Chang 1977b, 23–52.

 (ed.) 1977b. *Food in Chinese Culture: Anthropological and Historical Perspectives.* Yale University Press, New Haven.

Chen Guiting 陳貴廷 (ed.) 1992. *Bencao gangmu tongshi* 本草綱目通釋 (Classified *Materia Medica* Annotated). Xueyuan chubanshe, Beijing.

Chen Jiarui 陳家瑞 1978. 'Dui woguo gudai zhiwu fenleixue ji qi sixiang de tantao' 對我國古代植物分類學及其思想的探討 (A Preliminary Study on Plant Classification in Ancient China and [corresponding] Conceptions). *Zhongguo zhiwu fenlei xuebao* 中國植物分類學報 (Acta Phytotaxonomica Sinica) 16 (3), 101–12.

Chen Xinqian 陳新謙 et al. (ed.) 1985. *Li Shizhen yanjiu lunwen ji* 李時珍研究論文集 (Collected Essays of the Researches on Li Shizhen). Hubei kexue jishu chubanshe, Wuhan.

Cheng Chung-ying 1991. *New Dimensions of Confucian and Neo-Confucian Philosophy.* State University of New York Press, Albany.

Ching, Julia 1976. *To Acquire Wisdom: the Way of Wang Yang-ming.* Columbia University Press, New York.

Cooper, William C. and Sivin, Nathan 1973. 'Man as a Medicine: Pharmacological and Ritual Aspects of Traditional Therapy Using Drugs Derived from the Human Body'. In Nakayama and Sivin, 203–72.

du Halde, Jean Baptiste 1735. *Description géographique, historique, chronologique, politique et physique de l'Empire de la Chine et de la Tartarie chinoise.* 4 vols. P. G. Le Mercier, Paris.

Edkins, John 1898. *Opium: Historical Note on the Poppy in China.* American Presbyterian Mission Press, Shanghai.

Ellen, Roy 1993. *The Cultural Relations of Classification: an Analysis of Nuaulu Animal Categories from Central Seram.* Cambridge University Press, Cambridge.

Fung, Yu-lan (1952) 1973. *A History of Chinese Philosophy*, vol. I: *The Period of the Philosophers.* Transl. by Derk Bodde. Princeton University Press, Princeton.

Geerts, A. J. C. 1978. *Les produits de la nature japonaise et chinoise*, vol. I. C. Levy, Yokohama.

Gelman, S. 1988. 'The Development of Induction within Natural Kind and Artifact Categories'. *Cognitive Psychology* 20, 65–95.

Gerard, John (1633 edition as completed and enlarged by Thomas Johnson) 1975. *The Herbal or General History of Plants.* Dover, New York.

Germain de Saint-Pierre, Ernest 1870. *Nouveau dictionaire de botanique.* Baillière, Paris.

Gillispie, Charles C. (ed.) 1973. *Dictionary of Scientific Biography.* Charles Scribner's Sons, New York.

Greene, Edward L. and Egerton, Frank (eds.) 1983. *Landmarks of Botanical History.* Stanford University Press, Stanford.

Haas, William J. 1988. 'Botany in Republican China: the Leading Role of Taxonomy'. In J. Z. Bowers et al. (eds.), 31–64.

Keil, Frank C. 1986. 'The Acquisition of Natural Kind and Artefact Terms'. In Marras and Demopoulos, 133–53.

Lau, D. C. 1967. 'A Note on *ke wu*'. *Bulletin of the School of Oriental and African Studies* 30 (2), 353–7.

Laufer, Bertold 1919. 'Sino-Iranica: Chinese Contributions to the History of Civilisation in Ancient Iran; with Special Reference to the History of Cultivated Plants and Products'. *Anthropological Series* 15 (3), 185–630. Field Museum of Natural History, Chicago. Publication no. 201. Reprint: Ch'eng-wu, Taipei, 1967.

Legge, James 1861. *Confucian Analects, the Great Learning, and the Doctrine of the Mean. The Chinese Classics*, vol. I. Truebner, London.

Linnaeus, Carolus 1751. *Philosophia botanica in qua explicantur fundamenta botanica cum definitionibus partium, exemplis terminorum, observationibus variorum, adjectis figuris aeneis.* Godor Kiesewetter, Stockholm; Z. Chatelain, Amsterdam.

Liu Hongyao 劉洪耀 (ed.) 1994a. *Lidai mingren yu Wudang* 歷代名人與武當 (Famous Historical Figures and Wudang). *Wudang zazhi zengkan* 武當雜誌增刊.

 1994b. 'Li Shizhen Wudang caiyao xiu bencao' 李時珍武當採藥修本草 (Li Shizhen's Improved *Materia Medica* of the Flora and Pharmaca in Wudang), in Liu Hongyao 1994a, 137–8.

Lu Gwei-djen 1966. 'China's Greatest Naturalist: a Brief Biography of Li Shih-Chen'. *Physis* 8 (4), 383–92.

Ma Jixing 馬繼興 1992. *Mawangdui guyishu kaoshi* 馬王堆古醫書考釋 (Study of the Ancient Medical Works from Mawangdui). Hunan kexue jishu chubanshe, Changsha.

Marras, Ausonio and Demopoulos, William (eds.) 1986. *Language Learning and Concept Acquisition.* Ablex, Norwood, N.J.

Mei, Y. P. 1951. 'Hsun-tzu on Terminology'. *Philosophy East and West* 1 (2), 51–66.

Métailié, Georges 1981. 'La création lexicale dans le premier traité de botanique occidentale publié en chinois (1858)'. *Documents pour l'histoire du vocabulaire scientifique* 2, 65–73.

 1988. 'Des mots et des plantes dans le *Bencao gangmu* de Li Shizhen'. *Extrême-Orient Extrême-Occident* 10, 27–43.

 1989. 'Histoire naturelle et humanisme en Chine et en Europe au XVIe siècle: Li Shizhen et Jacques Dalechamps'. *Révue d'histoire des sciences* 42 (4), 353–74.

1990. 'Botanical terminology of Li Shizhen in *Bencao gangmu*'. In Said, 140–53.

1992. 'Des mots, des animaux, des plantes'. *Extrême-Orient Extrême-Occident* 14, 169–83.

1993. 'Plantes et noms, plantes sans noms dans le *Zhiwu mingshi tukao*'. *Extrême-Orient Extrême-Occident* 15, 139–48.

1995. 'Note a propos de citations implicites dans les textes chinois'. *Extrême-Orient Extrême-Occident* 17, 131–9.

1997. 'Ethnobotany in China'. In H. Selin, 312–15.

Nakayama Shigeru and Sivin, Nathan 1973. *Chinese Science: Explorations of an Ancient Tradition.* MIT Press, Cambridge, Mass.

Needham, Joseph and Lu Gwei-djen 1986. *Botany.* In Joseph Needham (ed.), *Science and Civilisation in China*, vol. VI, part 1. Cambridge University Press, Cambridge.

Needham, Joseph 1971. 'The Development of Botanical Taxonomy in Chinese Culture'. In Anon., 127–33.

Okanishi Tameto 1977. *Honzō kaisetsu* 本草概説 (Survey of Chinese Books on *Materia Medica*). Sōgensha, Osaka.

Pan Jixing 潘吉星 1984. 'Tan "Zhiwuxue" yi ci zai Zhongguo he Riben de youlai' 談植物學一辭在中國和日本的由來 (On the Origin of the Term 'Botany' in China and Japan). *Daziran tansuo* 大自然探索 3, 167–72.

Pei Shengji 1984. *Botanical Gardens in China.* University of Hawaii Press, Honolulu.

Qian Yuanming 錢遠銘 (ed.) 1984. *Li Shizhen yanjiu* 李時珍研究 (Researches on Li Shizhen). Guangdong keji chubanshe, Guangzhou.

Quanguo zhongyi tushu lianhe mulu 全國中醫聯合目錄 (Union Catalogue of the National Libraries for Chinese Medicine) 1991. Zhongguo zhongyi yanjiuyuan tushuguan 中國中醫研究院圖書館 (eds.). Zhongyi guji chubanshe, Beijing.

Read, Bernard E. 1936. *Chinese Medicinal Plants from the Pen Ts'ao Kang Mu.* 3rd edn. Peking Natural History Bulletin, Peking.

Said, Hakim Mohammed (ed.) 1990. *Essays on Science.* Hamdard Foundation Pakistan, Karachi.

Selin, Helaine (ed.) 1997. *Encyclopaedia of the History of Science, Technology, and Medicine in Non-Western Cultures.* Kluwer Academic, Dordrecht.

Shi Guanfen 施觀芬 and Wang Lingmin 王靈敏 1991. '*Bencao gangmu* chongyan tanxi' 《本草綱目》重言探析 (Preliminary Study on Reduplicated Terms in the *Classified Materia Medica*), *Shandong zhongyi xueyuan xuebao* 15 (5), 53–6.

Sivin, Nathan 1973. 'Li Shih-Chen'. In Gillispie, 390–8.

Unshuld, Paul U. 1986. *Medicine in China: a History of Pharmaceutics.* University of California Press, Berkeley.

Yu Ying-shih 1977. 'Han China.' In Chang 1977b, 53–83.

Zhongguo yiji tongkao 中國醫籍通考 (Comprehensive Examination of Chinese Medical Books) 1990–94. Yan Shiyun 嚴世芸 (ed.). 3 vols. Shanghai zhongyiyao daxue chubanshe, Shanghai.

Zhongyao dacidian. 中藥大辭典 (Dictionary of Chinese *Materia Medica*) 1977. Jiangsu xinyi xueyuan 江蘇新醫學院 (eds.). Shanghai kexue jishu chubanshe, Shanghai.

Zhongyi dacidian: yishi wenxian fence 中醫大辭典：醫史文獻分冊 (Great Dictionary of Chinese Medicine: Documents on the History of Medicine) 1981. Zhongyi dacidian bianji weiyuanhui 中醫大辭典編輯委員會 (eds.). Renmin weisheng chubanshe, Beijing.

8

Robust northerners and delicate southerners: the nineteenth-century invention of a southern medical tradition[1]

MARTA HANSON

The Chinese regard for classical precedent has often prompted a picture of medicine as a static art, its doctrines perfected early and merely elaborated later. Actually, Chinese medical doctrines changed regularly, perhaps more so than those of premodern Europe. Up to the end of the Ming dynasty, two canonical medical texts from the Han dynasty established the foundation for all later developments: the *Huangdi neijing: Suwen, Lingshu* 黃帝內經素問，靈樞 (Inner Canon of the Yellow Emperor: Basic Questions and Divine Pivot) compiled some time during the first century BC, and the *Shanghan zabing lun* 傷寒雜病論 (Treatise on Cold Damage and Miscellaneous Disorders) completed some time between the date of its preface in 196 AD and the death of its author in 219 AD. Traditionally, the Chinese have considered the *Huangdi neijing*, the most complex cosmological and medical treatise of the Han dynasty, to be the founding canon of Chinese medicine passed down from the legendary Yellow Emperor since unrecorded antiquity. With the extraordinary find in 1973 of the medical manuscripts from the third tomb at the Mawangdui archeological site, we now have evidence that an earlier stage of medical knowledge preceded and was related to the more complex concepts systematised in the *Huangdi neijing*.[2] Scholars have concurred for some time that the *Huangdi neijing*, which is now only extant in three recensions, was from the beginning a collection of interrelated short essays from different lineages

---

[1] This article is a revision based on the article by the same title published in *Positions: East Asia Cultures Critique* 6.3 (Winter 1998), 515–50. Revisions have been made to address more directly the theme of the book *Innovation in Chinese Medicine*.

[2] For a complete translation and fine study of these texts, see Harper 1998.

at different times, compiled most likely from sources written no more than a century before.[3]

The *Shanghan lun* is less shrouded in the mystery of undocumented Chinese antiquity. An official from Changsha in Hunan province, Zhang Ji 張機 (150–219 CE), wrote it in response to epidemics during the last decades of the Later Han dynasty.[4] Chinese physicians have traditionally considered the *Neijing* to be the foundation of medical theory and the *Shanghan lun* to be the basis for clinical practice. Up to the end of the Ming dynasty, medical practices based on these two treatises largely dominated Chinese medicine. Physicians regularly presented later innovations as supplements to these founding canons.

During the course of the Qing dynasty, however, a new tradition based on Warm-factor disorders (*wenbing* 溫病) was invented first as complementary and then increasingly in opposition to the cold-damage tradition.[5] In the *Shanghan lun*, the term *wenbing* originally referred to an insignificant type of cold-damage disorder (*shanghan* 傷寒) that occurred in the spring or summer. Among practitioners of traditional Chinese medicine (TCM) today, *wenbing* is the collective term for disorders that biomedicine classifies as 'acute febrile diseases', that is, diseases characterised by high fevers that are also often infectious, such as typhoid and typhus.[6] In classical doctrinal medical

[3] The three recensions are the *Suwen*, *Lingshu*, and *Taisu* 太素 (The Grand Basis), all of which Tang and Song editors revised, but of which the Taisu appears to be the least revised. According to Sivin, *Huangdi neijing* has been the collective title since the Northern Song for the first two recensions: the first part, *Suwen* or 'Basic Questions', focuses on theoretical and cosmological issues, and the second part, *Lingshu* or 'Divine Pivot', turns to clinical medicine, particularly the relationship between acupuncture and the circulation tracts. From this point on I will refer to the entire text, comprised of these two parts, simply as the *Neijing*. For the sources and argument supporting this consensus, see Sivin (1993), 196–9.

[4] The original version of this text no longer exists. It was lost by the late third century, and first reconstituted and revised by Wang Xi 王熙 (third century) at the end of the third century. Then it was edited again and significantly changed by Northern Song compilers within the period from 968 to 975. The same occurred again in 1064–65 when it was finally divided into three separate books. Since this text was rearranged and revised several times, I use *Shanghan lun* to refer to the whole of Zhang Ji's original *Shanghan zabing lun*. Since 1064–65 this text has been separated into *Shanghan lun* 傷寒論 (Treatise on Cold Damage), the *Jingui yuhan jing* 金匱玉函經 (Canon of the Golden Casket and Jade Cases), and *Jingui yaolüe fanglun* 金匱要略方論 (Essentials and Discussions of Prescriptions in the Gold Casket). For details of this textual history see Okanishi (1958), 19–32, and Ōtsuka (1966), 17–45. For a summary of this Japanese scholarship on recensions of the *Shanghan zabing lun*, see the bibliography in Sivin (1987), 460–1.

[5] The 'cold-damage tradition' refers to the textual commentary and compilations based on Zhang Ji's canonical *Shanghan zabing lun* starting with Wang Xi's recension and those edited during the Northern Song dynasty.

[6] See for example the following two textbooks published in the PRC, edited by Wu Yin'gen and Shen Qingfa (1991) and Meng Shujiang (1985).

texts such as the *Neijing* and the *Shanghan lun*, however, 'wenbing' encompassed a range of illnesses from the common cold to high fevers and epidemic diseases, all of which were characterised by acute fevers and hot sensations in the patient's body. Medical doctrine attributes these disorders to pathogenic heat of varying quality from warm (*wen* 溫) to hot (*re* 熱), which is characteristic of the climate in spring and summer respectively.

Certain Qing physicians, denying the universality of the *Shanghan lun* tradition, broadened the narrow meaning of *wenbing* to encompass a separate class of disorders that were more prevalent than cold damage throughout the year in the Jiangnan region, which included Jiangsu, Zhejiang, and Anhui provinces of central China. These physicians argued that this local class of disorders required medical responses that were different from the orthodox *Shanghan lun* tradition. Over the course of the nineteenth-century *wenbing* thus went from a subcategory of cold damage to a separate category of disorders with its own system of diagnoses, treatments, and canon of medical writings. Based in the south, on the lower reaches of the Yangzi River, in Jiangnan, for centuries the wealthiest and most influential region in every aspect of intellectual life, the *wenbing* movement transformed medical practice and its underlying rationales. Study of this movement reveals not only new theoretical departures but also resonances with broad social and cultural changes in late Imperial China.

By inventing a Jiangnan-centred medical tradition, nineteenth-century authors and publishers of *wenbing* texts reinforced a regional identity. They argued that southern bodies were distinct from and more delicate than the bodies of robust northerners. They not only mapped geography onto physiology, they asserted local knowledge over state-sanctioned universal orthodoxy. They implicitly but unmistakably challenged the universality of a political ideology that was defined and enforced in the capital far to the north.

Wenbing physicians borrowed the ancient concept of resonant local *qi* to commend their medical writings to Jiangnan patients. This concept of human variation does not fit well into modern Western categories of racial and biological determinism. Their division of bodies into southern and northern was remarkable in a culture built on monolithic generalisations about the Chinese Empire. Considering that medicine, political theory, and social mores were represented in ideology as part of a single ideological manifold throughout Chinese history, it is all the more significant to find *wenbing* emerging in the nineteenth century as a distinctly Jiangnan-centred medical tradition.

The first systematisers of a *wenbing* canon compiled scattered writings on *wenbing* that they found both in the Han medical canon and in the new texts that Qing physicians – mostly from Suzhou and its environs – wrote on disorders due to the local climate. In a famous 1852 publication titled *Wenre jingwei* 溫熱經緯 (Warp and Weft of Warm- and Hot-Factor Disorders), for example, the selections on *wenbing* from the *Neijing* and the *Shanghan lun* formed the warp (*jing* 經) and the new *wenbing* writings made up the weft (*wei* 緯) of a new synthesis.[7] This compilation presented the new *wenbing* writings not as displacing or replacing the cold-damage tradition but as the missing threads needed to complete the whole. For the first time, the editor remarked, he had woven the warp and weft of Chinese medicine – the past canon and present experience – into one textual fabric.[8]

By 1878, however, a new compilation titled *Nanbing biejian* 南病別鑑 (Discriminating Examination of Southern Diseases) presented the same Qing authors as constituting a southern tradition in opposition to an irrelevant northern cold-damage tradition. The status of *wenbing* writings before and after the Taiping Rebellion (1853–64) changed from supplementing the writings on *wenbing* in the Han medical canon to opposing the cold-damage tradition, now newly identified as 'northern'. This change in status of *wenbing* writings *vis-à-vis* the older canonical tradition signals that more was involved in the debate between the two than simply clinical medicine.

During the Taiping Rebellion, the Qing government had to rely on local elites and their militias, especially in Jiangnan, to destroy the Taipings and retain at least the appearance of one unified empire. The government's army, to clear out all possible opposition, used what later came to be called 'strategic hamlet' policy, which devastated many parts of the region. After the suppression of the Taipings in 1864, local power had considerably expanded over regions in Jiangnan that had previously been under central authority. The result was increasing regionalism[9] and, I argue, a heightened awareness of linguistic, regional, and ethnic differences. *Wenbing* writings translated these differences as well into physiological distinctions.

Beginnings

Innovations in medical practice do not appear in divine revelations, though those who practise them may believe they do. Nor are they specific milestones on the road toward

---

[7] The author of this compilation, Wang Shixiong 王士雄 (1808–68), was one of the most important early promoters of *wenbing* texts generally. For the full statement of his organising rationale, see Wang's preface, repr. *Zhongguo yiji tongkao* (1992), vol. II, 1751–2.

[8] See Bray (1995), 116–17. Bray analyses the layers of meaning for these two terms, which have cosmological, medical, and ritually significant connotations. They are used, for example, to translate longitude (*jing* 經) and latitude (*wei* 緯). 'Weft' (*wei*) also referred to the textual appendices to canonical texts. From the Han on, it referred to new non-canonical writings offered as revelations of a classic. This was how Wang Shixiong used it in his 1852 compilation of canonical and appended new writings on *wenbing*.

[9] For expanding regionalism, see Michael (1976), 198–9. For the anti-Manchuist aspects of the Taiping Rebellion, see Laitinen (1990), 33–4.

truth, though many practitioners and scholars affirm that they are. By producing medical texts, sharing experience, and consolidating support from members of the local elite, groups of practitioners form a consensus on new theories, diagnostic methods, and drug therapies.[10] These changes in medical practice can be fully understood only when we recognise the local circumstances in which they were conceived, recorded, and transmitted. In the minds of Chinese physicians themselves, specific geographic locales required distinct therapeutic interventions.

Some eighteenth-century physicians in the Suzhou region, for example, thought that because of the propensity of the soil in their region to emit warmer and damper *qi* than in the northern and western regions, their patients were most likely to suffer from warm- and damp-type illnesses. The six climatic excesses of *qi* (*liuyin* 六淫) – wind, cold, fire, summer heat, damp, and dry – which linked the seasons with illness in Chinese medicine were not evenly distributed across the Empire. This concept of local *qi* (*tuqi* 土氣 or *diqi* 地氣) united traditional conceptions of the environment, climate, and disease with a notion of self that was deeply rooted in native place. The related ideas of local *qi* and native place came together when the Chinese established native-place associations to secure a sense of self and community in business networks, urban culture, and local society in the Qing.[11] The nineteenth-century physicians who promoted *wenbing* styles of medical practice also borrowed both concepts to identify geographically resonant corporeal, physiological, and pathological characteristics. These physicians promoted their local tradition of medicine against the universalising claims of the self-proclaimed guardians of the cold-damage orthodoxy. They focused their works on the climatic excesses of *qi* (fire, summer heat, and damp) that they thought were endemic in the Jiangnan environment, but that had been largely ignored in previous medical texts.

The debate about cold-damage and warm-factor disorders during the nineteenth century reflected an epistemological shift that was integral with social developments. With the formation of this new group of physicians, the epistemological framework underlying medical practice shifted from the dominant cold-damage tradition, which promoted universal medical knowledge, continuity with antiquity, and the canonical authority of the Han medical classics, to a more pluralistic *wenbing* tradition, which promoted regional variation, discontinuity with the past, and locally tailored therapy for Jiangnan patients.

The nineteenth-century anthologists and publishers of *wenbing* texts challenged the universal authority of the cold-damage tradition primarily in order to convince local elites and patients that *wenbing* texts offered diagnostic methods and prescriptions tailored to southern bodies. Once considered ideal for all diseases, the cold-damage

---

[10] For theoretical approaches to the history of medicine in China and the USA, see Sivin (1995), Rosenberg (1979, 1992), and Wu Yiyi (1993–94).

[11] See, for example, Goodman (1995).

diagnostic methods and formulas now became relative and unsuitable for Jiangnan patients. Zhang Ji's Han-dynasty *Shanghan lun* could no longer satisfy the medical needs of All-Under-Heaven.

Two points on the trajectory toward a new tradition

Two texts that were published within a century of one another in Suzhou, one of the most urban cultural centres of the Jiangnan region, illustrate the situation before and after *wenbing* was defined as a southern medical tradition. The *Wuyi huijiang* 吳醫彙講 (Compilation of Lectures by Suzhou Physicians),[12] published in 1793 by Tang Dalie 唐大烈 (d. 1801), represents the situation before the writings on *wenbing* were anthologised and their authors identified as founders. On the other hand, the *Nanbing biejian* 南病別鑑 (A Discriminating Examination of Southern Diseases), first published in 1878 by Song Zhaoqi 宋兆淇 (late nineteenth century), presents early *wenbing* texts together and considers their authors to be founders of a new tradition of southern diseases.[13]

I first interpret two essays published in *Suzhou Physicians*. The essays' author, a scholar named Guan Ding 管鼎 (eighteenth century), voiced the positions of those who argued for the universal authority of the *Shanghan lun*. I then turn to the opposing perspective of the editor, Tang Dalie, who supported new developments in medicine. I next analyse the important issues regarding local medical knowledge discussed in the six prefaces to *Southern Diseases*, which were written for three different editions. Prefaces often reveal more than the contents of a book about the motivations underlying it. With this in mind, I read these prefaces as representative of a nineteenth-century opposition to the cold-damage tradition. The authors encouraged physicians in Jiangnan to use the methods published in *Southern Diseases* instead of those recorded in the *Shanghan lun*. Thus, *Suzhou Physicians* and *Southern Diseases* mark distinct points on a trajectory along which physicians in the Suzhou region invented the *wenbing* tradition.

Wuyi huijiang, 1793

The editor of *Suzhou Physicians*, Tang Dalie, was a physician from Changzhou, a prefectural capital east of Suzhou.[14] He wrote a great deal in his preface about how he organised the project. When acting as the principal of the prefectural medical school in

---

[12] Wu included cities around Suzhou such as Wuxi about 45 km to the north-west, Changshu about 37 km to the north, and Taicang about 50 km to the north-east.

[13] I refer to the first as *Suzhou Physicians* and the second as *Southern Diseases*.

[14] Tang Dalie wrote a few sentences about himself directly preceding the first group of essays he wrote in *Wuyi huijiang, juan* 2, 16. Tang records his medical title as *Suzhou fuyixue zhengke* 蘇州府醫學正科 (Principal of the Prefectural Medical School of Suzhou).

Suzhou, he asked local physicians to submit essays on medical topics. He then distributed among them copies of some of the submissions to solicit their criticism. He combined their comments with his own revisions before compiling the final draft. The resulting compilation contains ninety-four essays by forty-one authors, including many by Tang himself.

The diversity of opinions that Tang brought together made *Suzhou Physicians* the first compilation of its kind in Chinese medical history. Tang divided the essays by different authors into eleven separate sections (*juan* 卷), which roughly resemble the format of a journal.[15] Inspired by previous medical compilations organised chronologically, Tang gathered together for the first time essays on a wide range of medical issues by many physicians from only one region. He combined the genre of collected medical jottings and case records of famous physicians throughout history with the subgenres of the collected writings of a single physician and of case records from a single region.[16] *Suzhou Physicians* offers an unprecedented range of medical ideas, practices, and therapies in traditional China. In anticipation of a wide readership, the four essays of the first section addressed completely different subjects: an essay on praying to the medical gods; the seminal essay 'On Treating Warm-Factor Syndromes' (Wenzheng lun zhi 溫証論治) by Ye Gui 葉桂 (1667–1746); a short discourse on man as microcosm; and an explanation of how to use formularies. The remaining essays are similarly varied. Most importantly, we find in this compilation writings that represent the cold-damage tradition as well as some of the earliest extant versions of the writings of authors who wrote on *wenbing*.

Guan Ding: representative of the cold-damage tradition

Tang published the only four extant essays by Guan Ding, an eighteenth-century representative of the cold-damage tradition. Guan Ding was a disciple of Miao Zunyi 繆遵義

[15] Some Chinese medical historians have claimed that he published the eleven sections individually over nine years from 1792, the date of his preface, to his death in 1801. His son supposedly republished the serials as a book after Tang's death. See entry on the *Wuyi huijiang* in Qian Xinzhong (1987), 220. There is no evidence, however, to support these claims. The earliest extant edition shows that the entire compilation was completed and published in 1793, the date of the third preface. For confirmation of this conclusion, see Su Tiege (1993).

[16] Two comprehensive publications that recorded the theories of individual physicians and the various *pai* or 'currents of thought' from antiquity to the present impressed Tang Dalie. These were the *Mingyi lei'an* 名醫類案 (Classified Medical Case Histories of Famous Physicians) by Jiang Guan 江瓘 (1503–65) and the *Gujin mingyi fanglun* 古今名醫方論 (Treatise on the Prescriptions of Famous Physicians Past and Present) by Luo Mei 羅美 (1662–1722). Tang also mentioned that he used a collection of case histories from the Wu region titled *Wuzhong yi'an* 吳中醫案 (Case Histories from Suzhou) as a model for his own, but this text is no longer extant. See Tang Dalie, *Wuyi huijiang*, preface, 1.

(1710–93), a *jinshi* physician from Suzhou who wrote one of the prefaces to the first edition of *Suzhou Physicians*. Guan's arguments represent the sentiments of physicians who defended the canonical authority of the *Shanghan lun* against the challenges of critical physicians. Guan's first two essays present his opinion on theories concerning the increase since antiquity of illnesses caused by excessive fire *qi* (火氣), which Liu Wansu 劉完素 (1120–1200), one of the first critics of the Song medical orthodoxy, argued was the major cause of disorders of his era.[17] Liu believed that the climate had become hotter since antiquity and therefore more people suffered in his day from fevers and other symptoms of excessive heat than in the past. In the last two essays, Guan Ding refutes the attacks on the universality of the cold-damage tradition that were based on its temporal and seasonal limitations. I focus the following analysis on the latter two essays.

The critics of the cold-damage tradition used the idea of a decreasing endowment of primordial *qi* (*yuanqi* 原氣) to support their skepticism toward using the ancient cold-damage formulas to treat disorders in contemporary society. Primordial *qi* has both a cosmological and individual denotation:[18] it can refer to the 'undifferentiated potential of cosmic energy' in the world, or it can mean each human individual's innate constitution, as well as the potential *qi* that is gradually used up in the course of a life. In the third essay, Guan refutes the claim that the natural endowment of primordial *qi* in humans has decreased over time.[19] Physicians who followed this point of view believed that patients in antiquity required stronger formulas to expel heteropathic *qi* from their bodies because their endowment of primordial *qi* was greater than that of current patients.[20] Guan thinks there is no evidence for this claim and attempts to prove it:

> Physicians often cite these two statements as essential points in therapy: 'The environments of the five regions[21] [call for] different appropriate [measures]',[22]

---

[17] These essays are titled 'Qi you yu bian shi huo jie' 氣有餘便是火解 (Explanation of the Statement 'When there is a Surplus of *qi*, then it is Fire') and 'Dongyuan Jingyue lun xianghuo bian' 東垣景岳論相火辨 (Li Gao and Zhang Jiebin's Discussions on Ministerial Fire Differentiation). In *Wuyi huijiang*, *juan* 7, 84–5.

[18] The translation 'primordial *qi*' is from Porkert (1974), 173.

[19] This essay was titled 'Gujin yuanqi bu shen xiangyuan shuo' 古今元氣不甚相遠説 (On the [Endowment of] Primordial *qi* in the Past and Present not Greatly Differing). In *Wuyi huijiang, juan* 7, 86.

[20] For a seventeenth-century summary of this theory, see Li Zhongzi 李仲梓 'Gujin yuanqi butong lun' 古今元氣不同論 (On [the Endowment of] Primordial *qi* in the Past and the Present not Being the Same), *Yizong bidu* 醫宗必讀 (Essential Readings in the Medical Lineage), *juan* 1, 4a–b.

[21] The 'five regions' refer to the regions in the five cardinal directions north, south, east, west, and centre, which also correspond to the Five Phases.

[22] Locus classicus in *Huangdi neijing*, 'Yifa fangyi lun' 異法方宜論 (On Different Methods of Treatment Appropriate to the Region), *Suwen, pian* 12, 39–40.

and 'the [endowment of] primordial *qi* in the past and present is not the same'.[23] [They] believe that in the north and west [the land] is high, [climate] dry, and cold dominant; in the south and east, [the land] is low, [climate] damp, and heat dominant. [Because of the] high land and dry climate, the sinews and bones [of people who live in the north and west] are strong (*jingu jinqiang* 筋骨勁強); due to the low land and damp climate, the muscles and flesh [of the people who live in the south and east] are soft and weak (*jirou rouruo* 肌肉柔弱). This distinction is based on the hardness and softness of topography and not on any distinction between the [endowment of] original primordial *qi* [i.e., in humans in the past and present]. Thus the sages early on set out this [distinction] in detail in the *Neijing*'s 'Treatise on Different Methods of Treatment Appropriate to the Region', and 'Main Treatise on the Regulations for the Five Constants'.[24]

Guan Ding sets forth in these essays the conventional view that local *qi* creates contrasts in bodily constitutions and that the five geographic regions call for different therapeutic practices. In both essays from the *Neijing*, the porous skin was a permeable boundary between the body and its environment. The high land and dry climate of the northern and western regions made strong bodies; the low land and damp climate of the eastern and southern regions formed weak bodies. Geography and climate structured corporeal difference.

Although Guan agrees with the first statement that physicians should adapt their medical practice to regional variations in environment and body types, he rejects the second statement on the decreasing endowment of primordial *qi*. On the contrary, he argues, the endowment of primordial *qi* in present-day humans is no different from that of the ancients. The distinction between strong and weak constitutions only reflects the relative strength of the *qi* in any given topography (*xingshi* 形勢). It does not mean that the relative strength of the innate primordial *qi* (*benyuan qi* 本原氣) of the individual has decreased over time.

The remaining sections of Guan's third essay defend the universal applicability of cold-damage treatments. In the beginning of his rebuttal, Guan dismisses the common belief that in antiquity people lived for several centuries:

> I can explain [the statement] 'the [endowment of] primordial *qi* in the past and present are not the same'. During the era of the august ancients, it was said that

[23] This statement refers to a quotation attributed to a Jin dynasty doctor, Zhang Yuansu 張元素 (fl. 1100s), who believed that ancient methods were no longer best suited for new diseases. Locus classicus in *Jin shi*, *juan* 131, 2812.

[24] These are *pian* 12 and 70 of the *Huangdi neijing Suwen*. The sections on local *qi* are in *Suwen*, *pian* 70, 205.

[some] lives lasted for centuries or millennia. [Because the belief] may have been either difficult [for scholars] to discuss or there are gaps in the texts, perhaps it is not to be trusted? All of the contents of the *Book of Documents* from [King] Yao 堯 on are clear and can be examined. The so-called generosity of [endowment of] primordial *qi* has to be verified [by determining] longevity. Although the primordial *qi* of the ancients cannot be seen, their longevity can. During the time of Tang 唐 and Yu 虞 and the Three Eras (*sandai* 三代), we no longer hear of people living for several hundred years. Confucius 孔 and [his disciple] Yan 顏 are even clearer proof [because, although they were sages, their life spans were ordinary].

Having asserted that longevity is not notably different today than it was in the past, Guan turns his attention to the argument that Zhang Ji's formulas are too strong for treating contemporary patients. It is not that Zhang's patients had a stronger constitution founded on a greater endowment of primordial *qi* than people have today; rather, Zhang was more adept at making a diagnosis and so he knew exactly what drug to use for what illness. His patients recovered quickly, so they sometimes did not need to finish their entire prescription. Multiple doses per day meant the whole course could be prepared and brewed at one time. The quantity of drug may appear greater, but the amount taken was not. This is why, Guan argues, Zhang's formulas appear to be stronger than those used in contemporary practice.

Guan Ding then resumes his point that neither longevity nor primordial *qi* has changed since antiquity. He attributes variations in life spans to differing endowments of *qi* in individuals and not, as critics of the cold-damage tradition argued, to the decrease in everyone's endowment of primordial *qi* since antiquity. Since the bodies of humans in antiquity were no different than human bodies today, the ancient methods remain as effective to treat illness now as in the past:

> The ancients thought that one hundred was the upper limit of longevity. Seventy to one hundred years was considered old age [and anything less], premature death. From the Han down to the present has anyone had a different [view]? Now certainly in the whole of Heaven and Earth there has been no pattern of gradual decrease over long periods. Heaven and Earth are not concerned with the shaping and transforming forces [of *yin* and *yang*]. Humans are endowed with the *qi* of Heaven and Earth in order to be born, each person having enough for a hundred years. The fact that people have different [life spans] is due to the varying generosity of this endowment [of *qi*] in each person. The present and past [have followed] the same track. Were this not so, why would the Yellow Emperor and Qibo pass down teachings, and [Zhang Ji of] Changsha begin transmitting [the *Shanghan lun*] if they were appropriate for only one region or one era?

Physicians who, like Guan Ding, supported the canonical status of the *Shanghan lun* attached great significance to continuity with the past and rejected deviations from the Han canon.[25]

Whereas Guan's third essay attacks the claim that the endowment of primordial *qi* has decreased over time, his fourth essay refutes the argument that cold-damage methods are only effective for treating cold-damage disorders. Critics of the cold-damage tradition argued that because cold-damage disorders are initially caused by excessive cold *qi* (*hanqi* 寒氣), people suffer from them in the winter and not during any other seasons. Guan counters this claim by promoting the *Shanghan lun* as the ultimate authority on treatments for illnesses in all the seasons, owing to the six climatic excesses of *qi*. When Guan Ding argues that 'all four seasons have cold-damage [disorders]', he reasserts the temporal comprehensiveness of the *Shanghan lun*.[26] He challenges the limitations placed on the *Shanghan lun* by physicians who sought to legitimate their own emphases on disorders caused by either the remaining five climatic excesses in the environment or the various internal factors within the body. These physicians, Guan argues, misdiagnose syndromes when the cold heteropathy goes directly to the centre of the body instead of passing from the skin inward through the first two of the six warps (*liu jing* 六經), which represent the initial stages of penetration of climatic *qi* into the body.[27] Because of this misconception, Guan believes they wrongly think that cold-damage disorders do not occur in the south:

> The three *yang* warps in cold-damage [syndromes] all exhibit symptoms in the outer aspect [of the body]. As for the three *yin* [warps], they do not have symptoms in the outer aspect [of the body] on which to base [diagnoses]. Moreover [the cold heteropathy] is not necessarily transmitted from the mature *yang* warp on the first day to the *yang* brightness warp on the second day. It may suddenly go directly to the centre [of the body] without passing through a mature or immature [warp]. Now if someone suddenly exhibits a pulse pattern indicating a *yin*-warp dysfunction, a physician who examines him does not know how to classify the disorder and can-

---

[25] Before ending the essay, Guan made several points on prescriptions. He criticised alterations of canonical formulas. But he was not a rigid traditionalist and recommended a middle road. Doctors should use the ancient models and decrease dosages as necessary, but pay attention to how people today use prescriptions and increase them accordingly.

[26] See 'Sishi jie you shanghan lun' 四時皆有傷寒論 (On there Being Cold-Damage Disorders During All Four Seasons), in *Wuyi huijiang*, *juan* 7, 87.

[27] The six warps of the cold-damage tradition signify six stages of penetration of external stimuli (*waigan* 外感) into the body. The three *yang* warp stages of penetration are *yang* brightness, mature *yang*, and immature *yang*. The three *yin* warp stages of penetration are immature *yin*, mature *yin*, and attenuated *yin*. All six stages have characteristic symptoms associated with them: the three *yang* warps are characterised by more exterior-type disorders, and the three *yin* warps have relatively interior types. Guan refers here to the first two stages of the three *yang* warps.

not work out a treatment. Because of this, some say that there are no cold-damage disorders in the southern regions. It is not that there is no cold damage. Actually there is, but it is difficult to recognise and treat. Cold [*qi*] is one [type of] cosmic *qi*. The [author of] *Shanghan lun* selected one [type] to name his book. But as for its 113 formulas, surely they are not all formulas for treating disorders due to cold?

Guan then compares this misconception to believing that the use of *spring* and *autumn* in the title of *The Spring and Autumn Annals* (*Lüshi chun qiu* 呂氏春秋) from the Warring States period means that the *Annals* only covered events of these two seasons:

> This is comparable to the Historian Lü choosing only spring and autumn of the four seasons [in the title of his book to represent the entire year]. I venture to think that cold-damage [disorders] do not occur only during the period between the first frost and the beginning of spring. The other three seasons also have them. However, because of the different seasons, the names [of the disorders] change. For example, [there are] spring-warm and summer-heat [disorders].[28] The treatments for these syndromes, however, are all included in the 397 [cold-damage] methods.[29] The most important point for scholars is to be able to comprehend its [i.e., cold-damage disorders] transformations. The *Shanghan lun* is complete for treatments of disorders due to all of the six types of climatic configurations of *qi*.

Guan Ding rejects the idea that the knowledge preserved in the *Shanghan lun* is partial and incomplete. The febrile illnesses of the spring and summer, which other physicians claimed to treat with more appropriate drug therapies, are in fact transformed cold damage. The name of the disorder changes according to the season in which the latent cold *qi* manifests itself as an illness. This conception of a latent form of cold *qi* hiding in the body and waiting for an external stimulus to activate it represents a completely different conception of causation from the *wenbing* idea of seasonal and local varieties of *qi* that have an immediate effect on the body:

> Later [physicians] have focused on warm and hot [*qi*],[30] or have concentrated on the [diagnostic method] triple *jiao* (*sanjiao* 三焦),[31] or have emphasised the

---

[28] In the cold-damage conception, these syndromes were thought to be the spring and summer manifestations of heteropathic cold *qi* that had invaded the body in the winter. The cold *qi* remained latent in the body until the change in seasons stimulated it to manifest itself as an illness.

[29] There were originally 113 cold-damage formulas and 397 rules for treating disease.

[30] The reference is to followers of Liu Wansu who adhered to his doctrine: 'The six *qi* all come from changes in fire [*qi*]' (*liu qi jie cong huo hua* 六氣皆從火化). See p. 269.

[31] 'The triple *jiao*' refers to a division of the torso into three sections. It was a diagnostic method that divided the stages of penetration of external heteropathic *qi* vertically from the upper region of the body to the lower region. The first stage begins in the organ systems of the upper *jiao* (lungs and heart). If the heteropathic *qi* is not expelled from the upper *jiao*, it travels to the medial *jiao* (stomach and spleen) and, finally, to the lower *jiao* (kidneys and liver).

heart-constructive and lung-defensive sectors [of four-sectors diagnosis].[32] If they do not look beyond one [type of] *qi* or one warp [type of syndrome], [they] cannot 'see the leopard for its spots'. In reading texts, the most important thing is to understand [them]; one cannot be like a young novice bound by monastic rules.

In this essay, Guan Ding considers the trend among physicians to analyse illness in terms of one type of heteropathic *qi* or one type of syndrome to be reductionist. In his view, the new therapeutic emphases from the Song dynasty on were merely partial views of the patterns of disorders that had already been fully explained in the *Shanghan lun*.

The remainder of Guan's fourth essay returns to the three stages of *yin*-warp syndromes of the cold-damage tradition mentioned in his opening statement. In this last section he argues that none of the various ways physicians classify syndromes and prescribe medicines fall outside the categories established in the *Shanghan lun*. The so-called hot and purge syndromes (*rexia zheng* 熱下証) and warm and supplement syndromes (*wenbu zheng* 溫補証), he argues, can also be seen in the three *yin*-warp syndromes of the cold-damage tradition.[33]

Guan ignores the socio-geographic argument recorded nearly a hundred and fifty years earlier in an essay by the physician Li Zhongzi 李仲梓 (1588–1655) on different treatments for the wealthy and the poor.[34] Li explains that the different therapeutic emphases of the northerner Zhang Congzheng 張從正 (1156–1228) and the southerner Xue Ji 薛己 (1487–1559) were responses to the geographically determined contrasting constitutions of their patients. For Guan, however, these physicians merely call by a different name syndromes already analysed in the *Shanghan lun*. Proponents, such as Guan, of the cold-damage tradition did not believe that human bodies differed with respect to time, class, or place (north or south). If they had, they would have questioned

<hr />

[32] He refers to Ye Gui's four sectors (*sifen* 四分) diagnostic method in which Ye divided the degree of penetration of pathogenic heat into the body. The four sectors follow one another from the outer aspect of the body to the most inner aspect. The defensive *qi* sector (*weifen* 衛分) includes the most superficial level of penetration by pathogenic hot and warm *qi*. It is often associated with problems with the lung visceral system. The active *qi* sector (*qifen* 氣分) is the next level of penetration. It includes symptoms of hot and warm *qi* in the chest and diaphragm. The constructive *qi* sector (*yingfen* 營分) indicates the third level of penetration and therefore more severe illnesses of the heart visceral system and cardiac envelope junction (*xinbao* 心包). The blood sector (*xuefen* 血分) is the deepest level hot and warm *qi* can penetrate and represents the most serious stages of warm-factor disorders.

[33] Chinese physicians often named syndromes after the main function associated with the drugs used to treat the symptoms. The first two syndromes, for example, refer to the tradition of attacking and purging drug therapy associated with the Jin dynasty physician from Henan in the north, Zhang Congzheng 張從正 (1156–1228), who is considered the founder of the *gongxia pai* 攻下派 (attack and purge current of thought). The second pair of syndromes refers to the tradition of warming and supplementing drug therapy associated with Xue Ji 薛己 (1487–1559), who is considered the founder of the *wenbu pai* 溫補派 (warm and supplement current of thought).

[34] See Li Zhongzi, 'Fugui pinjian zhibing youbie lun' 富貴貧賤治病有別論 (On Treatments for the Wealthy and the Poor Being Different), *Yizong bidu, juan* 1, 4b–5b.

the universal validity of the six-warp diagnostic method and canonical formulas of antiquity. Guan concludes:

> Moreover, the [disorders] due to external stimuli (*waigan* 外感) do not fall outside the six warps [patterns][35] and [disorders] due to inner damage (*neishang* 內傷) do not go beyond the five visceral systems of function (*wu zang* 五臟).[36] The *Shanghan lun* also encompasses disorders caused by heterogeneous *qi* (*zaqi* 雜氣).[37] How could any time or place have been without them? The origin [of medicine] is traced to Changsha 長沙 [i.e., Zhang Ji].[38] [One] ought to immerse [oneself] in and read back and forth in his book. [One] must also think carefully about treatments for syndromes that are not [manifested] in the outer aspect [of the body]. 'Even though the palace wall may be high [i.e., mastering the *Shanghan lun* is hard], one can still peep into it.'

This passage contrasts two opposing perspectives on the *Shanghan lun*: it was either a comprehensive revelation whose deeper meanings required immersion, or simply a guide to practice that needed to be supplemented with new theories and therapies based on clinical experience.[39] Guan Ding's defence of the first view reveals many of the issues that proponents of the second raised. We see in his two essays a dissonance between physicians who believed in the universal authority of the cold-damage tradition and those people, such as followers of the influential medical thinkers of the Jin and Yuan dynasties,[40] who considered it to be biased, limited, and not in accord with their clinical experience.

---

[35] This statement is an attack on the *wenbing* physicians Ye Gui and Xue Xue 薛雪 (1681–1770) both of whom were thought to have used the four sector and three *jiao* diagnostic methods to differentiate syndromes due to warm *qi* (*wen qi* 溫氣) and damp *qi* (*shi qi* 濕氣). They both became posthumous members of the *wenbing xuepai* 溫病學派 (warm-factor disorders current of thought). See below.

[36] This is an attack on the ideas of Li Gao 李杲 (1180–1251) and Zhu Zhenheng 朱震亨 (1281–1358) who devised new approaches to illnesses due to internal causes. Li Gao is considered the founder of the *piwei pai* 脾胃派 (spleen and stomach current of thought) or *butu pai* 補土派 (replenish earth current of thought, i.e., on spleen and stomach disorders). Zhu Zhenheng is considered to be the founder of the *yangyin pai* 養陰派 (nourish the *yin* current of thought, i.e., disorders due to internal factors).

[37] This is an attack on the ideas of Wu Youxing. He argued in his *Wenyi lun* 瘟疫論 (Treatise on Warm-Factor Epidemics) that illnesses caused by heterogeneous *qi* fall outside the pattern of the six climatic excesses of *qi* (*liuqi* 六氣) and cannot be classified according to the six warps method of the cold-damage tradition.

[38] Changsha is Zhang Ji's literary name.

[39] For analyses of the relationship between texts and practice, see Farquhar (1992), Sivin (1995), and Hsu (1999).

[40] I refer to the 'Four Masters of the Jin and Yuan Dynasties' in recent Chinese medical historiography: Liu Wansu, Li Gao, Zhang Congzheng, and Zhu Zhenheng. The first references to the 'Four Masters' in the Ming dynasty, however, included Zhang Ji of the Han dynasty instead of Zhang Congzheng of the Jin dynasty. By at least the early nineteenth century, Zhang Congzheng had replaced Zhang Ji in this pantheon of medical masters. See essay on 'Yizong sidajia zhi shuo' 醫宗四大家之說 (The Doctrine of Four Masters of Medicine) in Luo Ji 羅浩, *Yijing yulun* 醫經餘論 (Leftover Discourses on the Medical Canon) (1812). Essay reprinted in Wang Xinhua and Pan Qiuxiang (1990), 549–50.

Early *wenbing* writings in *Wuyi huijiang*

Although Tang Dalie chose to include Guan Ding's essays in his *Suzhou Physicians*, several selections, including his own essays, make it clear that he did not agree with Guan's opinions. His point of view combines skepticism of the canons of antiquity with an emphasis on locality. Tang published, for example, Ye Gui's long essay 'Wenzheng lunzhi' 溫証論治 (On Working Out Treatment for Warm-Factor Syndromes).[41] In this essay Ye introduced the four-sectors diagnostic system referred to in Guan's fourth essay as a biased alternative to the six-warps diagnostic method of the cold-damage tradition. Guan explicitly opposed Ye's innovation. Four-sectors diagnosis, however, later became the preferred approach to identifying the stages of fevers and other symptoms in the *wenbing* tradition; *wenbing* physicians considered it more accurate to classify the levels of penetration of hot or warm factors in the body. Ye Gui summarises his four-sectors analysis – in which constructive (*ying* 營), defensive (*wei* 衛), active *qi* (*qi* 氣), and blood (*xue* 血) sectors[42] refer to increasingly interior penetration of hot or warm *qi* and severity of the illness – near the beginning of his essay: '[The analytic system of] differentiating the constructive *qi*, defensive *qi*, active *qi*, and blood sectors [of penetration of hot and warm *qi*], although similar to cold-damage [diagnosis], are related to treatment methods that are completely different [from] those for cold damage. The cold-damage heteropathy resides on the outer aspect [of the body] and later changes into hot [*qi*] to enter the inner aspect [of the body].'

Later in the same essay, Ye Gui takes a localist stance: 'The people in our Wu region (i.e., Suzhou) suffer most from damp heteropathies (*shixie* 濕邪).'[43] Ye's main themes are clinical, practical, and local. He focuses on disorders due to warm and damp factors because he believes that they are the most common causative factors in the Suzhou region. He relates symptoms to one of the four sectors, explains transformations from one manifestation type to another, and lists appropriate prescriptions for each variation. The essay contains a detailed analysis of the abnormalities of the tongue and teeth that indicate levels of penetration of pathogenic climatic factors. Ye does not refer to the six warps, nor does he use only the cold-damage formulas. He adapts formulas to changing circumstances instead of strictly adhering to the canonical prescriptions.

Tang Dalie's essay on 'Badajia lun' 八大家論 (Eight Masters of Medicine) presents a view of developments in knowledge that also opposes Guan Ding's position on the

---

[41] In *Wuyi huijiang*, *juan* 1, 3–11.

[42] In contrast to biomedical conceptions of blood as a separate substance, blood here refers to a kind of *qi* and the blood sector refers to the deepest level in the body reached by, and the most severe stage of an illness due to, pathogenic heat or dampness. See note 32.

[43] In *Wuyi huijiang*, *juan* 1, 5.

universality of the *Shanghan lun*. According to Tang, each innovative medical thinker in his synopsis of Chinese medical history adds to what his predecessors neglected to discuss: 'Liu Wansu went back [to Zhang Ji] and established teachings on spring-warm (*chunwen* 春溫) and summer-hot (*xiare* 夏熱) disorders. He added what Zhang had left incomplete. Li Gao clarified the differentiation of spleen and stomach inner damage (*piwei neishang* 脾胃內傷) disorders. They are different from disorders due to external stimuli [which Zhang and Liu discussed]. Li added what Zhang and Liu had not completed.'[44]

Tang Dalie does not agree with Guan Ding that these new developments are reductionist and limited. Earlier commentators on medical history also shared Tang's view that changes in medical practice redressed significant omissions in the medical canon. The sixteenth-century physician Wang Lun 王綸, for example, wrote about omissions in the *Shanghan lun* in an essay on the contributions of past physicians: 'It was not that Zhang Ji did not understand [disorders caused by] warm *qi* (*wen* 溫), summer heat (*shu* 暑), or inner damage (*neishang* 內傷);[45] [rather] his writings did not take them up.'[46] Wang Lun incorporated the new trends in medical thought into a pattern not yet realised, although implied, in the *Shanghan lun*. Neither Wang Lun nor Tang Dalie saw the innovations, however, as advances toward ever-expanding frontiers of medicine; rather, they saw them as filling in gaps within a finite body of knowledge. Thus according to Wang and Tang, medical knowledge develops by supplementing areas one's predecessors had not completely described and that are already latent in the classics. The innovative physicians during the Jin and Yuan dynasties, for example, wrote on disorders caused by external stimuli and internal damage until a more complete pattern of health and illness emerged. This process is neither reductive nor revolutionary, but accretive, accumulative, and progressive only in that sense.

Contrary to Guan Ding, in the same essay on 'Eight Masters of Medicine', Tang also supported Zhang Yuansu's idea that the endowment of primordial *qi* had decreased over time: '[Xue Ji] also thought that the *qi* from wind was not uniform [from past to present]. People today have a decreased endowment of [*qi*] so they should not be treated

---

[44] See essay by Tang Dalie, 'Zhang, Liu, Li, Zhu hou dangyi Xue, Zhang, Wu, Yu peiwei badajia lun' 張劉李朱后當以薛張吳喻配為八大家論 (Zhang Ji, Liu Wansu, Li Gao, and Zhu Zhenheng Ought to be Joined with Xue Ji, Zhang Jiebin, Wu Youxing, and Yu Chang 喻昌 [1585–?] to Make Eight Masters), *Wuyi huijiang*, *juan* 2, 18–19.

[45] 'Warm *qi*' and summer-heat' refer to Liu Wansu's focus on climatic factors not fully covered in the *Shanghan lun*; 'inner damage' refers to Li Gao's focus on internal causes.

[46] See Wang Lun, 'Zhongjing, Donghuan, Hejian, Danxi zhushu shuyou' 仲景東桓河間丹溪諸書孰优 (Which one of the various Books by Zhang Ji, Li Gao, Liu Wansu, and Zhu Zhenheng is the Best?), *Mingyi zazhu*, *juan* 1, 1.

with the cooling drugs [of the cold-damage tradition] but rather with [Xue Ji's] warming and supplementing drugs.'[47]

Although Tang Dalie viewed post-Han innovations in medical knowledge not as challenges to the authority of the Han medical canon but as a new genealogy descended from it, he still included essays by physicians such as Guan Ding, who disagreed. Tang and Guan represent profoundly different historiographical modes of thinking: whereas Guan posits antiquity as a totality and present knowledge as a fragment of this past whole, Tang sees antiquity as incomplete and is prepared to fill in with new approaches to current problems. Tang's aim was neither to secure the classical roots of medicine nor to establish the foundations for a Suzhou-style medicine. Rather, he sought to preserve the medical works of his local colleagues without preference for the canons of antiquity or, it seems, for one of the various lineages in the present.

Tang chose essays by Ye Gui, Xue Xue 薛雪 (1681–1770), and Xue Chengji 薛承基 (eighteenth century), for example, although they were not members of a cohesive group of physicians. Even though Xue Xue published several books on medicine,[48] Tang published only eight statements attributed to him. They are terse yet varied. The topics range from a statement on the use of ass-hide glue (*ejiao* 阿膠) in the *Shanghan lun* to how to apply the *Book of Changes* (*Yijing* 易經) to treatments for epidemic diseases.[49] Not one statement refers to the *wenbing* writings later attributed to him, nor is there evidence that Xue Xue intended for the jottings to be published. His great-grandson Xue Qiqian 薛啟潛 (eighteenth century) submitted the material to Tang Dalie for his compilation.[50] Tang states: 'Xue Xue was as famous as Ye Gui. Although something can be gained from both men and one is not better than the other, Xue did not like to think of himself as a physician and thus did not complete [his own medical] text.'[51] Tang included Xue's jottings because Xue was a Suzhou physician as famous as Ye, not because he belonged to a particular medical tradition.[52] In addition, the long text by Xue

[47] *Wuyi huijiang, juan* 2, 19.

[48] Xue helped edit one book on epidemic diseases and wrote three others on the medical canon. He also published a collection of his poetry and an anthology of Tang poetry. See note 63. His commentary to the *Book of Changes* is listed in the *Siku quanshu zongmu* 四庫全書總目 (Catalogue of the Complete Collection of the Four Treasuries), *juan* 10, 83.

[49] In this passage Xue does not refer to the *Wenyi lun* by Wu Youxing or even seem to know about his doctrines, even though later they would be associated with the same school of thought.

[50] For Xue Xue's 'Rijiang zaji' 日講雜集 (Miscellaneous Jottings from Daily Lectures), see *Wuyi huijiang, juan* 2, 14–15.

[51] See Tang's short note on Xue preceding Xue's jottings in *Wuyi huijiang, juan* 1, 14. Xue, on the contrary, published his commentary on two medical texts by other authors.

[52] The *wenbing* text attributed to Xue was the *Shire tiaobian* 濕熱條辨 (Systematic Determination of Manifestations of Damp- and Hot-Factor Disorders), but it was not widely available until the 1830s.

Chengji is a draft of a previous treatise in the cold-damage tradition.[53] Tang made no other associations between Xue Xue, Ye Gui, or Xue Chengji, all of whom Song Zhaoqi, however, later grouped together as authorities on southern diseases. At the end of the eighteenth century, these physicians had not yet been identified as *wenbing* authors, nor was there a *wenbing* tradition.

Nanjing biejiang, 1878

In 1878, Song Zhaoqi selected three previously published texts by Ye Gui, Xue Xue, and Xue Chengji: the 'Wenzheng lun zhi' 溫証論治 (On Treatments for Warm-Factor Syndromes) attributed to Ye Gui; the 'Shire tiaobian' 溼熱條辨 (Determination of Damp and Hot-Factor Disorders) attributed to Xue Xue; and the 'Shanghan gufeng' 傷寒古風 (The Ancient Style of [Treating] Cold-Damage Disorders) attributed to Xue Chengji. To these he added one of his own to complete his new compilation *Southern Diseases*.[54] He chose these three authors because he 'knew their methods were the best suited for the diseases of Jiangnan people' (*zhi qi yu Jiangnan ren bing zui wei hefa* 知其于江南人病最為合法).[55] Song no doubt also published these texts to preserve a family tradition in medicine, since both Xue Xue and Xue Chengji were his maternal ancestors. Xue Chengji was Xue Xue's great-great-grandson.[56] Song was the son of one of Xue Chengji's daughters.[57] In the concluding sentence of his preface, however, he stressed their writings' regional significance: 'I have called the book *Discriminating Explanation of Southern Diseases* to emphasise that these [illnesses] are different from northern diseases' (*wei yu beifang bing jiongyi ye* 謂與北方病迥異也).[58]

By this time the meaning of *wenbing* had metamorphosed from a general medical term denoting cold-damage-type febrile disorders that erupted in the spring and summer months to a broad bibliographic category designating the texts and authors of a local medical tradition. In contrast to the universal orientation of the writings of Guan Ding, the prefaces to the *Southern Diseases* of 1878 stress that cold-damage treatments are only effective for the body types and diseases of northern patients.

This final section uses the third edition of *Southern Diseases*, published in 1883, as an endpoint in the invention of the *wenbing* tradition. Its prefaces show that the

---

[53] More than half of the fifth chapter has Xue Chengji's draft of another physician's work on cold damage: 'Ni Zhang Lingshao *Shanghan zhijie*' 擬張令韶傷寒直解(Draft of Zhang Lingshao's 'Straightforward Explanations of Cold Damage Disorders'). See *Wuyi huijiang, juan* 4, 62–70.

[54] Only the text by Ye Gui was previously published in Tang Dalie's *Suzhou Physicians*.

[55] See Song Zhaoqi, *Nanbing biejian*, preface, 2.   [56] See Wu Runqiu (1984), 7–9.

[57] Evidence in Song Zhaoqi, *Nanbing biejian*, preface, 2.

[58] Song Zhaoqi, *Nanbing biejian*, preface, 2. Also in *Zhongguo yiji tongkao* (1990–94), 1777–8.

physicians who formed the *wenbing* corpus combined a renewed medical emphasis on local *qi*, southern geographic distinctiveness, and corporeal polarities with the native-place identities and regionalism widespread in nineteenth-century Qing society.

The essays Song Zhaoqi selected and attributed to Ye Gui and Xue Xue have complicated histories since both were published posthumously. In his 1793 compilation on Suzhou medicine, Tang Dalie writes that Ye dictated 'Wenzheng lunzhi' 溫証論治 (On Treating Warm-Factor Syndromes) to his disciple Gu Jingwen 顧景文 (eighteenth century) while on a boat touring Lake Tai, south-west of Suzhou.[59] It was first published in a 1764 collection of his medical cases[60] and later included in the first section of Tang's 1793 *Suzhou Physicians*. Extracts from Tang's version were republished in compilations from the 1820s to 1878, when it was included in *Southern Diseases*.[61] These recensions, though similar in theme and structure, are not exactly the same.

There is only one version of Xue Xue's 'Shire tiaobian' 濕熱條辨 (Systematic Determination of Damp- and Hot-Factor Disorders). Like Ye, Xue did not publish it himself. There is some doubt that he even wrote it. It first appears in *Yixue mengqiu* 醫學蒙求 (Medical Learning for Novices), a medical primer written in 1804 by Xu Xing 徐行 (late eighteenth century). Xu was a disciple of one of Xue's collaborators, Wu Meng 吳蒙 (late eighteenth century).[62] Thereafter, it was included in other compilations, increasingly, along with Ye's work, until both authors came to be seen as the main representatives of the *wenbing* tradition.

Following the convention that republished prefaces from previous editions, the third edition of *Southern Diseases*, published in 1883, has six prefaces, five compiled from the earlier editions (see table 8.1). The oldest preface (no. 5 in the third edition) was written in 1734 by Xue – not for this text, but for a collection of his writings on poetry.[63] Song Zhaoqi extracted Xue's preface and adopted it for his compilation. This editorial decision was not extraordinary; publishers valued prefaces sometimes more for their prestige than their content or relevance to the subject of the text. They were often the only sections of a text that showed the calligraphic hand of the author, an immediate

---

[59] See Tang Dalie, *Wuyi huijiang*, preface, 1.

[60] Hua Xiuyun 華岫雲 (eighteenth century) published it in a compilation of Ye Gui's medical case records titled *Linzheng zhinan yi'an* 臨證指南醫案 (Medical Case Histories as a Guide to Clinical Practice). This compilation gives Ye's essay the title 'Wenre lun' 溫熱論 (On Warm and Hot Factor Disorders).

[61] The transmission chart for Ye's 'Wenre lun' is charted in Ma Jixing (1990), 210–13.

[62] Xue Xue worked with Wu Meng on an edition of the *Wen re shu yi quanshu* 溫熱暑疫全書 (Complete Treatise on Warm-Factor, Hot-Factor, Summer-Heat, and Epidemic Disorders), by Zhou Yangjun 周揚俊 (eighteenth century). Evidence in 1754 original edition.

[63] This 1734 publication was titled *Yipiao shihua* 一瓢詩話 (Xue Xue's Anecdotes on Poetry).

Table 8.1. *Prefaces to the* Discriminating Examination of Southern Diseases

#	Date	Name	Relationship	Status
1	1883	Gu Wenbin 顧文彬	Member of local elite	Official
2	1879	Xu Kang 徐康	Song's acquaintance	Painter
3	1879	Bi Changqing 畢長慶	Song's patient	Local elite
4	1878	Song Zhaoqi 宋兆淇	Editor of text	Physician
5	1734	Xue Xue 薛雪	Author of text	Poet Physician
6	1829	Li Qingjun 李清俊	Published Xue Xue's text	Physician

visual expression of his personal and social distinction.[64] When a member of the local elite or literati wrote a preface for a text, his patronage signified as much as his opinions.

The ordering of the prefaces signified a social stratification. In the 1883 third edition, the official Gu Wenbin's preface (no. 1) came first, then that of the locally famous painter Xu Kang (no. 2).[65] Xu's preface was followed by a preface of one of Song's former patients, Bi Changqing (fl. late nineteenth century) wrote (no. 3). Song's preface (no. 4) followed. Finally, on the lower two rungs of the social hierarchy were the prefaces of the two physicians, Xue Xue (no. 5) and Li Qingjun (no. 6).[66] The order of these prefaces illustrates the social network and hierarchy that underlie the production of all texts. I discuss their contents in reverse order from the physician Li Qingjun to the official Gu Wenbin, leaving out Xue's preface (no. 5), which he wrote originally for a different book.

The physician Li Qingjun's preface

These prefaces not only reflect the social relationships supporting the publication of the *Southern Diseases*, they explain why Song Zhaoqi brought the three authors Ye Gui, Xue Xue, and Xue Chengji together and considered their works significant.[67] Li Qingjun's 1829 preface told local physicians why they should read Xue Xue's essay:

> Xue's 'Treatise on Damp- and Hot-Factor Disorders' was a secret book (*mishu* 密書) kept in [my] family. My father was well versed in medical principles, and especially treasured this book. Xue's analysis shows that the entire course (*yuan-wei* 原委) of illness is mostly via transmission from the *yang* brightness to major

[64] On the politics of calligraphy, see Kraus (1991).
[65] On Xu Kang's reputation as a painter, see *Qingdai zhuanji congkan* 1985, vol. 78, 62, and vol. 81, 20.
[66] Before Gu Wenbing wrote his preface to the 1883 edition, the first edition from 1878 listed the prefaces 2–5 in the same order, but did not include Li Qingjun's preface. The edition is at the China Academy of Traditional Chinese Medicine in Beijing.
[67] All six prefaces are reprinted in *Zhongguo yiji tongkao* (1990–1994), 1776–79.

yin warps as [the excessive climatic *qi*] is transmitted from the outer to the inner [aspects of the body]. His perspective on this is precise. His words on it are detailed. His treatments are appropriate in every case. [His methods] can be used as a model for future generations. No one has been able to exceed his scope.

Li then turns to localism to praise Xue's medical text. Because of the dominance of dampness and heat, he believes, patients in the Yangzi River region are more likely to come down with an illness related to the climatic and terrestrial *qi* of the locale.

> In our Suzhou, south of the Yangzi, the local *qi* is low and damp (*diqi beishi* 地氣 卑濕). Many suffer from this sickness. Physicians sometimes call [these illnesses] either damp-warm or cold-damage [disorders]. They are unable to differentiate them. Surely they do not realise, as the discussion says, that damp- and hot-factor disorders are not only not the same as cold-damage [disorders], they are also very different from warm-factor disorders. I did not dare to keep this a secret. I have perpetuated the book by having the wood blocks cut [for publication] so that [Xue's text] will be available generally to my colleagues. Thus those who ponder illness [will] no longer be divided or mistaken on this [matter].

The editor Song Zhaoqi's preface

In Song Zhaoqi's preface to the first edition of the *Southern Diseases*, written almost fifty years after Li Qingjun's preface, Song Zhaoqi repeats Li's statement on the prevalence of disorders due to damp and hot *qi* in the Jiangnan region, but he elaborates further on corporeal and regional distinctions. Cold-damage disorders afflict people living in the north; other disorders due to damp and hot *qi* afflict the people of Jiangnan. He further distinguishes strong northern bodies from weaker southern ones:

> Now [the] Arbiters of Fate [i.e. doctors], in addition to the four methods of diagnosis [looking, listening, questioning, and pulse taking], must furthermore [be able to] differentiate between place (*tudi* 土地) and individual constitution (*renqing* 人情). For example, the northern region is cold (*dihan* 地寒), the people are strong, and cold-damage disorders are the most common. That is why Zhang Ji established the prescriptions such as Ephedra and Cassia decoctions [to treat such disorders].[68] [For such cases] one could rely on [his] *Shanghan lun*. But south of the Yangzi the land is low, dampness is more prevalent, and the people's constitutions are soft and weak (*rouruo* 柔弱). Cases of cold damage are no more than one or two out of a hundred. But those who suffer from damp and hot [*qi* in the south] number eight or nine out of ten. Surely using therapies for cold damage to treat damp- and hot-factor disorders makes a great difference!

---

[68] Both drugs are identified with the cold-damage tradition.

Here Song expresses the view that the *Shanghan lun* cannot encompass illnesses associated with Jiangnan's hot and humid climate. Clearly, his *Southern Diseases* marks the culmination of a new Suzhou medical tradition in which the type of soil, dominant climatic excesses of *qi*, and local diseases interacted to fashion a southern body type so different from northern bodies that it required its own medicine.

The former patient Bi Changqing's preface

Song Zhaoqi had cured Bi Changqing of a serious case of insomnia ten years earlier. Perhaps to return the favour, Bi agreed to write a preface for Song's compilation. In his preface, Bi writes on a different theme by referring to a process of revising the canonical lineage to assimilate medical innovations and to link them to ancient origins. At the onset Bi states that although the writings of Ye Gui, Xue Xue, and Xue Chengji take a different approach, they still continue the lineage established by the founding texts of the Han medical canon:

> From the medical books *Lingshu* and *Jingui* onward,[69] each era had [writings by] famous men of worth. [These texts] 'made oxen sweat filling the [house] to the rafters' [because there were so many]. [When] one seeks [those who] have continued the genuine transmissions of Qibo and the Yellow Emperor to benefit later generations of scholars, they are hardly to be found. [When one] seeks the reason [for this], it [is clear] that they have ingested but not digested [the knowledge of] the ancients. As a result, they have made the subtle thought of the ancient writings obscure and difficult to understand. Some physicians are even more undisciplined, seeking strange theories and pretending genius. Some set up their own lineages, being fond of exoticisms. As for the division between the local *qi* of the north and south, and the difference between the hardness and softness of [human] constitutions, they generally ignore [these conceptions]. One can hardly be surprised that the way of medicine is a moribund field of study. Recently there have been Ye Gui's 'Treatise on Warm-Factor Syndromes', Xue Xue's 'Determination of Damp- and Hot-Factor Disorders', and Xue Chengji's 'The Ancient Winds of Cold-Damage Disorders'. [These] discussions are refined and rich. [Their] roots are penetrating and deep. [They] account for all changes using the Five Phases and distinguish appropriate [therapies for each of] the five regions. [They] truly continue the single vein of the *Lingshu* and *Jingui* as they greatly contribute to future generations.

In this statement, Bi suggests that the writings in *Southern Diseases* address two subjects that he believes previous physicians had ignored: the geographic division between

---

[69] Here *Lingshu* probably refers to both parts of the *Neijing*, the *Divine Pivot* and *Basic Questions*. *Jingui* here also probably refers to the two recensions of Zhang Ji's writings, the *Jingui yaolüe fanglun* and *Jingui yuhan jing*. See note 4.

north and south, and corresponding variations in bodily constitutions. Contrary to what critics in the cold-damage tradition would argue, by addressing both issues, Bi explains that these three authors in fact returned to, instead of diverged from, the orthodox medical lineage. Bi strategically places their writings both within the orthodox medical lineage of antiquity and poises them to meet the needs of physicians in the future.

The painter Xu Kang's preface

In the second of the six prefaces, the Changzhou painter Xu Kang favours Ye Gui, writing that he was the most influential physician of the three physicians whose works were compiled in *Southern Diseases*. Xu's preface marks a shift in emphasis from the clinical inadequacies of the cold-damage tradition to claims of a new tradition that started with Ye Gui's medical writings and continued through those of Xue Xue and Xue Chengji. Xu begins his short preface with the following statement:

> During the Kangxi reign (1662–1722), Ye Gui of Suzhou had the greatest medical reputation of his era. At the same time, Xue Xue was his successor. [He was] followed by the venerable Xue Chengji. [They] are called the three legs of the tripod [i.e., the foundation of medicine at that time]. Only Ye's [writings] were most widely considered as orthodox. [They are] worthy to serve as a model for later scholars. Of his available writings, all compiled by his disciples, his medical case records are the best known. 'Wenzheng lunzhi' is even clearer than his 'She jian' 舌鑒 (Tongue Examination) and 'She bian' 舌辨 (Tongue Differentiation).

In the remaining half of the preface Xu states that he was impressed with a copy he received of the *Southern Diseases* as well as with Song Zhaoqi's 'medical acumen and kinship to Xue Xue'. Xu considers Song's approach to medicine exceptional: '[Although] when treating illnesses his conscientiousness often surpassed people's expectations, [he remained] on the one path of orthodoxy.' These qualities led Xu to pay the publication costs of the second edition. By stressing Song's orthodoxy, Xu assimilates Ye's and the two Xues' writings into the orthodox lineage of medicine.

The official Gu Wenbin's preface

Southern Diseases had finally received wide enough distribution and sufficient recognition by its third printing in 1883 that the provincial official Gu Wenbin 顧文彬 offered his patronage by writing a preface.[70] Of all the men who prefaced this text, Gu crafted

---

[70] Gu received his *jinshi* in 1841. Because Gu Wenbin was a provincial official, biographical sources on him are comparatively rich. See *Qingdai zhuanji congkan* (1985), vol. 29, 481; vol. 33, 138; vol. 84, 377; vol. 121, 137; and vol. 125, 305.

the most penetrating analysis with respect to conceptions of space, disease, bodies, and local medicine. He elaborates on distinctions between northern and southern regions that go beyond topographical generalities and corporeal differences to include language, cultural preferences, and desires. All such differences, he argues, can be attributed to variations in local *qi*. This theory of resonant *qi* supports his argument for indigenous knowledge suited to local conditions. He begins by paraphrasing a quotation from the 'Kaogong ji' 考工記 (Artificer's Record), a subsection of the *Zhouli* 周禮 (Rites of Zhou).[71] The passage follows an assertion that four things must be brought together to ensure a finely crafted artefact: the right season, favorable local *qi*, the quality of the material, and the skill of the craftsman. If the material is of good quality and the craftsman is skilled but the result of his work is not good, this is because the craftsman did not choose the appropriate season and the artefact did not receive favourable local *qi*. Gu applies this analogy to physicians:

> The 'Artificer's Record' said: '[When] despite beautiful materials and ingenious skill, an artefact is not excellent, it was made in the wrong season or did not partake of the local *qi* (*diqi* 地氣). The [thin-skinned] tangerine [of the south], when it is planted across the Huai, becomes the [thorny-skinned] orange. The mynah bird does not cross the river Ji. The He [i.e., a badger-like animal] does not cross the river Wen.' [These examples] clarify the meaning [of the phrase]. 'Away from its native place a thing is not excellent.' Again and again [the 'Artificer's Record'] says 'this is due to the local *qi*'. Too true! If one does not [make one's products] partake of the local *qi*, one cannot become a fine craftsman. If one does not investigate the local *qi*, how can one become a fine physician?[72]

Edward Schafer's summary of the same account in *The Vermilion Bird: T'ang Images of the South*, reveals slight variations: 'Two millennia ago Chinese books pointed out that the jaunty and loquacious Crested Mynah (Aethiopsar cristellatus) could not be found in the Yellow River valley, and that the tangerine of the south gives way to the thorny lime of the north, each being the peculiar product of its own environment.' Schafer goes on to describe the Chinese conception of 'local *qi*' as 'a more homely and immediate agency' than the grand metaphysical schemes of Buddhist sects in Tang China. Chinese, he says, commonly attributed differences between fauna, flora, minerals, language, and culture to variations in the 'energetic emanations of local soil topography – the active principles of what we now call biomes'.[73]

---

[71] See 'Dongguan Kaogong ji' 冬官考工記 (Artificer's Record of the Winter Ministry), in the edition of the *Zhouli* with commentary, *Zhouli Zhengshi zhu* 周禮鄭氏注, *juan* 11, 278. For translation into French, see Biot, ((1851) 1969), vol. 2, 460.

[72] Gu Wenbin, *Nanbing biejian*, preface, 1, lines 1–3.

[73] For both quotations, see Schafer (1967), 119.

Scholars also employed the concept of 'local *qi*' – which Schafer translates as either 'land pneuma' or 'earth breath' – to explain cultural differences.[74] Gu referred to the political situation of divided states during the Warring States period to support his argument about the cultural differences between the people in the states to the north, Qi and Yan, and those in the states to the south, Chu and Yue. Regional differences, he suggests, have not changed notably since the Warring States:

> The languages [of the people in] the Qi and Chu states are not mutually comprehensible; their preferences differ accordingly. The languages [of the people of] Yan [north of Qi] and Yue [south of Chu] are [also] mutually incomprehensible; their preferences differ accordingly. What differs is the earth, namely [its] *qi*. Language and preferences are [due to] the normal *qi* [whereas] illness and disease are due to abnormal *qi*. I understand that it is hardly possible [to use] what can treat those in Qi to treat those in Chu. I [also] understand that [using] what can treat those in Yan [in the far north] to treat those in Yue [in the far south] will make [the disease] worse.[75]

According to Gu it was bad enough to use drugs meant to cure the diseases of the state of Qi in the north to treat those of the state of Chu to the south, and worse to use treatments appropriate in the Yan state to treat Yue subjects. Because these states were further apart along the north–south axis, their soils differed even more in their quality of local *qi*. Gu explains variations in culture, ecology, and nosology in terms of different manifestations of resonant local *qi*. Just as normal *qi* produces particular forms of culture, preferences, and desires, abnormal *qi* causes disease and other irregularities.

Gu drew his ideas from a philosophy of cultural difference based on a conception of resonant local *qi*, that can be traced back at least to the *Neijing*. He used this concept to promote, and in the process legitimate, a renewed ideal of local medical knowledge. Because each region or state has its own characteristic manifestations of order (i.e., culture, language, tastes, and desires) and disorder (i.e., diseases, syndromes, and illnesses), it should accordingly have medical treatments tailored to regional conditions. Gu uses historical references to support Song Zhaoqi's position that the diseases of China continue to differ along the north–south axis because of the prevalence of cold *qi* in the north and greater damp and hot *qi* in the south. This argument could also be used to bolster the special local expertise of Jiangnan doctors who were familiar with

---

[74] The locus classicus for medical views on the correlation between the five major geographic regions and different cultural habits, diseases, and therapeutic methods are two chapters in the *Huangdi neijing*: the 'Yifa fangyi lun' 異法方宜論 (see note 22) and the 'Wuchang zheng dalun' 五常政大論 (Main Discussion on the Rules of Phase Energetics). See *Suwen*, *pian* 12, 39–40; and *pian* 70, 201–4.

[75] Gu Wenbin, *Nanbing biejian*, preface, 1, lines 3–6.

the diseases of their patients. Gu re-emphasises that what is suited to the north is not true for the south:

> Cold-damage illnesses are diseases of the north. But when a southerner contracts an illness, why do we call it cold damage? Zhang Ji's book [i.e., *Shanghan lun*] is ubiquitous, so everyone memorises it; [they] forget differences in local *qi*. Does this differ from expecting to use treatments for [a patient in the state of] Qi to treat [a patient in the state of] Chu, or to use treatments for [a patient in the state of] Yan to treat [a patient in the state of] Yue? Would [the illness] improve or worsen?[76]

By thus localising medical knowledge, Gu challenges not only the universal authority of the cold-damage tradition but also that of all northern medical knowledge. By focusing on memorising the *Shanghan lun*, physicians had forgotten that they also must adapt to local conditions. Here, Gu puts forth a subtle critique of physicians who place authority in the medical canons of antiquity instead of in themselves. He concludes that of the many famous physicians in Suzhou, Ye Gui and Xue Xue were not only the most prolific, they were the first 'to discover that it is not suitable for the most part to use cold-damage methods to treat southerners'.

Gu concludes that Song Zhaoqi

> combined the three into one [book] and named [it] *Nanbing biejian*. [He] was about to turn it over to the printer when he asked me to write a preface. I do not understand medicine so I [can] only recommend this [work]. Based on [the principles stated in] the 'Artificer's Record', is not Song Zhaoqi himself someone adept at examining local *qi*? In medical practice, is he not superlative?

Gu returns in his conclusion to the points made in the beginning of his preface. Song Zhaoqi embodies the knowledge required to become both a good craftsmen and a fine physician: knowledge of the manifestations of *qi* in a given region and the superior skills of a seasoned practitioner. Both require attention to local *qi*.

Geography, lineage, and local medical knowledge

Two currents of medical thought from the Han medical canon influenced the physicians who invented the *wenbing* tradition: the study of local *qi* and disease based on the *Neijing* tradition and the thread of skepticism from at least the twelfth century toward the universality of the *Shanghan lun*. The geographic polarities of space and bodies in the *Neijing* provided a framework in which physicians could imagine a dichotomy

---

[76] Gu Wenbin, *Nanbing biejian*, preface, 1, lines 7–8.

between a northern cold-damage and southern *wenbing* tradition. Gu Wenbin mapped this dichotomy onto the bodies of robust northerners and delicate southerners. Gu's mapping of regional corporeal difference in his 1883 preface was done after the Taiping Rebellion revived anti-Manchu rhetoric and before the early Chinese nationalists refashioned the anti-Manchu thought for their own purposes in the 1890s.[77] Although the dichotomy between a weaker southern body and stronger northern body was not new, it re-emerged in the political climate after the Taiping Rebellion, which saw a resurgence of Han hostility, particularly in Jiangnan, toward Manchu rulership centred in the north, and expressed, most explicitly, a strengthened sense of regional character within this same climate.

The thread of skepticism toward the *Shanghan lun*, which began in the twelfth century, also reached fruition in the invention of *wenbing* tradition in nineteenth-century Jiangnan. The issues underlying the conflict between the cold-damage and *wenbing* traditions during the Qing dynasty reveal a transition from one epistemological framework to another. The change in the importance of *wenbing* – from an insignificant type of cold-damage disorder to a Jiangnan medical tradition – marked a breakaway from the traditional framework. Whereas previously, all symptoms were systematised within universal patterns recorded in antiquity, now the framework was a more relativist one that assumed variation, multiplicity, and adaptation to the present.

This epistemological shift from universal to local medical knowledge appears to parallel the political transition from centralised Qing power in the eighteenth century to the rise of regionalism in the latter half of the nineteenth century. Considering the myriad political and social meanings associated with definitions of disease, it is not surprising to find political subtexts embedded in medical discourse. Jiangnan physicians invented *wenbing* as a southern medical tradition within the context, first, of expanding regionalism, and then, possibly of increasing ethnic rhetoric. Their prefaces and those of their acquaintances gave cohesion and meaning to this new medical tradition; these prefaces, in fact, were the site of its invention.

References to premodern Chinese and Japanese works

Gujin mingyi fanglun 古今名醫方論 (Treatise on the Prescriptions of Famous Physicians Past and Present). Qing, printed in 1675. Luo Mei 羅美. Jiangsu keji chubanshe, Nanjing, 1983.
Huangdi neijing 黃帝內經 (Inner Canon of the Yellow Emperor). Han, *ca* 1st century BC. Anon. Tang, 762. Edited by Wang Bing 王冰. Cited from *Huangdi neijing zhangju suoyin* 黃帝內經章句索引

---

[77] For general background to anti-Manchu thought based on the writings of Zhang Binglin 章炳麟 (1868–1936); see Laitinen, (1990).

(Phrase Index to the Inner Canon of the Yellow Emperor), edited by Ren Yingqiu 任應秋. Renmin weisheng chubanshe, Beijing, 1986.

Jin shi 金史 (Official History of the Jin Dynasty). Song. Tuo Tuo 脱脱 (1313–55). Zhonghua shuju, Beijing, 1975.

Linzheng zhinan yi'an 臨証指南醫案 (Medical Case Histories as a Guide to Clinical Practice). Qing, editor's preface of 1766. Attributed to Ye Gui 葉桂, edited by his followers Hua Nantian 華南田 and Li Guohua 李國華. Shanghai keji jishu chubanshe, Shanghai, 1991.

Mingyi lei'an 名醫類案 (Classified Case Histories of Famous Physicians). Ming, author's preface of 1549, first printed in 1591. Jiang Guan 江瓘. In *Zhongguo yixue dacheng san bian*, vol. XI.

Mingyi zazhu 明醫雜著 (Miscellaneous Writings by Enlightened Physicians). Ming, compiled in 1502. Wang Lun 王綸. In *Zhongyi guji xiaocongshu*.

Nanbing biejian 南病別鑑 (Discriminating Examination of Southern Diseases). Qing, printed in 1878. Song Zhaoqi 宋兆淇. In *Zhongguo yixue dacheng*, vol. XV. Prefaces reprinted in *Zhongguo yiji tongkao*, 1776–79.

'Shanghan gufeng' 傷寒古風 (The Ancient Style of [Treating] Cold-Damage Disorders). Qing, 1878. Xue Chengji 薛承基. In *Nanbing biejian*.

Shanghan zabing lun 傷寒雜病論 (Treatise on Cold-Damage and Miscellaneous Disorders). Zhang Ji 張機. No definitive text of this work exists. Critical edition based on 4 recensions, including a Japanese manuscript of 1064–65. See Ōtsuka 1966.

'Shire tiaobian' 濕熱條辨 (Systematic Determination of Manifestations of Damp- and Hot-Factor Disorders). Attributed to Xue Xue 薛雪. In *Nanbing biejian*.

Siku quanshu zongmu 四庫全書總目 (Catalogue of the Complete Collection of the Four Treasuries). Qing, 1795. Yong Rong 永瑢 et al. (eds.). Zhonghua shuju, Beijing, 1983.

Wen re jingwei 溫熱經緯 (The Warp and Weft of Warm- and Hot-Factor Disorders). Qing, author's preface of 1852. Wang Shixiong 王士雄. In Lu Zheng 陸拯 et al. (eds.), 1–192.

Wen re shu yi quanshu 溫熱暑疫全書 (Complete Treatise on Warm-Factor, Hot-Factor, Summer-Heat, and Epidemic Disorders). Qing, author's preface of 1670. Zhou Yangjun 周揚俊. Shanghai keji weisheng chubanshe, Shanghai, 1959.

Wenyi lun 瘟疫論 (Treatise on Warm-Factor Epidemics). Ming, author's preface of 1642. Wu Youxing, 吳有性. In *Zhongguo yixue dacheng*, vol. XIII.

'Wenzheng lun zhi' 溫証論治 (On Treatments for Warm-Factor Syndromes). Qing, 1878. Attributed to Ye Gui 葉桂. In *Nanbing biejian*.

Wuyi huijiang 吳醫彙講 (Compilation of Essays by Suzhou Physicians). Qing, editor's preface of 1792; printed in 1793. Tang Dalie 唐大烈. Critical edition by Ding Guangdi 丁光迪. Shanghai kexue jishu chubanshe, Shanghai, 1983. Prefaces reprinted in *Zhongguo yiji tongkao*, 3112–16.

Wuzhong yi'an 吳中醫案 (Medical Case Histories from Suzhou). No longer extant. Cited in Tang Dalie's foreword to the *Wuyi huijiang, juan* 1, 1.

Yijing yulun 醫經餘論 (Leftover Discourses on the Medical Canon). Qing, author's preface of 1812. Luo Ji 羅洁. One original edition and manuscript still extant at the Library of the Shanghai College of Traditional Chinese Medicine. The essay 'Yizong sidajia zhi shuo' 醫宗四大家之説(The Doctrine of Four Masters of Medicine) is reprinted in Wang Xinhua and Pan Qiuxiang (eds.), 549–50.

Yipiao shihua 一瓢詩話 (Xue Xue's Poetry and Prose). Qing, author's preface of 1734. Xue Xue 薛雪. In Guo Shaoyu 郭紹虞 (ed.), 89–182.

Yizong bidu 醫宗必讀 (Essential Readings in the Medical Lineage). Ming, author's preface of 1637. Li Zhongzi 李仲梓. Zhongguo shudian, Beijing, 1991.

Zhouli 周禮 (Rites of Zhou). In *Zhouli Zhengshi zhu* 周禮鄭氏注 (Zheng's Commentary on the 'Rites of Zhou'). 2nd century AD, Later Han. Zheng Xuan 鄭玄. Shangwu yinshuguan, Shanghai, 1939.

References to modern works

Bates, Don (ed.) 1995. *Knowledge and the Scholarly Medical Traditions*. Cambridge University Press, Cambridge.

Biot, Edouard (1851) 1969. *Le Tcheou-li ou Rites des Tcheou*. 3 vols. L'Imprimerie nationale, Paris. Reprint Ch'eng-wen, Taipei.

Bray, Francesca 1995. 'Textile Production and Gender Roles in China, 1000–1700'. *Chinese Science* 12, 115–37.

Farquhar, Judith 1992. 'Time and Text: Approaching Chinese Medical Practice through Analysis of a Published Case'. In Leslie and Young, 62–73.

Goodman, Bryna 1995. *Native Place, City, and Nation*. University of California Press, Berkeley.

Guo Shaoyu 郭紹虞 (ed.) 1979. *Zhongguo gudian wenxue lilun piping kaozhu xuanji* 中國古典文學理論批評考著選輯 (Anthology of Ancient Chinese Literary Theory, Criticism, and Reference Sources). Renmin wenxue chubanshe, Beijing.

Harper, Donald 1998. *Early Chinese Medical Literature: the Mawangdui Medical Manuscripts*. The Sir Henry Wellcome Asian Series, 3. Kegan Paul, London/ New York.

Hsu, Elisabeth 1999. *The Transmission of Chinese Medicine*. Cambridge Studies in Medical Anthropology, 7. Cambridge University Press, Cambridge.

Kraus, Richard Curt 1991. *Brushes With Power: Modern Politics and the Chinese Art of Calligraphy*. University of California Press, Berkeley.

Laitinen, Kauko 1990. *Chinese Nationalism in the late Qing Dynasty: Zhang Binglin as an Anti-Manchu Propagandist*. Scandinavian Institute of Asian Studies Monograph Series, 57. Curzon, London.

Leslie, Charles and Young, Allan (eds.) 1992. *Paths to Asian Medical Knowledge*. University of California Press, Berkeley.

Loewe, Michael (ed.) 1993. *Early Chinese Texts: a Bibliographical Guide*. Society for the Study of Early China, Institute of East Asian Studies. University of California, Berkeley.

Lu Zheng 陸拯 et al. (eds.) 1987. *Jindai zhongyi zhenben ji: wenbing fence* 近代中醫珍本集：溫病分冊 (Collection of Rare Chinese Medical Books in Recent History: Warm-Factor Disorders). Zhejiang kexue jishu chubanshe, Zhejiang.

Ma Jixing 馬繼興 1990. *Zhongyi wenxian xue* 中醫文獻學 (Studies of Chinese Medical Literature). Shanghai kexue jishu chubanshe, Shanghai.

Meng Shujiang 孟樹江 (ed.) 1985. *Wenbing xue* 溫病學 (Warm-Factor Disorder Studies). Gaodeng yiyao yuan xiao jiaocai 高等醫藥院校教材 (Teaching Materials for Upper Division Medical and Pharmaceutical Colleges and Schools). Shanghai kexue jishu chubanshe, Shanghai.

Michael, Franz 1976. *The Taiping Rebellion: History and Documents*, vol. I: History, in collaboration with Chung-li Chang. Publications on Asia of the Institute for Comparative and Foreign Area Studies, 14. University of Washington Press, Seattle/London.

Okanishi Tameto 岡西為人 1958. *Song yiqian yiji kao* 宋以前醫籍考 (Studies of Medical Books through the Song Period). Renmin weisheng chubanshe, Beijing.

Oleson, Alexandra and Voss, John (eds.) 1979. *The Organization of Knowledge in Modern America, 1860–1920*. Johns Hopkins University Press, Baltimore.

Ôtsuka Keisetsu 大塚敬節 1966. *Rinsô ôyô Shôkanron kaisetsu* 臨床應用傷寒論解説. (Explanations of the Cold-Damage Treatise for Clinical Use). Sōgensha, Osaka.

Porkert, Manfred 1974. *The Theoretical Foundations of Chinese Medicine: Systems of Correspondence*. MIT Press, Boston.

Qian Xinzhong 錢信忠 (ed.) 1987. *Zhongguo yixue baike quanshu: yixue shi* 中國醫學百科全書：醫學史 (Encyclopaedia of Chinese Medicine: Medical History). Shanghai kexue jishu chubanshe, Shanghai.

Rosenberg, Charles E. 1979. 'Toward an Ecology of Knowledge: on Discipline, Context, and History'. In Oleson and Voss, 440–55.

1992. 'Framing Disease: Illness, Society, and History'. In Rosenberg and Golden, xiii–xxvi.

Rosenberg, Charles E. and Golden, Janet (eds.) 1992. *Framing Disease: Studies in Cultural History.* Rutgers University Press, New Brunswick, N.J.

Schafer, Edward 1967. *The Vermilion Bird: T'ang Images of the South.* University of California Press, Berkeley.

Sivin, Nathan 1987. *Traditional Medicine in Contemporary China: A Partial Translation of* 'Revised Outline of Chinese Medicine' *(1972) with an Introductory Study on Change in Present-day and Early Medicine.* Center for Chinese Studies, The University of Michigan, Ann Arbor.

1993. '*Huang ti nei ching*'. In Loewe, 196–215.

1995. 'Text and Experience in Classical Chinese Medicine'. In Bates, 177–204.

Su Tiege 蘇鐵戈 1993. '"Wuyi huijiang" wei lianxu chuban kanwu zhi zhiyi' 吳醫彙講為連續出版刊物 之質疑 ('Calling into Question the "Wuyi huijiang" as a Serial Publication'). *Zhongguo yishi zazhi* 23 (3), 145–8.

Wang Xinhua 王新華 and Pan Qiuxiang 潘秋翔 (eds.) 1990. *Zhongyi lidai yihua xuan* 中醫歷代醫話選 (Selection of Medical Anecdotes from the History of Chinese Medicine). Jiangsu kexue jishu chubanshe, Nanjing.

Wu Runqiu 吳潤秋 1984. 'Xue Shengbai shengping shiji yu zhixue fangfa' 薛生百生平事跡與治學方法 (Xue Xue's Life and Methods of Study). *Zhongguo yishi zazhi* 4 (1), 7–9.

Wu Yiyi 1993–94. 'A Medical Line of Many Masters: a Prosopographical Study of Liu Wansu and his Disciples from the Jin to the Early Ming', *Chinese Science* 11, 36–65.

Wu Yin'gen 吳銀根 and Shen Qingfa 深慶法 (eds.) 1991. *Zhongyi waigan rebing xue* 中醫外感熱病學 (Traditional Chinese Medicine Studies of Externally Stimulated Hot-Factor Disorders). Shanghai kexue jishu chubanshe, Shanghai.

Zhongguo yixue dacheng 中國醫學大成 (Complete Collection of Chinese Medicine) (1935) 1992. Cao Bingzhang 曹炳章 (ed.). Shanghai kexue jishu chubanshe, Shanghai.

Zhongguo yixue dacheng san bian 中國醫學大成三編 (The Third Series of the Complete Collection of Chinese Medicine) 1994. Qiu Peiran 裘沛然 (ed.). Yuelu shushe, Changsha.

Zhongguo yiji tongkao 中國醫籍通考 (Comprehensive Examination of Chinese Medical Books) 1990–94. Yan Shiyun 嚴世芸 et al. (eds.). 4 vols. Shanghai zhongyi xueyuan chubanshe, Shanghai.

Zhongyi guji xiaocongshu 中醫古籍小叢書 (Small Collectanea of Ancient Chinese Medical Books) 1985. Wang Xinhua 王新華 (ed.). Jiangsu kexue jishu chubanshe, Nanjing.

Zhou Junfu 周駿富 (ed.) 1985. *Qingdai zhuanji congkan* 清代傳記叢刊 (Collections of Biographies from the Qing Dynasty). Ming Wen, Taipei.

PART V

Medical case histories

Introduction

The late Ming is generally characterised as a time of important social changes that set the frame for the following four hundred years.[1] It is marked by the economic growth and the monetisation of silver, increased urbanisation and status mobility, growing complexity in the relations between the emergent merchant class and the traditional scholar-gentry, and a decline of the role of the state which affected also medicine.[2] Expansion of the school system enabled an unusually broad range of men from the literate population to take civil service examinations; the official career promised prestige and wealth, and education was considered the key to it. These economic and educational changes together with some advances in printing technology led to a thriving publishing industry.[3] The technology of wood print permitted decentralisation, and the printed book reached both urban and rural audiences; in medicine it became a generally recognised source of authority and guide to practice.[4]

Charlotte Furth remarks in chapter 9 that 'Although case histories were scattered through Chinese medical writings of all earlier periods, the individually authored and published case history collection was a Ming innovation.'[5] This finding is put forth also by Christopher Cullen in this volume. The medical case history genre (yi'an 醫案) forms but one of the many genres of medical writing that were increasingly printed and published in the Ming and Qing, and this phenomenon is generally explained to testify

[1] Rawski, Evelyne S. (1985), 'Economic and Social Foundations of Late Imperial Culture', in Johnson, David, Nathan, Andrew J. and Rawski, Evelyne S. (eds.), *Popular Culture in Late Imperial China*, University of California Press, Berkeley, 3–33.

[2] Leung, Angela (1987), 'Organised Medicine in Ming-Qing China: State and Private Medical Institutions in the Lower Yangzi Region', *Late Imperial China* 8 (1), 134–66; and Grant, Joanna C. (1996), 'Wang Ji's *Shi shan yi an*: Aspects of Gender and Culture in Ming Dynasty Medical Case Histories', PhD thesis in History, School of Oriental and African Studies, University of London.

[3] See for instance Elman, Benjamin (1984), *From Philosophy to Philology: Intellectual and Social Aspects of Change in Late Imperial China*, Harvard University Press, Cambridge, Mass., 139–69.

[4] Furth, Charlotte (1999), *A Flourishing Yin: Gender in China's Medical History, 960–1665*, University of California Press, Berkeley, 157.

[5] Furth (1999), 225.

to a shift in medical authority from the hereditary physicians, who had previously been in the majority, to the scholar doctors who increasingly populated the field. The former had claimed their authority and reputation through their family tradition, while the latter sought legitimacy largely through the writing of medical treatises.[6]

The *yi'an* genre detracted from the pre-eminence of the canons for medical practice,[7] and where the latter referred to the particular case by embedding it in prescriptive terms within the workings of the universe in general, the case histories emphasised the individuality of each illness event in accounts of past events. Where rule-governed philosophical treatises tended to underline the synchronicity of events by highlighting correlations between the spatio-temporal rubrics of microcosm and macrocosm, the case histories emphasised the diachronic aspect of an illness and its course.[8]

So far, analyses of the Chinese case history genre have emphasised narrative aspects, and the role of the narrative in the constitution of illness and lived experience: case histories are viewed as stories with a dramatic structure, and though they can be recounted many times to multiple 'readers', they always have an individual as author, activities and events being described alongside their significance for the author. And yet they are marked by indeterminacy and openness, particularly if authors change from, for instance, female patient and her oral complaints to male physician and his written jottings, and no final judgement can be made about their meaning. For the historian and anthropologist illness narratives provide clues to the popular cultural dimension of a certain time period, the assumption being that when people reason about illness, culture provides them the rationale for it.[9] In the light of the emphasis of recent scholarship on the individualistic and narrative aspects of medical case histories, the articles in this volume represent an important counterbalance: Christopher Cullen and Bridie Andrews both focus on the standardisation of the case history format.

Christopher Cullen's chapter (chapter 9) argues that *yi'an* as a genre of Chinese medical literature is an innovation of the Ming on the basis of both numerical data from outside observers and text excerpts that reveal the insiders' viewpoint: on the one hand he presents statistics that record the steady increase of compilations of medical case

---

[6] Another genre that became popular in the Ming was that on formulae (*fangji*), and also that of the medical primer. See Chao Yuan-ling (1995), 'Medicine and Society in Late Imperial China: a Study of Physicians in Suzhou', PhD in History, University of California, Los Angeles, 185–94, and in particular 188. On this issue, see also Bray, Francesca (1997), *Technology and Gender: Fabrics of Power in Late Imperial China*, University of California Press, Berkeley, 302–16.

[7] Furth (1999), 226.

[8] See for instance Farquhar, Judith (1991), 'Objects, Processes, and Female Infertility in Chinese Medicine', *Medical Anthropology Quarterly* 5 (4), 370–99; and Furth (1999), 226.

[9] Good, Byron (1994), *Medicine, Rationality and Experience: an Anthropological Perspective*, Cambridge University Press, Cambridge, 135–65.

records during the Ming and Qing dynasties and on the other hand he translates prescriptive essays outlining a format of writing case histories, which reflect the Chinese authors' self-awareness of this novel way of doing things. One of these essays, published in 1522 by Han Mao 韓懋, outlined 'six procedures' (*liufa* 六法): looking (*wang* 望), listening/smelling (*wen* 聞), questioning (*wen* 問), palpating [the pulse] (*qie* 切), reasoning (*lun* 論), and treatment (*zhi* 治). As translation for *yi'an*, Cullen therefore suggests not 'case history' but 'case statement'. This translation is also meant to underline the affinity of the medical case statement with the legal one, and Cullen cites text passages demonstrating that the Chinese themselves recognised the striking similarities between them.

Christopher Cullen explains the emergence of this new literary genre in two ways. First he looks at how a physician established his authority. Of course a physician had to convince his patient that his diagnosis and treatment were well founded, but it was also crucial to convince both the patient's family members, and the fellow practitioners – including those with whom he was in competition. By generating a document (*an* 案) that backed up the prescription (*fang* 方), the doctor provided a rationale for his therapy. Presuming an audience who judged the quality and cogency of these documents, Cullen suggests that for anyone who wanted to succeed as a physician it was important to learn to write convincing documents.

Secondly, Cullen considers demographic changes. He points out that in the seventeenth and eighteenth centuries, China's population more than doubled. Young men who found it increasingly difficult to gain entry into a civil service career may therefore have turned to other occupations like medicine, and Cullen suggests that the case statement genre offered a route, in fact, the quickest, to apparent expertise. His explanation for the emergence of this new literary genre, then, stresses how it served the interests of an individual wishing to establish his credentials.

In chapter 10 Bridie Andrews shows how records of medical cases could be used not simply to suggest the merits of an individual practitioner, but to build what we might call a profession. Despite the recommendations of physicians like Han Mao that cases should be standardised, the contents of early case records were highly variable, ranging from terse notes to long and detailed disquisitions (*biji* 筆記) on the merits of various therapies. But during the Republican period a new understanding arose: the new case history format adopted the biomedical model. It included entries on the patient, the disease name (*bingming* 病名), the disease cause (*bingyin* 病因), the symptoms (*zheng* 症候), a diagnosis (*zhenduan* 診斷), a treatment method (*liaofa* 廖法), prescriptions (*chufang* 處方), and results (*xiaoguo* 效果).

The formal requirements of the new genre did not draw a firm line between old and new. Old-style case records could often be reworked to fit the new genre. Andrews shows this in her example of the traditional-style didactic case record written by the famous Shanghai physician Ding Ganren 丁甘仁, which was originally included in his *Essentials of Throat-pox, Symptoms and Treatment* (Housha zhengzhi gaiyao 喉痧症治概要) and several years later republished by He Lianchen 何廉臣 in his *Classified Case Histories by Famous Chinese Physicians* (Zhongguo mingyi yan'an leibian 中國名醫驗案類編). One and the same case is here represented in a new 'case history' format.

Standardising medicine was part of a state-building project, and attempts at Chinese medical standardisation were generally supported by the government. Andrews explains that representing Chinese medical records according to a Western schema was not considered a capitulation to Western medicine. Rather it was felt that this kind of systematisation would help Chinese medicine to retain its unique character. Andrews points out that the 'case history' format requires that each drug in a prescription be named and the relative proportions given, that treatment methods be recorded, and that disorders be termed *bing* 病 rather than *zheng* 症. The significance of this, argues Andrews, is not that it transforms Chinese categories into those of Western medicine. Rather, its importance lay in providing schemas and nosological categories that could impose a sense of unity, a means for overcoming the internal factionalism that beset Chinese medicine at this vulnerable time. Contrary to what one might surmise, Chinese doctors did not consider this innovation as resulting from an assimilation of foreign values. Andrews suggests that it was an effort to overcome internal tensions and assert the value of the Chinese nation's knowledge.

9

Yi'an 醫案 (case statements): the origins of a genre of Chinese medical literature

CHRISTOPHER CULLEN

Introduction

In this chapter I shall discuss certain problems relating to the origins and purpose of the genre of Chinese medical literature known as *yi'an* 醫案, a term commonly rendered in English as '[medical] case histories', or as proposed here 'medical case statements'.[1] I shall concentrate here on the process of innovation through which this genre was created, and ask how this innovative process might be linked to wider social and intellectual changes.

What are *yi'an*? The answer seems obvious enough. They are individual records of the diagnosis and treatment of a single patient by a single physician. Large numbers of such records from the past few centuries are available in printed form, and they have begun to attract considerable scholarly attention in recent years.[2] There are two main reasons for this.

Firstly, scholars have rightly begun to be suspicious about the relations between medical literature and medical practice. There are plenty of prescriptive books about Chinese medicine extant, in which authors of the last two thousand years have told us

---

[1] When translating the Chinese term '*yi'an*' I attempt consistent use of the phrase 'medical case state-ment' rather than 'medical case history', since in my view 'case statement' is a more accurate reflection than 'history' of the etymology of the word *an* 案, and (more to the point) it better reflects the context in which it came to be used in the expression '*yi'an*': see below. When however I am discussing the liter-ary form taken by such medical records outside the Chinese context, I generally use the more familiar term 'case histories'.

[2] In recent years several scholars in Western countries have started to explore this resource. One might mention Charlotte Furth who has been looking at issues relating to the treatment of women in Late Imperial times: see Furth (1999). Francesca Bray has embarked on a more general study of certain Qing case histories, and at SOAS Joanna Grant has completed a PhD (University of London, 1997) which involved her in examining the case histories of the sixteenth-century physician Wang Ji 汪機 (1463–1529) from the perspective of issues of gender.

how curing ought to be done, but it is not clear how far we can treat such books as telling us what doctors really did. Prescription is only equivalent to description when the prescription is backed with adequate coercive authority – and as we know, medical practitioners in pre-modern China were not under the control of any equivalent of such British institutions as the Royal College of Physicians or more recently the General Medical Council. I am of course speaking of the great majority who were in private practice as economically independent individuals, as opposed to the much smaller group of medically expert bureaucrats in government employ, whose role was for the most part to provide services for the dwellers in the Imperial palace and for other officials. Secondly, scholars more interested in the social relations of curing than its technical aspects often find that prescriptive medical literature has little to say to them.

Case statements seem at first sight to offer us ways round both these problems. They are explicitly formulated as descriptions of how individual patients with specific illnesses were treated, and although general principles are often invoked and classic texts are often quoted we are still mostly told what was actually done for the patient, and what the result was perceived to be. Secondly, in many cases we hear a fair amount about the ways in which physicians related to their patients, to the patient's carers, and to their fellow-physicians attending the same bedside. This we just do not get from the rest of the medical literature, and through the study of this material we are beginning to get closer to an accurate picture of elite Chinese health care as it was in practice.

But if these case statement texts are to be so important in our study of the history of Chinese medicine, we must surely be cautious in the weight we place on them. Texts are produced by groups or individuals with purposes and under constraints that we would do well to reflect on before we use such writings for purposes of our own. If this applies to general prescriptive texts, it applies all the more strongly to texts which appear to be telling us what 'really happened', particularly if we are tempted to take them at their word.

We cannot turn to the literature of current scholarship in Chinese to perform the task of problematisation on our behalf. There are clear institutional reasons for this, which can be set out roughly as follows:

(1) Case statements play a recognised role in the modern practice of what is often called Traditional Chinese Medicine (TCM), and in the training of TCM practitioners. They are a part of a cultural complex which cannot be subtracted without damaging the whole, and are indeed seen as a particularly favourable part of the complex.
(2) Since case statements are seen as an essential part of TCM, the process of their evolution is normatively recounted as a story of progress leading up to the present situation, with the emphasis on the inevitability of progress on the one hand, and the early appearance of precursors and anticipations on the other.

Support for these two generalisations may easily be found in the works of Shi Qi (1994) and Chen Dawu (1994). As Chen puts it in the foreword to his book 'the case statements of Chinese medicine are an extremely important constituent of this subject, and from a number of points of view one may say that the value of case statements is considerably greater than that of [other types of] medical books'. The compiler of one modern collection of case records from the Song to the Qing goes further:

> A carpenter or a wheelwright can give someone a compass and setsquare, but cannot make him a skilled workman . . . [The medical classics] are the compass and setsquare of medical practice . . . [But] it is medical case statements that are the traces left by the good practitioner's use of his skill. The very essence of Chinese medicine is preserved in them.[3]

In the historical writing of such authors as Shi Qi, the organising force of the current view of case statements is projected back into the remotest past, and draws into itself everything that bears the possibility of assimilation. Thus we begin as long ago as the records of royal illnesses on Shang oracle bones. We continue through anecdotes of physicians and their patients amongst the feudal lords of the Spring and Autumn period in the eighth to fifth centuries BC, and on through the story of Chunyu Yi 淳于意 in the second century BC.[4] We continue for another 1,500 years, referring to many instances in which a physician (or perhaps someone else) tells us the circumstances of a particular patient's illness and how it was treated. Finally we reach the sixteenth century, and for the first time we find authors who give explicit instructions on how to write *yi'an* properly, together with the publication of the first specialist books devoted solely to *yi'an*.[5] At last the goal has been achieved, and fully developed *yi'an* take their place in the edifice of TCM, where they remain to this day.

But faced with this story of steady progress, one can only ask why it took so long for Chinese physicians to realise the benefits to be gained from studying books filled with the case statements of other physicians, and of publishing their own in their turn. The story as usually told is no doubt a worthy one, but it is very slow, and rather dull – a journey up a slowly ascending gradient, with no notable landmarks or sharp turnings until we reach our destination. If it is the job of the historian to analyse the process of change, and to seek for the peculiar circumstances which give rise to it, there would not seem to be much interest in the historical task of studying the origins of *yi'an*.

On the contrary, the position I shall put forward here sees the late Ming not as a time when a long and gradual process of growth reached (more or less) its culmination, but

---

[3] Yao Ruoqin (1933), preface, 1.   [4] See below for details of his case histories.
[5] See below on the work of Han Mao and Wu Kun.

as a time when changes specific to the Ming created what was a new genre of publication – the *yi'an*. This new genre was created through a change in perception of what purposes medical writing could serve, and explicitly invoked resonances with another new genre of writing from outside medicine. And what is more, I shall maintain that late Ming medical writers saw it that way too.

By way of background to setting out my position, I shall first review some of the ways in which physicians have left records of their practice in cultures outside China, and the way that these records have been used. Then I shall survey some of the ground gone over by Shi and Chen when they discuss what is from their point of view the pre-Ming development of *yi'an*. I shall then try to establish why what happened next should be seen as a radically new departure.

Physician's records world-wide

Documents from many premodern sources give us accounts, direct or indirect, of what passed between particular patients and particular physicians. It is worth pausing to ask how far such evidence may be relevant to the questions discussed here.

From ancient Egypt we have the Edwin Smith papyrus of *ca* 1600 BC, possibly containing material as old as 3000–2500 BC.[6] It describes 48 surgical problems with instructions for action under various circumstances. The cases are however considered as type examples, and are not presented as records of specific clinical experience. Undoubtedly this material could not have been composed without a background of a long experience of the treatment of many injured persons on the part of the individual or group concerned. But the element of particularity has been subsumed into generality. The individual case exhibits the tension between the particular and the general, whereas the typical case deliberately avoids it.

Thus the Egyptian scribe typically tells us: 'If you examine a patient who shows qualities A, B and C, then you shall say "it is a case of D", and you shall treat it using therapy E.'[7] But if we were presented with the case of an individual workman who had fallen off a wall, we might find that he did show qualities A and B in 'typical' mode, but failed to show C very clearly. It would be fascinating to know how the physician would have dealt with such a patient – presumably not by saying 'You do not fit anything in the text my teacher made me copy out – so I dare not venture to treat you!' But the Smith papyrus gives us no evidence on such points.

In Greece we may locate records relating to specific individuals in the Hippocratic corpus, particularly the *Epidemics*, but also in the inscriptions relating to cures

---

[6] Nunn (1996), 25 ff.   [7] See the discussion in Nunn (1996), 27–9.

performed at the shrine of Asclepius at Epidaurus *ca* 400 BC. A typical example of the latter runs as follows:

> Alketas of Haleis. This one, being blind, saw a dream. It seemed to him that the god came and drew apart his eyelids with his fingers and that he first saw the trees in the shrine. When day came he went out cured.[8]

In the *Epidemics*, we find such records as:

> At Larisa, a bald man suddenly had a pain in the right thigh. No treatment which he received did him any good . . . Fourth day: died about noon.[9]

The most obvious difference here is the outcome. Whereas the Epidaurian inscriptions are a record of complete (and often explicitly miraculous) success, the *Epidemics* record a death rate of nearly 60 per cent. But there are deeper and more significant differences here than the inevitable difference between the success rates of human and divine healers. Most importantly, the readerships envisaged for these accounts are completely separate. The Asclepian cures are taken from public inscriptions set up in the shrine by grateful worshippers in thank-offering for a cure. They were clearly addressed in part to other potential patients of the god, in addition to serving as a general public expression of thankfulness. There is no suggestion that either the god himself, or shrine personnel acting on his behalf, would find these records useful in informing their practice as healers.

The *Epidemics* on the other hand appear to originate from the records kept by Hippocratic physicians for their own purposes rather than as manifestos designed for public admiration. If this is the case, it may seem odd that hardly any therapy is mentioned in *Epidemics*, but some hint as to the purpose these records were meant to serve may be drawn from the emphasis laid on dispassionate observation of the passage of the illness, with particular attention to 'critical days'.[10] It is likely that the theoretical preoccupations of the group responsible for the text are at work here: what is observed and recorded is not a mere brute fact. But our evidence as to the purposes of those who compiled and preserved the *Epidemics* is still decidedly thin. Were young physicians intended to read these texts as part of their training? Were they intended as controversial ammunition for theoreticians engaged in debate with other groups? We simply do not know.

In Mediaeval Europe, however, we can find examples of case histories compiled for an explicitly didactic purpose. By the late thirteenth or early fourteenth century the European medical literature included collections of opinions on specific cases by

[8] Lang (1977), 20. [9] Lloyd (1983), 130–1. [10] Lloyd (1983), 32.

famous physicians (*consilia*). We have the *consilia* and writings on practice of some famous scholastic learned physicians of this period – Taddeo Alderotti, Guglielmo da Brescia, and Gentile da Foligno. University education in practical medicine included study of collections of *consilia* describing individual cases. Likewise in surgery anecdotal case histories were evidently designed as teaching devices, much as collections of *consilia* seem to have been for physicians.[11] We must be clear, however, that the explicit connection between case histories and formal medical training is not just a matter of the inevitable unfolding of progress in the use of the genre. It occurs in the specific context of the development of university medical curricula demanding standardised teaching texts. There is nothing natural or ineluctable in this, and if we want to trace the origins of innovation in the use of *yi'an* in China we shall have to be prepared to look for similar links with institutional change.

The written medical record in China

Early evidence of medical practice

The first pieces of Chinese writing that tell us anything about the health problems of individuals are undoubtedly found on Shang oracle bones. One quoted by Shi may serve as an example:

> Day renxu. Crackmaking. Diviner: Huan. [The king] has a sick tooth. It is [a case of] *chi* [= attack by demonic agency].[12]

As Shi notes, some scholars have gone so far as to see in such records all the 'essential' elements of *yi'an*: we know who the patient was (since it is nearly always the king who is the subject of divination), we know the practitioner (in the person of the diviner) and the date, and both the disease and its cause have been identified. Some oracle bones even mention ritual actions that might be taken as the 'treatment'. What more could one ask for – if this is indeed all that is needed to constitute a *yi'an*. But that is precisely the point: the view outlined by Shi is a *reductio ad absurdum* of the idea of looking for 'early forms' of any genre without reference to social or historical context. A definition of *yi'an* that can include both the oracle texts and the contents of sixteenth century case statement collections does not delimit any concept likely to be helpful in the historical analysis of change. The reasons for the creation of a text, and the uses to which it is put are surely as essential to defining its identity as its formal content. So many things are lacking from the context of the oracle record. For instance, there are no signs that the

---

[11] Siraisi (1990), 175.   [12] Shi Qi (1994), 138.

creator of the record is anything like the later *yi* 醫 (which I translate conventionally as 'physician') in the sense of being a specialist mostly concerned with the sickness of his patients conceived very largely in naturalistic and rationalistic terms. A given diviner may enquire about royal concerns ranging from warfare to the prospects of the harvest, and the king's toothache is only one uncertainty to be resolved amongst many. Further, it is utterly obscure to whom (if anyone) the text is addressed. Did it indeed have an intended human readership at all, once the divination was over and the plastron or scapula had been filed away in its storage pit?

Medicine and bureaucratic structures

Perhaps the earliest suggestion that Chinese physicians might keep systematic records of their dealings with patients is to be found in the *Zhouli* 周禮 (Rites of the Zhou), an idealised account of government structure and the duties of officials perhaps compiled some time around the third century BC.[13] Recent rumours of an excavated text of the Warring States period promise more certain knowledge on this point. This document is certainly not to be taken as a description of what was actually done by physicians in state employ at this period, or indeed at any period, but its author's ideas of what physicians might be asked to do by an ideal ruler is unlikely to be completely disconnected from reality. At any rate, we are told in the *Zhouli*:

> The Master of Medicine (*yishi* 醫師) has charge of the governance of medicine. He assembles all potent drugs in order to provide a common resource for physicians. Should there be any state in which sicknesses or sores break out, he sends physicians to identify and treat them. At the end of each year he looks into medical work, to regulate salaries. Ten [cures] out of ten is ranked first; next comes one failure out of ten; next comes two failures out of ten; next comes three failures out of ten, and last comes four failures out of ten.[14]

What happens to anyone scoring below that is not recorded, but the implication is clear that it is considered reasonable for a physician to be expected to produce systematic documentary evidence of the results of his treatment. Elsewhere in this section of the *Zhouli* the role of writing is made explicit:

> When there is any sickness amongst the people [the Pestilence Physician *jiyi* 疾醫] identifies and treats it. If there are fatalities, in each case he writes down the cause of death, and submits it to the Master of Medicine.[15]

---

[13] Boltz (1993), 24–32.   [14] *Zhouli, juan* 5, 1a–1b.   [15] *Zhouli, juan* 5, 7a.

So by the late first millennium BC we have the notion (if no more than that) of bills of mortality and of payment by results. We cannot guess at the background from which such ideas sprang, but they are unlikely to have been pulled from the empty air.

Much later in Chinese history we have evidence of something like the *Zhouli* system being put into practice – or at least laid down in actual administrative rules, which may or may not have been observed. Thus the Song dynasty regulations for students of medicine provide that they should annually submit for inspection the official 'stamped papers' (*yinzhi* 印紙) bearing the records of cases treated during the past year for inspection and grading. Those with a cure rate of less than 70 per cent had to repeat the course, and those with a cure rate below 50 per cent were expelled from the college.[16]

Their presence from early times as private documents

But of course what we really need is some indication of what sort of documents physicians actually produced. Fortuitously, we do have some very good evidence from the early Han dynasty in the second century BC. This is to be found in chapter 105 of the *Shiji* 史記, a universal history completed around 90 BC by Sima Qian 司馬遷 (*ca* 145–86 BC). There he records the troubles suffered by a physician called Chunyu Yi 淳于意, who had built up a busy practice amongst the elite of the princedom of Qi 齊 in the north-east of the Han empire. In connection with various political upheavals he was called in for questioning by Imperial order:

> Yi was resident at home, [when] an Imperial order summoned [him to be] asked [about] those on whose behalf he had treated diseases [for whom] there was verification of death or life [as the outcome], how many persons [there had been] and which were the principal names [amongst them].[17]

In my view a great deal of what follows is basically a transcription of the text of the annotated interrogatory from official files, all of which would have been available to Sima Qian, whose responsibilities included those of court archivist:

[16] *Zizhi tongjian changbian jishi benmo* 資治通鑑長編紀事本末, 81, 14a (2605). In view of the claim made later in this discussion that the term *yi'an* is of sixteenth-century creation, it is noteworthy that the formal prose of the Song regulations does not refer to what the students record as being *yi'an*, but simply says they must record 'the illnesses they diagnose, and whether the disease results in a cure or a fatality'. Compare however Lü Kun's 呂坤 use of the term in his late sixteenth-century guide for bureaucrats – see below.
[17] *Shiji*, juan 105, 2796. Compare the different interpretation of this and subsequent passages by Nathan Sivin (1995), 178 ff.

The order questions the former Granary Intendant, the vassal Yi: Special methods in which you excel? Also [types of] sick persons you are able to treat? Do you have the [relevant] books or not? In each [speciality] from where did you receive training? For how many years were you trained? When you have proved successful in practice, of what county and hamlet were the people [you treated]? What illnesses? When the medical treatment and drugs were done with, in each case what was the state of the illness? Give detailed and complete answers.

The vassal Yi replies: [twenty-five case histories then follow] . . . As for others whom I have examined and fixed the term for death or life, or those I have treated who were already ill are very many, and due to the lapse of time I have forgotten them. I cannot give a complete account, and hence do not dare to reply concerning them.[18]

How, we may wonder, was Chunyu Yi able to give such detailed replies (and we must remember that Sima Qian may well not have copied the entire file for us)? Chunyu Yi tells us:

In every case where your vassal has conducted a medical consultation, he has always made a consultation record (*zhenji* 診籍).[19]

So for the first time a Chinese physician confirms that he routinely writes case histories – and as I have said we have twenty-five of them before our eyes. They make fascinating reading but Chunyu Yi's story cannot be followed further here. We may note however, that despite the fascinating detail of this text, Chunyu Yi tantalisingly fails to say *why* he kept these records. We can perhaps rule out the notion that he kept them in case the authorities should demand them of him – but apart from that we have no idea what the purpose of his record keeping might be.

Appearance in literature

Chunyu Yi's brush with the authorities was no doubt stressful for him, but it is fortuitous for us. We have no other Western Han examples of systematic medical records, but since Chunyu Yi's appearance in history was not apparently due to any uniqueness in his practice there seems no reason to think that he was alone in keeping written notes of at least some cases. In fact we have other evidence to suggest that such records existed. Thus from the third century AD we have detailed accounts of cases treated by the physician Hua Tuo 華佗 (*ca* AD 141–208) in both the *Sanguo zhi* 三國志 (*ca* AD 290) and the *Hou Han shu* 後漢書 (*ca* AD 450). Here are summary notes of the details given in the

[18] *Shiji, juan* 105, 2796–813. For discussion of the twenty-five case histories, see Hsu (this volume) and Harper (this volume).
[19] *Shiji, juan* 105, 2813.

Sanguo zhi, which is the earlier of the two accounts.[20] For the present discussion, it is the existence and level of detail of these records that is significant rather than their technical medical content.

(1) Sex of dead foetus is predicted by position in belly; it is expelled after Hua Tuo prescribes an unspecified decoction.

(2) Man suffers from limb pain, dry mouth, dislike of hearing speech, stoppage of urine. Hua Tuo suggests attempting to induce sweating by hot food; predicts death in three days if this fails; no sweating takes place, death occurs as predicted.

(3) Two men suffer from identical symptoms of headache and fever. Hua Tuo says one must be purged and the other sweated on the grounds that the one suffers from outer repletion and the other from inner repletion. Hence the treatments are different. Both cases are cured.

(4) Hua Tuo meets someone and enquires how he feels. The man says he feels quite well. Hua Tuo says that he can tell from his face that he is acutely ill from excess of alcohol. Shortly afterwards the man is taken ill and dies.

(5) Hua Tuo feels the pulse of someone just recovered from illness. Says he is still depleted and must not exhaust himself, particularly through sexual intercourse. He predicts that tongue will protrude several inches on point of death. Man has intercourse and dies as predicted.

(6) Man complains of pain after acupuncture by a third party. Hua Tuo says liver channel must have been pierced in error. Predicts death if food is not reduced within five days. Prediction verified.

(7) Hua Tuo diagnoses child as suffering from effects of mother's cold. Prescribes medicine, child recovers in ten days.

(8) Woman bitten by insect during night visit to privy. Hua Tuo prescribes heat treatment which cures her.

(9) Hua Tuo meets a person invalided out of the army on his way home. Hua Tuo regrets that there has been no earlier meeting, predicts death in five days; verified.

(10) Hua Tuo meets sick man on road on way to see doctor. Prescribes garlic puree which expels worm. Sufferer visits Hua Tuo's house and sees several of these hanging over wall.

(11) Hua Tuo cures man by angering him so that he vomits blood.

(12) Hua Tuo advises man that surgery will remove illness but he will die in ten years, however illness is not fatal in itself. Man cannot bear pain, submits to surgery and dies in ten years.

---

[20] *Sanguo zhi*, juan 29, 799 ff.

(13) Man suffers from chest discomfort, red face, lack of appetite. Hua Tuo diagnoses worms caused by eating rotten food. Administers a decoction which expels worms. Predicts return of illness; this occurs, but Hua Tuo then not alive, and man dies.

(14) Hua Tuo cures the ruler of headache through acupuncture.

(15) Hua Tuo feels the pulse of woman and says dead (twin) foetus still to be expelled. At first disbelieved, then summoned back on recurrence of illness. He expels foetus through decoction and needling.

(16) Hua Tuo's refusal to attend on ruler; his consequent death in prison; ruler's regret for this when he is ill himself, and when his son dies for lack of proper treatment.

(17) A man who vomits pus and blood is cured by drugs prescribed by Hua Tuo, but dies when unable to obtain a further supply after Hua Tuo's death.

There are significant differences in structure and genre in these records from those of Chunyu Yi. Hua Tuo's cases are presented as if narrated by the historian, with no indication of how the data were assembled. Nor is there the insistence shown by Chunyu Yi on his diagnostic reasoning, or for that matter on the central importance of the pulse. Nevertheless this material does suggest the existence of a written source in which someone, perhaps one of Hua Tuo's disciples, had recorded notable cases treated by the master. In addition it is clearly different in tone from other material on Hua Tuo recorded in later commentaries to the text discussed here in which he is represented as a wonder-worker whose bizarre therapies set him outside the range of normal human physicians. But while we undoubtedly know something about Hua Tuo's practice, as in the case of Chunyu Yi we do not know why we know it: the reason why someone wrote down the original records behind the *Sanguo zhi* text is quite unclear.

After Chunyu Yi and Hua Tuo it is many centuries before we again find more than a handful of records of individual cases. That is not to say that we have any reason to think that physicians ceased to make such records, or that they were markedly less attentive to the lessons to be drawn from the particularities of practice. No-one who reads the *Shanghan lun* 傷寒論 (Treatise on Cold Damage Disorders) of Zhang Ji 張機 (*ca* AD 200) could fail to be convinced that Zhang's work is the result of deep and systematic reflection upon many individual cases, and the same is true of the writings of other physicians in succeeding centuries. But the nature of the written record from the period of division does not permit us to go into greater detail.

By the time that the flow of surviving literature grows with the rise of the Tang dynasty in the seventh century, we find for the first time instances where records of medical cases are included in texts for an obvious purpose. Early but typical examples are found in the *Beiji qianjin yaofang* 備急千金要方 (Emergency Prescriptions Worth a

Thousand Gold Pieces) of Sun Simiao 孫思邈 (*ca* 581–682). After giving a prescription for the treatment of ulcerous swellings, Sun continues:

> In the fourth year of the Zhengguan reign period (AD 630) an ulcerous swelling suddenly appeared at the corner of my mouth. I made a *ganzi chenmu* 甘子振母 plaster, but there was no improvement after ten days. I anointed [the lesion] with the [above] prescription and obtained a cure. Thereafter I constantly used this medicine to help others, and none failed to be cured.[21]

No physician could give a more forceful or effective recommendation than one based on his own self-treatment. Other Tang physicians likewise appealed to the test of experience in support of their prescriptions, although the experience was more commonly that of their patients rather than their own. In addition to this use of actual cases in support of specific therapies, we also find authors citing such cases in support of broader theoretical contentions. Once more we may find an early example in the writing of Sun Simiao. In a general discussion of the disorder known as *xiaoke* 消渴 (which is clearly linked with what we would nowadays call diabetes) Sun cites as evidence the story of the illness and death of an official in AD 636.[22] In succeeding centuries it is easy to find many other examples of authors citing cases in both of these ways – to recommend a prescription or to support a theoretical position.[23]

One striking instance is the *Shanghan jiushi lun* 傷寒九十論 (Ninety Theses on Cold Damage Disorders) of Xu Shuwei 許叔微 (1079–*ca* 1154). Here ninety cases are given, carefully sequenced and each followed by a discussion in which a general point is made. As an instance of this, we may summarise the sixth and seventh cases and their subsequent discussions:

> Case 6: A Mr Li suffers from *shanghan* (傷寒 cold damage); pulse is floodlike, large and prolonged; body is hot, constipated, no sweating. Classified as *yangming* 陽明 syndrome in accordance with the scheme of Zhang Ji's *Shanghan lun*. Purge prescribed. Reluctance on part of patient to take purge on grounds of age; when purge is taken and has effect, patient recovers. Warned that 'tonic' medicines will bring back the heat and must not be taken. Discussion: Hot toxins must always be purged out whatever the patient's age; cold evil may likewise be treated by warming drugs in all cases. If one does not accord with the nature of the illness, there may be fatal results.

> Case 7: Another patient suffers from *shanghan*: heat and spontaneous sweating, constipation, normal urination, lassitude and sleepiness, pulse prolonged, large and depleted. Classified as *yangming* 陽明 syndrome. Brother of patient asks if this is not just the same as Mr Li's case, so should it not be treated with a purge?

---

[21] *Beiji qianjin yaofang, juan* 22, 391.   [22] *Beiji qianjin yaofang, juan* 21, 374.
[23] See Shi Qi (1994), 142–4, for examples and discussion.

Xu points out that there is the vital difference of sweating and normal urine flow, so that body fluids are being exhausted. Under such circumstances one should use honey suppositories rather than a purge. This is done and patient is cured. Discussion: It is essential to observe the small but significant differences between instances of the same major syndrome, as indicated by the presence of sweating and urination, and the state of the pulse. This is similar to the case of fate divination, where simply using the year, month, day and hour of birth fails to show up the factors which change from moment to moment and make all the difference to the fortunes of individuals.[24]

To sum up the situation so far: we have established that at least some Chinese physicians kept written records of the patients they treated from the beginning of the Imperial age, and that they found it natural to cite such records in support of their general writing on medical matters. But towards the end of the Ming, and as we move into the Qing, the medical case ceases to serve as a mere adjunct to other forms of writing, and takes on a new and different role. It is to this process of transformation that we will now turn our attention.

The appearance of *yi'an* as a special printed genre

In the sixteenth century, we find the beginning of an increasing stream of publications consisting solely of the collected *yi'an* (case statements) of notable physicians, a genre without precedent in the bibliography of Chinese medicine up to that time. The first book in the new genre appears to have been the *Shishan yi'an* 石山醫案 (Case Statements of Master Shishan) published by the disciples of the physician Wang Ji 汪機 in 1531. Later in the century we have the first volume giving a classified anthology of the significant cases of many famous physicians of the past, the *Mingyi lei'an* 名醫類案 (Classified Case Statements of Eminent Physicians) printed in 1591 after at least forty years of work by its compilers Jiang Quan 江瓘 and his son Jiang Yingsu 江應宿. Both were subsequently reprinted in many editions, and thereafter the number of such books grows steadily. We are obviously seeing the appearance of a new genre of literature, which goes on to become an increasingly important constituent of medical publication. Previously cases had been put into print in the context of other types of writing, because they served to support the contentions of an author who wished to make general points about medical theory or the validity of a particular therapy. Now the case statements apparently appear as ends in themselves. The trend towards publishing more and more works of this type appears clearly in the graph in figure 9.1, which indicates the numbers of new *yi'an* collections published in each twenty-year period from 1500 to 1800.[25]

[24] *Shanghan jiushi lun*, 151–3.   [25] Data are drawn from Xue Qinglu (1994), 627 ff.

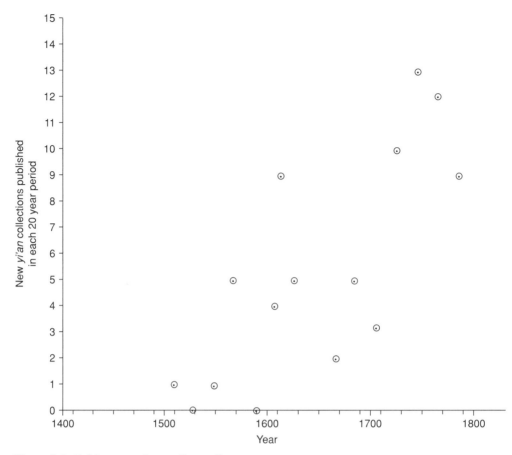

Figure 9.1. *Publication of new* yi'an *collections*

Before 1500 there were no specialist case collections, and after that date the steady growth trend of the new genre from a zero base-line is obvious.

Something has happened to the way records of cases are viewed by medical writers and their readers – but what? One of the keys to the answer lies in the very titles of the new collections of cases, which all contain the phrase *yi'an* 醫案 above rendered as '[medical] case statements'. In fact this is a new phrase, which so far as I am aware is not found before the sixteenth century. Chunyu Yi did not refer to his case histories as *yi'an* but as *zhenji* – consultation records. Xu Shuwei – whose ninety case histories occupy most of the text of *Shanghan jiushi lun* – does not find it necessary to use a special term for them at all. They are just there as evidence.

Three sixteenth-century books give us independent evidence for the significance of the new term. They are, in chronological order:

(1) *Hanshi yitong* 韓氏醫通 (Mr Han's Generalities on Medicine) by Han Mao 韓懋 (fl. sixteenth century). Preface dated 1522.

(2) *Shishan yi'an* 石山醫案 (Case Records of [Master] Stone Mountain) containing collected cases of Wang Ji 汪機 (1463–1539). Preface dated 1531.

(3) *Mai yu* 脈語 (Pulse Discourses) of Wu Kun 吳崑 (1552–*ca* 1620). Printed in 1584.

Han Mao is usually given the credit for laying down 'a standard format for writing *yi'an*'[25] – a formulation which assumes that he was meeting a perceived need (but were Chinese physicians really lamenting the chaos of medical record formats?), and that what he wrote was in some way normative (but what institution could have acted as the enforcement agency?). In fact an inspection of what Han actually wrote reveals a different picture. It is therefore worth quoting from it at some length:

> Medical books contain the doctrine of [diagnosis through] looking, listening/ smelling, questioning, and touching. This matter has been recklessly commented on by the recent [writer] Xiong Zongli [fl. *ca* 1450].[26] I have therefore set out my *liufa jianshi zhi an* 六法兼施之案 '[model] case statement [showing] combined application of the sixfold [diagnostic] procedure'. It may be that this will show fully the practice of the divine sages and artful practitioners.

> Format: In place X [relating to] person Y on date Z [I] fill out [this] medical case-statement *yi'an*, one instance.

> Looking at form and appearance:

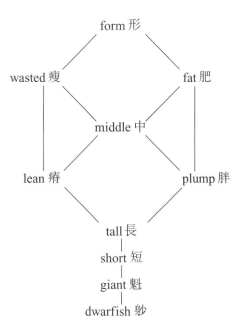

---

[26] See for instance Shi Qi (1994), 145.

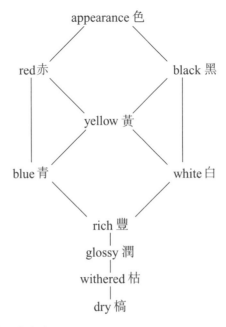

Listening to sound and pitch

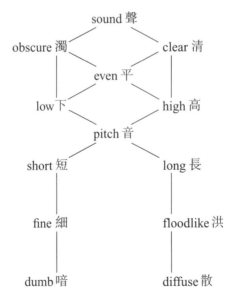

Asking about circumstances

What places are painful?
What brought this about?
On what day did this start?
Day or night – which is worse?

Cold or heat – which is predominant?
Like or dislike for what things?
What drugs have been taken?
What places have been visited?

Taking pulse patterns:

[There then follow labelled spaces for indicating eighteen pulse readings – three positions at three 'depths' on each wrist]

Reasoning out the source of the disease

What customarily predominates in this person's makeup?
In what category can the disease be placed at present?
Superficial or radical – in which aspect is it?
How will it end up? [Note in original: *this phrase refers to good or ill fortune, normal or perverse development, and whether easy or difficult to treat*]

Methods for treatment:

What is the principal method to be used in treatment?
What sequence of prescriptions will be used?

The 'six procedures' are looking, listening/smelling , questioning, touching, reasoning and treatment. Whenever you treat any disease, make a case statement on a piece of paper in this format (*fan zhi yi bing, yong ci shi yi zhi wei an* 凡治一病 用此式一紙為案). At the head fill in the place and date, and look into the climate, soil and what is appropriate for the season. Then perspicuously perform looking and listening/smelling, and do not scruple to question in detail. Thus one examines the externals. Then take the pulse; reason out the judgement and settle the prescription – and you will attain the truth. One should note down everything. Then as the patient's condition develops you will not commit the fault of 'changing the commander in the face of the enemy'. If the doctor gives his full attention in this way, every case will be a success.

When I had written out [one of my] 'combined procedure forms', a criminal law specialist (*xingming jia* 刑名家) was passing and he said 'Your "looking" and "listening" is like when the two parties are both ready – when you carefully examine what is said and look at appearances, that is taking the depositions. Taking the pulse is like conducting an examination of all closely connected persons. And the discussion of origins and the treatment are like sending in the judgement and finishing off [the case]'. Even though he was only joking, what he said was worth noticing.

Someone asked 'This "combined application of the six procedures" – isn't it bound to be over-fussy?' I answered 'Medicine is a matter of life and death. If one did not concentrate on planning treatment, one would not be practising the "humane art" ' . . . In the instance of a trivial complaint, it does not matter if one does not fill out a case statement (*sui bu tian an ke ye* 雖不填案可也). But to dispense with them altogether because one finds them fussy is no idea of mine![27]

[27] *Hanshi yitong* 1, 5–9. In *Zhongguo yixue dacheng.*

A number of points emerge at once from this text. In the first place, Han is quite explicit as to the purpose of the activity he describes here. The discipline of filling out documents in the format he prescribes is to be undertaken because that way the physician will do a better job – he will not omit to attend to any essential point, particularly in diagnosis, and reference back to his original notes will enable him to maintain a consistent line of treatment. Nothing is said about anyone else reading his notes for some aim unconnected with the patient's treatment. Rightly structuring the physicians' discourse about his patient will ensure that treatment is also rightly structured.

Secondly, it now emerges what the term *an* 案 really means in the context of Han's *yi'an*: it is in essence a structured presentation of data in a predetermined format. It is a 'record', certainly, but a record in the special sense found nowadays in connection with an electronic database, not simply a free-form notation of 'what happened' but a series of data fields whose existence enforces a particular pattern of observation and recording. It is also a 'form' in the sense of a bureaucratic form, designed to demand certain forms of information and exclude others.

Han's proposal is one which emerges naturally enough from a culture which has one of the world's longest and richest traditions of bureaucracy. More particularly, it is clear from Han's anecdote about the legal specialist that Han sees himself as drawing on the special traditions of the judicial bureaucracy in his proposal to formalise medical practice. The term *an* 案 – particularly in the phrase *gong'an* 公案 (see below) – had borne the sense of 'formal statement of a law case' for centuries, as well as bearing the more general sense of a formal and official setting out of a state of affairs, or more trivially a 'form' of the type that one fills in.

Leaving Wang Ji aside for the moment and passing directly to Wu Kun, we find the point made very clearly.

> Format for pulse case statements (*mai'an geshi* 脈案格式)
>
> I have taken the expression '*mai'an* 脈案' [pulse case statement] from the idea of '*gong'an* 公案' [legal case statements]. In medicine, one makes an investigation into the circumstances of the disease, so that the evil behind the disease will not be able to escape one's prescription. When the drug gets to work and the disease hides away, [one must act like] an old legal official hearing a case, who cites the law and fixes the penalty (*yuanlu dingxing* 援律定刑) so that the guilty have no place to flee to.
>
> 1. Write down the year, month, place and person.
>
> 2. Write down the age of the person, and whether their physique is fat or lean, tall or short, whether their appearance is dark or light, withered or sleek, whether their speech is clear or thick, drawn-out or clipped.
>
> 3. Write down their likes and dislikes, and how the illness began, and on what day.

4. Write down what drugs were taken on the initial manifestation of the illness, and what drugs were taken thereafter, and what drugs were taken repeatedly, what drugs had some effect and what drugs had no effect.

5. Write down whether things are worse during the day or during the night, whether cold or heat predominates, what things are liked or disliked, and the nature of [readings] from the three sections and nine-fold observations of the pulse.

6. Adduce classical authorities to determine the name of the illness; which manifestation is superficial and which is radical; which manifestation is acute and should be treated first, and which is chronic and should be treated later; which viscus should be supplemented and which should be drained.

7. Write down what [standard] prescription should be used, and how it is to be modified by the increase or decrease of which drugs; which drug is to supplement which viscus and which drug is to drain which viscus; how they are classified in accordance with the patterns of ruler, minister, assistant and envoy, and the intended effect in terms of vomiting, purging, sweating, or harmonising.

Write down all these things in exhaustive detail. At the end, write 'Written by Dr XY of Z prefecture'.

[Explanatory notes:]

Recording the cyclical characters for the year, and recording the season in which the month falls is for predicting the evolutionary phase. Recording the place is for judging what suits the locale. Writing down age, physique, sound and appearance is for use in aligning these with the pulse. Writing down likes and dislikes is for judging the seven emotions. Writing down the day it started is for judging whether prolonged or recent. Systematically asking about the manifestations of the illness and medicinal substances taken, and recording whether they were effective, is in order to evaluate what has already appeared. Recording day and night, hot and cold, is in order to distinguish the vital forces. Writing down what things are liked or disliked is in order to examine [which of] the *yin* and *yang* viscera [are involved]. Writing down the appearance of the pulse is in order to align it with the age, physique, sound, appearance and disease manifestation. Writing down classical authorities is like when legal specialists cite the laws, so that [their judgements] shall be firm and inescapable. Writing down the name of the disease: 'one uses drugs as one uses military forces' and when a general is sent forth he urgently needs to know the name [of his adversary]. Writing down what is superficial and what radical is in order to know what is trivial and what is serious. Writing down the pattern of ruler and minister in the drugs used in the prescription is in order to make the patient understand and try it. Writing one's name at the end is because one wishes the patient to remember it, so that he will attest one's humble labours.

When one is attending on the sickness of a prince, a grandee, a high minister or a scholar, one should write out such a case statement (*bi shu ci yi an* 必書此一案),

without the slightest negligence, and then one may truly be counted as a real physician.[28]

We shall now not be in the slightest surprised when we read in the preface to Wang Ji's *Shishan yi'an*, the first book of the new genre:

> When those who come after peruse these [case histories] is this not just like the use made by legal experts of settled cases (*duan'an* 斷案)?[29]

It seems quite clear, in the light of what these sources have to say, that it was the model of the legal case statement that provided the impetus for the creation of the new *yi'an* concept – the idea of a structured and indeed bureaucratised account of a case – as well as the name for the case statement itself. It is appropriate that the country which created the world's longest-lived bureaucracy should have made a distinctive contribution to medicine by inventing a form for physicians to fill in.

So far the advocates of creating medical *an* have all been physicians. By the end of the sixteenth century others were already seeing the creation of *yi'an* as desirable means to ensure that physicians did their job properly. Lü Kun 呂坤 (1536–1618), a senior Ming bureaucrat who rose to be Governor of Shanxi province, wrote a series of texts designed to help those charged with the task of governance at all levels. One section of his writing makes suggestions as to how the conscientious official should deal with medical matters amongst the population under his care.[30] It includes the following paragraph:

> Those who are able to recite some portion of the medical scriptures may be permitted by the medical officer (*yiguan* 醫官) to treat people. Every [such] physician is to be given a volume of *yi'an*. Their patients are to fill them in personally. They must make it clear what condition the patient was suffering from, and what medicine was used to cure them. Every quarter the sealing official (*changyin guan* 掌印官) shall check over the *yi'an*. Those who have cured over thirty people shall be given one picul of grain. Those who have cured over one hundred people shall be given lifetime tax exemption. Those who have cured more than three hundred people are honoured by the erection of a laudatory tablet. Should there be any falsification, the patients are called in for investigation, and if a single one is found to be inauthentic, then even if there are ten authentic patients the whole batch is excluded from the reckoning.[31]

It seems quite clear that for Lü Kun it is the form (in both senses) rather than the content that makes the *yi'an*, since this term is used for the book of blanks handed to the physician to be filled in by his patients. We have no means of telling whether any such measure was ever put into practice; Lü Kun's writings on administration were advisory

---

[28] *Mai yu, juan* 2, 651–2. In *Zhongguo yixue dacheng.*   [29] *Shishan yi'an*, preface.
[30] I owe this reference to Dr Joanna Grant.   [31] *Shizheng lu, juan* 2, 71a–71b.

rather than normative. It is however highly interesting to find an official suggesting that all physicians should be made to observe procedures that had been suggested as good practice over sixty years earlier.

Bureaucratic compulsion apart, the compiling of *yi'an* certainly served as a useful self-discipline for the physician who composed such documents. But we may reasonably ask why it should have begun to seem useful to *publish* collections of such statements for others to read. The prefaces of early *yi'an* collections are not strikingly helpful in answering this question. Once the flow of literature has begun, it seems largely to be taken for granted by those who compile them that such things should be published, and that they are a Good Thing. The compiler of the *Mingyi lei'an* does give us some help when he notes that his collection should be helpful to those studying medicine in isolation from regular clinical experience:

> Living in some retired place in the mountains, from where is one to gain broad experience? So I have widely gathered the traces left by the treatment methods and unusual experiences of the worthies of ancient and modern times.[32]

The aim is evidently to help those with a taste for medical learning to study on their own, without benefit of the usual apprenticeship to a senior physician. But such observations are not common. We may certainly take it that once the publication of *yi'an* collections became accepted as a common form of publication, there would have been all the usual drives in terms of local patriotism, and the wish to boost the reputation of one's teacher.

But are there any possible explanations in terms of wider social factors, or of changes in medical practice? I want to propose a tentative hypothesis.

Let us begin by asking ourselves who might be wanting to learn how to compete in medical practice at the elite level in the period from the late Ming through the Qing. As ever, there would be physicians who learned their skills in the context of hereditary medical practice, or perhaps through a system of apprenticeship which effectively mimicked the way skill was transmitted from father to son. Such men would presumably learn how to draft case statements by seeing it done, and doing it themselves under supervision.

But in addition, I suspect there was a demand for readily assimilable medical expertise from another direction. By this I mean that there are grounds for expecting that more and more literate males with no family backgrounds in medicine may have been drawn to attempt to make a living from medicine during the period in question. We know that China's population more than doubled during the seventeenth and eighteenth centuries. Much of the impact of this growth was borne at the lower levels of society

---

[32] *Mingyi lei'an*, preface, 8a.

as peasants sank to subsistence level and below. But the pressure was felt amongst the literate elite as well. Young men from gentry families found it more and more difficult to gain entry into the civil service career which was the only really respectable route to success, since neither the statutory number of government posts nor the quotas for academic degrees were expanded in relation to the burgeoning population.[33] They had few alternatives. They could become teachers, and hence help others attempt to scale the heights they had failed to climb themselves. They could hang on to the coat-tails of the successful by joining the supernumerary assistants who increasingly infested yamen offices and made a living by extorting fees for bureaucratic services. They might become legal pettifoggers, *songkun* 訟棍, or rather more respectably act as legal assistants to magistrates.[34] But it was proverbial that medical practice was the most obvious resort for a scholar whose career was not flourishing: 'If you can't become a good prime minister, become a good physician.'[35]

The effects of such literati career blockage on the publishing industry are not difficult to guess: there was always a ready sale for anything that could hold out the hope of increasing one's chances of passing the civil service examinations. One highly popular genre was the model examination essay, ready to be learned by heart and regurgitated at need. In that well-known depiction of late Imperial literati life the *Rulin waishi* 儒林外史 (Unofficial History of the Literati) one character turns down a dubious publishing proposition saying that what he would really like to handle would be a collection of examination essays – those always sell well.[36] In addition, books paralleling the medical case history collections were also being produced in increasing numbers for those interested in more or less respectable legal careers. These were compilations of decisions in legal cases (also called *an* 案).[37] The numbers of these published are much smaller than the numbers of medical case history collections, which is no surprise given that the number of yamen legal clerks would necessarily be much smaller than the number of aspirant physicians. As a consequence we are dealing with the statistics of smaller numbers, and the picture will be fuzzier. But Zhang's data suggest that the picture of the growth of a genre during the sixteenth to nineteenth centuries – with a beginning not long after 1500 – is not inconsistent with what we saw in medicine.[38]

So it seems that the circumstances of the historical period we are discussing may help us to make sense of the phenomenon of the origin and growth of the specialised *yi'an* collection. In times of increasing career stress the publication of more and more

[33] Twitchett and Fairbank (1978), 110–13.   [34] On legal careers for literati, see Chang Wejen (1994).
[35] See for instance *Hanshi yitong, juan* 1, 390.
[36] On officially sponsored collections of examination essays, see Chow (1994), 193.
[37] For a listing see Zhang Weiren (1976).   [38] Zhang Weiren (1976), 804–13.

medical case statements can be seen as a response to competition in two ways: firstly a good way to boost one's own reputation is to boost that of one's master by publishing his case statements. That would relate particularly to such books as the *Shishan yi'an*, which contain the cases of a single physician. Secondly a young man trying to break into a medical career might well find the case history genre his quickest route to apparent expertise. In the same way that it was to his advantage to have examination essays at his fingertips, or to have ready-made legal precedents to hand, what could be more useful as a quick route to apparent expertise than a collection of authoritative medical case statements? It will be recalled that the compiler of the *Mingyi lei'an* collection hinted that his book would be particularly useful to aspiring autodidacts without access to much clinical experience. And of course the preface to Wang Ji's collection states explicitly that it is intended to serve in precisely the same way as a *legal* case history collection. Could anything be clearer than this?

One remaining point to be settled is exactly how the ability to write a good *yi'an* is helpful to an aspiring young physician, apart from the possibility put forward by Han Mao that the discipline of writing *yi'an* will simply make him a more effective healer. If we turn back to Wu Kun, however, we can see clear hints that some of the purposes of writing case statements related to the possible effects of seeing such documents on the patient – who evidently did see them. At the end of the passage quoted, we may recall that he told us:

> Writing down the pattern of ruler and minister in the drugs used in the prescription is in order to make the patient understand and try it. Writing one's name at the end is because one wishes the patient to remember it, so that he will attest one's humble labours.
>
> When one is attending on the sickness of a prince, a grandee, a high minister or a scholar, one should write out such a case statement (*bi shu ci yi an* 必書此一案), without the slightest negligence, and then one may truly be counted as a real physician.

So writing a case statement is clearly intended to act on the patient in two ways. Firstly, the carefully structured rationale of diagnosis and prescription, backed by classical authorities, is intended to persuade the patient to follow the advice given. Secondly, Wu Kun clearly expects that the patient will be reminded of the skills of the physician by his name on the statement. To a modern doctor it may seem slightly strange that the physician should be anxious lest the patient should not follow his advice, or that he should feel the need to leave a documentary reminder of his visit. But the fact is that this was a typical feature of the pre-modern Chinese doctor–patient relationship. To illustrate this point, I shall give an example from the records of a late Qing and early Republican physician, Xiao Bozhang 蕭伯章. He was born in the late nineteenth century and was active in the early part of the twentieth century in moves to bring about a rapprochement between Eastern and Western medicine. In the first instance, Xiao is called in to examine a patient with a painful swollen belly.

> He was variously treated by physicians for over ten days, but the illness became more severe, and I was invited to diagnose and treat him. When I arrived three medical gentlemen were already seated. We introduced ourselves to each other, and the master of the house asked us to come into the private apartments . . . I looked through the prescriptions he had previously taken: they were mostly random and unsystematic. When I had done this the master of the house drew me into another room. He called for brush and paper and requested me to make a statement of the case (*li'an* 立案) and draft a prescription. He also told me that the three physicians outside had already acceded to his request to do this. Now I had the benefit of some acquaintance with the patient's elder brother, so I laughed and asked the master of the house 'Sir, are you really holding an examination for medical students today? If not, why all this? Now I treat sick people, and an examination doesn't scare me. But who will grade the papers?'
>
> The master of the house replied 'I am not the sort of person who understands medicine. My idea is to wait until all the doctors have written their case statements (*an* 案) and then compare them. Then I shall follow the points in which they agree, letting the majority decide. I don't know what else to do – what do you think, Sir?'
>
> I said 'That is well enough in theory, but is no good in practice. Most physicians nowadays have little real grasp of their subject. All they can do is to prescribe some remedy that is relatively harmless but cannot do any good either. If by chance they agree it will only be because they have all fallen into the same error. If you ask them for an explanation all you will get will be mere obfuscation. So let me see what they have written, and I can give you an evaluation at once. If they turn up their nose at what I have said, please let us have a face to face debate about it.'
>
> The master of the house did as I had asked. In a little while I wrote out my own case statement, and drafted a prescription for a strong purgative. Then I looked at what the others had written. All were for ineffectual treatments. I wrote out a criticism of each, and the master handed them to the physicians in question. They all departed without a word.[39]

The story continues: in fact Xiao's prescription is not used immediately, because of pressure from family members anxious that the medicine may be too violent. Eventually the patient insists on it and a cure ensues. Subsequently Xiao expounds his views further in the course of a debate with the family tutor. Now it is increasingly common ground

---

[39] *Xiao Zhuoru yi'an* (Medical Case Statements by Xiao Bozhang). In Yao Ruoqin (1933), vol. II, 1–3.

amongst scholars that for the pre-modern Chinese physician the locus of debate where he must establish his authority is the patient's bedside – and he will have to argue with family members as well as with fellow practitioners. Unlike the nineteenth-century European physician, the Chinese healer has not succeeded in establishing a right to dictate as a 'man of science', who is entitled to withdraw in a huff if his expertise is called into question – and unlike an ancient Greek physician he does not expect to debate in public. Xiao's case exemplifies this very well. But it also describes a situation in which as well as taking part in private oral debate it is expected that the physician will generate a document (*an* 案), which backs up the prescription (*fang* 方) by giving a diagnosis and rationale for therapy. It is clear from Xiao's example that the quality and cogency of these documents determines whose advice is followed, and hence determines the vocational success of the physicians who generate them in competition with each other. It would therefore be important for anyone who wanted to succeed as a physician to learn to generate effective and convincing *an* 案, just as Wu Kun had suggested centuries earlier. A nineteenth-century British observer, Benjamin Hobson (1816–73), confirms the testimony given by Xiao Bozhang on the practice of providing written *an*:

> If the patient is an officer of the government or a wealthy person, the nature of the disease, prognosis and treatment are written out for the inspection of the family.[40]

It is striking how closely this echoes the advice given by Wu Kun as to the class of patient who should be given an impressive *an* by which to remember the physician.

No single-factor approach can be adequate to explain the growth of *yi'an* publication in Late Imperial China. Clearly any attempt to understand what was going on must also look anthropologically at the ways in which authority in medicine was claimed, validated, and transmitted through documentary means. We must also look at changing trends in the uses of literature for practical purposes in this period, and see how the citation of exemplary instances may have become more fashionable in fields ranging from historical studies to practical handbooks. In pointing to the influence of the legal case statement as a model for format and publication I am no doubt offering only a partial answer to the problem. But given the greatly increased attention that the Chinese case history is drawing, it is essential for us to be aware of how its origins may condition its usefulness, and it is as a contribution to that awareness that I offer the observations and conjectures in this essay.

---

[40] Hillier and Jewell (1983), 4–6.

References to premodern Chinese and Japanese works

Beiji qianjin yaofang 備急千金要方 (Emergency Prescriptions Worth a Thousand Gold Pieces). Tang, 652. Sun Simiao 孫思邈. Facsimile of a Ming print. Zhonghua shuju, Beijing, 1955.

Hanshi yitong 韓氏醫通 (Mr Han's Generalities on Medicine). Ming, preface of 1522. Han Mao 韓懋. Ming, early 16th century. In *Zhongguo yixue dacheng* 中國醫學大成.

Lügong shizheng lu 呂公實政錄 (His Excellency Lü's Notes on Effective Governance). Ming, 1598. Lü Kun 呂坤. Wenshizhe chubanshe, Taibei, 1971.

Mai yu 脈語 (Pulse Discourses). Ming, 1584. Wu Kun 吳崑. In *Zhongguo yixue dacheng* 中國醫學大成.

Mingyi lei'an 名醫類案 (Classified Case Statements of Eminent Physicians). Ming, 1591. Jiang Quan 江瓘, with additional work by his son Jiang Yingsu 江應宿. Renmin weisheng chubanshe, Beijing, 1957.

Sanguo zhi 三國志 (History of the Three Kingdoms). Western Jin. Chen Shou 陳壽 (d. 297) et al. Zhonghua shuju, Beijing, 1959.

Shanghan jiushi lun 傷寒九十論. Song. Xu Shuwei 許叔微. In *Xu Shuwei Shanghan lun zhu san zhong*. Renmin weisheng chubanshe, Beijing, 1993.

Shiji 史記 (Records of the Historian). Han, *ca* 90 BC. Sima Qian 司馬遷. Zhonghua shuju, Beijing, 1959.

Shisanjing zhushu 十三經注疏 (Commentary on the Thirteen Canons). Qing, 1816. Ruan Yuan 阮元. Reprint, Taipei, 1972.

Shishan yi'an 石山醫案 (Case Statements of Master Stone Mountain). Ming, preface 1531. Wang Ji 汪機 and disciples.

Zhouli 周禮 (Rites of the Zhou). Late Warring States. Anon. Textual references to *Zhouli zhushu*. *Shisanjing zhushu* 十三經注疏.

Zizhi tongjian changbian jishi benmo 資治通鑑長編紀事本末 (Sequential Record of Events from the Long Draft of the Comprehensive Mirror for Aid in Government). Song. Annotated by Yang Zhongliang 楊仲良. Wenhai chubanshe, Taibei, 1967.

References to modern works

Bates, Don (ed.) 1995. *Knowledge and the Scholarly Medical Traditions*. Cambridge University Press, Cambridge.

Boltz, William G. 1993. 'Chou Li'. In Loewe, 24–32.

Chang Wejen [Zhang Weiren] 1994. 'Legal Education in Ch'ing China'. In Elman and Woodside, 292–339.

Chen Dawu 陳大舞 1994. *Lidai mingyi yi'an xuanjiang* 歷代名醫醫案選講 (Selected and Commented Case Statements of Eminent Physicians of Successive Ages). Shanghai zhongyiyao daxue chubanshe, Shanghai.

Chow Kai-wing 1994. 'Discourse, Examination, and Local Elite: the Invention of the T'ung-Ch'eng School in Ch'ing China'. In Elman and Woodside, 183–219.

Elman, Benjamin A. and Woodside, Alexander (eds.) 1994. *Education and Society in Late Imperial China, 1600–1900*. University of California Press, Berkeley.

Furth, Charlotte 1999. *A Flourishing Yin: Gender in China's Medical History, 960–1665*. University of California Press, Berkeley.

Grant, Joanna C. 1997 'Wang Ji's *Shishan Yi'an*: Aspects of Gender and Culture in Ming Dynasty Medical Case Histories'. PhD thesis in History, University of London.

Hillier, S. M. and Jewell, J. A. 1983. *Health Care and Traditional Medicine in China, 1800–1982*. Routledge and Kegan Paul, London.

Lang, Mabel 1977. *Cure and Cult in Ancient Corinth*. American School of Classical Studies, Athens, Princeton, NJ.

Lloyd, G. E. R. (ed.) 1983. *Hippocratic Writings*. Penguin, Harmondsworth.

Loewe, Michael (ed.) 1993. *Early Chinese Texts: a Bibliographical Guide*. Society for the Study of Early China, Berkeley.

Nunn, John F. 1996. *Ancient Egyptian Medicine*. British Museum Press, London.

Siraisi, Nancy G. 1990. *Mediaeval and Early Renaissance Medicine: an Introduction to Knowledge and Practice*. University of Chicago Press, Chicago.

Shi Qi 施杞 1994. *Zhongyi bing'an xue* 中醫病案學 (Case Histories in Chinese Medicine). Zhongguo dabaike quanshu chubanshe, Shanghai.

Sivin, Nathan 1995. 'Text and Experience in Classical Chinese Medicine'. In Bates, 177–204.

Twitchett, Denis and Fairbank, John K. (eds.) 1978. *The Cambridge History of China*, vol. X: *Late Ch'ing, 1800–1911*, part 1. Cambridge University Press, Cambridge.

Xue Qinglu 薛清錄 1994. *Quanguo zhongyi tushu lianhe mulu* 全國中醫圖書聯合目錄 (National Union Catalogue of Books on Chinese Medicine). Zhongyi guji chubanshe, Beijing.

Yao Ruoqin 姚若琴 1933. *Song, Yuan, Ming, Qing mingyi lei'an* 宋元明清名醫類案 (Classified Case Histories of Eminent Physicians of the Song, Yuan and Ming Dynasties). Xuanfeng chubanshe, Taipei.

Zhang Weiren 張偉仁 1976. *Zhongguo fazhishi shumu* 中國法制史書目 (A Bibliography for the History of Chinese Law). Institute of History and Philology, Academia Sinica, Taipei.

Zhongguo yixue dacheng 中國醫學大成 (Complete Collection of Chinese Medicine). 50 vols. Cao Bingzhang 曹炳章 (ed.). Shanghai kexue chubanshe, Shanghai, 1992.

10

From case records to case histories: the modernisation of a Chinese medical genre, 1912–49[1]

BRIDIE J. ANDREWS

This study of the modernisation of medical case records is one example of how Chinese physicians during the 1920s and 1930s attempted to make Chinese medicine more 'scientific'. Modernisation was intended to facilitate the creation of a new, eclectic medicine that would combine the best of both western and Chinese traditions. Beyond demonstrating what great changes have occurred in the creation of the new Chinese medicine, I also want to explore some of the motives for this restructuring of medical case records in the Republican period.

Throughout most of Chinese history, physicians made records of their consultations. In Late Imperial China, it was normal practice for a visiting physician to write down his diagnosis and analysis of a patient's case along with the recommended prescription. This record, or case report, *an* 案, was left with the patient, who chose whether or not to act on its recommendations. (In Chinese, the phrase for this action is *tou an* 投案, literally, 'submit' or 'present a case report'.) There are many cases on record of families inviting (and presumably also paying) several physicians in turn to submit their analyses, and then choosing which to follow. The doctors themselves frequently described this process in their own collections of case records, clearly with the aim of explaining why their own analysis was the best. We shall examine a record of this type below.

The historian's access to case records is rarely mediated by patients or their families: our sources are overwhelmingly drawn from published collections of physicians' own records. Since most of these are compiled either by the physicians themselves, or by

[1] This work received generous support in the form of a studentship from the Wellcome Trust for the History of Medicine, Ref. No. 034026/Z/91. I would also like to thank Andrew Cunningham, Chang Chia-feng, Chang Che-chia, Elisabeth Hsu, Angela Ki-che Leung, Ma Kanwen, Volker Scheid, Nathan Sivin, and the external referees for their helpful comments on earlier versions of this article.

their close relatives or personal students, there is a strong bias in the available literature towards cases that offer a display of the practitioner's virtuosity. Cases of failure are relatively rare, and death is most often recorded in order to demonstrate the veracity of the physician's powers of prognosis. In recent years, professional historians in China have supplemented these highly selective collections by publishing all the available case records of famous doctors for whom the material is still available. These supplementary records make it possible to gain an insight into both the kinds of ailment and therapy considered particularly interesting by the individual physician and those so mundane as to not merit a full record.[2]

Since such case record collections are necessarily the products of the educated elite, they also create an image of Chinese medicine in the past that is distorted in favour of mainly secular, 'Confucian' medicine. 'Folk' and 'popular' medical practices usually only appear when a doctor finds cause to criticise the family for employing this kind of treatment previously. Regrettably, case records are also silent on the crucial matter of the physician's compensation. On the plus side, case records provide unique historical access to patient–physician interactions. In the many case records which cover repeated visits to a particular case, they are also a valuable guide to the therapeutic process in Chinese medicine.

The structure of these records varies tremendously, the simplest being a brief note to remind the doctor of the treatment dispensed in particular cases. Here is an example from a collection of the 'unpublished' case records of the famous Qing dynasty physician Ye Gui 葉桂, styled Tianshi 天士 (1667–1746). It consists of only two lines of text in Chinese:

> Left *cun* [pulse] accelerated (*zuocun shuo* 左寸數)
> *Radix Rehmanniae Praeparata; Radix Asparagi;* sweetened Northern *Radix Glehniae; Sclerotium Poriae Cocos Pararadicis; Herba Dendrobium off.;* roasted, loose *Radix Ophiogonis*
> (*shudi* 熟地, *tiandong* 天冬, *tianbei shashen* 甜北沙參, *fushen* 茯神, *huohu* 霍斛, *chaosong maidong* 炒松麥冬 (reading 鬆 *song*, 'loose' for 松).[3]

---

[2] All the collections of case records first published before 1949 and still extant in China are listed in the National Union Catalogue, *Quanguo zhongyi tushu lianhe mulu* 全國中醫圖書聯合目錄 (1991), 627–59. Two publications that collect together particular physicians' case records are Shi Nianzu ((1991) 1957) and He Shutian (1994).

[3] Reproduced in Shi Ji and Su Mincai (1994), 153. There are several reference handbooks of Chinese *materia medica* available for translating between Chinese and Latin botanical nomenclature: I used *Zhongyao dacidian* (1986). Such equivalences depend on a one-to-one correspondence between named drugs and plant species, which does not always exist. In particular, regional variations in plant substitutions for particular drugs were very common in pre-modern China, as is well attested by the alternate entries in handbooks of *materia medica* such as that referred to above.

Although this record is little more than the physician's notes to himself, there is a great deal of information embedded in it.[4] For instance, the accelerated pulse indicates *yang* (陽), with associated heat (*re* 熱). The index finger position on the left wrist (*cun* 寸) correlates to the pulses of the heart (*xin* 心) and small intestine (*xiaochang* 小腸). The principal drug, *Radix Rehmanniae Praeparata* (*Shudi* [*huang*], 熟 地 [黃]) is attributive to the heart, liver, and kidney tracts (*xin, gan, shenjing* 心肝腎經), the pulses of all of which are felt on the left wrist, and this drug has the effect of nourishing *yin* (*zi yin* 滋陰) and replenishing the blood (*bu xue* 補血). Already we may deduce that Ye Tianshi considered the excess of *yang* influence manifested in the accelerated pulse to be due to a deficiency of *yin* (*yinxu* 陰虛), and his mention of the specific pulse site indi-cates that the organ most affected was the heart. This deduction is borne out by examining the properties of the other drugs: *Radix Asparagi, Radix Glehniae, Herba Dendrobium*, and *Radix Ophiogonis* are all found in handbooks of Chinese *materia medica* under the heading of 'drugs that nourish *yin*' (*yang yinyao* 養陰藥 or *bu yinyao* 補陰藥). Most are also used to moisturise dryness, specifically lung-dryness (*feizao* 肺燥) in three out of the four cases. Two out of the four drugs also clear away heat (*qing re* 清熱) or 'heart-fire' (*xinhuo* 心火), a typical sign of general depletion. The last drug, *Sclerotium Poriae Cocos Pararadicis*, is a specific for heart depletion (*xinxu* 心虛) and has the effect of calming the spirit (*an shen* 安神). So, working backwards from the very terse case record it is possible to deduce that Ye Tianshi was treating a case of *yin*-depletion which had damaged the body fluids and heart; signs of this included the accelerated pulse, and most probably also low fever and lung-dryness symptoms such as a hacking cough, with possibly other symptoms related to heart tract disease such as insomnia or over-anxiety. Although two or more of the *yin*-replenishing drugs often appear together in standard prescriptions, this particular combination of drugs seems to have been Ye's own invention.

To work all this out, I have had access to several modern reference works in English and Chinese.[5] Such systematic reference works were not available in the early Qing dynasty, so any case descriptions as brief and highly embedded as this would only have been of use to other physicians with substantial experience and knowledge of the medi-cal canon. The prescription also omits to give the relative proportions of the drugs, again underlining the importance of tacit knowledge in the interpretation of this kind of case record.

At the other end of the spectrum we find long and detailed disquisitions on the merits of various therapies used on a single patient over time, or on several patients with

---

[4] I am grateful to Judith Farquhar for suggesting that it would be useful to see just how much information can be squeezed out of such minimal case records.

[5] For instance, *Zhongyao dacidian* (1986) and Ou Ming (1989).

similar symptoms. The discursive kind of case record is often called the 'notebook' (*biji* 筆記) form of case record, and was written down after the consultation, perhaps using notes taken there, but relying mainly on the physician's (or the physician's student's) memory. This is the kind of case record most often used to advance particular theoretical standpoints. Such records are also often used to explain how particularly complicated cases were worked out and treated, and as such are valuable guides to the processes of inference and deduction used in Chinese therapy, as well as attesting to their author's great skill and erudition.[6]

Somewhere between these two extremes lies the kind of case record recently analysed by Judith Farquhar.[7] We could call this the 'didactic' case record. To be of use to a physician's students, a case record needed to include basic information about the patient, information derived from diagnostic procedures, an account of the treatment applied, and a record of the effect of that treatment. Even more usefully, a record might also explain how the diagnosis was reached and explain why a particular therapy was chosen. It is the standardisation of this kind of 'didactic' case record that I want to examine in more detail here.

The following is an example of a traditional style didactic case record from the early twentieth century by the famous Shanghai physician, Ding Zezhou 丁澤周, usually known by his style of Ganren 甘仁 (1865–1926). None of the contents of Ding Ganren's writings that I have seen show the slightest trace of western diagnostic methods or of western therapeutics. This particular case concerns an epidemic disease known in Chinese as *housha* (喉痧; lit. 'throat-rash'),[8] the symptoms of which overlap with the western disease entity known as scarlet fever. The case is labelled: *Throat-rash with high fever, aversion to cold and difficulty in swallowing*[9]

> [Mr] Fu, aged 20-odd, had been suffering from throat-rash for eight days. He had a high fever without sweating, and had a slight aversion to cold. The rashes were dispersed and indistinct. His face was purple and dark, and the throat was swollen

---

[6] In Shi Ji and Su Mincai (1994), 152 and 162–7, case records are classified as clinical (*linzheng* 臨症) and notebook style (*biji ti* 筆記體), respectively. See also Wang Xinhua (1993), preface.

[7] Farquhar (1992).

[8] *Sha* 痧 is an infrequent disease term in both the canonical medical literature and in modern usage. In Late Imperial China it was current and had several meanings, some of which still survive in the vernacular. The basic medical meaning of *sha* (沙) is 'a granular rash', as in this case, and derived from the word's original meaning of 'sand'. *Housha* is also referred to by its longer disease name *lanhou dansha* (爛喉丹痧 sore/inflamed throat and red rash). An inflamed throat and red body rash that turns white under finger pressure are signs of scarlet fever in western medicine. *Shazi* 痧子 was and is a Shanghai dialect variant for *mazhen* 麻疹, measles. Another meaning of *sha* was of a disease similar to cholera, with vomiting, diarrhoea, and twisted limbs (nowadays explained as caused by acute fluid loss and electrolyte imbalance in the muscles). Some authors collapsed *sha* into *huoluan* 霍亂, a classical disease term with similar symptoms, long used by western translators to convey cholera. Others distinguished between the two.

[9] The entire Chinese text of this case record is included in the appendix to this chapter.

and putrid. He had trouble swallowing even trickles of water, and experienced restlessness and nausea, with no respite day or night. The Fu family had several households, but only [this] one son,[10] so his old mother and young wife were weeping bitterly as they begged me to save him. I said: 'Although the condition is critical, his normal *qi* (*zhengqi* 正氣) is not yet defeated, so he could still recover.' On diagnosis his pulse was obstructed, accelerated, and not clearly distinguishable; the tongue coating was greasy and yellow; when I read the prescriptions he had taken earlier, sure enough, they were [mistakenly] of the 'nurturing *yin* and clearing the lungs decoction' type. Thereupon I prescribed 'decoction for penetrating rash and dispelling poison', with added *Fructus Aurantii Immaturus* (immature orange fruits) and *Caulis Bambusae in Taeniam* (bamboo shavings), two doses to be taken every 24 hours. I also let blood from the *shaoshang* 少商 point [specific for fever, fainting, and sore and swollen throats] in order to open up the blockage and let out the fire. After taking the medicine, he succeeded in sweating profusely, and the rash gradually dispersed. His facial colour changed to red, and the throat swelling and pus began to recede. After taking several doses, he was cured in three to four days. 'Cases of throat-rash will survive if they sweat' – experience shows this to be true.[11]

This is a fairly transparent 'didactic' case record. The nature of the ailment is stated, together with the external symptoms. Diagnosis at the pulse allows the physician to assess the condition of the patient's normal *qi* and to correct previous false diagnoses. From this information the physician is able to offer a hopeful prognosis. This is then realised using a named drug decoction and bloodletting at a named site. The effects of the treatment are noted, as is the duration of the treatment, resulting in a full recovery. There is even a little rhyming couplet at the end to aid retention of the didactic message, which is that cases of *housha* (throat-rash) must be made to sweat.[12] A student studying this record would need to know only where to look up the composition of the named decoction if they had not memorised it already, and the position and effects of the named acupoint.

Compare this case with the following rendering of the same case, this time deliberately rendered in a case history format similar to that used to record western-medical case histories:

---

[10] For one family to have several households means that the patient's grandfather had had several sons who were now married, but that the patient's father was the only one in his generation to have borne a son (all his brothers having failed to do so).

[11] From Ding Ganren's *Housha zhengzhi gaiyao* (喉痧症治概要 Essentials of Throat-rash, Symptoms and Treatment), republished from a mimeographed text from the early Republican period in Lu Zheng (1994), 565–84, at p. 574.

[12] I have been unable to versify the rhyming couplet at the end satisfactorily; suggestions include 'Cases of throat-rash will get better, if the patient is a sweater' (Christopher Cullen, with thanks), or 'In throat-rash there's no need to fret, if the patient can be made to sweat.'

A case of wind-poison throat-rash[13]

Patient:	Mr Fu, aged in his twenties, resident of Tangshan Road, Shanghai.
Disease:	Wind-poison throat-rash.
Causes of disease:	Caught by contagion eight days ago. Prescriptions left by doctors consulted previously were all of the 'nurture *yin* and clear the lungs decoction' type.
Symptoms:	High fever, no sweat, slight aversion to cold, rash dispersed and indistinct. Facial appearance was purple and dark, the throat swollen and putrid, and there was difficulty in swallowing even trickles of water. [The patient] experienced restlessness and nausea, with no respite day or night.
Diagnosis:	The pulse was obstructed, accelerated and not clearly distinguishable, the tongue coating was greasy and yellow. I said: 'This is [a case of] throat-rash that has been misdiagnosed as *baihou* [白喉; lit. 'white throat'; symptoms similar to the western disease entity of diphtheria].'
	The Fu family had several households, but only [this] one son, so his old mother and young wife were weeping bitterly as they begged me to save him. I responded, saying: 'Although the condition is critical, his normal *qi* is not yet defeated, so he could still recover.'
Therapy:	Accordingly I prescribed 'decoction for penetrating rash and dispelling poison', with added *Fructus Aurantii Immaturus* (immature orange fruits) and *Caulis Bambusae in Taeniam* (bamboo shavings) to facilitate penetration [of the drugs] and to open up [obstructions]. I also let blood from the *shao shang* point in order to open up the blockage and let out the fire.
Prescription:	*Herba Schizonepetae*, 1.5 *qian*; *Periostracum cicadae*, 8 *fen*; powdered *Radix puerariae*, 2 *qian*; green *Fructus Forsythiae*, 2 *qian*; *Herba Spirodelae*, 3 *qian*; fried *Fructus Arctii*, 2 *qian*; roasted *Bombyx Batryticatus*, 3 *qian*; young *Rhizoma Belamcandae*, 1 *qian*; *Lasiosphaeraseu Calratia*, 8 *fen* (wrapped, then decocted); *Fructus Aurantii immaturus*, 1.5 *qian*; *Caulis Bambusae in Taeniam*, 2 *qian*; fresh *Radix Glycyrrhizae*, 5 *fen*; *Radix Peucedani*, 1.5 *qian*.[14]

---

[13] The full Chinese text of this version is given in the appendix.

[14] One *fen* 分 is one-tenth of a *qian* 錢, which is one-tenth of a *liang* 兩 (Chinese ounce). International weight units were introduced by the Republican government in China, and if this is the scale referred to, one *fen* equals 1 g, one *qian* equals 10 g, and one *liang* equals 100 g. The kilogramme is called *gongjin* 公斤. In the most common Chinese weight system before this, there were 10 *fen* to the *qian*, 10 *qian* to the *liang*, and 16 *liang* to one *jin* 斤. See the tables of weights and measures appended to the 1947 edition of the *Sea of Words* (Cihai 辭海) dictionary, for example.

Results: After taking two doses of the medicine in the first twenty-
                            four hours, he succeeded in sweating profusely, and the rash
                            gradually dispersed. His facial colour changed to red, and
                            the throat swelling and pus began to recede. After taking
                            several doses, he was cured in three to four days. 'Cases of
                            throat-pox will survive if they sweat' – experience shows
                            this to be true.[15]

Although the details of the case are largely unchanged in these two versions, there are
some significant differences. Most striking is the organisation under specific rubrics in
the second version. The use of the heading on causes of disease (*bingyin* 病因) prompts
the additional information that the affliction was caught by infection (*chuanran* 傳染).
Although there is plenty of evidence for the notion of the contagiousness of particular
diseases in pre-modern China,[16] I think it is significant that the use of the rubrics of
western case histories prompts the further use of explanations compatible with western
medicine. Similarly, the heading on disease names (*bingming* 病名), forces precise
classification, in this case as wind-poison throat-rash (*fengdu housha* 風毒喉痧), an
identification that was omitted in the first version.

Under the rubric 'prescription' (*chufang* 處方), the terse reference to a prescription
in the first case record has been replaced in the case history with a detailed list of all the
drugs in the decoction, including some information on the quality of drug required. (For
instance, for *Rhizoma Belamcandae* the prescription specifies that the original plant
material should be young.)

The first version of this case was taken from a book by Ding Ganren specifically on
the disease entity of throat-rash (*housha*), the second is the same case as it appears in
a compilation of model medical case histories in Chinese medicine compiled in 1927
by He Bingyuan 何炳元, who published under his style as He Lianchen 何廉臣
(1861–1929). Ding Ganren and He Lianchen were two of the leading figures in the modernisation of Chinese medicine in the early years of this century. He Lianchen came
from Shaoxing in Zhejiang province, where he was one of the founders of the Shaoxing
Medical and Pharmaceutical Association (*Shaoxing yiyao xuehui* 紹興醫藥學會). From
1908, he was also editor of the *Shaoxing Journal of Medicine and Pharmacy* (*Shaoxing
yiyao xuebao* 紹興醫藥學報), a journal which became the leading organ of discussion
as to the future development of Chinese medicine until it changed format in 1922, thereafter concentrating on the serial publication of rare medical works.[17] During his time as

[15] He Lianchen ((1927) 1969), 301–3.
[16] I have dealt with one of these, *lao* 勞／癆 or consumptive disorders, in Andrews (1997).
[17] Zhao Hongjun (1989), 92–4. For brief biographies of He Lianchen and Ding Ganren, see Zhang
      Xiaoping (1991), 41–7 and 32–40. Ding Ganren's career is further described in He Shixi (1991).

editor of this journal, He Lianchen advocated using western medicine to improve Chinese medicine in specific ways.

Concerning the Chinese case records genre, He complained that there was no agreement on the amount of detail necessary to constitute a good case record; that they had no standard structure, making them difficult to interpret; that the information given in them was often incomplete; that they seldom reported the success or failure of the treatment; and that they were often long on rhetoric and short on facts.[18] In particular, He Lianchen objected to the great popularity enjoyed by Ye Tianshi's collection of cases, the *Linzheng zhinan yi'an* 臨証指南醫案 (Case Records as a Guide to Clinical Practice), first published in 1766, which exemplified many of these faults.

He Lianchen decided that by following the example of western medical case histories (as opposed to Chinese case records or reports), Chinese physicians would be able to strengthen their case for Chinese government support, and that far from giving ground to western medicine, this would help Chinese medicine to retain its unique character. In other words, He Lianchen wanted to standardise this aspect of Chinese medicine in order to define it, in the hope that once clearly defined, it could then be effectively defended and propagated. It is easy to see how this might be an effective tactic in the then current atmosphere of widespread scientism in China, and antipathy towards such 'old and corrupt' elements of Chinese culture as Chinese medicine, with its associations of unhygienic practices and superstition.[19] It is also fairly easy for us to see that this kind of medical innovation created a Chinese medicine that was very largely a new invention.

In any case, He Lianchen's approach to the modernisation of Chinese case records, which he promoted in the pages of the *Shaoxing Journal of Medicine and Pharmacy*, won the approval of many of his colleagues. As we have seen, Ding Ganren gave permission for He Lianchen to rewrite his (Ding's) case records to accord with the new standard format. Ding was not only a famous and respected traditional physician, but was also a co-founder of the only government-licensed college of Chinese medicine, the Shanghai Technical College of Chinese Medicine (*Shanghai zhongyi zhuanmen xuexiao* 上海中醫專門學校).[20]

He Lianchen did not only rewrite Ding Ganren's case records into case histories; he also took case records from the famous and venerable physicians of the medical

---

[18] Summarised in Shi Ji and Su Mincai (1994), 150. For specifics, see Xia Yingtang's 夏應堂 (1871–1936) preface to He Lianchen ((1927) 1969), 1–2, and He's own preface, pp. 3–4.

[19] For evidence of this scientism and associated vilification of Chinese medicine, see Croizier (1968), 70–80, and Kwok (1965), *passim*.

[20] Zhao Hongjun (1989), 142–5. The government licence was issued by oversight by the Ministry of Education during the administrative chaos of the Beiyang period, in 1915. Ding's school was therefore the only college of Chinese medicine licensed by central government until the 1930s.

classics and reorganised them under his new rubrics. What were the consequences of
this reorganisation?

First of all, the prescription. In the first example above, we are just given the name of
the prescription, without being told where it comes from, or what its constituents were.
The presumption seems to have been that well-educated *literati* would have memorised
sufficient medical texts to at least recognise the provenance of the prescription, so that
even if they did not have its contents off by heart, they would at least know where to look
it up. By contrast, the systematically reorganised case history contains very detailed
information about the contents of the prescription, not only naming every drug, but
also giving the relative proportions used. Very often, even the prescriptions given in
the classic texts did not give drug proportions. This, then, is one way in which He
Lianchen's innovative use of western-style systematisation in case records resulted in
the creation of a new corpus of standardised prescriptions. The two versions of Ding
Ganren's case exemplify this nicely.

Secondly, by insisting on the rubric 'therapy' (*liaofa* 療法), He Lianchen was insisting on the relevance of theory to practice. One of the most frequently cited opinions
about Chinese medicine in this period was that Chinese medical theory was unscien-
tific and full of superstition. Several of the most prominent Chinese physicians of the
time, including He Lianchen himself, and also Ding Ganren, Zhang Xichun 張錫純
(1860–1933), and Zhu Weiju 祝味菊 (1884–1951) avoided referring to the Five Phases
(*wuxing* 五行) in their writings. This was not just because they were afraid of being
criticised by others – they genuinely believed that a modern Chinese medicine would
be better off without this particular theory, which they regarded as an obsolete relic.

For instance, in a 1940 collection of Chinese medical case histories by a leading
advocate of medical syncretism, Shi Jinmo 施今墨 (1884–1968) neatly encapsulated
prevailing attitudes in the 'Organising Principles' (Fanli 凡例) section at the front of the
book:

• This book is organised according to the categories of western medicine, for convenience of reference.
• The systematic organisation of this book is exceptionally clear, and there is also no
  mention of the mysterious theories of the Five Phases, so it is very suitable for patients
  to consult for themselves.[21]

Many people, following the Japanese example, would have happily done away with
it all, retaining only the drugs and prescriptions for use based on simple empirical

---

[21] Shi Jinmo ((1940) 1994). In Lu Zheng (1990), 967–1103 at p. 971.

observations of their effectiveness. Others stressed the need for chemical and pharma-cological analysis of Chinese drugs, so that they could be used as alternatives to western drugs, but within a western-medical theoretical framework. This would in effect have meant the creation of western drugs out of Chinese prescriptions, lifting Chinese phar-macy out of its theoretical context. This was the option favoured by Yu Yan 余巖, styled Yunxiu 雲岫 (1879–1954), who is notorious for having tried to pass a law forbidding the practice of Chinese medicine in 1929.[22] Yet others defended the Five Phases in the name of preserving the essential elements of Chinese culture in the face of encroaching westernisation. They, too, found it necessary to redefine what Five Phases theory was to mean for Chinese medicine. For example, two of the articles in Wang Shenxuan's 王慎軒 1932 compilation of new essays in Chinese medicine redefine the Five Phases: the first as different kinds of force; electrical, electrostatic, gravitational, heat, and chemical attraction; the second explains them as metaphors for the seasons.[23]

By insisting that Chinese-medical physicians explain their reasons for employing a particular therapy, He Lianchen was defending the relevance of Chinese-medical views of the etiology of disease, at the same time as defining the terms on which comparisons between Chinese and western medicine should be made. The same point can also be made about his use of the rubric 'causes of disease' (*bingyin*).

Finally, these new case histories were organised under their respective disease names (*bingming*) rather than by their symptoms or symptom-complexes (*zheng* 症), indicat-ing a perceived need to classify Chinese disease entities in such a way that they could be meaningfully compared with western disease terms.

He Lianchen's new format for Chinese-medical case histories, first published as a compilation of model case histories in book form in 1927, was followed in 1931 by Zhang Xichun 張錫純. The case records in the first five instalments of Zhang's famous book *Yixue zhong zhong can xi lu* 醫學衷中參西錄 (The Assimilation of Western to Chinese in Medicine), published serially from 1918, had been detailed examples of the didactic kind of case record, usually also specifying the exact proportions of the drugs in each prescription. This level of detail was necessary because about half of the prescriptions listed by Zhang were his own inventions. Starting with the sixth instal-ment, published in 1931, Zhang further modernised his case records, changing the format to western-style case histories with clearly demarcated headings almost ident-ical to those proposed by He Lianchen. As the title of Zhang Xichun's work suggests, his aim was to use western medicine to justify and confirm Chinese medicine, but for

---

[22] Jin Shiying (1993).
[23] See Wang Shenxuan ((1932) 1992), 33–40: essays by Yuan Fuchu 袁復初 and Yun Tieqiao 惲鐵樵.

him as for He, to do this it was necessary to redefine just what should count as Chinese medicine.[24]

   To summarise, we see that an attempt to identify and standardise the essential features of Chinese medicine resulted in quite large changes to its theory and practice. I would like to argue that the Chinese-medical community gained more than it lost. At a time when attempts were being made to standardise many aspects of Chinese society – the standardisation of pronunciation in order to create a national language, the creation of a single national currency, and the adoption of international weights and measures all spring to mind – standards had to be found by which Chinese physicians and Chinese-medical practice could be assessed. A Chinese-medicine based on secret remedies and individual reputations was not consistent or measurable enough to count as modern or scientific. By adapting the genre of Chinese case records (*yi'an* 醫案) into the western case history model of describing disease (*bing'an* 病案). He Lianchen and his colleagues in the late 1920s and early 1930s not only provided a useful standard around which to organise medical practice and teaching, but they also created a theoretical framework which encouraged, and to some extent presupposed, theoretical coherence. As Elisabeth Hsu has observed, for Chinese medicine to have any chance of counting as sufficiently 'scientific' in the new China, it had first to be systematised and made internally consistent.[25] The reworking of case records into western-style case histories in the Republican period was one part of this creation of internal consistency.

Appendix: Ding Ganren's case of 'throat-pox' in Chinese

1. Original, 'case record' genre

喉痧壯熱畏寒滴水難咽

傳左。年廿余歲。患喉痧八天，壯熱無汗，微有畏寒，痧麻隱約，布而不顯，面色紫暗，咽喉腫腐，滴水難咽，煩躁泛惡，日夜不安。傳氏數房，僅此一子，老母少妻，哭泣求救。余曰：症雖凶險，正氣未敗，尚可換回。診其脈鬱數不揚，舌苔膩黃。閱前服之方，竟是滋陰清肺湯等類。隨投透痧解毒湯，加枳實、竹茹，一日夜服兩劑，兼刺少商出血，開閉泄火。服藥後，即得暢

---

[24] For Zhang's adoption of the western-style case-history format, see Zhang Xichun ((1918–34) 1984). Publication dates of successive instalments are noted in the editor's preface. For Zhang's biographical details, see Zhao Hongjun (1991), 214–18. Zhang is almost certain to have learned most of his western medicine from Japanese medical textbooks, since he was living in Shenyang, the capital of the Japanese informal empire in Manchuria at this time.

[25] Hsu (1999), 186–98.

汗，痧麻漸布，面色轉紅，咽喉腫腐亦減。連進數劑，三四日即愈。喉痧之症，有汗則生，驗之信然。

2. *As rewritten as a modern 'case history' by He Lianchen*

風毒喉痧案

病者：　傅君。年廿余歲。住上海塘山路

病名：　風毒喉痧

病因：　傳染而得，已有八天。前醫之方，皆是養陰清肺湯等。

症候：　壯熱無汗，微有畏寒，痧麻隱約，布而不顯，面色紫暗，咽喉腫腐，滴水難咽，煩躁泛惡，日夜不安。

診斷：　脈鬱數不揚，舌苔黃膩。余曰：此喉痧誤認白喉也。傅氏數房，僅此一子，老母少妻，哭泣求救。余對之曰：症雖凶險，正氣未敗，上可換回。

療法：　隨投透痧解毒湯，加枳實、竹茹，疏達開豁，兼刺少商出血，開閉泄火。

處方：　荊芥穗 錢半　淨蟬衣 八分　粉葛根 二錢　青連翹 二錢　紫背浮萍 三錢　炒牛蒡 二錢　灸僵蚕 三錢　嫩射乾 一錢　輕馬勃 八分（包煎）小枳實 錢半　鮮竹茹 二錢　生甘草 五分　前胡 錢半。

效果：　一日夜服兩劑後，即得暢汗，痧麻漸布，面色轉紅，咽喉腫腐亦減。連進數劑，三四日即愈。喉痧之症，有汗則生，驗之信然。

References

Andrews, Bridie J. 1997. 'Tuberculosis and the Assimilation of Germ Theory in China, 1895–1937'. *Journal of the History of Medicine and Allied Sciences* 52, 114–57.

Croizier, Ralph C. 1968. *Traditional Medicine in Modern China: Science, Nationalism and the Tensions of Cultural Change*. Harvard University Press, Cambridge, Mass.

Ding Ganren 丁甘仁 (n.d.) *Housha zhengzhi gai yao* 喉痧症治概要 (Essentials of Throat-rash Symptoms and Treatment). In Lu Zheng 1994, 565–84.

Farquhar, Judith 1992. 'Time And Text: Approaching Chinese Medical Practice through Analysis of a Published Case'. In Leslie and Young, 62–73.

He Lianchen 何廉臣 (1927) 1969. *Zhongguo mingyi yan'an leibian* 中國名醫驗案類編 (Classified Case Histories by Famous Chinese Physicians). Minglang chubanshe, Hong Kong.

He Shixi 何時希 1991. 'Menghe Ding shi sandai mingyi' 孟河丁氏三代名醫 (Three Generations of Famous Physicians of the Ding Family from Menghe). In Shanghaishi wenshi ziliao weiyuanhui (Shanghai Literary and Historical Materials Committee), 1–11.

He Shutian 何書田 1994. *Qingdai mingyi He Shutian yi'an* 清代名醫何書田醫案 (Case Records of the Famous Qing Dynasty Physician He Shutian). Shanghai kexue jishu chubanshe, Shanghai.

Hsu, Elisabeth 1999. *The Transmission of Chinese Medicine*. Cambridge University Press, Cambridge.

Jin Shiying 1993. 'Riben fan feizhi Han fang [kanpō] yu Zhongguo fan feizhi zhongyi zhi douzheng ji qi bijiao' 日本反廢止漢方與中國反廢止中醫之鬪爭及其比較 (Comparison of the Japanese and Chinese Opposition to the Abolition of Traditional Medicine). *Zhonghua yishi zazhi* 中華醫史雜誌 23, 45–51.

Kwok, David W. Y. 1965. *Scientism in Chinese Thought, 1900–1950*. Yale University Press, New Haven.

Leslie, Charles and Young, Allan (eds.) 1992. *Paths to Asian Medical Knowledge*. University of California Press, Berkeley.

Lu Zheng 陸拯 (ed.) 1990. *Jindai zhongyi zhenben ji: yi'an fence* 近代中醫珍本集：醫案分冊 (Valuable Works of Modern Chinese Medicine: Medical Case Records). Zhejiang kexue jishu chubanshe, Hangzhou.

    1994. *Jindai zhongyi zhenben ji: wu guan ke fence.* 近代中醫珍本集：五官科分冊 (Valuable Works of Modern Chinese Medicine: Volume on the Five Sense Organs). Zhejiang kexue jishu chubanshe, Hangzhou.

Ou Ming 1989. *Chinese–English Manual Of Common-Used [Drugs] in Traditional Chinese Medicine*. Joint Publishing (H.K.), Hong Kong.

Quanguo zhongyi tushu lianhe mulu 全國中醫圖書聯合目錄 (Chinese National Union Catalogue of Library Holdings in Chinese Medicine) 1991. Zhongguo zhougi yanjiuyuan tushuguan 中國中醫研究院圖書館. Zhongyi guji chubanshe, Beijing.

Shanghaishi wenshi ziliao weiyuanhui 上海文史資料委員會 (eds.) 1991. *Haishang yilin* 海上醫林 (Physicians of Shanghai). Shanghai renmin chubanshe, Shanghai.

Shi Ji 施杞 and Su Mincai 蕭敏材 1994. *Zhongyi bing'an xue* 中醫病案學 (Study of Chinese Medical Case Histories). Zhongguo baike quanshu chubanshe, Shanghai.

Shi Jinmo 施今墨 (1940) 1994. 'Shi Jinmo yi'an' 施今墨醫案 (Shi Jinmo's Case Records). In Lu Zheng, 967–1103.

Shi Nianzu 石念祖 (1919) 1957. *Wangshi yi'an yizhu* 王氏醫案繹注 (Wang [Shixiong]'s Case Records, Annotated and Explained). Shangwu yinshuguan, Shanghai.

Wang Shenxuan 王慎軒 (1932) 1992. *Zhongyi xinlun huibian* 中醫新論匯編 (Compilation of New Essays in Chinese Medicine). Shanghai shuju, Shanghai.

Wang Xinhua 王新華 1993. *Zhongguo lidai yi'an xuan* 中醫歷代醫案選 (Selected Medical Case Records in Chinese History). Jiangsu kexue jishu chubanshe, Nanjing.

Zhang Xiaoping 張笑平 1991. *Xiandai zhongyi gejia xueshuo* 現代中醫各家學説 (Doctrines of Modern Chinese Medical Physicians). Zhongguo zhongyi chubanshe, Beijing.

Zhang Xichun 張錫純 (1918–34) 1984. *Yixue zhong zhong can xi lu* 醫學表中參西錄 (The Assimilation of Western to Chinese in Medicine). 3 vols. Hebei kexue jishu chubanshe, Shijiazhuang.

Zhao Hongjun 趙洪鈞 1989. *Jindai zhongxiyi lunzheng shi* 近代中西醫論爭史 (History of the Polemics between Modern Chinese and Western Medicine). Anhui kexue jishu chubanshe, Hefei.

Zhao Hongjun 趙洪鈞 1991. 'Zhang Xichun nianpu' 張錫純年譜 (Chronological Biography of [the Life of] Zhang Xichun). *Zhonghua yishi zazhi* 中華醫史雜誌 21, 214–18.

Zhongyao dacidian 中藥大辭典 (Encyclopaedic Dictionary of Chinese *Materia Medica*) 1986. Jiangsu xinyi xueyuan 江蘇新醫學院 (eds.). Shanghai kexue jishu chubanshe, Shanghai.

PART VI

Medical rationale in the People's Republic

Introduction

If one accepts that Chinese medicine was canonised by the elite of the Western Han when the Imperial bureaucracy first became institutionalised, one would expect that with the abdication of the last Emperor in 1911 and the political repercussions that preceded and followed it, medical practice and doctrine would have been, like other aspects of Chinese society, subject to drastic transformation. Twentieth-century China saw the fall of the Empire, feuds between warlords, the institution of a Republican government (1928–37), the Sino-Japanese War from 1937 to 1945, the ensuing civil war, the victory of the Communists in 1949 and the building up of a Socialist state, which at intervals was shaken by nation-wide mass movements and drastic economic reforms. This testifies to a century of social upheaval. Indeed, traditional Chinese historiography gives a picture of continuity until 1911, interrupted occasionally by the rise and fall of dynastic houses, and historians of the PRC, or for that matter also some Western ones, are inclined to view the political changes occurring this century as more dramatic than any previous ones. Nevertheless, it is doubtful whether the two thousand years preceding it were by comparison more stable: the articles in this final section highlight both radical changes and continuities with the past.

In the first half of the twentieth century, initiatives of Chinese physicians to institutionalise Chinese medicine were not infrequent but remained localised, and despite governmental promotion Western medical provisions remained fairly limited. Both Chinese and Western medical doctors aimed at forming their own profession of elite medicine, but with varying success.[1] It was only in the second half of the twentieth

---

[1] Andrews, Bridie J. (1996), 'The Making of Modern Chinese Medicine, 1895–1937', PhD thesis in History, University of Cambridge. See also Croizier, Ralph C. (1968), *Traditional Medicine in Modern China: Science, Nationalism, and the Tensions of Cultural Change*, Harvard University Press, Cambridge, Mass.; Zhao Hongjun (1989), *Jindai zhongxi yi lunzheng shi* 近代中西醫論爭史 (History of the Polemics between Chinese and Western Medicine in Modern Times), Anhui ke xue ji shu chubanshe, Hefei; and Ma Boying et al. (1993), *Zhongwai yixue wenhua jiaoliu shi* 中外醫學文化交流史 (The History of Intercultural Medicine Communication between China and Foreign Countries), Wenhui chubanshe, Shanghai.

century, after the Communist government had established itself and could ensure state control throughout its territory, that it was possible, alongside large-scale implementation of Western medicine, to institutionalise Chinese medicine on a nation-wide scale, a process which went hand in hand with a reinterpretation of medical doctrine and practice.[2]

Chapter 11, by Kim Taylor, concerns a short-lived doctrine that exemplifies the above conviction that changes in Chinese medicine were more drastic than ever before. She shows that the nation-wide institutionalisation of Chinese medicine in the Socialist state had its beginnings in times of guerrilla warfare in the rural areas of Yan'an (1945–49). Mao Zedong 毛澤東 (1893–1976) had called for the 'co-operation of Chinese and Western medical doctors' (*zhongxi yi hezuo* 中西醫合作) in Yan'an in 1944, using the guidelines of the revolution – new (*xin* 新), scientific (*kexue* 科學), and unified (*tuanjie* 團結) – laid out in the key speech 'On New Democracy' (Xin minzhu zhuyi lun 新民主主義論) in 1940. This meant that the promotion of Chinese medicine under the Communist Party was begun not by traditional doctors but by Western medical doctors who were dedicated Party members.

Zhu Lian 朱璉 (1909–78), a Western medical doctor who at that time was deputy director of the Yan'an China Medical University, was a zealous follower of Mao and in 1951 she published *The New Acumoxa* (Xin zhenjiuxue 新針灸學). Yet by the mid-1950s medical professionals had distanced themselves from this work. Political commitment in Zhu Lian's 'new acumoxa' is obvious, and although Taylor does not suggest this, this may explain why her innovation was ephemeral and why, even if Zhu Lian continues to be mentioned in medical dictionaries, some PRC medical historians have given her scarcely any attention.

Acumoxa was chosen to represent this 'new' medicine because of its practicalities within wartime conditions. Its wide embrace by both Chinese medical practitioners scattered across the base areas and Western medical personnel, meant that it satisfied the criteria of 'unified'. However, it also had to be rendered 'scientific', and Taylor points out how Zhu Lian's political loyalties influenced her choice of science. In particular, Zhu Lian availed herself of the Soviet scientist Pavlov's theory of the higher function of the nervous system (*gaoji shenjing lun xueshuo* 高級神經論學說), to replace the reasoning in terms of *mai* 脈 and *qi* 氣 as explanation for the therapeutic effects of acu-

[2] On medical politics in the PRC, see Lampton, David L. (1977), *The Politics of Medicine in China: the Policy Process 1949–1977*, Dawson, Folkestone. On traditional medicine in government institutions, see Farquhar, Judith (1994), *Knowing Practice: the Clinical Encounter of Chinese Medicine*, Westview, Boulder; Scheid, Volker (1997), 'Synthesis and Plurality in Contemporary Chinese Medicine', PhD thesis in social anthropology, University of Cambridge; and Hsu, Elisabeth (1999), *The Transmission of Chinese Medicine*, Cambridge University Press, Cambridge, 168–223.

moxa. Zhu Lian also approved of the Soviets' 'great discovery' in tissue therapy (*zuzhi liaofa* 組織療法), and disapproved of recent Western researches into cell pathology (*xibao bingli xue* 細胞病理學). The former was said to put emphasis on the collective and the latter on the individual; it thus was associated with the capitalist economies of the West. Likewise, the Communists' ambivalence towards Japan was reflected in Zhu Lian's critical remarks on Japanese research into Chinese medicine.

Political motivation is also reflected in Zhu Lian's portrayal of the body. She did away with the concept of the twelve *jingluo* which, linked together, formed a circuit and distributed blood and *qi* throughout the body. Instead, she divided the body into separate sections (*bu* 部), divisions (*qu* 區), and lines (*xian* 線), terms reminiscent of the military jargon then prevalent in the base areas. The most innovative of these were the 'divisions'. In the main they were on the head, neck, and shoulder, and with four or five straight lines they formed polygons, which enclosed a number of stimulation points (*ciji dian* 刺激點). This echoed the social reality of liberated areas (*jiefang qu* 解放區) or border regions (*bianqu* 邊區) and reflected the Communist Party's wartime geography.

To go beyond the investigation of the overtly proclaimed, at the end of the article Taylor analyses Zhu Lian's description of a disease entity, relapsing fever (*huigui re* 回歸熱), and the treatment recommended. In this way, she exposes continuities with the Chinese medical canons and the assimilation of Western medical aetiology. Zhu Lian is thereby revealed to have adopted knowledge for medical practice from sources from which she explicitly distanced herself in the preface. Her new medical theory is shown to be incompatible with medical practice, her medicine internally incoherent.

Taylor's approach follows the permutation of the slogan 'co-operation of Chinese and Western medical doctors' downwards through the social hierarchy from the highest policy making levels, through the intermediate levels of policy interpreters and implementers, and down to the final product itself, medical practice and theory. In this way, she demonstrates how considerations of medical efficiency were subordinated to Party criteria, and it comes as no surprise that the 'new acumoxa' was short-lived.

Volker Scheid's chapter (chapter 12) is a study of Chinese medicine in the PRC fifty years later, and it provides insight into integrated Chinese and Western medicine (*zhongxi yi jiehe* 中西醫結合) as practised in the urban metropole Beijing. His article consists of a comparison of two physicians whom he considers exemplary in respect of their professed attitude towards Western medicine. One was a senior physician who could trace his medical lineage back nine generations and was known to be a more traditionally minded conservative (*baoshou* 保守). The other, a generation younger, belonged among the first to graduate from a college of Traditional Chinese Medicine (TCM) and considered himself a moderniser (*xiandaihua* 現代化). Like most other cadres trained in government colleges, he was not from a family of medical learning, and like many other middle aged cadres of the 1990s, he had been sent, as a young man, down to the village (*xia xiang* 下鄉) and, as a postgraduate, out of the country (*chu guo* 出國). Scheid shows that although the two doctors claimed to have a different attitude to Western medicine, both integrated Western medical rationale into their Chinese medical practice.

The senior physician attributed a condition of what in translation can be approximated as a headache or dizziness (*touyun* 頭暈) not to a depletion of the kidneys (*shenxu* 腎虛), as in textbooks, but to a 'heart disease' (*xinzang bing* 心臟病). The formula he prescribes strengthens the gathering *qi* (*zongqi* 宗氣) in the chest (which includes not only the region of the lungs but also that of the heart). Simultaneously it is a formula that has recently gained in importance for treating biomedically diagnosed heart disease. It is complemented by herbs that are considered to free the blood vessels (*tong mai* 通脈) and in biomedical jargon have a positive effect on blood circulation. Scheid's point is that Chinese medical doctrine does not make blood stasis (*yuxue* 瘀血) responsible for dizziness. Hence the doctor's treatment must be grounded in the Western medical explanation that increased blood circulation reduces dizziness.

The second example also concerns dizziness (*xuanyun* 眩暈), a dizziness that the progressive government-trained doctor attributes to Menière's disease. This younger doctor, who is a specialist for Menière's disease, has developed a formula that is now industrially produced and marketed throughout China and Japan. The formula is derived from reasoning that equates the Chinese notion phlegm (*tan* 痰) to the biomedically recognised fluids of the endolymphatic system in the ear. These fluids are known to increase the endolymphatic pressure in the ear and for reducing this pressure, Western trained doctors attempt to diminish the total amount of body fluids, sometimes by treating Menière's disease with intravenous diuretics. This doctor is shown to have added to a formula for directing down *qi* (*jiang qi* 降氣) and transforming phlegm (*hua tan* 化痰) an ingredient that is known to enhance urinating: Semen Plantaginis (*cheqianzi* 車前子) which 'disinhibits water' (*li shui* 利水). Evidently this doctor understands the Chinese concept *li shui* (disinhibiting water) to embrace the Western notion 'diuresis' and thereby combines Chinese and Western medical rationale in a treatment that, in addition to directing down *qi* and transforming phlegm, enhances urination.

Scheid stresses that such processes of change are individually based. Individual doctors, interested in improving therapeutic efficacy and success, are seen as selecting different treatment strategies and combining them into innovative ones. His two examples show that it is possible to combine medical knowledge effectively across apparently incommensurable paradigms. The vagueness of Chinese medical concepts permits them to include new meanings, and if a complaint allows for an ambiguous interpretation, a doctor can understand a Chinese medical term to embrace the meanings of both the Chinese and the Western medical concept. The two examples that Scheid gives show that Western medical considerations have become part of Chinese medical reasoning and that they can determine the application of Chinese herbs.

Both articles in this part focus on individuals who were eclectic and innovative. They reveal that innovative theories and practices arose not only from integrating the different sources of knowledge that the individuals themselves professed to have used, but also from ways of acting and thinking that were not made explicit. Regardless of the motivation attributed to these individuals, whether it arose from political fervour or individualistic strategies, their innovations were based on selectively combined knowledge and practice. This knowledge and practice came from various Chinese medical lineages and also from different traditions of non-Chinese modern scientific research: Soviet research in the 1950s and Western research since the 1980s. The juxtaposition of the two articles accentuates the contrast between the political engagement in the Communist base areas and the early years of Socialist construction, on the one hand, and the pluralism that marked the urban PRC of the 1990s, on the other. Important changes that have taken place in the PRC are thereby highlighted, while these two accounts with which this book ends also point out continuities with the canonical doctrine.

11

A new, scientific, and unified medicine: civil war in China and the new acumoxa, 1945–49[1]

KIM TAYLOR

The Civil War (1945–49) was the culmination of a twenty-year-long conflict between the Nationalist and Communist Parties in mainland China, which resulted in the unexpected triumph of the militarily inferior Chinese Communist Party (CCP). The CCP, however, possessed a well-structured ideological framework which extended to include large areas of the local populace, and this was to prove a significant advantage over the Nationalist Party. An important period in the development of this ideology had occurred ten years earlier in Yan'an, as pressure both within and without of the CCP forced Mao Zedong 毛澤東 (1893–1976) to strike out from the Soviet-guided faction of the Party and put forward his own interpretation of the direction of the Communist struggle. War with Japan (1937–45), and the deterioration of the United Front with the Nationalist Party (1937–41), threatened the existence of the CCP should it become an isolated force without significant foreign or national backing. This made it necessary by the end of 1939 for Mao to rethink the strategies of the CCP, if they were to succeed in leading China independently from the Nationalist Party. The CCP needed to convince the people in the base areas that they had a policy program capable of guiding China to victory through the present state of war, and capable also of providing a strong and consolidated government in the future. Such a plan for the future was presented by Mao in his key text 'On New Democracy' (Xin minzhu zhuyi lun 新民主主義論), published on 19 January

---

[1] An initial version of this article was first presented at the 8th International Conference on the History of Science in East Asia, held in Seoul, Korea, in August 1996. Since then it has been substantially revised and reworked with the encouragement of Elisabeth Hsu. I am also indebted to Andrew Cunningham, Hans van de Ven, and Bridie Andrews for their valuable comments on earlier versions of this article. The contents of this article constitute the first chapter in my PhD thesis.

1940 in the debut edition of the CCP journal *Zhongguo wenhua* 中國文化 (Chinese Culture).[2]

Mao's concept of the new democratic revolution was to finally give him credence amongst his critics as a viable theoretician, and this text was to define the Communist revolution for the next ten years. The ensuing Rectification Movement (*zheng feng yundong* 整風運動) (1942–43), during which ideological impurities were eliminated from the Party, saw Mao emerge in March 1943 as chairman of the Secretariat and Politburo of the CCP. This rectification campaign placed Mao's words on the Party agenda and served to widen the distribution of Mao's works within the local populace. The sociological effect of this manner of ideological indoctrination was to cause greater allegiance to Mao's thought, and as such the influence of works like 'On New Democracy' was substantial. The Communist principles on which this article is based thus stem from this formative period of Maoist Communism. Society in the base areas was so fraught with revolution that the influence of Mao was to penetrate Party life to the extent that it affected even the medicine itself, as shall be shown later in this article.

In 'On New Democracy' Mao reaffirmed Socialism as the Party's ultimate goal, and appealed to the wider public to join the Communists in their efforts to rebuild China. He defined China's revolutionary path and the role played by the Communist Party in this revolution. Mao stated that 'We want not only to change a politically oppressed and economically exploited China into a politically free and economically prosperous China, but also to change a China which has been ignorant and backward under the rule of the old culture into a China that will be enlightened and progressive under the rule of a new culture. In a sentence, we want to build up a new China'.[3] Mao was thus suggesting not merely political and economic reform, but an entire upheaval of cultural roots to produce a free-thinking and independent 'new democratic culture' which would transform Chinese society and give rise to an enlightened and prosperous new China.

In Mao's definition of the creation of this 'new democratic culture', he was to use three words which were to describe its development. These were 'new' (*xin* 新), 'science' (*kexue* 科學), and 'unity' (*tuanjie* 團結). The term 'new' implied free from superstition and the heavy links of a feudal past. Instead the components of the new culture would have to be forward-moving and enterprising. Mao advocated that such

---

[2] Reprinted in Mao Zedong (1952), 633–82. Wylie (1980), 159–60, describes 'On New Democracy' with the words 'as great a work as any Mao was to produce in the future . . . It was offered in 1940 as a polished, comprehensive synthesis of Mao's thinking on the Chinese revolution, and it had a dramatic impact at the time on both Chinese and foreign audiences.' Schram (1989), 101, mentions that 'On New Democracy' was used as a basic study material in political education classes during the early 1950s.

[3] Mao Zedong (1952), 634.

a change would be possible through the use of 'science'. By 'science' Mao was not so much referring to the science linked with the Western interpretation of a quantifiable methodology, but more to the Marxist ideal of science as the criteria for true knowledge. 'Unity' was the third criterion in the building up of a new China. Everybody had to join together and fight for the same cause, and this included all classes of Chinese society, from the upper bourgeoisie to the peasantry, so long as their beliefs were not against those of the Party. It also implied a unity of knowledge, and this had particular implications for the revolutionary intellectual. Mao stated that 'This type of new democratic culture is scientific. It is opposed to all feudal and superstitious ideas; it stands for seeking truth from facts, it stands for objective truth and for unity between theory and practice'.[4]

Four years after his speech 'On New Democracy', Mao's concept of 'unity' within the 'new democratic culture' expanded to include the traditional, folk aspects of the land the Communist Party was occupying. On 30 October 1944 Mao addressed the Shaanxi–Gansu–Ningxia border region with a speech entitled 'The United Front in Cultural Work' (Wenhua gongzuo zhong de tongyi zhanxian 文化工作中的統一戰線). This meeting was to be of great significance to the medical world, and Mao's support of Chinese medicine is today traced back to this speech.[5] Yet this speech was not originally intended to promote the study of Chinese medicine; rather it was delivered to point out some of the conditions in the countryside which were hindering the development of the 'new democratic culture'. And Chinese medicine just so happened to be one of these 'hindering factors'. Mao's strategy in overcoming these factors was to 'unite' with them, and 'remould' them, so that they could become part of the revolutionary movement, and not stand in the way of it.

In this speech Mao pointed out that although work towards constructing a 'new democratic culture' had already begun in the revolutionary base areas (*geming genjudi* 革命根据地), there were still many traces of feudalism remaining. He identified these traces of feudalism as those of illiteracy (*wenmang* 文盲), superstition (*mixin* 迷信), and unhygienic habits (*buweisheng de xiguan* 不衛生的習慣), and he called them 'the enemies inside the minds of the masses' (*qunzhong naozi li de diren* 群眾腦子里的敵人). He complained that, 'It is often more difficult to fight these enemies than to fight the Japanese imperialists. We must tell the masses that they should wage a struggle against their own illiteracy, superstitions and unhygienic habits'.[6] In order to educate the masses in such ways, Mao stressed the need of an united front:

---

[4] Mao Zedong (1952), 679.
[5] Reprinted in Mao Zedong (1953), 1031–3. Croizier (1972), 8, describes this speech as 'legitimising at the highest level' the use of indigenous medicines.
[6] Mao Zedong (1953), 1031.

In the Shaanxi–Gansu–Ningxia border region the mortality rate of men and live-stock is high, and still many of the people believe in witchcraft. In these circumstances, if we only rely on the new medicine (*xinyi* 新醫), we will not be able to solve our problems. Of course the new medicine is superior to the old medicine (*jiuyi* 舊醫), but if they [the doctors of the new medicine] are not concerned about the sufferings of the people, do not train doctors to serve the people and do not unite with the thousand old doctors and veterinarians of the old school in the border region in order to help them to improve, then they will be actually helping the practitioners of witchcraft by callously observing the death of a large number of men and livestock. There are two principles of the united front: one is unity (*tuanjie* 團結) and the other is [comprised of] criticism (*piping* 批評), education (*jiaoyu* 教育) and remoulding (*gaizao* 改造). In forming a united front, capitulation is wrong, and sectarian intolerance and arrogance are also wrong. Our task is to unite with all the old style intellectuals (*jiu zhishifenzi* 舊知識分子), old style artists (*jiu yiren* 舊藝人) and old style doctors (*jiu yisheng* 舊醫生) who can be used, and to help, educate and remould them. In order to remould them we must first unite [with them]. Only if we act appropriately will they welcome our help.[7]

This was one of the few speeches in which Mao addressed the field of medicine before Liberation, and he was referring to both doctors and veterinarians. He never mentioned the term Chinese medicine (*zhongyi* 中醫) in his speech, yet called it the 'old medicine'. Western medicine was the 'new medicine' and the present task was to update the 'old' with the 'new'.[8] However, Mao pointed out that even though the 'new' was clearly superior to the 'old', if the 'new' was unwilling or even unable, to serve the masses, then it was necessary to use the 'old'. Mao wanted a 'broad united front' and this in medical terms meant 'criticising, educating and remoulding' the 'useful' parts of the 'old medicine' to produce a consolidated form of medicine which could satisfy the health needs of the nation. These were the revolutionary guidelines which he presented to medical workers in Yan'an, and medical policy did not become any more specific until the mid-1950s. Yet these few words were to have a huge impact on those members of the Communist Party with a medical background.

Zhu Lian's 'new acumoxa'

Shortly after Mao's speech on 'The United Front in Cultural Work', Yan'an regional government officials called for an informal discussion between Western and Chinese medical doctors of the border region. During this meeting two slogans were formed,

---

[7] Mao Zedong (1953), 1032.
[8] The terms old (*jiu* 舊) and new (*xin* 新) stem from concepts within dialectical materialism. Croizier (1968), 152, relates modern medicine to the 'new antithesis' overcoming the 'old thesis' of Chinese medicine.

namely 'the scientification of Chinese medicine and the popularisation of Western medicine' (*zhongyi kexuehua, xiyi dazhonghua* 中醫科學化，西醫大眾化). These called for Chinese medicine to be better integrated with modern science, and for Western medicine to be brought down to the level of the people, such as in the forms of basic hygiene and sanitation. During this meeting, the Chinese medical doctor Li Dingming 李鼎銘 (1881–1947),[9] who is renowned for healing Mao Zedong and other leading members of the CCP, led the way in calling for cooperation between Chinese and Western medical practicners (*zhongxiyi hezuo* 中西醫合作).[10] At the meeting various folk healers pledged their services to the Communist cause, such as Ma Rulin 馬汝林 (twentieth century), who offered up two secret prescriptions,[11] and Ren Zuotian 任作田 (1886–1950), who offered to teach Western doctors acumoxa so that these Western doctors could better investigate its curing properties.[12] Several doctors signed up after the meeting, including Zhu Lian 朱璉 (1909–78).

Of all the doctors who were to participate in this movement, Zhu Lian's resolve continued until well after Liberation. She was also one of the few to publicise the results of her work,[13] and we are able to study her contribution to this period largely through her book *Xin zhenjiuxue* 新針灸學 (The New Acumoxa),[14] first published by the People's

---

[9]   Ma Boying, Gao Xi, and Hong Zhongli (1993), 575. Ma Boying does not mention Zhu Lian 朱璉 in his description of this period.

[10] The slogan of 'the co-operation between Chinese and Western medical practitioners' is the first in a series of Communist government slogans on the relationship between Chinese and Western medicine. It is interesting to note that the slogans start out advocating 'co-operation'. During the 1950s this slogan changed to that of the uniting of Chinese and Western medicine (*zhongxiyi tuanjie* 中西醫團結), and from the end of the 1950s until today, the slogan has been one of the integration of Chinese and Western medicine (*zhongxiyi jiehe* 中西醫結合). See also Scheid (chapter 12, this volume).

[11] Ma Boying, Gao Xi, and Hong Zhongli (1993), 575.

[12] Guo Shiyu (1989), 292. I have chosen to translate the term *zhenjiu* 針灸 as 'acumoxa', thereby comprising within one term the dual connotations of both acupuncture and moxibustion.

[13] A colleague to Zhu Lian, Lu Zhijun 魯之俊 (1911–), was the head of the Bethune Memorial International Peace Hospital in Yan'an (*Yan'an Baiqiu'en guoji heping yiyuan* 延安白求恩國際和平醫院). He is accredited in her preface as being a strong motivating force in her decision to begin studying acumoxa. Also originally a Western medically trained doctor, Lu Zhijun published the *Xinbian zhenjiuxue* 新編針灸學 (Newly Revised Acumoxa) in July 1950. By June 1956 it was in its fourteenth edition. However, he includes a minimum of medical theory in his book, and therefore is only a peripheral figure in this study of the medicine of the revolution. Few other participants in this new acumoxa movement are recorded in Chinese medical histories of this period. See for example, Xiao Shaoqing (1997), 521–4.

[14] I have only had access to the second edition of her book, published by the Renmin weisheng chubanshe in 1954, and therefore quotes from her work all refer to this second edition. However, the prefaces to the first edition, plus the unique theoretical content of her book, were published in two separate articles in the *Renmin Ribao* 人民日報" (People's Daily). These were 'Myself and Acumoxa' (Wo yu

Publishers in March 1951.[15] *The New Acumoxa* is invaluable to the history of acumoxa in twentieth-century pre-Liberation China, for in her writings Zhu Lian goes into great detail, not only about the theory and application of the 'new acumoxa', but also about her motivation in researching this 'new acumoxa'. The ideas which she puts forward are not necessarily unique to Zhu Lian, but she can be credited with the role of propagator. Zhu Lian's political connections gave her a high profile in the early years of Liberated China, and while her work was later to be much criticised,[16] she can be acknowledged with creating some of the regard with which Chinese medicine came to be treated by Communist leaders.[17]

Zhu Lian was a Western trained doctor who joined the Chinese Communist Party in 1935 and served the Party as deputy leader of the General Health Department of the 129th Division of the Eighth Route Army. During the time of Yan'an (1935–47), Zhu Lian served as Deputy Director of the Yan'an China Medical University (*Yan'an Zhongguo yike daxue* 延安中國醫科大學), Head of the General Health Department Outpatient Section of the Eighteenth Group Army in Yan'an, Advisor on Child Welfare to the People's Government of the Shaanxi–Gansu–Ningxia Border Region, and acted as Head of the People's Government Ministry of Health in the Shaanxi–Hebei–Shandong–Henan Border Region and director of the hospitals in this border region. After Liberation, Zhu Lian was to become Deputy Director of the Maternity and Child Hygiene Section of the Ministry of Health. She was also to become Deputy Director of the Beijing Traditional Chinese Medical Research Institute (*Beijing zhongyi yanjiuyuan* 北京中醫研究院) soon after it was set up in 1955,[18] and head of

---

zhenjiushu 我與針灸術) (14 March 1949) and 'The Importance of Acumoxa Therapeutics and its Principles' (Zhenjiu liaofa de zhongyaoxing ji qi yuanli 針灸療法的重要性及其原理) (17–18 February 1951). All quotes given in my article have been double-checked with these parallel publications and are thus verbatim contained within the first edition, unless otherwise stated. In addition, a student of Zhu Lian's, Tang Xuezheng 唐學正, promoted her work by producing an annotated edition of *The New Acumoxa* (1951). His details, however, cannot be found in modern medical biographies and it would appear that his status as a disciple of Zhu Lian did not enhance his later career.

[15] The publication of *The New Acumoxa* was announced in the *Renmin Ribao* (15 April 1951), 6.

[16] See Zhao Rong ((1956) 1987), 325–6; and Zhao Qinxuan ((1957) 1987), 328–31.

[17] One of her more influential allies was Dong Biwu 董必武 (1886–1975), chairman of the Finance and Economic Committee of the Huabei People's Government (1948–49), who encouraged her to take her manuscript to Beijing for publication (see second preface in *The New Acumoxa*). Dong Biwu also penned an introductory preface to her book, praising her research work on acumoxa.

[18] Lu Zhijun was at the same time to become director of the Beijing Traditional Chinese Medical Research Institute. Such a position appears to have been granted more through his political leanings than his medical prowess, for his education in Chinese medicine was informal and he was not a prolific writer.

the Acumoxa Research Centre at the same school. She held these positions until 1960 when she was transferred to the Guangxi Autonomous Region to work in the public health service.[19]

Western medical resources available to the Communist Party were extremely limited during the Civil War.[20] By 1945 there were five main medical teaching schools serving the CCP in the revolutionary base areas. These were the Yan'an China Medical University set up in 1940 in Yan'an, the North-east Pharmaceutical College (*Dongbei yao xueyuan* 東北藥學院) set up in 1942 in Yan'an, the Shaanxi–Chahar–Hebei Bethune Hygiene School (*Jin Cha Ji Baiqiu'en weisheng xuexiao* 晉察冀白求恩衛生學校) set up in 1939 in the Shaanxi–Chahar–Hebei military region, the New Fourth Army Military Medical School (*Xin sijun junyi xuexiao* 新四軍軍醫學校) set up in 1945 in Shandong province, and the Yan'an Outskirts Medical College (*Yanbian yike zhuanmen xuexiao* 延邊醫科專門學校) set up on the borders of Yan'an in 1945.[21] These schools all produced Western medical trained doctors to work in the revolutionary base areas. Between 1939 and 1945 the Bethune Hygiene School trained 928 medical workers, only 386 of whom were army doctors.[22] In order to supplement these numbers, short-term training programs were set up in every military region, however, the number of adequately trained doctors remained desperately small. Hospital facilities were to be found dotted across the base areas, and the *History of China's Military Medicine* gives a total of eighty-two Western medical hospitals serving the CCP in the five main military regions.[23] The first department of acumoxa to serve the Communist areas was opened in April 1945 at the Yan'an Bethune International Peace Hospital.[24]

Zhu Lian stayed in Yan'an until 1947. Then she moved to Pingshan county in the Huabei Military Region,[25] where she became the first deputy director of the Huabei People's Government's Ministry of Health (*Huabei renmin zhengfu weishengbu* 華北人民政府衛生部) and in the following year set up the Huabei Health School. Here

---

[19] These details are taken from *Zhongyi renmin cidian* (1988), 172; and Huang Wendong (1983), 260–1. It would appear that she was transferred to Guangxi province to accompany her husband.

[20] Details of the CCP's health care administrative program in the Shaanxi–Gansu–Ningxia border region are given by Hsia (1972), 109–35. A more general account is given by Minden (1979), 299–315.

[21] Zhu Chao and Zhang Weifeng (1990), 2–4.

[22] Liu Liangfu (1989), 36. [23] Gao Yaoguo (1996b), 335. [24] Guo Shiyu (1989), 292.

[25] This coincided with the move of the Military Health Section (*Junwei weishengbu* 軍委衛生部) to the city of Xibopo 西柏坡 in Pingshan county in Hebei province. The Huabei military region was a new North China Liberated Area, formed from the amalgamation of the two border regions, the Shaanxi–Chahar–Hebei region and the Shaanxi–Hebei–Shandong–Hebei region in May 1948. This became the new centre, after the flight from Yan'an, for the Communist's military, governmental, and Party organs in North China. Taken from Gao Yaoguo (1996a), 315–18.

she combined teaching with the scientific research of acumoxa. Zhu Lian was generally known as a tireless worker, who despite frequent cases of ill health, would rarely take leave off work. She propagated acumoxa wherever she went.[26] The Huabei Health School offered short-term training courses including maternity and child hygiene, and midwifery. Each course included a class in acumoxa. Students with either Western or Chinese medical backgrounds had to have a minimum of three years medical experience. Those taking a full-time course in acumoxa were also taught aspects of Western medicine such as the basics of anatomy and physiology, hygiene and sanitation, pathology and diagnostics.[27] The acumoxa classes were taught mainly by Zhu Lian. She had no teaching materials available, but worked from an outline provisionally compiled, and made notes as she taught. Together with a group of editors whom she lists in the preface to her book, Zhu Lian compiled *The New Acumoxa*, completing the final draft in the summer of 1949.

The military metaphor in Zhu Lian's description of the body

By the time *The New Acumoxa* was completed, the Communists had won the Civil War. From the inception of the concept of a 'new acumoxa' to its handing over in book form to the publishers, China was at war with itself. In fact, from the time the Communists were forced into the countryside in 1927 to their eventual triumph in 1949, there were twenty-two years of unmitigated military struggle. The first generation of leaders of the CCP were the generals of the People's Army in pre-Liberation China, and Mao Zedong rose to power in the Party when the existence of the Party could no longer be negotiated through diplomatic tactics but instead had to rely on military tactics.[28] Thus the administration of war was integral to the administration of government over the revolutionary base areas. American political records note that 'the organisation of the Chinese Communist Army is closely linked with the political organisation of the Communist Party and the political organisation of the territory controlled by the Communists'.[29] The Communist Party's position during these years has been described as 'existing in significant measure as a soul or parasite in the body of the army'.[30] However, the last

---

[26] Professor Li Jingwei 李經緯 of the Research Institute for the History of Chinese Medicine and Medical Literature at the Chinese Medical Research Academy (*Zhongguo zhongyi yanjiuyuan, Zhongguo yishi wenxian yanjiusuo* 中國中醫研究院，中國醫史文獻研究所) in Beijing; interview, 7 November 1997.

[27] Zhu Lian (1954), xvii.

[28] Saich (1996), xliii, points out that military leaders were the first to support Mao and propel him up the Party ranks. Their support came through their identification with, and approval of, Mao's military strategies.

[29] van Slyke (1968), 182.   [30] Schram (1989), 44.

four years of Civil War were especially intense, as the number of peasants involved in the CCP movement increased and radical social reforms caused conflict within the structure of villages in the border regions. Such military circumstances influenced the make-up of the 'new acumoxa'.

War was thus a part of life in the revolutionary base areas. To such an extent, in fact, that it was classified as 'work'.[31] If war was such a major theme of life during the years 1945–49, then it would seem that much of society must have been affected by it, including medicine. Zhu Lian described acumoxa as a weapon (*wuqi* 武器) for launching (*kaibi* 開辟) sanitation work in the countryside.[32] In his postscript to Zhu Lian's death, her fellow colleague Lu Zhijun used similar analogies to illustrate the revolutionary fervour with which he perceived their role in utilising acumoxa to serve the Party. His language was rich with symbolism of the medical battle field in which acumoxa was on the offensive. Scientification he described as revolutionary (*gemingxing* 革命性) when he said 'Physiology and pathology are rich in the revolutionary theory of neuro-pathology' (*shengli binglixue shang fu you gemingxing de shenjing bingli xueshuo* 生理病理學上富有革命性的神經病理學説). He also described acumoxa as a 'powerful weapon which combats disease' (*tong jibing zuo douzhengde you li wuqi* 同疾病作斗爭的有力武器).[33] In this way acumoxa is portrayed as playing not only a very revolutionary but also a militant role in the battle for Liberation.

These military metaphors are no coincidence. They are the imprint of a new society on an old medicine. The medicine of correspondence with which we are familiar today was first arranged into a coherent system during the last three centuries BC. Soon after China had been united under the first Emperor, reforms were imposed to link all parts of China and have it function as a standardised, interrelated whole. Just as a new system of government was formed, so were new technologies and philosophies. Each influenced the other, and vocabulary was shared. Paul Unschuld explains that 'the symbolic value of the newly structured social and economic environment may have been significant enough to have been transferred, consciously or unconsciously, by thinkers concerned with health and illness to an understanding of structure and function of the human organism; hence the physiological and pathological basis of the medicine of systematic correspondence accurately reflected these structural innovations'.[34] And in this context Unschuld, for example, translates the *zang* (臟) and *fu* (腑) as 'depots or granaries' and 'palaces',[35] thus assigning these bodily structures a functional position in the social administration of the body. Nathan Sivin links the social body of Chinese medicine not only with the state, but also with the cosmos to prove that the conceptualisation of the

---

[31] Schurmann (1966), 425.   [32] Zhu Lian (1954), xviii.   [33] Lu Zhijun (1987), 323–5.
[34] Unschuld (1985), 80.   [35] Unschuld (1985), 81.

body at this time is intimately linked with the conceptualisation of the state and of the universe in general. He writes that the 'Political and somatic microcosms resonate in harmony with the macrocosm because the ensemble of dynamic processes circulate *qi* (氣) throughout all three. The influence runs not only downward but upward, and between state and body as well'.[36] In this way cognisance of the cosmos contained a similar mental framework to the man-made systems of government administration and the understanding of the functioning of the human body.

The perception of the body as a reflection of bureaucratic structure is shown in the famous chapter 3, section 8 of the *Huangdi neijing Suwen* 黃帝內經素問 (Basic Questions in the Yellow Emperor's Inner Canon), where internal body parts are ascribed a bureaucratic role in the functioning unit of the body.[37] The hierarchy of the government administration is thus apparent, and relevant, in the hierarchy of the governing of the body. Elaborations of government administrative analogies that border on military strategical reasoning are given by Erhard Rosner. They concern, for example, the similarities between treating external and internal diseases both in the body and in the nation.[38] Thus the classical term for government (*zhi* 治) is homophonous, and to a certain extent synonymous, with the term to cure (*zhi* 治). In other words, a disease is cured by restoring internal harmonies and a country is governed by keeping harmony within itself.[39] Rosner also discusses how a disorder on the surface of the body is not considered as serious as a disorder of one of the core internal organs. In the same way, disorder in a key state is much more serious than disorder in a peripheral state.[40]

With the passage of time, despite continuing to be rooted in a government system which encouraged the perpetuation of the ancient medical texts, the terminology used has lost much of its original meaning. Thus the same terms are being used but they are no longer being read with the same force, and although communicating the same medical meaning, they are no longer connected to the same social and philosophical innuendos. As the old social system falls away, a new system replaces it and in such a situation, the old medicine is put to new uses. As it is put to new uses, it will carry the values, customs, hierarchy, and vocabulary of the new society, for whose purposes it is being reshaped. This can mean that either the old vocabulary will have new meanings, or there will be some new vocabulary as well. The terms organs (*zang* 臟) and bowels (*fu* 腑) in TCM no longer have the connotations of the pre-Han bureaucratic roles of 'depots and granaries' or 'palaces'. Doctors in contemporary China tend to compare

---

[36] Sivin (1995), 25.   [37] *Huangdi neijing Suwen, juan 3, pian 8*, 56–7.   [38] Rosner (1991), 22.
[39] Likewise the term for illness (*bing* 病) can mean disorder in both a governing state and the human body. See Hsu (this volume).
[40] Rosner (1991), 22–31.

them with the organs (*zangqi* 臟器) described in Western biomedicine. Elisabeth Hsu points out that such direct translations, however, fail to represent their functional and spacial interrelatedness, which she compares with that of the interrelatedness of 'compartments' within an administrative unit, such as the Socialist work unit (*danwei* 單位). Such a conceptualisation of the Chinese medical terms of *zang* and *fu* stresses their existence in relation with one another, a connection which cannot be derived from the Western biomedical model.[41]

The New Acumoxa is rich in terms such as 'division of labour' (*fengong* 分工), 'leadership' (*lingdao* 領導), 'to allocate' (*zhipei* 支配), 'to regulate' (*tiaojie* 調節), and 'to command' (*zhihui* 指揮). Such terms were interchangeable with the military and administrative terms of the day. This can be seen for example in the phrase 'to appropriately allocate the working force' (*heli zhipei laodongli* 合理支配勞動力) and Zhu Lian's 'to be allocated by the nervous system' (*you shenjing xitong zhipei* 由神經係統支配). However, although administrative metaphors are evident, Zhu Lian's military metaphors are more distinct in this medicine. The military slogans of 'everything [to be done] for victory at the front line' (*yiqie weile qianxian shengli* 一切為了前線胜利) and 'the inner sections and the outer sections of the army units in the liberated areas' (*zai jiefangqu junduei de neibu he waibu* 在解放區軍隊的內部和外部) and also 'to thoroughly exterminate the Japanese invaders' (*chedi xiaomie Riben qinlüe zhe* 澈底消滅日本侵略者)[42] all contain vocabulary which are 'borrowed' by Zhu Lian to describe key features in her medicine. Zhu Lian describes the body as 'a unified and complete entity characterised by division of labour and leadership' (*you fengong you lingdao de tongyi de wanzhengti* 有分工有領導的統一的完整體)[43] and here the parallel is obvious for Zhu Lian is attributing a state of health to a physiological system which functions through an administration of 'division of labour' and 'leadership'.

The representation of the body in *The New Acumoxa* uses a large military and political vocabulary, which in itself is a direct reflection on the society of the revolutionary base areas.[44] Zhu Lian divided the human body into sections (*bu* 部), marked by lines (*xian* 線), and into divisions (*qu* 區). The 'sections' to which Zhu Lian refers can be alikened to an army unit or a government ministry. For example, army troops (*budui* 部隊), the department of health (*weishengbu* 衛生部), the inner section (*neibu* 內部), and the outer section (*waibu* 外部). The term 'division' to which Zhu Lian refers abounds in military allegory. There are the liberated areas (*jiefangqu* 解放區), the military areas

---

[41] Hsu (1999), 206–10. [42] Mao Zedong (1953), 1078.
[43] Zhu Lian (1954), 11. This wording is given only in the second edition.
[44] Saich (1996), xliv, writes that 'the military nature of the Chinese revolution has deeply affected the language of the CCP. While Marxism . . . is punctuated by the language of struggle, particularly that of class, the terminology of the CCP is one of war.'

(*junqu* 軍區), or border areas (*bianqu* 邊區). The term 'lines', too, was used regularly in military and political jargon. There were the interior lines (*neixian* 內線) and the exterior lines (*waixian* 外線), the front line (*qianxian* 前線), the united front line (*tongyi zhanxian* 統一戰線), and many more. Although, as has already been described, the usage of administrative and governmental terms in medicine is by no means novel, the large proportion of military terms is a result of the intensity of war in the revolutionary base areas, and as such is of particular relevance to the study of medicine in this period.

The body is not portrayed as a whole, and makes no allusion to 'holism'. Instead Zhu Lian presents the body in sections and depicts each of these separately. She divides the body into eight sections. In the table of contents to her book she lists a head and neck section (*toujingbu* 頭頸部), back and shoulder section (*beibu ji jianjiabu* 背部及肩胛部), chest section (*xiongbu* 胸部), abdominal section (*fubu* 腹部), two lateral (*ce* 側)[45] chest and abdominal sections (*xiongfubu* 胸腹部), upper limbs section (*shangzhibu* 上肢部) and lower limbs section (*xiazhibu* 下肢部). The body is then further subdivided into divisions. Again, there are eight divisions in all – the eye division (*yanqu* 眼區), ear division (*erqu* 耳區), mouth and nose division (*koubiqu* 口鼻區), temple division (*niequ* 顳區), cheek division (*jiaqu* 頰區), front of the neck division (*jingqianqu* 頸前區), back of the neck division (*jinghouqu* 頸后區), and shoulder division (*jianjiaqu* 肩胛區).

The divisions are a concept unusual to Chinese medicine. While previous Chinese medical reformers such as Cheng Dan'an 承澹庵 (1899–1957) had also portrayed the body in sections and presented them separately, in general they adhered to the theory of twelve individual channels (*jingluo* 經絡) of *qi* running along the length of the body.[46] Zhu Lian did not organise her acumoxa points[47] along such channels. In areas of the body where there was a cluster of acumoxa points which were difficult to arrange on lines, she enclosed the area with a number of joined, straight lines and called it a division. For example, the temple division (*niequ* 顳區) contains acumoxa points, from different channels, all found within the temple area. These are *touwei* 頭維 (stomach 8), *lugu* 率谷 (gall bladder 8), *hanyan* 頷厭 (gall bladder 4), *xuanlu* 懸顱 (gall bladder 5), *xuanli* 懸厘 (gall bladder 6), *shangguan* 上關 (gall bladder 3) and *taiyang* 太陽 (point outside the tract version).[48] The concept of division appears analogous to the unique

[45] The term *ce* 側 is also a specialist military term meaning 'flank', such as *ceji* 側擊, 'to make a flank attack'.
[46] In Cheng Dan'an (1932). More about his reforms can be found in Andrews (1996), 273–80, and Lu Gwei-djen and Needham (1980), 9–10.
[47] *xuewei* 穴位, translation discussed below, in note 58.
[48] Such a numbering system complies with a later international standardisation of acumoxa points and can be found, for example, in the index of Zhenjiu gaiyao bianji xiaozu (1964).

Communist innovation of a base area, described as 'central to the Chinese approach to rural revolution and guerrilla warfare'.[49]

Those acumoxa points which were not arranged in divisions were then arranged on lines. And unlike illustrations of channels in previous centuries, these were very straight lines, resembling the front lines of an army. The front lines are labelled either according to their position in that particular section of the body or in relation to one another. In all, she names a total of thirteen front lines. Each section of the body could have one or more front lines, and in total Zhu Lian draws twenty-eight separate front lines along the body. The head and neck, back and shoulders, chest and abdominal sections all contain a central front line (*zhengzhong xian* 正中線) and three parallel front lines known as the first, second, and third lateral front lines (*diyi, dier, disan cexian* 第一，第二，第三側線). The upper and lower limb sections contain anterior (*qian* 前) central front lines, external lateral front lines, or internal lateral front lines (*zhengzhong xian, waice xian, neice xian* 正中線，外側線，內側線), and vice versa for the posterior (*hou* 后). In addition there are also two lateral (*ce* 側) chest and abdominal front lines (*xiong fu xian* 胸腹線) which run along the two lateral chest and abdominal sections.

The front lines which Zhu Lian draws on the body are usually straight, or in some cases curved, but they do not meander. They are also not very long, being limited to the length of any one section, and therefore never linking two sections together. A particular example is the lines in the head and neck section.[50] This section shows most vividly Zhu Lian's positioning of the acumoxa points. It includes four front lines and seven divisions. Zhu Lian herself mentions that she had spent some time simplifying the representation of the acumoxa points on the head, in order to facilitate the study of the points in this section.[51] Acumoxa points on the head and neck section have been arranged to lie neatly on three parallel front lines called the central front line of the top of the head (*toudingbu zhengzhongxian* 頭頂部正中線), the first lateral front line of the top of the head (*toudingbu diyi cexian* 頭頂部第一側線), the second lateral front line of the top of the head (*toudingbu dier cexian* 頭頂部第二側線), and the third lateral front line of the top of the head section (*toudingbu disan cexian* 頭頂部第三側線). These front lines accord roughly to the directing (*ren* 任), governing (*du* 督), bladder (*pangguan*g 膀胱), and gall bladder (*dan* 膽) channels, but the positioning of these acumoxa points does not necessarily accord with that in the medical canons.[52] Zhu Lian attempts to place the points on the parallel front lines in line with one another. Her written descriptions of the positioning of these points all support their relative positions on her diagram.

---

[49] Selden (1971), 59. [50] See Zhu Lian (1954), diagram no. 1.

[51] Zhu Lian (1954), xxii. This further simplification is unique to the second edition.

[52] See for instance *Zhenjiu dacheng* 針灸大成, *juan* 6, *pian* 10, 828–9.

Zhu Lian's system of disease was very different from the medicine of correspondence still evident in writings of contemporaries, and this too, had an impact on her conception of the body. The Chinese medical world (*zhongyi jie* 中醫界) at this time was largely based in and around the south-eastern provinces of Jiangsu and Zhejiang.[53] Although these doctors, too, had been involved in the reformation of acumoxa since the beginning of the century, Zhu Lian's motives were mostly based on revolutionary fervour. This meant that Zhu Lian's medicine was aimed at an audience more lowbrow than was the case with those Chinese medical physicians who had to compete with Western medical clinics for customers. Books produced during the Civil War period were few.[54] They included, for example, the *Zhenjiu miji gangyao* 針灸秘笈綱要 (Essentials of Acumoxa Secret Books) (1947) by Zhao Erkang 趙爾康 (1913–), who was a disciple of Cheng Dan'an. In this book he went into great detail on the anatomical positioning, main curing properties, and acumoxa hand techniques for each respective acumoxa point. The points were arranged around the channel system and medical cures largely based on information from the Chinese medical archive. Lu Shouyan 陸瘦燕 (1909–69) published the controversially titled *Zhenjiu zhengzong* 針灸正宗 (Orthodox Acumoxa) (1951), which produced in meticulous detail a Western medical description of disease, but which relied upon acumoxa points and hand techniques for their cure. Lu also advocated the channel system, and in 1948, after much research into existing illustrated manuals of acumoxa, produced his own revised model of the acumoxa channels and points.[55]

Zhu Lian abandoned the age old concepts of *qi* (氣), *yin* (陰), and *yang* (陽) and the Five Phases (*wuxing* 五行). She based her theory of disease on the nervous system, and this determined much of her understanding of bodily functions and acumoxa treatment: it was the object of acumoxa to stimulate and adjust the regulatory and controlling function of the body's internal nerves.[56] The acumoxa points thus did not lie along channels of energy, which linked internal organs to the surface of the body. Zhu Lian considered such a method of arranging the acumoxa points contrived (*qianqiang fuhui* 牽強附會)[57] and she found it necessary to be more scientific (*kexuede* 科學的) in explaining the healing functions of acumoxa on the body. Zhu Lian referred to the acumoxa points as 'stimulation points' (*cijidian* 刺激點), and not with the conventional *xuewei* (穴位).[58]

---

[53] This can be seen, for example, in Andrews (1996), where her description of Chinese medicine in China between the years 1895–1937 is mainly situated in south-east China.

[54] Statistics give a total of 39 Chinese medical books published between 1945–49, out of a total of 884 Chinese medical books published between 1911–49. In *Minguo shiqi zong shumu* (1995), 407–80.

[55] *Zhongyi dacidian* (1995), 840.   [56] Zhu Lian (1954), 11.   [57] Zhu Lian (1954), xv.

[58] Accordingly, I translate *xuewei* 穴位 as 'acumoxa points', and not as '*loci*' or 'holes'. I refer to *xuewei* purely as areas where the techniques of acupuncture or moxibustion can be applied, and do not wish to include any broader connotations.

This appeared to be a more 'scientific' use of terminology, which again alienated any allusion to the channel system. Another feature to note is that in her book Zhu Lian gives detailed information of 370 acumoxa points, the names of 360 of which correspond to those in the channel system. The extra ten belong to a vast array of points known as 'extra-meridional points'. However, there is one point from the channel system of 361 points which she does not include and this is *meichong* 眉沖 (bladder 3). It is uncertain why she omits this point, for it is one of the more well-known acumoxa points, used especially in the case of headache (*toutong* 頭痛) and blocked nose (*bisai* 鼻塞), as recorded by Cheng Dan'an[59] and Yang Jizhou 楊繼洲 (1522–1620).[60]

Zhu Lian also 'discovered' two acumoxa points of her own which are described in her book. These points are recorded in the *Chinese Medical Dictionary* as originating from *The New Acumoxa*,[61] yet they have not been included in later standardised textbooks of acumoxa.[62] The two new points are labelled *xinjian* (新建) and *xinshe* (新設). Just as *loci* named in the *Huangdi neijing* and Mawangdui medical manuscripts can be linked to the landscaping of the body at the time, such as the sea of *qi* (*qihai* 氣海) and the gushing spring (*yongquan* 涌泉),[63] the names given to these two points clearly mark the period during which they were discovered. Both start with the prefix *xin*, meaning 'new'. Both words are similar in meaning and, in fact, the two suffixes, when put together form one word *jianshe* (建設) which means to 'build, construct', as one would build and construct a new society.[64] The first one means 'the new construction' and the second one means 'the new establishment'. All very suitable names for acumoxa points in a medicine which was aiming to be part of the 'new democratic culture'.

A new, scientific, and unified medicine

To be part of the 'new democratic culture', Zhu Lian's medicine would have to fulfil Mao's criteria of new, scientific, and unified. Just how she applied these conditions to her medicine depended upon her interpretation of Mao's words. Zhu Lian's acumoxa was 'new' in that she did not identify it with the acumoxa currently being practised in the countryside. Zhu Lian complained that 'Ordinary acupuncturists of today when practising acumoxa do not stress cleanliness and sterilisation and many inject through clothes; they do not understand physiology and anatomy, some of them are not even sure

---

[59] Cheng Dan'an (1932), 134. [60] *Zhenjiu dacheng, juan* 6, *pian* 10, 828.
[61] *Zhongyi dacidian* (1995), 1636. [62] See for instance Zhenjiuxue gaiyao bianji xiaozu (1964).
[63] See Lo (this volume).
[64] See for instance Mao Zedong (1953), 1078, 'to construct new China' (*jianshe xin Zhongguo* 建設新中國). I am aware that this terminology was used similarly by the Nationalist Party, however, in the revolutionary base areas it is likely that such language was linked primarily with the goals of the CCP.

how to find acumoxa points, to the degree where they do not pay attention to acumoxa points, and they randomly [place the] needles and moxa'.[65] Acumoxa was not the only form of Chinese medicine available at the time, but Zhu Lian felt that acumoxa had the right qualities to serve the needs of the Communist Party in wartime China. She emphasised just how self-sufficient the system of acumoxa could be. All you needed were needles, alcoholic spirits, cotton-wool, moxa, and an explanatory handbook! Acumoxa was cheap, effective, very portable, and, if the instructions in her book were followed carefully, it was a very safe form of treatment as well. In the face of the existing medical conditions in the countryside, Zhu Lian believed that acumoxa could help.

However, Zhu Lian's attempts to create a 'new acumoxa' had to extend beyond the Huabei Health School. The simple creation of a novel and functioning medical system could not hope to exist if it was not also guaranteed a place in society. Her medicine could only be perpetuated if there were many other participants, among whom this medicine would continue to interact. Bruno Latour speaks of the importance of 'enrolling' others, 'so that they believe, buy it and disseminate it across time and space'.[66] To some extent, the Communist environment in which it was shaped automatically made the medicine belong. Yet this medicine was the result of an individual effort, and as such did not have the institutional or financial backing necessary to implant it in society on a large enough scale to be noticed. Rather, Zhu Lian had to convince others of the suitability of her 'new acumoxa', if it was ever to become a representative form of Chinese medicine. Latour writes that there were three main conditions involved in motivating people to support the claims of an innovator. These were to show that (1) the main road is clearly cut off, (2) the new detour is well signposted, and (3) that the detour appears short.[67] Zhu Lian satisfied all three of these conditions.

Clearly, both ideologically and practically speaking, Western medicine was not a medical system the Communists could rely on in the wartime guerrilla base areas. Zhu Lian herself pointed out 'The sanitation and medical problems of China's population of six hundred million are not going to be solved by a handful of Western medical doctors'.[68] Thus the main road of using Western medicine was quite literally cut off. However, there was a detour of using the folk, or 'old', medicine available in the countryside. Mao had already pointed out this route, and he had also specified how this 'old' medicine had to be joined with the 'new', to become scientific and unified. In this way the detour was well signposted. That the detour should appear short meant that this new medicine had also to be easy to learn and readily available. Zhu Lian saw her task as not only to upgrade the scientific content of this medicine, but also to simplify it and present it as an easily digestible whole. This meant that Zhu Lian's new medicine was not so

---

[65] Zhu Lian (1954), 6.   [66] Latour (1987), 121.   [67] Latour (1987), 111–12.   [68] Zhu Lian (1954), 5.

much aimed at existing medical practitioners, but more at the layman. It would be a medical textbook presented in colloquial speech (*baihua* 白話) and laid out with clearly defined chapters, to allow the uninitiated to supplement the limited numbers of trained medical personnel in wartime China.

Her medicine would be part of an as yet under-developed section of the national welfare network, that of a primary health care system. Zhu Lian advocated that because of the problem of a lack of high level cadres responsible for medical work, a large number of middle level public health workers should be trained. She thought that acumoxa could be learnt quickly by 'people of a low cultural level' and she suggested that, 'If we could at the same time send some adequately trained doctors down to the factories and countryside to teach, research, diagnose and treat complicated illnesses, in this way, it would indeed enable medical prevention work to gradually improve on a universal basis. This also conforms with the present day needs of the broad masses of workers and peasants and our cultural and financial conditions.'[69] This medicine was therefore meant to serve the masses. It had a primary health care function and was aimed at the countryside.

Unification was stressed in her medicine, for not only was the 'new acumoxa' to work to build a united front between Western and Chinese medicine, it was also to unite with the peasants and in this way allow it to more easily penetrate the countryside and facilitate the sanitary health care movements. Zhu Lian wrote that 'Experience has proven that the masses are accustomed to acumoxa, [and] it is the cheapest [of medical treatments]. Due to its welcome among the broad masses of the people, through the use of acumoxa as a curing method, we can quickly gain the trust of the people, and in this way can successfully further develop mass sanitation movements.'[70] Unification was to be a key process in the upgrading of acumoxa and its dissemination through the rural areas.

The scientification of acumoxa was more complicated. As has been explained before, Mao's use of the term 'science' referred to the Marxist sense of the word, which implies the search for 'true knowledge' and as such is not restricted to any particular nation or discipline. In this way, Zhu Lian did not automatically turn to the West for guidance in making her medicine more scientific. Western anatomy and physiology had long made inroads into Chinese medicine and these Zhu Lian also integrated into her medicine, but Zhu Lian herself did not make any new innovations in the use of Western medical sciences within Chinese medicine. Rather, Zhu Lian believed that 'Reform does not mean that Chinese medicine should drop all its original theories, nor does it mean study Western methods. Instead we need to choose those areas of ancient

---

[69] Zhu Lian (1954), 5.   [70] Zhu Lian (1954), xviii.

medicine which are appropriate, drop those areas which are not appropriate, use scientific methods, sort out the experience [of the ancient medicine], so as to improve its
scientific theory'.[71] In this way Zhu Lian's 'new acumoxa' would rely neither on
Chinese medical theory, nor on Western medicine to cure disease. The 'new acumoxa'
would have a new, scientific theory of its own.

Science in the 'new acumoxa'

Zhu Lian had a very eclectic approach to the use of science in her medicine. Available
at the time were a number of different scientific influences and Zhu Lian appears to have
used a bit of everything. She saw many of the concepts in the canonical medical doctrine
as out of date. She also did not feel that they properly explained the therapeutic effects
of acumoxa. In her own words she said, 'Practitioners know the effects [of acumoxa]
but they do not know the reasons for these effects'. She went on to say that today there
was still no medical theory which could properly explain the principles behind acumoxa's therapeutic effects, and because of this 'Some people believe that acumoxa
being capable of treating diseases is just ridiculous, and [they] refuse to investigate
any further'.[72] In her book, Zhu Lian compounded Chinese medical acumoxa points
with Western biomedical anatomy and physiology. However, her theory of disease was
based largely on relatively new scientific innovations being made in the realm of Soviet
science.

  As the product of a fellow Communist nation, Soviet science was a politically acceptable foundation for her medicine. Zhu Lian was thus able to draw heavily on Soviet
resources to support her new medicine. Zhu Lian based her interpretation of acumoxa
on Soviet innovations in the medical theory of neuro-pathology. She studied the latest
experiments made by the then Soviet Union to regulate health through the stimulation of
the nerves, often through stimulus of the spinal nerves by injection of fluids or electrical
stimulation. Zhu Lian largely based her interpretation of acumoxa on the Russian scientist Pavlov's theory of the advanced function of the nervous system (*gaoji shenjing
huodong* 高級神經活動). Zhu Lian wrote that 'The theory of the advanced function of
the nerves provides the explanatory key for the mystery surrounding acumoxa's therapeutic effects'. Pavlov (1849–1936) had carried out ground-breaking research in the
neural control of the circulation of the blood, beating of the heart and the regulating of
the pancreas, and considered the cerebral cortical control of the nerves to rely on the
processes of inhibition and excitation.[73] Zhu Lian also linked acumoxa with the Soviet

---

[71] Zhu Lian (1954), 6.   [72] Zhu Lian (1954), 6.
[73] For Ivan Petrovich Pavlov's life and research, see Gray (1979).

scientists' creation of tissue therapy (*zuzhi liaofa* 組織療法).[74] She saw the removal of a small section of human tissue in researching a regulatory function of the nerves as similar to scarring moxibustion and piercing acupuncture.[75] Soviet influence was to become stronger in the years after Liberation, as ties between the two nations strengthened, and the second edition of her book placed even more emphasis on research by Russian doctors on the role of the nervous system in health regulation.

If Soviet science was being lauded in China at this time as ground-breakingly modern, the Japanese, too, had been carrying out a significant amount of Western scientific research on acumoxa since the beginning of the century. However, unlike earlier reformers of Chinese medicine such as Cheng Dan'an, Zhu Lian appears to have been reluctant to incorporate Japanese science into her medicine. No doubt politically ice-cold relations due to the atrocities of the second Sino-Japanese War (1937–45) from which China had only just emerged, discouraged dealings with Japan at this time. Japanese doctors appear to have concentrated in particular on the therapeutic effects of moxibustion[76] but they too had taken steps towards simplifying the complexities of the canonical medical literature.[77] Zhu Lian, however, criticised their analysis of acumoxa, saying that Japanese scientific research on acumoxa 'still lacked the medical outlook of materialistic dialectics' and added that, 'it is also thought that its effects on the regulating and controlling of the higher function of the nerves in the internal body is not enough'.[78] Thus Soviet science was to dominate in her medicine.

In a similar vein, Zhu Lian did not approve of the recent innovation in Western medical science of cell pathology (*xibao binglixue* 細胞病理學). Western science, too, was not politically in favour in China, for the Communists were at this time condemning the Americans for assisting the Nationalists in the Civil War, and the animosity was to be exacerbated with the onset of the Korean War (1950–53). Cell pathology was thus linked with the capitalist (*zibenzhuyi* 資本主義) West and, apparently, it was only after the end of the Cultural Revolution in 1979 that this theory was able to be applied freely to the medicine.[79] Zhu Lian wrote that

[74] Tissue therapy was proclaimed as 'a great discovery in the modern medical world' in '*Zhongyang renmin zhengfu weishengbu guanyu zuzhi tuixing "zuzhi liaofa" de zhibiao*' 中央人民政府衛生部關于組織推行《組織療法》的指標 (The Central People's Government Ministry of Health's directives concerning the organisation of reaching the targets set for the "treatment method of tissue therapy"). *Renmin Ribao* (6 March 1951), 3.

[75] Zhu Lian (1954), 15.

[76] See Li Jie (1952), 55–76. The same essay is also reproduced in the appendices to *The New Acumoxa*.

[77] Andrews (1996), 173, discusses the relocation of acumoxa points and channels by Japanese researchers, and mentions how the number of acumoxa points was limited to only 70.

[78] Zhu Lian (1954), 31.

[79] Dr Han Gang 韓剛, lecturer in the history of medicine at the Beijing University of Traditional Chinese Medicine and Pharmacology (*Beijing zhongyiyao daxue* 北京中醫藥大學), interview, 3 November 1997, Beijing.

cell pathology has not emphasised enough the effect of the nerves within the body; it believes that all pathological phenomena are due to certain stimuli (e.g. bacterial toxins, or stimuli from chemicals or physics) which cause harm to the cells. Therefore, in pathology, the main research is on every aspect of change in cell organisation (e.g. denaturation of fats, protein, and tissue, inflammation, sores with pus, ulcers etc.). They believed that these changes were the direct result of stimulation to the cells. This is a biased and isolated outlook which only sees the outer appearance and does not see the inner essence.[80]

Zhu Lian's attitude can be identified with a Communist device of not putting the emphasis on the individual (such as the individual cell), but rather on the group (such as tissue structures). The Chinese term here for 'tissue' is *zuzhi* (組織) which also means 'organisation' and was used in Communist political language, to describe group gatherings.

To validate her medicine during these politically sensitive times, Zhu Lian placed great emphasis on the Soviet medical system. However, in the actual diagnosis and categorisation of illnesses, Zhu Lian utilised the Western medicine that had become part of the Chinese health care system. For the treatment of disease, she prescribed very few Western-medical drugs but utilised almost exclusively the techniques of acumoxa. But curing a Western-medical disease with Chinese-medical acumoxa points inevitably gives rise to conflicting theories of the causation of disease. Zhu Lian dealt with this 'problem' by keeping the Chinese-medical content in her medicine to a minimum – the hand techniques of acupuncture and moxibustion, and the location of the acumoxa points. Zhu Lian then listed individually the therapeutic values of each acumoxa point, and illnesses were to be addressed in this way.

Zhu Lian described her acumoxa as being 'effective' (*youxiao* 有校) in the treatment of most diseases. In fact, in the majority of cases, acumoxa was used to alleviate symptoms (*jianqing zhengzhuang* 減輕癥狀). In *The New Acumoxa* acumoxa points were chosen to relieve pain (*zhen tong* 鎮痛), reduce inflammation (*xiao yan* 消炎), build up the resistance to disease (*zengqiang dikangli* 增強抵抗力), promote blood circulation (*cujin quanshen xuexing* 促進全身血行), stop vomiting (*zhi tu* 止吐), and so on. Such a superficial approach to disease is generally seen as a Western-medical trait. In China today it is still considered that Western medicine cures the symptoms while Chinese medicine cures the root of the disease (*xiyi zhibiao, zhongyi zhiben* 西醫治標，中醫治本). As an example of a typical wartime disease caused by insanitary conditions, relapsing fever (*huiguire* 回歸熱), is given.[81] The disease itself is a Western-medical disease, made specific by the *Borrelia* spirochaete which causes it. In Chinese medicine, how-

[80] Zhu Lian (1954), 14.
[81] More details of relapsing fever as a major infectious disease affecting the base areas are given in Lun Shaohua (1996), 357.

ever, the symptoms are such that they could be related to a number of Chinese-medical disease categories. Zhu Lian defines the disease in Western medical terms and prescribes acumoxa to help relieve some of the symptoms. If we then compare Zhu Lian's description with the description given in the Chinese edition of William Osler and Thomas McCrae's *The Principles and Practice of Medicine*, printed in Shanghai in 1931 at around the same time that Zhu Lian was studying Western medicine herself in Suzhou, we can see that theirs is a somewhat more detailed description than that which Zhu Lian gives, but the main criteria remain the same (in the following extracts, emphasis is added by the author).

Relapsing Fever in *The New Acumoxa*
This disease is caused by *spirobacteria*. The symptoms include aversion to cold, *shivering and high fever*,[82] as in the initial stages of malaria. The fever is intermittent, however it does not subside after a few hours, but more usually *lasts for six to seven days*. After *profuse sweating, the body temperature will then drop* and the patient himself will feel better. Between four to fourteen days later, there will be a recurring attack. Before the temperature drops after the recurring bout, the temperature will rise even higher, the pulse will race (*can reach 120–140 beats per minute*); *the spleen will quickly swell*, and the liver will also at the same time swell. However, once the body temperature has returned to normal, the liver and the spleen will both shrink again. The whole body is without strength, the complexion is pale, *gradually turning to a yellow colour. The muscles ache*, and especially the gastrocnemius muscle (calf muscle) will hurt when pressed. These are all characteristic features of relapsing fever.

這病的病原體是螺旋菌。癥狀也是惡寒戰慄與高熱，像瘧疾開始一樣。發徵熱是間歇性的，不過不是几小時就退熱，通常是發熱六，七天，出大汗后，體溫才下降，病人自己覺得是好了；再經四至十四天中，又重復發作。發作后的降熱前，體溫更高，脈搏極快（每分鐘可達一百二十到一百四十次）；脾臟也是迅速腫大，肝臟也同時腫大，不過在體溫正常的時候，肝臟，脾臟又縮小；全身無力，皮膚蒼白，逐漸轉為黃膽色；肌肉疼痛，尤其是腓腸肌（腿肚子）有厭痛；這些都是回歸熱的特征。[83]

Relapsing Fever in *The Principles and Practice of Medicine*
Suddenly there is *shivering and fever*, and the small of the back and the *four limbs ache* tremendously; if young people get this disease, there can sometimes be vomiting with convulsions; the fever rapidly rises, and during the first night [it] can sometimes reach up to 104 degrees [Fahrenheit] (40 [Celcius]); *often there is sweating*, and *the pulse is rapid reaching around 110–130 [beats per minute]*. When the fever is high it can fluctuate, *the spleen will quickly swell up* and *there is jaundice*; stomach symptoms can become exacerbated, [and this is] sometimes accompanied by cough. At times there are herpes blisters, pompholyx [eruption

---

[82] The phrases in italics are found in both texts.   [83] Zhu Lian (1954), 326.

of vesicles esp. on feet and hands] or petechiae [a minute reddish or purplish spot containing blood that appears in skin or mucous membrane] and only very rarely are there symptoms of the intestinal tract. During the fever, often tests will show parasites in the blood, and an increase in the number of white blood cells. *The fever can last for five to six days*; during the final stages of the illness, in just a few hours the temperature can return to normal or below normal temperature.

陡起寒戰發熱，腰及四肢大痛；年少者患之，或吐并驚厥；熱速升第一夜或升至百零四度（四零）；常出汗，脈搏速至百一十或百三十不等，熱高時或譫妄，脾早腫大，黃疸；胃病狀或甚重，或咳嗽，時或顯皰疹，汗皰，瘀點等，惟罕有腸病狀。發熱時常可於血中查見寄生蟲，白血球加多，熱之高度延至五六日之久；達病終期后，則數小時內即可退至常度或常度以下.[84]

Thus we can see the parallels in the description of the disease. Although Zhu Lian's description contains a lot of data visible to the five senses, the details recorded are not equivalent to those determined by a standard Chinese medical examination.[85] For example, she refers to the pulse as *maibo* instead of *maixiang* (脈象), and describes it as *jikuai* instead of *shuo* (數), *shuo* being a specialised term for denoting a rapid pulse. In the same way, she also describes the patient's colouring as *pifu cangbai*, i.e., the skin is pale, rather than using the Chinese idom *se cangbai* (色蒼白), i.e., the complexion is pale. In addition, a Chinese medical examination would determine the condition of the organ systems indirectly through pulse diagnosis and examination of the appearance of the tongue and stool, information that is not detailed in either of the above diagnoses. In continuation with her description of the disease in Western medical terms, Zhu Lian prescribes acumoxa to confront this disease in a Western medical way as she explains that 'treatment with acumoxa can strengthen the immune system and reduce the symp-

---

[84]   Osler and McCrae in translation (1931), 237. Compare with Osler ((1892)1930), 262:

> The invasion is abrupt, with chill, fever, and intense pain in the back and limbs. In young persons there may be nausea, vomiting, and convulsions. The temperature rises rapidly and may reach 104 degrees on the evening of the first day. Sweats are common. The pulse is rapid, ranging from 110 to 130. There may be delirium if the fever is high. Swelling of the spleen can be detected early. Jaundice is common in some epidemics. The gastric symptoms may be severe, but intestinal symptoms are rare. Cough may be present. Occasionally herpes is noted, and there may be miliary vesicles and petechiae (i.e., a minute reddish or purplish spot containing blood that appears in skin or mucus membrane). During the paroxysm the blood invariably shows the spirochaetes and there is usually a leucocytosis (i.e., an increase in the number of leucocytes in the circulating blood). After the fever has persisted with severity or even with an increasing intensity for five or six days the crisis occurs. In the course of a few hours, accompanied by profuse sweating, sometimes by diarrhoea, the temperature falls to normal or even subnormal.

[85]   Although at this period there was no standard form of Chinese medicine, its various strands share certain features.

toms, and there have been several cases of positive results'.[86] Acumoxa points are thus chosen to reduce the symptoms of relapsing fever, and not chosen to deal with the 'root' of the disorder. As the main symptom of relapsing fever is indeed the fever, it is no surprise that most of the acumoxa points she chooses here are aimed at reducing the temperature of the patient.

However, by doing this she is trying to perform with the treatment methods of acupuncture and moxibustion, the roles of a Western medical drug. Osler himself recommended the use of the drugs Salvarsan (*sa'erfasan* 薩耳乏散) and neo-Salvarsan (*xin sa'erfasan* 新薩耳乏散), both of which are anti-syphilitic drugs used often for the treatment of spirocheatal diseases. Osler also suggested a few other drugs to be used for the relief of symptoms. In the case of great weakness he suggested the use of some strong stimulants such as Digitalis (*dijitali* 狄吉他利) – i.e. foxglove, a powerful cardiac stimulant and diurectic, used especially in the treatment of congestive heart failure – and for an aching back and limbs, Osler prescribed doses of ipecac opium (*yegen yapian* 葉根鴉片) or the injection of morphine.[87]

Zhu Lian's selection of points were *quchi* 曲池, *zusanli* 足三里, *jiquan* 極泉, *xingjian* 行間, *feishu* 肺俞, *ganshu* 肝俞, *pishu* 脾俞, *tianshu* 天樞, *dazhui* 大椎, *neiguan* 內關, *laogong* 勞宮, *neiting* 內庭. With the exception of *jiquan* (heart 1) and *tianshu* (stomach 25), whose therapeutic effects are not especially related to that of heat reduction or of supplementing energy, it is possible to understand why the other points were chosen.[88] *Zusanli* (stomach 36) is an overall strengthening point which in Zhu Lian's understanding would be used to boost the immune system. The *shu* (俞) points of the lung, liver, and spleen run parallel to the spinal cord and are believed to have a direct connection with the organ after which they are named. Stimulation of these points will directly boost the organ in question and thus she chose to boost the lung, liver, and spleen. The points *quchi* (large intestine 11), *neiguan* (pericardium 6), *dazhui* (governing 14) and *neiting* (stomach 44) are all attributed heat-clearing properties in Chinese medicine. *Laogong* (pericardium 8) and *xingjian* (liver 2) belong to a category called *ying* (榮) points, which are used specifically to cool heat. Thus we find that she has chosen points which are intimately linked with a Chinese medical concept of pathological heat (*re* 熱), and that the majority of these points have the function of releasing excess heat (*qing re* 清熱).[89] Consequently, in *The New Acumoxa*, Zhu Lian uses an unusual amalgam of Western medical science to explain the pathology of disease and

---

[86] Zhu Lian (1954), 326.   [87] Osler and McCrae (1931), 238.

[88] In examining these points I consulted both the *Zhenjiu dacheng*, passim, and Cheng Dan'an's *Xiuding zhongguo zhenjiu zhiliaoxue*.

[89] For the analysis I have chosen to only represent one healing aspect, that of cooling heat, in this discussion. I am aware that the therapeutic possibilities inherent in a selection of acumoxa points are far more intricate.

Soviet science for the theory of her medicine, but when it comes to the essence of her curing skills, it would appear that the 'new acumoxa' is imbued heavily with a Chinese medical theory.

Summary

The new, scientific, and unified medicine was thus created to satisfy the conditions of war in the Communist rural base areas. However this medicine was not created solely to cure the masses. It contains enough elaborate justifications on the merits of acumoxa to suggest that Zhu Lian was aiming her medicine at the Party leadership as well; in which case political credibility was an important point. Zhu Lian followed Mao's guidelines of 'new', 'scientific', and 'unified' to produce a medicine which was shaped by Party criteria, wartime conditions, and the practicalities of healing. Certainly, as this chapter has shown, social influences played a key role in determining which elements could be accepted into the 'new acumoxa'. This encompassed everything from terminology used within the medicine, to the physical portrayal of the body, and to the degree of foreign input in its medical theory. Thus the 'new acumoxa' embodies how the scope of intellectual freedom was significantly narrowed by Communist Party political guidelines, to the extent that medical efficiency was subordinated to party objectives.

The CCP was the first ruling government in China to officially recognise the medical discipline of acumoxa in over a century. Alongside bonesetting (*zhenggu* 正骨) and massage (*anmo* 按摩), acumoxa represented Chinese medicine in the Chinese medical improvement schools (*zhongyi jinxiu xuexiao* 中醫進修學校) set up nationwide soon after Liberation. The 'new acumoxa', which by this time was no longer unique to Zhu Lian, was to form the core of these acumoxa classes. However, such an educational system was to come under heavy criticism after 1954 and, once again, the 'improvement' of Chinese medicine was to take a different path. Zhu Lian's impact was the cause of some interest in medical circles in the 1950s, and her name is in general still remembered today by those involved with Chinese medicine during that period. However, her impact was small and her 'new acumoxa', which attempted to reflect the social, economic, and political conditions of the Civil War in China, was short-lived.

References to premodern Chinese and Japanese works

Huangdi neijing Suwen 黃帝內經素問 (Basic Questions in the Yellow Emperor's Canon). Han, *ca* 100 AD. Anon. References to Guo Aichun 郭靄春 (ed.), *Huangdi neijing Suwen yuyi* 黃帝內經素問語譯 (Interpretation of the Basic Questions in the Yellow Emperor's Inner Canon). Renmin weisheng chubanshe, Beijing, 1992.

Zhenjiu dacheng 針灸大成 (Great Compilation of Acumoxa). Ming, 1601. Yang Jizhou 楊繼洲.
References to *Heilongjiangsheng zuguo yiyao yanjiusuo* 黑龍江省祖國醫藥研究所 (ed.), *Zhenjiu dacheng xiaoshi* 針灸大成校釋 (Teaching Edition of the Great Compilation of Acumoxa). Renmin weisheng chubanshe, Beijing, 1995.

References to modern works

Andrews, Bridie J. 1996. 'The Making of Modern Chinese Medicine 1895–1937'. PhD thesis in History, University of Cambridge.

Cheng Dan'an 承澹庵 1932. *Xiuding Zhongguo zhenjiu zhiliaoxue* 修訂中國針灸治療學 (Revised and Enlarged Edition of China's Acumoxa Therapeutics). Qianjingtang shuju, Shanghai.

Croizier, Ralph C. 1968. *Traditional Medicine in Modern China: Science, Nationalism and the Tensions of Cultural Change*. Harvard University Press, Cambridge, Mass.

 1972. 'Traditional Medicine as a Basis for Chinese Medical Practice.' In Quinn, 3–21.

Gao Yaoguo 高耀國 1996a. 'Weisheng gongzuo zuzhi jigou' 衛生工作組織機構 (Organisational Structure of Sanitation Work 1945–49). In Zhu Kewen, Gao Enxian, and Gong Chun, 315–24.

 1996b. 'Yiyuan gongzuo' 醫院工作 1945–49 (Hospital Work 1945–49). In Zhu Kewen, Gao Enxian, and Gong Chun, 334–41.

Gray, Jeffrey A. 1979. *Pavlov*. Harvester, Brighton.

Guo Aichun 郭靄春 (ed.) 1987. *Xiancun zhenjiu yiji* 現存針灸醫籍 (Existing Acumoxa Medical Records). Hunan kexue jishu chubanshe, Changsha.

Guo Shiyu 郭世余 1989. *Zhongguo zhenjiu shi* 中國針灸史 (The History of Chinese Acumoxa). Tianjin kexue jishu chubanshe, Tianjin.

Hsia, Tao-tai 1972. 'Laws on Public Health'. In Quinn, 109–35.

Hsu, Elisabeth 1999. *The Transmission of Chinese Medicine*. Cambridge University Press, Cambridge.

 1996. 'Innovations in Acumoxa: Acupuncture Analgesia, Scalp and Ear Acupuncture in the People's Republic of China'. *Social Science and Medicine* 42 (1), 421–30.

Huang Wendong 黃文東 (ed.) 1983. *Zhuming zhongyi xuejia de xueshu jingyan* 著名中醫學家的學述經驗 (Scholarship and Experience of Famous Chinese Medical Experts). Hunan kexue jishu chubanshe, Changsha.

Latour, Bruno 1987. *Science in Action*. Harvard University Press, Cambridge, Mass.

Li Jie 李解 1952. 'Riben dui zhenjiu de kexue yanjiu' 日本對針灸的科學研究 (Japanese Scientific Research of Acumoxa). In Xinan xingzheng weiyuanhui weishengju, 55–76.

Liu Liangfu 劉良富 1989. *Baiqiu'en yike daxue xiaoshi* 白求恩醫科大學校史 (A History of the Bethune Medical University). Sichuan renmin chubanshe, Chongqing.

Lu Gwei-djen and Needham, Joseph 1980. *Celestial Lancets: a History and Rationale of Acupuncture and Moxa*. Cambridge University Press, Cambridge.

Lu Shouyan 陸瘦燕 1951. *Zhenjiu zhengzong* 針灸正宗 (Orthodox Acumoxa). Qianjingtang shuju, Shanghai.

Lu Zhijun 魯之俊 1950. *Xinbian zhenjiuxue* 新編針灸學 (Newly Revised Acumoxa). Chongqing renmin chubanshe, Chongqing.

 1987. 'Lu Zhijun ba' 魯之俊跋 (Postscript by Lu Zhijun). In Guo Aichun, 323–5.

Lun Shaohua 倫少華 1996. 'Sanitation and Anti-Epidemic Work 1945–49' (*Weisheng fangyi gongzuo* 衛生防疫工作 1945–49). In Zhu Kewen, Gao Enxian, and Gong Chun, 350–60.

Ma Boying 馬伯英, Gao Xi 高晞 and Hong Zhongli 洪中立 1993. *Zhongwai yixue wenhua jiaoliushi* 中外醫學文化交流史 (The History of Intercultural Medicine Communication between China and Foreign Countries). Wenhui chubanshe, Shanghai.

Mao Zedong 毛澤東 1952. *Mao Zedong xuanji di er juan* 毛澤東選集第二卷 (Selected Works of Mao Zedong), vol. II. Renmin chubanshe, Beijing.

1953. *Mao Zedong xuanji di san juan* 毛澤東選集第三卷 (Selected Works of Mao Zedong), vol. III. Renmin chubanshe, Beijing.

Minden, Karen 1979. 'The Development of Early Chinese Communist Health Policy: Health Care in the Border Regions, 1936–1949'. *American Journal of Chinese Medicine* 7 (4), 299–315.

Minguo shiqi zong shumu 民國時期總書目 (Complete Catalogue of Books from the Republican Period). 1995. *Beijing tushuguan* 北京圖書館 (eds.). Shumu wenxian chubanshe, Beijing.

Osler, William (1892) 1930. *The Principles and Practice of Medicine*. 11th edition revised by Thomas McCrae. Appleton, New York.

Osler, William and McCrae, Thomas 1931. *Oushi neikexue* 歐氏內科學 (The Principles and Practice of Medicine). China Medical Association, Shanghai. Transl. Philip B. Cousland.

Perry, Elizabeth J. 1980. *Rebels and Revolutionaries in North West China 1845–1945*. Stanford University Press, Stanford, Calif.

Quinn, Joseph R. (ed.) 1972. *Medicine and Public Health in the PRC*. US Department of Health, Education and Welfare, Washington, D.C.

Rosner, Erhard 1991. *Die Heilkunst des Pien Lu. Arzt und Krankheit in bildhaften Ausdrücken der chinesischen Sprache*. Franz Steiner, Stuttgart.

Saich, Tony (ed.) 1996. *The Rise to Power of the Chinese Communist Party: Documents and Analysis*. Sharpe, Armonk.

Schram, Stuart 1989. *The Thought of Mao Tse-tung*. Cambridge University Press, Cambridge.

Schurman, Franz 1966. *Ideology and Organization in Communist China*. University of California Press, Berkeley.

Selden, Mark 1971. *The Yenan Way in Revolutionary China*. Harvard University Press, Cambridge, Mass.

Sivin, Nathan 1995. 'State, Cosmos and Body in the Last Three Centuries BC'. *Harvard Journal of Asiatic Studies* 55 (1), 5–37.

Tang Xuezheng 唐學正 1951. *Xuexi xin zhenjiuxue* 學習新針灸學 (A Study of the New Acumoxa). Xinhua shudian, Beijing.

Taylor, Kim 2000. 'Chinese Medicine in Early Communist China 1945–1963'. PhD thesis in History, University of Cambridge.

Unschuld, Paul. U. 1985. *Medicine in China: a History of Ideas*. University of California Press, Berkeley.

van Slyke, Lyman P. (ed.) 1968. *The Chinese Communist Movement: a Report of the United States War Department, July 1945*. Stanford University Press, Stanford.

Wylie, Raymond F. 1980. *The Emergence of Maoism: Mao Tse-tung, Ch'en Po-ta, and the Search for Chinese Theory 1935–1945*. Stanford University Press, Stanford.

Xiao Shaoqing 蕭少卿 (ed.) 1997. *Zhongguo zhenjiuxue shi* 中國針灸學史 (A History of China's Acumoxa). Ningxia renmin chubanshe, Yinchuan.

Xinan xingzheng weiyuanhui weishengju 西南行政委員會衛生局 (ed.) 1952. *Xin zhenjiuxue luncong* 新針灸學論叢 (A Collection of Essays on the New Acumoxa). Chongqing renmin chubanshe, Chongqing.

Zhao Erkang 趙爾康 1947. *Zhenjiu miji gangyao* 針灸秘笈綱要 (Essentials of Acumoxa Secret Books). Qianjingtang shuju, Shanghai.

Zhao Qinxuan 趙琴軒 (1957) 1987. 'Wo ye ping *Xin zhenjiuxue*' 我也評《新針灸學》 (My Comment on *The New Acumoxa*). *Guangdong zhongyi* 9 廣東中醫 (Guangdong Traditional Chinese Medicine 9). References to Guo Aichun 1987, 328–31.

Zhao Rong 趙榮 (1956) 1987. 'Dui Zhu Lian zhu *Xin zhenjiuxue* de jidian yijian' 對朱璉著《新針灸學》的幾點意見 (A Few Comments on Zhu Lian's '*The New Acumoxa*'). *Zhonghua yishi zazhi* 2 中華醫史雜志 (Journal on China's Medicine 2). References to Guo Aichun 1987, 325–26.

Zhenjiuxue gaiyao bianji xiaozu 針灸學概要編輯小組 (eds.) 1964. *Zhongguo zhenjiuxue gaiyao* 中國針灸學概要 (Outline of China's Acumoxa). Renmin weisheng chubanshe, Beijing.

Zhongyi dacidian 中醫大辭典 (Chinese Medical Dictionary) 1995. Li Jingwei 李經緯 and Deng Tietao 鄧鐵濤 (eds.). Renmin weisheng chubanshe, Beijing.

Zhongyi renmin cidian 中醫人民辭典 (Biographical Dictionary of Chinese Medicine) 1988. Li Yun 李雲 (ed.). Guoji wenhua chubangongsi, Beijing.

Zhu Chao 朱潮 and Zhang Weifeng 張慰豐 1990. *Xin Zhongguo yixue jiaoyu shi* 新中國醫學教育史 (A History of Medical Education in New China). Beijing yike daxue and Zhongguo xiehe yike daxue, Beijing.

Zhu Kewen 朱克文, Gao Enxian 高恩顯 and Gong Chun 龔純 (eds.) 1996. *Zhongguo junshi yixue shi* 中國軍事醫學史 (A History of China's Military Medicine). Renmin junyi chubanshe, Beijing.

Zhu Lian 朱璉 1954. *Xin zhenjiuxue* 新針灸學 (The New Acumoxa). 2nd edition. Renmin weisheng chubanshe, Beijing. (1st edition 1951, with Renmin chubanshe, Beijing).

12

Shaping Chinese medicine:
two case studies from contemporary China

VOLKER SCHEID

Ever since China embarked on its course of modernisation at the end of the Imperial era, pressure was exerted on traditional physicians to modernise (*xiandaihua* 現代化) and render scientific (*kexuehua* 科學化) their medicine, adjusting it to rapid social and economic change.[1] Recent scholarship has afforded much insight into the resultant multiple and complex transformations of Chinese medicine, ranging from new forms of professional organisation, communication, and self-representation to novel ways of teaching and transmitting medical knowledge.[2] One particularly fascinating field of study which has not yet received the detailed attention it deserves is the rich history of strategies and tactics by which Chinese medical practitioners have utilised biomedical knowledge and technologies within the context of their own practices.[3]

Contemporary physicians of Chinese medicine look back on a century of sustained effort in this area. During an initial period, from the late nineteenth century to the end of the Republican era, members of a heterogeneous group of practitioners collectively referred to today as the 'School of Merging [Chinese and Western Medicine]' (*huitong pai* 匯通派) put forward and practised their individual suggestions for integration. Their efforts ranged across a wide spectrum from assimilation of certain Western ideas to

---

[1] For descriptions and analyses of the struggles which shaped Chinese medicine over the last century, see Andrews (1996), Chen (1989), Croizier (1986), Jia Dedao (1993), 328–45, Hillier and Jewell (1983), Lampton (1977), Ma Boying, Gao Xi and Hong Zhongli (1994), 469–601, Maldener (1995), Ots (1990), Sivin (1987), Unschuld (1985), 249–62, Xu (1997), and Zhao Hongjun (1989). Unschuld (1992) deals particularly with the issue of legitimisation.

[2] For exemplary scholarship in this area see Andrews (1996, 1997), Farquhar (1986, 1994), Hsu (1992, 1999), Sivin (1987), Unschuld (1992). Zhang Weiyao (1994) is a mine of information on changes in Chinese medicine particularly since 1949.

[3] In the author's opinion, the study of medical practice should be analysed as *practice* in the manner defined by Rouse (1996), 125–57, rather than as a system of beliefs, knowledge, or technologies.

Chinese medicine to the use of biomedical knowledge to instigate total reform of Chinese medicine.[4]

A second period, lasting from the establishment of the People's Republic in 1949 to the late 1970s, witnessed politically motivated imposition from above of integration strategies onto Chinese medicine subsuming all such individual endeavours. Initially, the Chinese Communist Party under the leadership of Mao Zedong merely called for the cooperation of Chinese and Western health personnel under the political slogan *zhongxiyi tuanjie* 中西醫團結 ('Chinese and Western medicine [should] join together'). From the mid-1950s onwards, the actual integration of the two medical systems was promoted under the new slogan *zhongxiyi jiehe* 中西醫結合 ('Chinese and Western medicine [should] be integrated').[5] Such fusion was further accelerated during the Cultural Revolution (1966–76) when integrated Chinese and Western medicine (*zhongxiyi jiehe*) became the only ideologically correct way by which a revolutionary new medicine (*xinyi* 新醫) might be developed.[6]

A third period, starting in the late 1970s and lasting until today, is characterised by an officially plural health care system on the basis of the so-called 'three paths' (*san tiao daolu* 三條道路) policy. This states that Chinese medicine, Western medicine, and integrated Chinese and Western medicine should have equal status. Furthermore, Chinese medicine should be the starting point for work towards integrating Chinese and Western medicine.[7] The practical result is that while Chinese medicine can once again assert its traditional independence, there has, in fact, been a wholesale import of biomedical

---

[4] Jia Dedao (1979), 335–9, subdivides the movement into three factions. The first faction, under the leadership of physicians such as Tang Zonghai 唐宗海 (1862–1918), Zhang Xichun 張錫純 (1860–1933), and Yang Zemin 楊則民 (1893–1948) advocated the primacy of Chinese medicine. The second faction, under the leadership of physicians such as Ding Fubao 丁福保 (1874–1952) and Lu Yuanlei 陸淵雷 (1894–1955), favoured rendering Chinese medicine scientific through the guidance of Western science. The third faction, exemplified by physicians such as Yun Shujue 惲樹珏 (1878–1935), Zhu Weiju 祝味菊 (1884–1951), and Zhu Peiwen 朱沛文 (1805–?), argued that the strengths and weaknesses of both should be recognised. For a different analysis of some of the issues involved, see Andrews (1996).

[5] See Ots (1990), 18.

[6] 'Lü Bingkui cong yi liu shi nian wenji' bianji weiyuanhui (1993), 11–12; Ma Boying, Gao Xi and Hong Zhongli (1994), 573–601.

[7] This principle was developed in the late 1970s by traditional physicians under the leadership of Lü Bingkui 呂炳奎 (1914–), former director of the Chinese Medicine Bureau (*Zhongyisi* 中醫司) within the Ministry of Public Health (*Weishengbu* 衛生部), to counteract what they saw as the detrimental effects on Chinese medicine of the Cultural Revolution period's integrationist policies. Their principle was adopted in December 1982 at a conference sponsored by the Ministry of Public Health in Shijiazhuang, Hebei Province. It was confirmed as the official party line in 1985 and has remained in force ever since. See 'Lü Bingkui cong yi 60 nian wenji' bianji weiyuanhui (1993), 12–13; Zhang Weiyao (1994), 16–17; and Zhonghua renmin gongheguo weishengbu zhongyisi (1985).

knowledge and technology into its clinical domain. Public spending, furthermore, demonstrates a distinctly unequal support for the various sectors of the health care system, with Chinese medicine being at a clear disadvantage.[8]

The tensions intrinsic to this situation are reflected in contradictory perceptions of modernisation – sometimes by the same informants. Thus, on the one hand, there are multiple indicators suggesting a gradual corrosion of Chinese medicine's vital force. Students at colleges and universities of Chinese medicine in Beijing told me that a considerable number of their classmates as well as some of their teachers no longer believed in Chinese medicine. Senior physicians lamented the fact that levels of clinical expertise were gradually declining. Few contemporary texts were held in high esteem. Meanwhile patients bemoaned the fact that hardly any doctor nowadays is able to diagnose and prescribe from the pulse alone.

On the other hand, most doctors and students of Chinese medicine I spoke to also believed that their discipline, following the general trend in China, was undergoing a phase of accelerated development. They claimed that important new discoveries were being made, that treatments were becoming more effective, and that previously unclear concepts were now being clarified. They experienced Western medicine not as adversary, but as the source of the technologies and of the impetus necessary for lifting traditional medicine onto a higher plane. They perceived the 'Chinese medicine fever' (*zhongyi re* 中醫熱) currently sweeping the West as evidence that 'the 21st century will be the century of Chinese medicine'.[9]

The negative tenor of Western analyses of modernisation in Chinese medicine corresponds more closely to the first view. While acknowledging that Chinese medicine has resisted the hegemony of biomedicine over a remarkably long period, most authors suggest this achievement was possible only at the price of surrendering intellectual autonomy. A 'loss of creative vitality'[10] is detected in such tell-tale signs as diminishing conceptual integrity, 'an increase of incoherence', and the piecemeal assimilation of 'bits and pieces of modern medicine . . . onto the traditional structure' without, however, 'being guided by any overall plan of alteration'.[11] For many the deployment of traditional medical technologies is perceived to be legitimate only if it can be explained by biomedical science.[12]

---

[8] In 1986 hospitals of modern medicine received 39 per cent of government recurrent health expenditure, hospitals of traditional medicine (including those of integrated Chinese and Western medicine) only 6 per cent. Since both outpatient and inpatient care in Chinese cities is hospital based, this figure can be taken to reflect the unequal state support for medical systems that are only rhetorically equal. World Bank cited in Tang Shenglan et al. (1994), 64.

[9] Wang Ji (1993); Zhang Weiyao (1994), 14.   [10] Unschuld (1992), 46.

[11] Sivin (1987), 197–9. See also Sivin (1990).   [12] Rosenthal (1981) and (1987).

This essay is an attempt to demonstrate that the development of Chinese medicine by its leading practitioners in contemporary China is only partially represented by such descriptions. The reality constituted by biomedicine and modern technology inside and outside of China's consulting rooms is undoubtedly a major driving-force of change and innovation, though by no means the only one.[13] There is sufficient evidence to suggest that change will not necessarily lead to a weakening of the intellectual foundations of traditional medical practice. On the contrary. The century-old vision of physicians such as Zhang Xichun 張錫純 (1860–1933) that aspects of biomedicine might fruitfully be assimilated to Chinese medicine without threatening the integrity of traditional knowledge is still being fulfilled.

For this purpose, I will describe and compare the clinical practice of two outstanding but very different doctors: Professors Qian and Zhu.[14] My case studies are based on participant observation during twelve months of fieldwork in Beijing in 1994. Since I had already practised Chinese medicine in the West for over 10 years myself, I was then accepted by both doctors as an advanced student (*jinxiusheng* 進修生). Like my fellow Chinese students, I copied case histories, prescriptions, and our teacher's comments. Later I analysed these for their treatment strategies, compared them with those of other doctors past and present, and discussed them with friends and other teachers. This process, which relies on the hermeneutic ability to read prescriptions as much as on explicit teaching, is the way by which doctors of Chinese medicine even today develop and refine their clinical skills.

I intend to address the problem outlined above via a case-study approach choosing these two particular cases for several reasons. First, I concur with Farquhar's opinion that 'much of the intellectual life of Chinese medicine revolves around the reading and writing of prescriptions'.[15] Prescriptions are not primarily theoretical reflections (though they can be) and thus emphatically constitute medicine as practice. They reflect practitioners' affiliations to teachers and medical traditions, aesthetics, and even political commitments. The prescriptions of Professors Qian and Zhu thus provide a convenient, if somewhat technically demanding, focus for the examination of their clinical agency and the manner in which they cultivate their tradition.

Second, I wish to demonstrate by means of these two cases some of the real and rhetorical oppositions that I constantly encountered in conversation with Chinese medical physicians: oppositions between [traditional] Chinese medicine (*zhongyi* 中醫) and integrated Chinese and Western medicine (*zhongxiyi jiehe* 中西醫結合);

---

[13] See Farquhar (1994, 1996) for descriptions of two very different kinds of contemporary Chinese medical practice.
[14] The names of both physicians have been changed.   [15] Farquhar (1994), 190.

oppositions between different generations of medical practice, especially between physicians with pre- and post-revolutionary training and between septuagenarian and octogenarian *laozhongyi* 老中醫 (senior Chinese physicians) and their younger contemporaries; and oppositions between modernisers of various kinds (*xiandai pai* 現代派) and more traditionally minded conservatives (*baoshou pai* 保守派). I believe that these oppositions and the continuities on which they build furnish important insights into how Chinese medicine is changing in an environment characterised by rapid modernisation.

Third, both of the doctors whose practice I analyse are highly respected practitioners and influential teachers. I therefore feel entitled to present them as exemplary individuals – exemplary with respect to the level of their knowledge and clinical skills, yet also in regard to the oppositions outlined above. My access and relation to the two teachers was not of the same order, though. I had much greater opportunities to observe Professor Zhu in clinical practice and to converse with him at first hand. My contact with Professor Qian was more formal and my information was often gained from his students and writings rather than directly from him. Nevertheless, given normal student experience, I consider my analysis of the prescribing practice of both professors equally valid.

Professor Qian: senior Chinese physician

Professor Qian was 72 when I studied with him from August to December 1994. The son of a famous physician from Jiangsu Province, he traces his medical lineage back nine generations.[16] His medical education began at the age of five or six when he began to learn by heart the *Shanghan lun* 傷寒論 (Discussion of Cold Damage) and continued as apprentice to his father. In 1947 he qualified as a state-registered physician by passing recently established state examinations. In 1951 he completed a one-year evening class in Western medicine at his local hospital in Nantong, Jiangsu Province. In 1956 Professor Qian became leader of the Formula Teaching and Research Group at the then Chinese Medicine Vocational College (*Zhongyi jinxiu xuexiao* 中醫進修學校) in Jiangsu Province. By 1957 he had moved to Beijing where he was appointed chairman of the Formula Teaching and Research Office at the newly established Chinese Medicine College (*Beijing zhongyi xueyuan* 北京中醫學院). Today he is life professor at the Beijing University of Chinese Medicine and Pharmacology (*Beijing zhongyiyao daxue* 北京中醫藥大學), a position bestowed on only a very small number of teachers,

---

[16] This figure was indicated to me by his students.

and one of the *laozhongyi* who have helped to shape the development of Chinese medicine over recent decades.[17] Given his descent, teaching, and practice, Professor Qian is widely regarded by students and colleagues as a traditionalist.

Professor Qian still runs a surgery most days of the week, treating up to seventy patients during a typical morning session. Unlike many younger doctors, he does not specialise in the treatment of a narrow range of problems, but professes to be versed in the miscellaneous diseases of internal medicine (*neike zabing* 內科雜病), warm factor diseases (*wenbing* 溫病), gynaecology (*fuke* 婦科), and paediatrics (*erke* 兒科). He holds surgeries in the outpatient clinic attached to the Beijing University of Chinese Medicine and Pharmacology, the Beijing Municipal Hospital of Chinese Medicine (*Beijing shi zhongyi yiyuan* 北京市中醫醫院), and in his flat in the university compound. Demand for consultations with Professor Qian far exceeds his available time and all too often patients have to be turned away. Individual consultations, therefore, rarely last longer than five minutes. They usually begin with Professor Qian examining pulse and tongue. He then asks a few questions concerning symptoms, medical history and previous treatments before writing out a herbal prescription and maybe dispensing some advice regarding diet and life-style.

In spite of the little time Professor Qian has available for each patient, he still finds a few moments to speak to his audience of patients and students on topics such as the differences between Western and Chinese medicine. These reflections may be triggered off by a patient's request to learn more about the diagnosis, or comment about personal experience with Western medicine. Professor Qian identifies Chinese and Western medicine as distinct types of esoteric knowledge which require special study. Without being disparaging he tells patients that it would be quite useless to give them a detailed explanation, since they lack prerequisite background knowledge.

In the discourse with his patients Professor Qian never calls into question the use of Western medicine *per se*. He does however challenge its lack of understanding of many of the relationships existing within the human organism or between human beings and their environment. Possessed of such an understanding he is able to effect cures where biomedical therapy has failed to draw a definite dividing line between the two styles of medical practice. He also points out that he knows Western medicine and uses it to enlarge his personal understanding of disease, but that most doctors of Western medicine disdain Chinese medicine. Yet, for all his assertions, Professor Qian seems little interested in biomedical information beyond disease names or basic diagnostic data such as blood pressure, blood sugar levels, or liver function tests. Patients regularly

---

[17] On the role of these senior doctors in the development of Chinese medicine see Farquhar (1994), 14–17.

bring along their hospital files, CT scans, X-rays, and lab reports, but he usually pays them scant attention. His terse entries into the patients' case records make little or no reference to biomedicine beyond the occasional biomedical disease category. Professor Qian's young post-graduate students, by contrast, eagerly read these records and copy down the results noted in laboratory reports.

It thus appears that for Professor Qian, biomedicine mainly fulfils the role of a dialogic other against which he can more clearly mark out and define his own position. For instance, to a patient complaining of dizziness (*touyun* 頭暈), he explained: 'There is blood stasis (*xueyu* 血瘀), so your brain function is insufficient (*nao gongneng buzu* 腦功能不足), but what Western medicine does not know is that there is also phlegm (*tan* 痰).' This type of rhetorical opposition is quite typical and phrases such as 'Western medicine says . . . but Chinese medicine says' (*xiyi shuo . . . , danshi zhongyi shuo . . .* 西醫說 . . . 但是中醫說 . . .) are frequently heard in Professor Qian's surgery. A position in which Chinese medicine is externally set apart form an intrinsically different Western medicine certainly accords with the historical experience of Professor Qian's generation of doctors, who, after all, had to fight for the institutional survival of Chinese medicine in face of opposition from this Western medical other. Yet, beneath such surface antagonism, clinical practice admits of a more subtle and complex dialogue.

Professor Qian's use of biomedical knowledge

Many of Professor Qian's diagnoses and treatments make no reference at all to biomedicine. Occasional traces of biomedical terms and concepts do however lead on to the discovery of deeper levels of interaction. In both verbal and written discourse, Professor Qian employs in ways resembling Chinese medical terminology concepts taken from or alluding to biomedicine. In the statement quoted above, for instance, the idiom 'the brain function is insufficient' (*nao gongneng buzu* 腦功能不足) stands halfway between standard idioms from the Chinese medical lexicon such as 'spleen *qi* is insufficient' (*piqi buzu* 脾氣不足) and biomedical terms referring to organ vitality such as 'liver function' or 'kidney function' (*gan gongneng* 肝功能, *shen gongneng* 腎功能). Similarly, Professor Qian may state that 'the function of the heart blood is insufficient' (*xinxue gongneng buzu* 心血功能不足) or that 'the heart is [in a] bad [condition] and the kidneys are deserted' (*xinzang buhao, shen kui* 心臟不好，腎虧).

The borrowing of biomedical terms to describe entities or functions in Chinese medicine has become standard practice in contemporary China. Modern Chinese medical texts commonly refer to 'heart function' (*xinzang gongneng* 心臟功能) or the 'physiological function of spleen and stomach' (*piweide shengli gongneng* 脾胃的生理功能) when they wish to explain visceral function as described in the canonical literature.[18] Distinctive of this practice is the manner in which the boundaries between biomedical organs and Chinese medical viscera (*zangfu* 臟腑) is blurred. *Shen kui* in the above statement repeats classical terminology and thus clearly is a premodern concept. *Xinzang buhao*, however, is a colloquial expression which could refer to Chinese as well as Western medical reasoning.

The same impression is given by Professor Qian's explanation of the aetiology of dizziness in a fifty-three-year-old male patient. In his intake interview consisting of a series of brief questions and the examination only of pulse and tongue, the patient indicated that, according to the diagnosis of his local hospital, he had been suffering from 'heart disease' (*xinzang bing* 心臟病) for two years. His main complaint was 'dizziness' (*touyun* 頭暈), 'much worse after exertion' (*yundong yihou geng lihai* 運動以後更利害) but 'generally not occurring in the evenings' (*wanshang yiban mei fazuo* 晚上一般沒發作). He also suffered from 'palpitations' (*xinhuang* 心慌) which were 'somewhat relieved by lying down' (*wochuang hao yixie* 臥床好一些). The tongue, according to Professor Qian, was reddish with thin and insufficient fur (*she hong, tai bo bugou* 舌紅苔薄不夠). The pulse was thin and wiry (*mai xi xuan* 脈細弦). After a brief enumeration of symptoms, the entry in the patient's case history as noted down by Professor Qian reads: 'This is vacuity of the gathering *qi* [of the chest], the vessels are inhibited, the brain loses its nourishment' (*ci wei zongqi xu, mai buli, nao shi yang* 此為宗氣虛，脈不利，腦失養). There was no further interaction and the patient left with the following prescription after little more than ten minutes.

Magnetitum (*cishi* 磁石)	25 g
Rhizoma Gastrodiae Elatae (*tianma* 天麻)	3 g
Radix Ligustici Chuanxiong (*chuanxiong* 川芎)	3 g
Radix Achyranthis Bidentate (*huainiuxi* 怀牛膝)	10 g
Radix Rehmanniae Glutinosae (*shengdihuang* 生地黃)	25 g
Flos Carthami Tinctorii (*honghua* 紅花)	9 g
Semen Persicae (*taoren* 桃仁)	9 g
Radix Salviae Mitiorrhizae (*danshen* 丹參)	15 g
Lumbricus (*dilong* 地龍)	6 g
Radix Codonopsitis Pilosulae (*dangshen* 党參)	20 g
Tuber Ophiopogonis Japonici (*maimendong* 麥門冬)	12 g
Fructus Schisandrae Chinensis (*wuweizi* 五味子)	3 g
Cortex Albizziae Julibrissin (*hehuanpi* 合歡皮)	12 g

[18] Random examples exist in the modern literature. See for instance Beijing zhongyi xueyuan (1986), Liu Bingfan (1993), 5, or the entries under the various organs in the *Zhongyi dacidian: neike fence* (1987).

While the root of the problem in Professor Qian's diagnosis seems to be located firmly within premodern Chinese medical models (vacuity of the gathering *qi* of the chest), the proximal cause of the condition is phrased in terms linked semantically, structurally, and practically to biomedically defined pathologies. According to traditional understanding, the brain is, after all, associated with the marrow (*sui* 髓) and the kidneys (*shen* 腎) which store essence (*jing* 精), rather than with the blood (*xue* 血) or the vessels (*mai* 脈).[19] Even though Professor Qian leaves open the question of what nourishment is lacking and which vessels exactly are obstructed, there is a strong suggestion of biomedical models of blood circulation and an assumed lack of blood supply to the head. I make this assertion on two grounds. First, one of Professor Qian's doctoral students informed me explicitly on several occasions that to the best of his knowledge, in this as in other cases, Professor Qian was integrating biomedical ideas about the structure and function of the organism into his prescribing practices. Second, the prescription employed by Professor Qian to treat this problem indicates that not merely the *qi*, blood and essence as understood in classical Chinese medicine are treated here, but also the vascular system and the brain derived from Western anatomy and physiology.

The prescription may be divided into three parts. The first of these, consisting of the drugs Radix Codonopsitis, Tuber Ophiopogonis, and Fructus Schisandrae, corresponds to the classical formula *Shengmai san* 生脈散 (Generate Pulse Powder).[20] This is a formula devised by Li Gao 李杲 (1180–1251) for the treatment of summer-heat damaging the original *qi* (*yuanqi* 元氣) in patients with pre-existing spleen and stomach vacuity causing fatigue, heaviness and shortness of breath.[21] Some authors attribute its composition to Zhang Yuansu 張元素 (1151–1234), Li Gao's teacher. They point to a formula of the same name and ingredients in Zhang's *Yixue qiyuan* 醫學啟源 (On the Origins of Medicine) of 1186, which according to its author 'supplements insufficiency of the original *qi* within the lung' (*bu feizhong yuanqi buzu* 補肺中元氣不足).[22] Throughout subsequent centuries physicians associated with competing medical traditions emphasised the importance of the formula for the supplementation of *qi* and *yin* vacuity (*qixu* 氣虛, *yinxu* 陰虛) conditions.[23] Diverse scholar-physicians provided complementary but nevertheless different interpretations of what was actually supplemented by the prescription. For some it was lung *yin* (*feiyin* 肺陰), for others the origi-

[19] Porkert (1974), 162–3.
[20] The original formula has Radix Ginseng (*renshen* 人參) which is commonly substituted today by Radix Codonopsitis Pilosulae (*dangshen* 党參). The latter is less expensive and thought by some physicians to be more effective in the treatment of heart disease.
[21] *Neiwai shang bian huo lun, juan* 3, 25–6.   [22] Xu Jiqun and Wang Mianzhi (1995), 246.
[23] Zhang Weiyao (1994), 402, lists Xu Dachun 徐大椿 (1693–1772) as an exemplary proponent of the use of *Shengmai san* belonging to the cold damage school (*shanghan xuepai* 傷寒學派) and Xue Xue 薛雪 (1681–1770) and Wang Mengying 王孟英 (1808–67) as equally influential proponents from the warm factor disease school (*wenbing xuepai* 溫病學派).

nal *qi* within the lung (*feizhong yuanqi* 肺中元氣), and for yet others the pulse and/or vessels (*mai* 脈). As a *qi* supplementing (*buqi* 補氣) prescription within the larger category of supplementing and boosting formulae (*buyiji* 補益劑), it has been integrated into the teaching of formulas at contemporary Chinese colleges. Modern textbooks (to which Professor Qian is a prominent contributor) list as *Shengmai san's* basic functions: it 'benefits the *qi* and astringes the *yin*, produces fluids and nourishes the heart' (*yi qi lian yin, sheng jin yang xin* 益氣斂陰生津養心).[24] Its pharmacological properties and actions have been widely researched since the early 1960s and it is administered today not only in the traditional form of decoction (*tang* 湯) or powder (*san* 散) but intravenously or orally in specially prepared formulations as a cardiotonic and circulatory stimulant.[25] It has also been adopted in contemporary China as one of the main formulas in the treatment of heart disease based on disease differentiation (*bianbing* 辨病) rather than pattern differentiation (*bianzheng* 辨証).[26]

To this formula Professor Qian has added several drugs which quicken blood (*huoxue* 活血) and which free the vessels and quicken the collaterals (*tong mai huo luo* 通脈活絡): Semen Persicae, Flos Carthami, Lumbricus, Radix Ligustici, Radix Salviae and Radix Achyranthis. Radix Rehmanniae supports this function by enriching *yin* (*zi yin* 滋陰) and cooling blood (*liang xue* 涼血), thereby preventing stagnation caused by heat and dryness. The combination of these drugs is a common strategy in treating problems diagnosed as blood stasis in Chinese medicine.

Blood stasis, referred to in some texts as blood amassment (*xuxue* 蓄血) is defined as '[the] blood fluid stagnates and binds [and] does not flow' (*xueye yujie buxing* 血液瘀結不行).[27] It is thought to cause a wide variety of problems from pain and bleeding to loss of memory and manic behaviour. The pattern was first discussed by Zhang Zhongjing (145–208) in both the *Shanghan lun* 傷寒論 and the *Jingui yaolüe* 金匱要略 (Essentials from the Golden Cabinet).[28] However, it was Wang Qingren 王清任 (1768–1831) who most influenced the contemporary treatment of these patterns.[29] Indeed, as figure 12.1 shows, Professor Qian's prescription can be interpreted as a variation of Wang Qingren's flagship formula *Xuefu zhuyu tang* 血府逐瘀湯 (Decoction for Expelling

---

[24] Xu Jiqun and Wang Mianzhi (1995), 244.

[25] For a detailed discussion of both modern and classical uses of *Shengmai san* see Shi Zaixiang (1981) and Xu Jiqun and Wang Mianzhi (1995), 244–8.

[26] In contemporary Chinese medicine the term *bianbing* can refer to a discrimination according to either traditional Chinese and/or modern biomedical disease categories. It designates a diagnostic practice with complex and ambivalent relations to the entirely Chinese *bianzheng*. See Scheid (1997), 149–79.

[27] Xie Guan ((1921) 1988), vol. IV, 3842.

[28] See for instance *Shanghan lun* 傷寒論, *tiao* 106, 163; *tiao* 124–6, 166–71; *tiao* 239, 342; and *tiao* 257, 343. *Jingui yaolüe, pian* 16, 456–78.

[29] On Wang Qingren see Andrews (1991) and Qiu Peiran and Ding Guangdi (1992), 654–62.

Stasis from the Blood Mansion) where *Shengmai san* has been substituted for *Sini san*
四逆散 (Counterflow Cold Powder) in the original formula.[30]

Several of the early proponents of the integration of Western and Chinese medicine,
notably Tang Zonghai 唐宗海 (1862–1918) and Zhang Xichun, as well as influential
teachers of the post-revolutionary period such as Pu Fuzhou 蒲輔周 (1888–1975) further emphasised the treatment of blood stasis patterns and established them as a core
concern of modern Chinese physicians.[31] Blood (*xue*) in Chinese medicine denotes, as
Porkert points out, 'but one of several forms of energy occurring in the microcosm, not
simply a moving fluid'.[32] However, to Chinese medical thinkers it offered more convenient analogies to Western medicine than did concepts such as *qi*, where no ready-made
counterpart exists in the world of biomedicine. Research on vascular pathologies constitutes a major focus of modern Chinese medical research and was allocated priority status in the eighth Five-Year Plan.[33] Such research has variously examined the
effects of blood enlivening herbal medicines such as Radix Ligustici Wallichii and
Radix Salviae Militiorrhizae on blood rheology and attempted to establish objective
indicators in the diagnosis of blood stasis.[34]

The remainder of the prescription comprises the synergistic drug combination
(*duiyao* 對藥) of Magnetitum and Rhizoma Gastrodiae and the calming drug Cortex
Albizziae.[35] The combination of Magnetitum and Rhizoma Gastrodiae is used by

---

[30] *Xuefu zhuyu tang* is presented by Wang Qingren in his *Yilin gaicuo* 醫林改錯 (Correction of Errors
among Physicians), *juan* 1, 61. Flagship formula implies: (i) that the formula serves as the basis for a
number of other formulas; (ii) that this is the formula for which Wang Qingren is today most widely
remembered. *Sini san* is a formula from the *Shanghan lun* and consists of the four drugs Radix Bupleuri
(*chaihu* 柴胡), Radix Paeoniae (*shaoyao* 芍藥), Fructus Citri seu Ponciri Immaturus (*zhishi* 枳實), and
Radix Glycyrrhizae Uralensis (*gancao* 甘草). It is employed in Wang Qingren's *Xuefu zhuyu tang* as
that aspect of the formula which moves *qi*. Building up new formulas by combining older ones and sub-
stituting drugs or drug groups in a formula with others so as to produce a new formula with a different
set of indications is an established practice in Chinese medicine that can be traced back as far as the
Shanghan lun. For discussion of the composition of *Xuefu zhuyu tang* and *Sini san*, see Xu Jiqun and
Wang Mianzhi (1995), 118–20 and 398–401.

[31] Professor Xu Zhu 許杼, Beijing, personal communication. The work of Tang Zonghai and Zhang
Xichun and its influence on Chinese medicine is assessed in Qiu Peiran and Ding Guangdi (1992),
708–36. A biography of Pu Fuzhou can be found in Li Yun (1988), 906. For his treatment style see
Zhongguo zhongyi yanjiuyuan (1979). For an example of the kind of syntheses currently produced in
the field see Yu Junsheng (1995).

[32] Porkert (1974), 186.   [33] Du Ruzhu (1994).   [34] Shi Yongde (1981).

[35] According to some of my informants the use of synergistic drug combinations is derived from Shi
Jinmo 施今墨 (1881–1969). Shi Jinmo was one of Beijing's *si da mingyi* 四大名醫 (four famous
physicians) during the first part of this century and an important figure, both intellectually and politically, in preparing the way for the integration of Chinese and Western medicine. See Qian Zifen,
Zhang Yuxuang and Gao Saishan (1993), 135. *Duiyao* are discussed independently by Qin Bowei
((1962) 1983) and their use dates back much further. Shi Jinmo is thus more important as a populariser
than as an inventor.

Professor Qian in many cases of headache (*toutong* 頭痛) and dizziness. The fixed combination of these two drugs as a constantly recurring pattern in Professor Qian's prescriptions marks them as an integral aspect of his own clinical experience and/or the strategies of his medical lineage.[36] Finally, Cortex Albizziae is a drug which calms the spirit and resolves depression (*an shen jie yu* 安神解鬱). As Chinese medicine postulates a close connection between blood and spirit, drugs that have an action on the spirit are sometimes included in blood quickening formulas. Cortex Albizziae is an obvious choice because it is a spirit calmer which has the secondary action of quickening the blood.[37] Figure 12.1 traces the genealogy of the entire formula and its various links to the archive of Chinese medical treatment strategies and formulas.

Having briefly presented the prescription, I now wish to analyse via the clinical response the pathomechanism that Professor Qian has diagnosed in this case. My purpose is to elucidate the way in which Professor Qian adapts Chinese medical practice to biomedical knowledge and the consequences thereof.

We may recall that the core problem diagnosed by Professor Qian was vacuity of *zongqi* or 'gathering' *qi* which, in his prescription, is clearly addressed via the supplementing action of *Shengmai san*. *Zongqi* is described in modern textbooks as a synthesis of the clear *qi* of the environment assimilated by the lungs, and the *qi* assimilated from food and drink by the spleen and stomach. *Zongqi* is said to accumulate in the chest and via its connection to the lungs (*fei* 肺) and the heart (*xin* 心) to influence breathing and the movement of *qi* and blood.[38] Professor Qian connects the depletion of *zongqi* in this particular patient to his complaint of dizziness, which he ascribes more proximally to an undernourishment of the brain. Though Professor Qian does not specify exactly what is lacking in the brain when he writes 'the brain loses its nourishment' (*nao shi yang* 腦失養), his use of terminology allows us to make some retrospective assumptions. The verb *yang* 養, 'to nourish', is used in Chinese medical discourse to refer to the physiological or therapeutic supplementation of *yin* or structive aspects of the body or specific organs.[39] Thus, one 'nourishes' *yin*, blood, essence, fluids as well as such organs as the heart, the liver, and the stomach which are involved in the physiology of these substances. Supplementation of *qi*, on the other hand, is described by terms

---

[36] While the distinction between treatment strategies derived from personal experience and those that have been passed down a medical lineage is an important one, in the present case it was beyond the resources available to me to differentiate between the two.

[37] On blood and spirit (*shen* 神) in Chinese medicine see Wang Miqu et al. (1986), 13–33. A historical precedent for the use of spirit calmers in blood stasis formulas is the inclusion of Cinnabaris (*zhusha* 朱砂) in the formula *Qili san* 七里散 (Seven Li Powder). See Xu Jiqun and Wang Mianzhi (1995), 403–4. For Cortex Albizziae, see Yan Zhenghua (1991), 669–70.

[38] Beijing zhongyi xueyuan (1986), 50.

[39] Strictly speaking the noun *yang* (nourishment) in Professor Qian's statement is not the same lexeme as the verbal *yang* used by Chinese physicians who nourish the blood (*yang xue*).

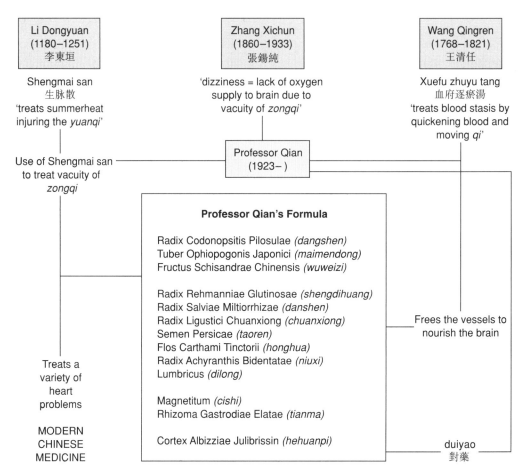

Figure 12.1. *The genealogy of Professor Qian's formula*

such as *yi* 益, 'to benefit'. Professor Qian's diagnosis implies that dizziness is here due to a lack of *yin* or structivity of some kind. One possibility would be a depletion of essence (*jing* 精), with which the brain is associated via the kidneys. But as the prescription contains no essence-nourishing drugs (*yangjing yao* 養精藥), this possibility must be discounted. The only alternative, therefore, is a lack of blood.

Professor Qian's prescription has been shown to be a variation of Wang Qingren's *Xuefu zhuyu tang*. This formula contains drugs that enliven blood and others that move *qi*, based on the adage that '*qi* can move blood' (*qi neng xing xue* 氣能行血).[40] In Professor Qian's prescription the *qi*-moving aspect of the formula (i.e. *Sini tang*) has been substituted by drugs for supplementing *qi*, specifically *zongqi* (i.e. *Shengmai san*),

---

[40] Beijing zhongyi xueyuan (1986), 54.

Professor Qian's Formula	Wang Qingren's *Xuefu zhuyu tang*
Shengmai san 生脉散 (supplements *qi* 补氣)	*Sini san* 四逆散 (regulates *qi* 理氣)
Radix Ginseng *(renshen)* here substituted by Radix Codonopsitis Pilosulae *(dangshen)* Tuber Ophiopogonis Japonici *(maimendong)* Fructus Schisandrae Chinensis *(wuweizi)*	Radix Bupleuri *(chaihu)* Fructus Citri seu Ponciri Immaturus *(zhishi)* Radix Paeoniae *(shaoyao)* Radix Glycyrrhizae Uralensis *(gancao)*
+	+
Radix Rehmanniae Glutinosae *(shengdihuang)* Radix Achyranthis Bidentatae *(niuxi)* Radix Ligustici Chuanxiong *(chuanxiong)* Semen Persicae *(taoren)* Flos Carthami Tinctorii *(honghua)*	Radix Rehmanniae Glutinosae *(shengdihuang)* Radix Achyranthis Bidentatae *(niuxi)* Radix Ligustici Chuanxiong *(chuanxiong)* Semen Persicae *(taoren)* Flos Carthami Tinctorii *(honghua)*
Radix Salviae Miltiorrhizae *(danshen)* Lumbricus *(dilong)*	Radix Angelicae Sinensis *(danggui)*
+	+
Magnetitum *(cishi)* Rhizoma Gastrodiae Elatae *(tianma)* Cortex Albizzia Julibirissin *(hehuanpi)*	Radix Platycodi Grandiflori *(jiegeng)*

Figure 12.2. *A comparison of Professor Qian's formula with Wang Qingren's* Xuefu zhuyu tang 血府逐瘀汤

as indicated in Figure 12.1.[41] The prescription as a whole still treats blood stasis, but a stasis which is envisaged to arise from *qi* vacuity rather than *qi* stagnation.[42]

Professor Qian is thus most likely treating dizziness as a problem of blood circulation. This is an important innovation, for neither classical strategies for the treatment of dizziness nor modern textbooks make any reference to blood stasis patterns.[43]

---

[41] Another important change is the omission of Radix Platycodi Grandiflori (*jiegeng* 桔梗). This is used in the original formula to guide the entire formula to the chest where, according to Wang Qingren, the blood mansion (*xuefu* 血府) is located. It would appear that this drug can be omitted by Professor Qian because *Shengmai san* (unlike *Sini san*) already unfolds its action in the chest.

[42] Regarding the role of *zongqi* in the causation of blood stasis cf. *Huangdi neijing Lingshu* 黃帝內經靈樞, *pian* 75, 494: 'Therefore, [if there is] reverse [frigidity of] the feet, the *zongqi* does not descend, the blood in the vessels congeals and gets stuck.'

[43] Neither of the following texts which comprehensively review contemporary and classical treatments for dizziness cite blood stasis: Han Guangmei (1993); Wang Letao (1993), 567–70; Zhang Baiyu, Dong Jianhua and Zhou Zhongying (1988), 439–50. See also Ots (1990), 147, for a phenomenologically grounded discussion of dizziness in contemporary China as a culturally impregnated bodily experience characterised by a sensation of nausea.

Furthermore, it is a revealing insight into how such innovation proceeds in contemporary Chinese medicine. Professor Qian's pathology of dizziness conjoins proximal brain function and distal circulatory insufficiency and obstruction. Both of these perceived causes suggest an influence from biomedicine. One possible channel through which biomedical influence may have reached Professor Qian was the work of Zhang Xichun. Zhang was an early proponent of the integration and convergence of Chinese and Western medicine, whose enduring influence on subsequent generations of physicians is clear from the number of his formulas that have entered contemporary formularies, including those to which Professor Qian has contributed.[44] Early this century, Zhang had already researched into the relationship between problems of brain function (indicated by symptoms such as dizziness) and insufficiency of the *zongqi*.[45] This research had been stimulated precisely by differences between Western accounts of brain function and Chinese medicine's view of brain and marrow as 'little more than accessories' to the kidneys.[46] Professor Qian's prescription can be seen as moving Zhang's convergence, which had focused on similarities between the Chinese concept of *qi* and the Western notion of oxygen, towards an even closer symmetry by bringing into play analogies between the circulation of *xue* 血 and blood. A second source of influence is modern research covering blood stasis, *Shengmai san* and, especially, disease differentiation, with which Professor Qian, as head of the formula department at the university, is intimately familiar. This influence is shown by the fact that *Shengmai san* was the Professor's formula of choice whenever a patient with the biomedical label 'heart disease' (*xinzangbing*) presented in one of his surgeries, irrespective of the Chinese medical pattern diagnosed.

Professor Qian's treatment approach thus skilfully interweaves three strands of learning: first and foremost, knowledge gained through reading and memorising the traditional medical archive; second, experience accumulated and handed down within his family tradition and therefore not available in the literature; finally, biomedical concepts reinterpreted and rewrought to fit in with traditional theory and practice. The dizziness of

---

[44] About ten (the exact figure varies from textbook to textbook) of the 176 new prescriptions composed by Zhang Xichun in his medical essays published between 1900 and 1934 under the title *Yixue zhong zhong can xi lu* 醫學衷中參西錄 (Records of Heart-felt Experiences in Medicine with References to the West) are among the 200 or so formulas taught today in elementary courses on formulas. These include *Zhangan xifeng tan* 鎮肝息風湯 (Sedate the Liver and Extinguish Wind Decoction), *Shoutai wan* 壽胎丸 (Foetus Longevity Pill), and *Huoluo xiaoling dan* 活洛效靈丹 (Phantastically Effective Pill to Invigorate the Collaterals). See Xu Jiqun and Wang Mianzhi (1995) and Yang Yiya (1994). In the explanations to these formulas, Zhang (1991) shows explicitly how their composition is inspired by the advances of Western medicine. Pertinent examples are the influence of Western notions of apoplexy in the formulation of *Zhengan xifeng tang* and of diabetes in the formulation of *Zengye tang* 增液湯 (Increase Fluids Decoction).
[45] Zhang Xichun ((1900) 1991), vol. II, 193–4.   [46] Porkert (1974), 163.

his patient is assumed to be due to a lack of nourishment to the brain (apparently of *xue* but also, perhaps of biomedical blood), caused by a vacuity of *qi* in the chest (which includes the function of the heart) and a resultant stasis of *xue* (or blood) in the vessels. Treatment is via a formula that strengthens the gathering *qi* in the chest, but that is *also* a modern formula for the treatment of a variety of heart problems. It is complemented by strategies to free the vessels based on the composition of traditional formulas, but uses herbs which are *also* known today to have an effect on (Western medical) blood circulation.

Professor Qian's treatments, like the terminology he employs, are replete with ambiguities which obscure the dividing lines between Western and Chinese medical knowledge. A patient with heart disease is identified, by means of Chinese medical pattern differentiation (*bianzheng* 辯証), as suffering from the Chinese pattern gathering *qi* vacuity (*zongqi xu* 宗氣虛) which suggests using *Shengmai san*. On the other hand, following the well-established practice of disease differentiation (*bianbing* 辯病), the 'heart disease' leads to the same formula. While Professor Qian would not prescribe herbs for blood stasis unless they were indicated by signs denoting their presence, one important sign in contemporary practice is that a prescription works where other treatment strategies have failed.[47] This means that blood-quickening prescriptions are often employed simply because everything else has failed, but also that blood stasis indicates deep-seated and long-standing conditions such as, for instance, heart disease.

Hence, Professor Qian's style of innovation leads out of and is marked by two important and mutually supportive characteristics of the Chinese medical tradition: the inherent polysemy of its concepts and the plurality of treatment strategies available to physicians in its medical archive. Medical authorities throughout the ages agreed that the movement of *qi* and *xue* through the body is controlled and influenced by various visceral systems and types of *qi* (such as *daqi* 大氣 or *zongqi* 宗氣) located in the chest. No unequivocal view ever existed, however, regarding the precise nature of these entities or their relation to each other. Important physicians such as Yu Chang 喻昌 (1585–1664),[48] Zhang Zhicong 張志聰 (1610–74),[49] and Chen Shiduo 陳士鐸 (fl. 1650)[50] all put forward different theories about the relationship between lungs (*fei* 肺), heart (*xin* 心), pericardium (*xinbaoluo* 心包洛), chest centre (*danzhong* 膻中),[51] great *qi* (*daqi* 大氣),[52]

---

[47] Anonymous (1983). Personal observations confirm this statement.

[48] *Yimen falü* 醫門法律 (Precepts for Physicians), *juan* 1, 277–9.

[49] Mentioned in Qiu Peiran and Ding Guangdi (1992), 710.   [50] Mentioned in Unschuld (1985), 206–8.

[51] *Danzhong* 膻中 is (i) the name of the acumoxa point CV17 located in the midline of the sternum on the level of the fourth intercostal space on the *ren* channel (*renmai* 任脈); (ii) the place in the chest where the *zongqi* accumulates, also known as the 'upper sea of *qi*' (*shang qihai* 上氣海); (iii) another name for the pericardium. Beijing zhongyi xueyuan (1986), 55, note 17.

[52] The *daqi* is by some equated with the *zongqi* (see Zhang Weiyao's (1994), 261, interpretation of Yu Chang), while by others it is an entity in its own right (see the reading of Yu Chang by Mao Juntong 毛俊同 and Ding Guangdi's 丁光迪 in Qiu Peiran and Ding Guangdi (1992), 606–7).

and gathering *qi* (*zongqi* 宗氣) and how their pathologies should be treated. In the case of Zhang Xichun, as outlined above, such thinking was already influenced by a Western-medical understanding of body function. Such diversity of opinions, however, never kept physicians from building on each other's work.[53] Furthermore, in a context where clinical efficacy rather than the coherence of theoretical concepts is paramount, such ambiguity and openness may be perceived as facilitating rather than as constraining successful medical practice. It allows physicians to formulate their own ideas, yet never ties them down to any one single set of clinical strategies.[54]

Many younger doctors, however, feel that Professor Qian represents an approach that cannot for much longer meet the demands made on Chinese medicine. These doctors openly accept the need for scientific explanation in modern Chinese society and conse-quently in Chinese medicine.[55] Their goal is to transform Chinese medicine by muster-ing the resources of medical science and technology and to create an integrated Chinese and Western medicine (*zhongxiyi jiehe* 中西醫結合). What exactly is meant by this term is difficult to ascertain. It seems that any practice which combines something from both Chinese and Western medicine can call itself *zhongxiyi jiehe*: the use of anti-viral herbal extracts by biomedical physicians and the prescribing of antibiotics in a Chinese medicine ward; the addition of herbs with anti-hypertensive action to a Chinese herbal formula prescribed on the basis of pattern differentiation for a patient with high blood-pressure; the development of new treatments such as scalp acupuncture using Chinese medical technology based on cerebral anatomy; and the assessment of Chinese medicine by means of biomedical research paradigms.

Professor Zhu: physician of integrated Chinese and Western medicine

Professor Zhu is fifty-five years old; he is one generation younger than Professor Qian. His life has been lived almost entirely in post-liberation China with a very different edu-cational background. Professor Zhu is the first physician of Chinese medicine in his immediate family, though one of his uncles did practise medicine. He graduated in 1965 from the newly established Nanjing College of Chinese Medicine (*Nanjing zhongyi*

---

[53] Zhang Xichun's innovative understanding of the *daqi*, for instance, was influenced by previous Chinese physicians such as Yu Chang and by Li Gao. See Scheid (1995).

[54] This openness, flexibility, and adaptability of Chinese medicine has been identified as one of its key characteristics by both Western and Chinese commentators. See Farquhar (1994), Unschuld (1992), and Wang Xudong (1989), 133–50.

[55] Zhang Weiyao (1994), 1–4, is an eloquent example for this line of thought, though he describes inte-grated Chinese and Western medicine (*zhongxiyi jiehe*) as merely one aspect of a wider modernisation process in Chinese medicine he calls modern Chinese medicine (*xiandai zhongyixue* 現代中醫學).

xueyuan 南京中醫學院) with the highest marks in his class. He spent the following years, the period of the Cultural Revolution, treating peasants in the countryside, studying with older doctors from renowned medical lineages and getting to know biomedical diagnostic techniques while collaborating with physicians at a Western medicine hospital in Shanghai. Following the reopening of universities, he studied for a Master's degree in Integrated Chinese and Western Medicine in the late 1970s at the Beijing College of Chinese Medicine. After two more years of postgraduate specialisation in cardiology at a medical school in Japan, he took up work in Beijing at the China–Japan Friendship Hospital (*Zhong Ri youhao yiyuan* 中日友好醫院), which has become a key institution for the integration of Chinese and Western medicine and is under the direct control of the Ministry of Health. Today, Professor Zhu is chief consultant of an internal medicine ward specialising in the treatment of heart and kidney disease (*xinshen neike bingfang* 心腎內科病房)[56] and professor of integrated Chinese and Western medicine at the Beijing University of Chinese Medicine and Pharmacology next door.

The direct care of patients on Professor Zhu's ward is in the hands of ordinary consultants and junior physicians. Professor Zhu's main task is to manage the ward and supervise student research. He has few inpatients of his own, but conducts a twice weekly ward round to supervise the clinical work of his staff. Professor Zhu also holds a surgery at the hospital's outpatient clinic twice a week, treating between ten and fifteen patients during a four hour morning session.[57] Most patients in Professor Zhu's care are seriously ill. Many have passed through a number of different clinics and hospitals before attending his surgery. A good number come from outlying districts or even from provinces as far away as Shanxi and Shandong.

Professor Zhu, who describes himself as a practitioner of integrated Chinese and Western medicine, claims to utilise the most advanced scientific knowledge in addition to the broadest range of resources from the Chinese medical archive. He eschews linkage with any one school or doctrine of Chinese medicine, yet holds that integration is best advanced from a firm foundation within Chinese medicine: *zhongyi xuexi xiyi* 中醫 學習西醫 (practitioners of Chinese medicine studying Western medicine) rather than Mao Zedong's original *xiyi xuexi zhongyi* 西醫學習中醫 (practitioners of Western medicine studying Chinese medicine) formulation.[58] Accordingly, in the majority of

---

[56] This term is an example of the ambiguous use of terms in contemporary Chinese medicine. *Xinshen* refers here to cardiology and urology as much as to the heart and kidneys of Chinese medical discourse.

[57] Throughout my period of observation in 1994, the demand for Professor Zhu's services was considerably greater, but he had specifically instructed the reception desk to limit the number of patients to a maximum of ten (a number that was always exceeded in the end) because he wished to have ample time for each consultation.

[58] Ma Boying, Gaoxi and Hong Zhongli (1994), 580.

cases he pays close attention to patients' biomedical diagnoses and case histories. Besides examination by the four methods of Chinese diagnosis (*sizhen* 四診), he routinely orders ECGs, blood and urine tests, X-Rays and CT scans. Biomedical physical examinations are carried out whenever considered necessary. On the ward and in the outpatient clinic, patients are sometimes treated by either biomedicine or Chinese medicine alone, though in the majority of cases a combined approach is used.[59] The explanations Professor Zhu gives to his patients about their illness, like his treatments, draw on both Chinese and biomedical reasoning. Comparisons between Chinese and Western medicine constitute a recurring theme. As an advocate of the integration of Chinese and Western medicine, Professor Zhu directs his rhetoric against two adversaries at the same time: conventional biomedicine which understands much about isolated areas, but little about complex processes, and the conservative (*baoshoude*) Chinese medicine of the *laozhongyi* which, in his opinion, fails to develop the valuable knowledge it possesses in the light of ever advancing scientific progress.

Individual treatment strategies depend on how Professor Zhu assesses he can most effectively manage the patient's complaint. Where Professor Zhu assumes that biomedicine has little or not more to offer than Chinese medicine (e.g. insomnia, menstrual irregularity, some types of headache, certain heart conditions, common colds) Chinese medicine is used alone. A few problems are treated with biomedical drugs alone, either for reasons of convenience (e.g. minor skin rashes where a steroid cream works quicker and is more convenient than bitter decoctions) or to manage a problem where Chinese medicine is considered a less effective therapeutic modality (e.g. in the management of severe hypertension). Where he considers that neither approach would be sufficient on its own, patients receive both Chinese herbs and biomedical drugs. Professor Zhu always follows a clear plan when using this approach. In some cases biomedical drugs are deployed to manage a particular symptom that is usually biomedically defined (e.g. hypertension), while Chinese medical drugs are prescribed to deal with the underlying cause which is specified in terms of Chinese medical theory (e.g. kidney *yin* vacuity with ascendant hyperactivity of liver *yang*: *shenyin xu, ganyang shangkang* 腎陰虛，肝陽上亢). Sometimes biomedical drugs are chosen to achieve a quick effect in the initial stages of treatment, with herbal medicines following to consolidate the effect. These treatment strategies recall popular stereotypes of Western medicine rapidly treating surface manifestations, while by contrast Chinese medicine excels at treating the root of a problem, even though it may take considerable time (*zhongyi zhi ben, xiyi zhi biao* 中醫治本，西醫治標).

---

[59] For a more detailed examination of the heterogeneous multiplicity of this combining, see Scheid (1997), 83–111.

When I asked Professor Zhu why he thought it important to assimilate Western medical knowledge to Chinese medicine he gave two reasons. His first reason concerned efficacy. As the essence of medicine is to help people get better, it matters little *how* patients are cured provided they *are* cured. However, there are particular advantages to Chinese medicine. Not only can it frequently help where Western medicine fails. If used correctly it also has no side-effects.[60] Thus, where both systems offer treatments for a given problem, Chinese medicine is always preferable. Chinese medicine must not merely be kept alive but should be developed to treat ever more problems successfully.

Professor Zhu's second reason concerned social and technological change. He argued that biomedicine presents Chinese medicine with a vast array of new data which cannot be ignored. Chinese medicine must integrate modern technologies and the data they produce within its modes of practice or run the danger of being left behind in the society China is constructing. Like all his colleagues, Professor Zhu is daily confronted with the fact that while traditional medical theory does not speak of proteinuria, blood sugar levels, and occluded arteries, modern Chinese patients certainly do. Progressivist doctors have long argued for the necessity of bringing such data within the scope of Chinese medical theory and practice. They claim that in some instances, the reality of Western medicine transcends that of Chinese medicine. A patient may suffer from proteinuria without having any subjective symptoms. Relying solely on pulse diagnosis and tongue inspection betrays not only ignorance but, more importantly, it fails the requirements of the patient.

Professor Zhu is representative of these progressivist physicians. For the last twenty years he has applied himself to projects ranging from biochemical research into the action of herbal drugs, such as measuring the effects of particular drug constituents on platelet agglutination and other aspects of blood rheology, to the redefinition of theoretical concepts in the classical literature such as a novel interpretation of the concept of *wuxue* 污血 (polluted blood). He has engaged in various clinical trials and clinically applied historical studies such as an exploration of the use of the formula *Shengmai san*. He has become a national expert in his speciality which is the treatment of *yuxue* 瘀血 (static blood) and has been awarded several national prizes for his achievements. Besides, he is a man of wide interests, in art and philosophy, as well as medicine, who emphasises the need for the wide-ranging perspective and combination of modern and traditional thought and practice which his profession and hobbies have taught him.[61]

---

[60] Professor Zhu is aware that Chinese medical drugs can, of course, have side effects. But in contradistinction to biomedical treatment where such side effects are accepted as a routine aspect of therapy, they are considered as signs of the inappropriate use of drugs in Chinese medicine.

[61] See Hay (1994) and Liscomb (1993) for investigations into the relationship between art and medicine in the Chinese tradition.

Menière's disease (*Meini'erbing* 美尼爾病)

Menière's disease, affecting the inner ear, is characterised by bouts of vertigo, nausea, and vomiting. These are accompanied by tinnitus, partial loss of hearing, a sensation of fullness in the ear, and sometimes a continued rapid oscillation of the eyeballs (nystagmus). Biomedicine describes its pathology, a progressive distension of the endolymphatic fluid, but determining its precise cause has proved more elusive and treatments to date remain palliative.[62] Contemporary Chinese medical textbooks place Menière's disease under the classical disease category 'dizziness' (*xuanyun* 眩暈) even where they are organised according to biomedical diseases.[63] The standard therapeutic approach is to use different treatments for different patients according to a pattern differentiation of dizziness.[64] Textbooks of integrated Chinese and Western medicine break up the disease into several types (*xing* 型) such as 'ascendant liver *yang* type' (*ganyang shangkang xing* 肝陽上亢型) or 'phlegm turbidity obstructing the middle type' (*tanzhuo zhongzu xing* 痰濁中阻型) which are derived from (and sometimes identical to) the more traditional patterns.[65] Professor Zhu criticises the variety of 'types' of Menière's disease put forward in the literature. His argument that it is possible to discover a much closer match between Western and Chinese descriptions of the disease leads to a novel method of treatment. The following analysis of his reasoning is derived from extensive discussions and the observation of six cases of Menière's disease treated by Professor Zhu.

In Professor Zhu's opinion over 80 per cent of all patients diagnosed as suffering from Menière's disease also exhibit a consistent pattern of disharmony according to Chinese medicine. Not only do these patients have a stable set of symptoms (nausea, vertigo, tinnitus, and/or deafness), they also show a wiry and slippery pulse (*mai xianhua* 脈弦滑) and a greasy tongue fur (*ni tai* 膩苔). The wiry pulse indicates phlegm (*tan* 痰) and/or wind (*feng* 風) as pathogenic *qi* (*xieqi* 邪氣) and points to impaired functions of liver (*gan* 肝) and/or gall bladder (*dan* 膽). Professor Zhu argues that the biomedical

---

[62] Edwards and Bouchier (1991), 843.
[63] Li Anmin and Long Yurong (1993); Zhang Baiyu, Dong Jianhua and Zhou Zhongying (1988), 439–50; Zhang Enqin (1990), 954–60.
[64] Different textbooks arrive at different patterns for dizziness. The *Zhongyi dacidian* (1987), 286, for instance, states that there are at least eight principal patterns which can be further subdivided: *fengyun* 風暈 (wind dizziness), *shiyun* 濕暈 (dampness dizziness), *tanyun* 痰暈 (phlegm dizziness), *zhongshu xuanyun* 中暑眩暈 (summerheat dizziness), *zaohuo xuanyun* 燥火眩暈 (dry fire dizziness), *qiyu xuanyun* 氣鬱眩暈 (*qi* depression dizziness), *ganhuo xuanyun* 肝火眩暈 (liver fire dizziness), and *xu yun* 虛暈 (vacuity dizziness).
[65] The use of the term *xing* (type) rather than the more traditional *zheng* (pattern) is common in clinical papers which take biomedical disease categories as their starting point. In practice, patterns are often designated as types, though types are stable whereas patterns are ephemeral. Clinical research is thus often carried out on the basis of types.

localisation of the problem in the inner ear, as well as the symptoms of tinnitus and impaired hearing also indicate a liver/gall bladder problem. The ear relates to the foot lesser *yang* gall bladder vessel (*zu shaoyang danjing* 足少陽膽經) which stands in an internal–external relation (*biaoli guanxi* 表里關係) to the foot attenuated *yin* liver vessel (*zu jueyin ganjing* 足厥陰肝經). 'The liver opens into the eyes' (*gan kai qiao yu mu* 肝開竅于目), explains why there should be nystagmus. Dizziness and loss of coordination signify internal wind (*neifeng* 內風) caused by ascendant liver *yang* (*ganyang shangkang* 肝陽上亢) and/or liver fire (*ganhuo* 肝火) which are, according to Chinese medical theory, closely related to each other.[66] This liver pathology is complicated by phlegm as indicated by the nausea, dizziness, and greasy tongue fur.

According to Professor Zhu, Menière's disease is the consequence of disordered ascending and directing-downward (*shengjiang shichang* 升降失常)[67] involving *jueyin* (attenuated *yin* or the liver visceral system) and *yangming* (*yang* brightness or the stomach visceral system). As ascending and directing downward involve many other visceral functions apart from liver and stomach, their specification as core of the present problem is a crucial aspect of Professor Zhu's diagnosis.[68] Here, he draws in particular on theories about ascending and directing-downward which have been developed by Li Gao 李杲 in the Jin Dynasty and Zhang Xichun in the early twentieth century. The liver is often in abundance (*gan chang you yu* 肝常有餘) while the stomach governs downward movement of the turbid (*wei zhu jiang zhuo* 胃主降濁). If the relationship between the two is disturbed, it can lead to an upward surge of *qi* (*qi shangchong* 氣上冲) and harm due to turbid pathogen (*zhuoxie* 濁邪) in the head and particularly the inner ear. Phlegm is the actual manifestation of this turbidity. Its presence is explained here both by the disordered function of the middle (*zhong* 中), namely the stomach or the *yang* brightness, and by a disturbed *qi* dynamic due to an abnormal upsurge of liver *qi*. Professor Zhu cites Pang Anshi 龐安時 (1044–99), who is usually known by his literary name Anchang 安常: 'Those who treat phlegm well do not treat phlegm but *qi*. [Once] the flow of *qi* is normalised the fluids of the entire body follow the *qi* and [their flow] is also normalised.'[69]

---

[66] Deng Tietao (1987), 426–39. Contemporary understandings of liver disorders are derived, in the main, from the three principles (*san gang bianzheng* 三綱辨証) of liver *qi*, liver fire, and liver wind as proposed by the Qing physician Ye Tianshi 葉天士 (1667–1746). See Li Xiaohai (1988) for an overview of Ye Tianshi's theories and their influence on other Qing physicians.

[67] For *shengjiang* theory see Kou Huaxing (1990).

[68] In both verbal and written discourse Chinese physicians sometimes use terms that would (strictly speaking) refer to a particular channel and/or to one of the six stages in the *shanghan* model of disease when they mean the organ or visceral system (*zangfu*) and its associated channel as in the present case. They can, of course, make the necessary distinction between the two if they so choose.

[69] This quotation, widely cited today, is attributed to Pang Anshi in the *Zhengzhi zhunsheng* 証治準繩 (Standards of Patterns and Treatments), vol. I, section 1, 203.

Thus far, the analysis includes only one element of biomedical knowledge: an awareness of the anatomical location of the disorder in the cochlear and vestibular sensory apparatus of the inner ear. In Menière's disease the excessive pressure and dilation of the endolymphatic system causes damage to these organs. The definition of phlegm and its relation to other substances such as water (*shui* 水), rheum (*yin* 飲), and dampness (*shi* 濕) in the classical literature is far from precise, while modern textbooks define it as a pathological body fluid. Without a great leap of imagination Professor Zhu now relates the phlegm, which manifests itself in vertigo, nausea, a wiry pulse, and greasy tongue fur, to a dysfunction of the fluids of the endolymphatic system, thereby establishing a conceptual link between the anatomical body of biomedicine and the functional body of Chinese medicine.

This link is important to Professor Zhu because he perceives it as resolving the problematic tension in contemporary Chinese medicine between tangible or formed (*youxing* 有形) and intangible or formless (*wuxing* 無形) phlegm. The former can be seen on expectoration, while the presence of the latter is deduced from symptoms and signs such as numbness of the extremities, lumps in various locations of the body, a sense of disorientation, mania, depression, and, in many cases, greasy tongue fur.[70] The structural opposition between tangible and intangible phlegm seems to be of quite recent origin. In the classical literature, phlegm was defined patho-physiologically as a process of condensation and congealing. The new interpretation perhaps reflects modern theoreticians' desires to move Chinese medicine closer to a reality capable of objective representation rather than delineation as a process.[71]

Professor Zhu explained to me on several occasions that the phlegm which causes dizziness and is described as intangible phlegm in contemporary Chinese texts, in fact, possesses a form, which in the case of Menière's disease presents as the thickened lymphatic fluid in the inner ear. This is made visible by modern scientific technology. In our discussions, Professor Zhu used this as one example to demonstrate to me that biomedical technology does not of necessity stand in opposition to Chinese medicine. Rather, it can affirm and strengthen it. Something previously related functionally by analogical reasoning can now be seen to be related in a visibly materialistic sense. In a social context where objective knowledge is frequently equated with the perceptually visible and where there is pressure on Chinese medicine to increase its objectivity, Professor Zhu thinks that this affirmation is no small achievement.

---

[70] Deng Tietao (1987), 377.

[71] The opposition between the tangible or formed (*xing*) and the intangible or formless (*wu xing*) is a recurrent topos of Chinese medicine, but is applied to phlegm for the first time in Chinese medical textbooks of the late 1950s (Steve Clavey, personal communication). See also Hsu (1999), 220–2.

Based on his analysis, Professor Zhu has also developed a herbal formula for the treatment of Menière's Disease which reads as follows:[72]

Haematitum (*daizheshi* 代赭石)
Spica Prunellae Vulgaris (*xiakucao* 夏枯草)
Radix Scutellariae Baicalensis (*huangqin* 黃芩)
Sclerotium Poriae Cocos (*fuling* 茯苓)
Rhizoma Pinelliae Ternatae (*banxia* 半夏)
Rhizoma Arisaematis (*tiannanxing* 天南星)
Semen et Fructus Trichosanthis (*quangualou* 全瓜蔞)
Semen Plantaginis (*cheqianzi* 車前子)

The main action of this formula is to direct *qi* downward (*jiangqi* 降氣) by regulating the *jueyin* and *yangming*. Its secondary action is to transform phlegm (*huatan* 化痰). It thereby reconstitutes harmony between ascending and directing downward and re-establishes the correct balance between the clear (*qing* 清) and the turbid (*zhuo* 濁). The formula draws inspiration in its selection of specific drugs from a variety of sources: (i) from Zhang Xichun, the deployment of Haematitum as sovereign drug (*jun* 君) to direct *qi* downward;[73] (ii) from established classical strategies, treating phlegm with Sclerotium Poriae, Rhizoma Pinelliae, and Rhizoma Arisaematis and treating liver disorders with Spica Prunellae and Radix Scutellariae Baicalensis;[74] (iii) from Professor Zhu's interest in the integration of Chinese and Western medicine, the use of Semen Plantaginis, and from his own clinical experience, the use of Semen et Fructus Trichosanthis.[75] A genealogy of the formula is graphically displayed in figure 12.3.

[72] It is common practice not to specify amounts but to leave these to the discretion of individual practitioners.

[73] An important antecedent formula frequently employed by Professor Zhu in which Haematitum is used for this purpose is *Zhengan xifeng tang* 鎮肝熄風湯 (Settle the Liver and Extinguish Wind Decoction) which was composed by Zhang Xichun (1991), vol. I, 312–18, and vol. II, 42–55. For the different roles drugs can assume in Chinese medical formulas see Xu Jiqun and Wang Mianzhi (1995), 14–15; Farquhar (1994), 181–4; or Métailié (this volume).

[74] The chief antecedent formulas here are *Erchen tang* 二陳湯 (Two Cured Decoction) and its variation *Daotan tang* 導痰湯 (Guide [Out] Phlegm Decoction). The former was first mentioned in the *Taiping huimin hejiju fang* 太平惠民和劑局方 (Prescriptions of the Public Pharmacy of the Era of Great Peace and of the Bureau of Medicines), *juan* 4, *fang* 19, 141, published after 1078, and has since become the representative formula for drying dampness and transforming phlegm (*zao shi hua tan* 燥濕化痰). The latter is a variation first mentioned in the *Jisheng fang* 濟生方 (Formulas to Benefit the Living) of 1253, cited in Xu Jiqun and Wang Mianzhi (1995), 529–32.

[75] There is a certain degree of overlap between these categories. Semen et Fructus Trichosanthis, for instance, is a drug for treating phlegm and Rhizoma Pinelliae also directs *qi* downwards. My presentation simplifies more complex relations.

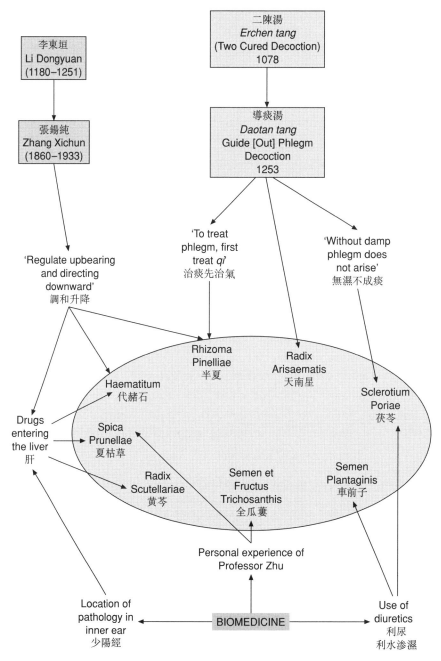

Figure 12.3. *The genealogy of Professor Zhu's formula*

The exact composition of Professor Zhu's formula need be of no further concern beyond the deployment of Semen Plantaginis as another example of the integrative reasoning by means of which Professor Zhu and many of his colleagues are currently developing Chinese medicine. Classical and modern *materiae medicae* give as the main actions of Semen Plantaginis its capacity to disinhibit water (*li shui* 利水)[76] and to dispel dampness and clear heat (*qu shi qing re* 祛濕清熱). Although some sources state that it transforms or dispels phlegm, it is not usually considered a primary drug for this purpose. Where the literature indicates its use in phlegm disorders, it refers to cough with a copious sputum, especially where this is due to lung heat.[77] As indicated above, phlegm constitutes a problematic and not clearly defined entity in Chinese medical theory. Like dampness, phlegm is an excessive accumulation of the turbid and is discussed under the rubric of fluid physiology and pathology.[78] Both phlegm and dampness are sometimes seen as having their cause in rheum. Rheum is often described as a fluid accumulation less dense than phlegm with which it combines in the paired term phlegm-rheum (*tanyin* 痰飲).[79] Phlegm is also described as originating from damp. Thus, it is sometimes said that 'without [the prior existence of] dampness phlegm does not arise' (*wu shi bucheng tan* 無濕不成痰).[80]

If, as biomedicine holds, Menière's disease is due to increased endolymphatic pressure, temporary relief at least may be attained by reducing the total amount of fluid in circulation. Some biomedical authorities administer intravenous diuretics to achieve this effect.[81] Professor Zhu explained that this was one reason why he used Semen Plantaginis. I had observed previously that Professor Zhu employed Semen Plantaginis, Herba Leonuri Heterophylli (*yimu cao* 益母草), Radix Achyranthis Bidentatae (*niu-xi* 牛膝), Herba Lycopi Lucidi (*zelan* 澤蘭), and other drugs with a known diuretic effect as assistant (*zuo* 佐) drugs in the treatment of essential hypertension. I had also observed a similar choice of drugs when studying with a physician from Chengdu in the late 1980s. This physician explained to me that his strategy was derived from the biomedical use of diuretics in the treatment of hypertension. Professor Zhu also

---

[76] Wiseman (1990), xxxvii–xxxviii, provides a detailed etymological analysis of the term *li shui* and its rendering into English as 'disinhibiting water'.

[77] Cheng Shao'en et al. (1990), 154–5; Yan Zhenghua (1991), 334–6; Zang Kuntang and Wu Keqiang (1990), 59–61; *Zhongyi dacidian: zhongyao fence* (1982), 65.

[78] Deng Tietao (1987), 377, for instance, quotes the first chapter of the Qing dynasty *Cuncunzhai yi hua gao* 存存齋醫話稿 (Notes on Medicine from the Hall of Actuality) as saying 'phlegm belongs to damp, it is a transformation of the fluids' (*tan shu shi, wei jinye suo hua* 痰屬濕，為津液所化).

[79] This is the most common view today, though there are quite different interpretations such as those of Cheng Menxue 程門雷 (1902–72), former Principal of the Shanghai College of Chinese Medicine. See Cheng Menxue (1986), 76–83. All of these refer back to *Jingui yaolüe*, *pian* 12, cited above.

[80] *Zhongshan yiyuan 'zhongyi fangji xuanjiang' bianxiezu* (1983), 232.

[81] Edwards and Bouchier (1991), 843.

admitted to the influence of biomedicine. Both physicians pointed out, however, that the drugs chosen were not selected because of their diuretic effects alone. Rather, they were integrated into a prescription because they combined a diuretic action with others that were important from a Chinese medical point of view, such as enlivening blood (*huo xue*), directing *qi* downward (*jiang qi*), or because they entered into a particular vessel (*gui jing* 歸經).

According to modern Chinese textbooks Semen Plantaginis belongs among the drugs which disinhibit water and percolate damp (*lishui shenshi yao* 利水滲濕藥). The capacity of a drug to 'disinhibit water' seems to encompass that of biomedical diuretics (*liniaoyao* 利尿藥, lit. drugs [to] disinhibit urine) while extending its effects to a wider fluid metabolism. Thus, these drugs have the biomedical function 'of increasing the volume of urine, promoting and extending urinary flow', and also the Chinese medical function of 'expelling water damp stagnating and accumulating in the interior of the body'.[82] Inducing diuresis is thus not only biomedically indicated, but just one further aspect of the Chinese medical 'disinhibition of water and percolation of damp'.

An increase in urination has long been one of the most important methods for removing the turbid from the body in Chinese medicine. Thus, in a second step which takes the action of Semen Plantaginis in Professor Zhu's prescription even further away from its use as a simple 'diuretic', the drug is integrated into a treatment strategy informed by traditional assumptions about the cooperation of drugs within a formula as sovereign (*jun* 君), minister (*chen* 臣), assistant (*zuo* 佐), and envoy (*shi* 使). Here, Semen Plantaginis, in its 'disinhibition of water and percolation of damp', assists the more important phlegm-transforming action of Rhizoma Pinelliae and Rhizoma Arisaematis. It has been noted that dampness is widely assumed in Chinese medical thinking to be a source of phlegm. Traditional formulas to treat phlegm therefore often include drugs which disinhibit damp (*li shi* 利濕) in order to assist their principal phlegm-transforming drugs. Both *Erchen tang* (Two Cured Decoction) and *Daotan tang* (Guide [Out] Phlegm Decoction), which are important influences on the formulation of Professor Zhu's own prescription, employ Sclerotium Poriae for this purpose. In the words of a contemporary teaching manual:

> Phlegm is engendered from dampness, [while] dampness itself comes from the spleen. Therefore, one uses Sclerotium Poriae as an assistant to strengthen the spleen and disinhibit damp, so [as to achieve that when] dampness has gone the spleen becomes effulgent and the phlegm has nothing from which it might be engendered.[83]

Semen Plantaginis is added to Sclerotium Poriae in Professor Zhu's formula primarily for this effect but *also* because it can be understood as a diuretic in the biomed-

---

[82] Yan Zhenghua (1991), 327.   [83] Xu Jiqun and Wang Mianzhi (1995), 531.

ical sense. In addition, it enters the liver (*gui gan* 歸肝) and brightens the eyes (*ming mu* 明目) and thus supports the dynamic of the entire formula both physiologically and symptomatically.

To sum up, we can say that in his treatment of Menière's disease, Professor Zhu collates symptoms and signs into a pattern of disharmony which is accessible to manipulation via treatment strategies recorded in the archives of the Chinese medical tradition. He also adds to this archive by strategically employing biomedical knowledge where connections can be established between the two frames of reference. Biomedicine is used as a tool which confirms Chinese medical knowledge, but also as one which makes possible new ways of reacting to a complex and ever-changing world. Furthermore, the above strategies here applied to Menière's disease are not an isolated effort by a single physician. Studying with different doctors at different institutions I came across many similar attempts to develop Chinese medicine. Some examples are: the interpretation of proteinuria (abnormal protein in the urine) as loss of essence (*jing* 精); formulas for female infertility based on an understanding of oestrogen and progesterone cycles; the treatment of male infertility based on investigations of sperm counts and sperm motility; and the use of ultrasound as an essential aspect of Chinese medical diagnosis. Physicians regularly include drugs in their prescriptions because they are anti-viral, spasmolytic, or anti-hypertensive. Neither is this a historically new phenomenon. Professor Zhu's training experience relates him to physicians in Shanghai in the 1950s who developed now-classical formulas such as *Tianma gouteng yin* 天麻鉤藤飲 (Gastrodia and Uncaria Beverage) for the treatment of biomedically defined problems such as hypertension;[84] and even further, to Zhang Xichun at the turn of the century. Zhang himself not only integrated biomedical knowledge into his clinical strategies, but also used biomedical drugs whose actions he had translated into Chinese medical functions.[85]

Professor Zhu has subtle strategies for appropriating from biomedicine that which he perceives as desirable because efficacious, while not surrendering what he values in his own tradition. Contrary to certain interpretations of and analogies with other traditional medicines, the import of Western knowledge into Chinese medicine is not bound to result in the gradual corruption of traditional practice.[86] On the contrary, what anthropologists have documented for other Asian medicines also holds true for contemporary China. Syncretisms abound while relationships between different medical practices can be, at one and the same time, complementary and conflicting, facilitating as well as competitive.[87]

[84] Xu Jiqun and Wang Mianzhi (1995), 445–6.
[85] On biomedical drugs, see Zhang Xichun (1991), vol. II, 141–65. Zhang employed biomedical theories in his understanding of the *sanjiao* 三焦 (pp. 194–6) or in the formulation of novel prescriptions for wasting thirst (*xiaoke* 消渴) which he equated with diabetes. See vol. I, pp. 76–8.
[86] Sivin (1987, 1990), Unschuld (1992), Last (1992).
[87] For related ethnographies of syncretism in the development of Chinese and Ayurvedic medical practice see Obeyesekere (1992) and Hsu (1995).

Integration as adaptation

Professor Qian's and Professor Zhu's integration of Chinese and Western medicine certainly represents a heterogeneous and unfinished project. At the simplest level a combination of the two medicines is practised concurrently but without any noticeable degree of interpenetration. In as much as such practice must be structured to be usable, it seems to be guided by Chinese medical concepts about the relationship between root (*ben* 本) and branch (*biao* 標). Wherever a more self-conscious interpenetration takes place, Professor Zhu and Professor Qian marshal the resources of biomedicine within a process of emergent *adaptation*. This process conjoins two interrelated mechanisms: assimilation and accommodation. Assimilation refers to those structures and practices which convert phenomena into experience that is intelligible. Accommodation is the restructuring of assimilation itself as it encounters new phenomena in the course of a person's development.[88]

The concept of adaptation well describes certain important features of the ongoing 'development' of Chinese medicine. The brain treated by Professor Qian and the cochlear and vestibular sense organs treated by Professor Zhu are neither entirely the brain or vessels of the *Huangdi neijing* 黃帝內經 (The Inner Classic of the Yellow Lord) and other canonical works, nor are they what a neurologist or ENT specialist would see, though they can be either. They are constituted by a mode of reasoning which has assimilated biomedical ideas of blood circulation to the *qi* movements, of endolymphatic fluid to Chinese medical ideas of phlegm, and of the inner ear to the lesser *yang* vessel. The body of Professor Qian's and Zhu's patients is still recognisable as the body of viscera and vessels. It is still brought to life by the metabolic transformation of *qi*, blood, and body fluids. Yet it also approximates the body that is revealed by biomedical technology. This body is accepted simultaneously as an important external reference point and as an object to be assimilated. The self-same process of adaptation occurs on the level of treatment formulation. Biomedical ideas about pathology are assimilated to Chinese treatment strategies and classical prescriptions. The concepts on which these prescriptions were built remain operative, but the formulas themselves have accommodated to a reality of disease made visible by a medical technology which was not available to the authors of the Han or the Yuan.

---

[88] The concepts of adaptation, accommodation, and assimilation I am using here have been developed by Piaget in the context of cognitive development. For accounts of this theory, see Flavell (1963) and Piaget (1988). I eschew, however, the notion (implicit in Piagetian structuralism) of a fixed environment relative to which an organism evolves in favour of a co-determinative development as outlined by neo-Darwinian theorists such as Lewontin (1983).

What I describe as adaptation is not, however, a process controlled by any single determining factor. As I have shown elsewhere, it emerges via the interaction of heterogeneous elements which include the biological characteristics of specific diseases, the various tools a physician has at hand and all the many other elements that partake of or intrude into the domain of medicine and healing – from patient demands to political process.[89]

There remains one further issue that deserves attention. It might be argued that the adaptive strategies I have described are evidence of the increasing domination of Chinese by Western medicine rather than of the independent survival of the former. I would concur with such a view in so far as science in general and biomedicine in particular constitute reference points of such power in contemporary China that traditional physicians simply cannot ignore them. However, the outcome of this confrontation is no foregone conclusion. As I have shown, the local is not simply dominated by the global, but rather has the power to make the global local by assimilating it to itself.

Professor Zhu, in particular, shows that the clinical gaze of biomedicine is not the natural outcome of viewing the body through the instruments of biomedical technology. As we know from Foucault and others, it is the result of distinctive disciplinary practices. Practitioners of Chinese medicine in contemporary China have learned to subject themselves to these disciplines but also know how to escape from them. The inner ear is filled with endolymphatic fluid, but it can also be full of phlegm. The chest is not only the seat of the heart, but also the place where the *zongqi* gathers. To argue that contemporary Chinese physicians are losing, or may already have lost, touch with 'traditional' medicine misses a more significant point: that it is possible to communicate effectively across apparently incommensurable paradigms, that horizons are essentially open, that plurality is practisable. Even though – or rather because – it emerges from a position of weakness, the adaptation of the Chinese medical body (corporeal as well as social) to that constructed by biomedicine teaches us much about how to engage with the other without abandoning the integrity of the self.

References to premodern Chinese and Japanese works

Huangdi neijing Lingshu 黃帝內經靈樞 (The Inner Classic of the Yellow Lord: Spiritual Pivot). Anon. Warring States and Han. Ren Yingqiu (ed.), *Huangdi neijing zhangju suoyin* 黃帝內經章句索引 (A Concordance of the Inner Classic of the Yellow Lord). Renmin weisheng chubanshe, Beijing, 1986.

Jingui yaolüe 金匱要略 (Essentials from the Golden Cabinet). Zhang Zhongjing 張仲景. Eastern Han. Based on edition of Wang Shuhe 王叔和. Re-edited in the Song, 1065. Li Keguang 李克光. (ed.) Renmin weisheng chubanshe, Beijing, 1989.

[89] See Scheid (1997). The concept of emergence attached above to that of adaptation is meant to further restrict the notion of self-evident agents acting in relation to a given environment in favour of a view which attempts to analyse the two as mutually unfolded and enfolded into and from each other.

Neiwai shang bian huo lun 內外傷辨惑論 (Clarifying Doubts about Injuries from Internal and External Causes). Li Gao 李杲. Jin, 1247. In Ding Guangdi 丁光迪 & Wang Kui 王魁 (eds.), *Dongyuan yiji.* 東垣醫集 (The Collected Medical Works of [Li] Dongyuan). Renmin weisheng chubanshe, Beijing, 1993, 1–50.

Shanghan lun 傷寒論 (Discussion of Cold Damage). Zhang Zhongjing 張仲. Eastern Han. Based on edition by Wang Shuhe 王叔和. Re-edited in the Song, 1065. Li Peisheng 李培生 and Liu Duzhou 劉渡舟 (eds.). Renmin weisheng chubanshe, Beijing, 1987.

Taiping huimin hejiju fang 太平惠民和劑局方 (Prescriptions of the Public Pharmacy of the Era of Great Peace and of the Bureau of Medicines). Song, 1078. Liu Jingyuan 劉景源 (ed.). Renmin weisheng chubanshe, Beijing, 1985.

Yilin gaicuo 醫林改錯 (Correction of Errors Among Physicians). Wang Qingren 王清任. Qing, 1830. References to Shanxisheng zhongyi yanjiuyuan 陝西省中醫研究院 (eds.), *Yilin gaicuo pingzhu* 醫林改錯評注 (Correction of Errors Among Physicians with Notes and Annotations). Renmin weisheng chubanshe, Beijing, 1976.

Yimen falü 醫門法律 (Precepts for Physicians). Yu Chang 喻昌. Qing, 1658. Si ku yixue congshu 四庫醫學叢書. Shanghai guji chubanshe, Shanghai, 1991.

Zhengzhi zhunsheng 証治準繩 (Standards of Patterns and Treatments). Wang Kentang 王肯堂. Ming, 1602–8. Ni Hexian 倪和憲 (ed.), Renmin weisheng chubanshe, Beijing, 1991.

References given in citations only

Cuncunzhai yihua gao 存存齋醫話稿 (Notes on Medicine from the Hall of Actuality). Zhao Qingchu 趙晴初. Qing. Cited by Deng Tietao 鄧鐵濤 (ed.) 1987.

Ji sheng fang 濟生坊 (Formulas to Benefit the Living). Yan Yonghe 嚴用和. Song, 1253. Cited by Xu Jiqun 許濟群 & Wang Mianzhi 王綿之 (eds.) 1995.

Yixue qiyuan 醫學啟源 (On the Origins of Medicine). Zhang Yuansu 張元素. Song, 1186. Cited by Xu Jiqun 許濟群 & Wang Mianzhi 王綿之 (eds.) 1995.

References to modern works

Aijmer, Göran (ed.) 1995. *Syncretism and the Commerce of Symbols*. Institute for Advanced Studies in Social Anthropology, Göteborg.

Andrews, Bridie J. 1991. 'Wang Qingren and the History of Chinese Anatomy.' *Journal of Chinese Medicine* 36, 30–6.

 1996. The Making of Modern Chinese Medicine, 1895–1937. PhD thesis in History, University of Cambridge.

 1997. 'TB and the Assimilation of Germ Theory in China, 1895–1937'. *Journal of the History of Medicine and Allied Sciences* 52, 114–57.

Anon. 1983. 'Zhongxiyi jiehe yanjiuhui diyice quanguo huoxue huayu xueshu huiyi ding' 中西醫結合研究會第一次全國活血化瘀學術會議訂 (Conference Proceedings of the First National Conference on Enlivening Blood and Transforming Stasis of the Research Council for the Integration of Chinese and Western Medicine). *Zhongxiyi jiehe zazhi* 中西醫結合雜誌 3.

Beijing zhongyi xueyuan 北京中醫學院 (ed.) 1986. *Zhongyi jichu lilun* 中醫基礎理論 (Basic Theory of Chinese Medicine). Zhongyi guji chubanshe, Beijing.

Chen, C. C. 1989. *Medicine in Rural China: a Personal Account*. University of California Press, Berkeley.

Cheng Menxue 程門雪 1986. *Jingui pianjie* 金匱篇解 (Interpreting the [Essentials of the] Golden Casket). Renmin weisheng chubanshe, Beijing.

Cheng Shao'en 程紹恩, Xu Baofeng 徐寶丰, Mei Guohui 美國輝 and Xia Yuehui 夏月輝 1990. *Zhongyao xinfa* 中藥心法 (The Essence of the Chinese *Materia Medica*). Beijing kexue jishu chubanshe, Beijing.

Clavey, Steve. 1995. *Jin Ye: Fluid Physiology and Pathology in Chinese Medicine*. Churchill Livingstone, Edinburgh.

Croizier, Ralph C. 1968. *Traditional Medicine in Modern China: Science, Nationalism and the Tensions of Cultural Change*. Harvard University Press, Cambridge, Mass.

Deng Tietao 鄧鐵濤(ed.) 1987. *Zhongyi zhenduanxue* 中醫診斷學 (Chinese Medical Diagnosis). Renmin weisheng chubanshe, Beijing.

Du Ruzhu 杜如竹 1994. 'Zhongyiyao "ba wu" keji zhengguan xinxi' 中醫藥 '八五' 科技政關信息 (Report on TCM Research Programs in the Eighth Five-Year Plan). *Zhongguo zhongyiyao xinxi zazhi* 中國中醫藥信息雜誌 1, 35–6.

Edwards, Christopher R. W. and Bouchier, Ian A. D. (eds.) 1991. *Davidson's Principles and Practice of Medicine*. Churchill Livingstone, Edinburgh.

Farquhar, Judith 1986. 'Knowledge and Practice in Chinese Medicine'. PhD thesis in Social Anthropology, University of Chicago.

 1994. *Knowing Practice: the Clinical Encounter in Chinese Medicine*. Westview, Boulder.

 1996. 'Market Magic: Getting Rich and Getting Personal in Medicine after Mao'. *American Ethnologist* 23, 239–57.

Feierman, Steven and Janzen, John M. (eds.) 1992. *The Social Basis of Health and Healing in Africa*. University of California Press, Berkeley.

Flavell, John H. 1963. *The Developmental Psychology of Jean Piaget*. Van Nostrand, Princeton.

Han Guangmei 韓廣妹 (ed.) 1993. *Zhongyi neike zhiyan* 中醫內科治驗 (Effective Treatments in Chinese Internal Medicine). Guizhou keji chubanshe, Guiyang.

Hay, John 1994. 'The Body Invisible in Chinese Art?' In Zito and Barlow, 42–77.

Hillier, Sheila M. and Jewell, J. A. 1983. *Health Care and Traditional Medicine in China, 1800–1982*. Routledge and Kegan Paul, London.

Hsü, Elisabeth 1992. 'Transmission of Knowledge, Texts and Treatment in Chinese Medicine'. PhD thesis in Social Anthropology, University of Cambridge.

 1995. 'The Manikin in Man: Culture Crossing and Creativity'. In Aijmer, 156–204.

 1999. *The Transmission of Chinese Medicine*. Cambridge University Press, Cambridge.

Jia Dedao 賈得道 1979. *Zhongguo yixueshi lüe* 中國醫學史略 (A Synopsis of the History of Medicine of China). Shanxi kexue jishu chubanshe, Taiyuan.

Kou Huasheng 寇華勝 1990. *Zhongyi shengjiangxue* 中醫升降學 (Ascending and Directing Downward in Chinese Medicine). Jiangxi kexue jishu chubanshe, Nanchang.

Lampton, David L. 1977. *The Politics of Medicine in China: the Policy Process 1949–1977*. Dawson, Folkestone.

Last, Murray 1992. 'The Importance of Knowing about not Knowing: Observations from Hausaland'. In Feierman and Janzen, 393–406.

Leslie, Charles and Young, Allan (eds.) 1992. *Paths to Asian Medical Knowledge*. University of California Press, Berkeley.

Lewontin, Richard (1983). 'The Organism as the Subject and Object of Evolution'. *Scientia* 118, 63–82.

Li Anmin 李安民 and Long Yurong 尤玉榮 1993. *Zhongxi canzhao neike bingzheng zhiliaoxue* 中西參照內科病証治療學 (A Cross-reference Manual of Chinese and Western Internal Medicine Diseases and Patterns, and their Treatment). Tianjin keji fanyi chubanshe, Tianjin.

Li Xiaohai 李曉海 1988. *Lun Qingdai de ganbing sangang bianzhi xueshuo* 論清代的肝病三綱辨治學說 (A Discussion of Qing Theories Regarding the Three Rubrics for Differentiating and Treating Liver Disorders). *Beijing zhongyi xueyuan xuebao* 北京中醫學院學報 11, 40–1.

Liscomb, Kathleen M. 1993. *Learning from Mt. Hua: a Chinese Physician's Illustrated Travel Record and Painting Theory*. Cambridge University Press, Cambridge.

Liu Bingfan 劉炳凡 1993. *Piweixue zhenquan* 脾胃學真詮 (A Reliable Commentary on Theories on Stomach and Spleen). Zhongguo guji chubanshe, Beijing.

'Lü Bingkui cong yi 60 nian wenji' bianji weiyuanhui 呂炳奎從醫60年文集編輯委員會 (eds.) 1993. *Lü Bingkui cong yi 60 nian wenji* 呂炳奎從醫60年文集 (Festschrift for Lü Bingkui's 60th Anniversary as a Physician). Huajia chubanshe, Beijing.

Ma Boying 馬伯英, Gao Xi 高晞 and Hong Zhongli 洪中立 1994. *Zhong-wai yixue wenhua jiaoliu shi* 中外醫學文化交流史 (A History of Intercultural Exchange in Medicine between China and the West). Wenhui chubanshi, Shanghai.

Maldener, Clara 1995. 'Grundzüge des chinesischen Gesundheitswesens (I und II)'. *ChinaMed* 5 & 6, 17–23.

Obeyesekere, Gananath 1992. 'Science, Experimentation, and Clinical Practice in Ayurveda'. In Leslie and Young, 160–76.

Ots, Thomas 1990. *Medizin und Heilung in China*. 2nd edn. Dietrich Reimer, Berlin.

Piaget, Jean 1988. *Einführung in die genetische Erkenntnistheorie*. Suhrkamp, Frankfurt am Main.

Porkert, Manfred 1974. *The Theoretical Foundations of Chinese Medicine: Systems of Correspondence*. MIT Press, Cambridge, Mass.

Qian Zifen 錢自奮, Zhang Yuxuan 張育軒 and Guo Saishan 郭賽珊 (eds.) 1993. *Zhu Chenyu linchuang jingyan ji* 祝諶予臨床經驗集 (The Collected Clinical Experiences of Zhu Chenyu). Beijing yike daxue and Zhongguo banhe yike daxue, Beijing.

Qin Bowei 秦伯未 (1962) 1983. 'Mantan chufang yong yao' 漫談處方用藥 (A Discussion of Drug Usage in Drawing Up Prescriptions). In Wu Dazhen and Wang Fengqi, 267–84.

Qiu Peiran 裘沛然 and Ding Guangdi 丁光迪 (eds.) 1992. *Zhongyi gejia xueshuo* 中醫各家學說 (Doctrines of Physicians of Chinese Medicine). Renmin weisheng chubanshe, Beijing.

Rosenthal, Marilyn M. 1981. 'Political Process and the Integration of Traditional and Western Medicine in the People's Republic of China'. *Social Science and Medicine* 15A, 599–613.

1987. *Health Care in the People's Republic of China: Moving Toward Modernization*. Westview, Boulder.

Rouse, Joseph 1996. *Engaging Science: How to Understand its Practices Philosophically*. Cornell University Press, Ithaca.

Scheid, Volker 1995. 'The Great Qi: Zhang Xichun's Reflections on the Nature, Pathology and Treatment of the *daqi*'. *Journal of Chinese Medicine* 49, 5–16.

1997. 'Synthesis and Plurality in Contemporary Chinese Medicine'. PhD thesis in Social Anthropology, University of Cambridge.

Shi Yongde 施永德 1981. 'Xueyu de shiyan yanjiu' 血瘀的實驗研究 (Experimental Research on Blood Stasis). *Zhejiang zhongyi zazhi* 浙江中醫雜誌 16(2), 92–6.

Shi Zaixiang 史載祥 1981. 'Shengmai san de linchuang ji shijian yanjiu' 生脈散的臨床及實驗研究 (Clinical and Experimental Research on *Shengmai san*). *Zhongyi zazhi* 中醫雜誌 22(12), 947–51.

Sivin, Nathan 1987. *Traditional Medicine in Contemporary China: a Partial Translation of* Revised Outline of Chinese Medicine (*1972*) *with an Introductory Study on Change in Present-day and Early Medicine*. Center for Chinese Studies, University of Michigan, Ann Arbor.

1990. 'Reflections on the Situation in the People's Republic of China, 1987'. *American Journal of Acupuncture* 18, 341–3.

Tang, Shenglan, Bloom, Gerald, Xushen Feng, Lucas, Henry, Xingyuan Gu and Segall, Malcolm (with Gail Singleton and Polly Payne) 1994. *Financing Health Services in China: Adapting to Economic Reform*. Institute for Development Studies, IDS Research Report 26.

Unschuld, Paul U. 1985. *Medicine in China: a History of Ideas*. University of California Press, Berkeley.

1992. 'Epistemological Issues and Changing Legitimation: Traditional Chinese Medicine in the Twentieth Century'. In Leslie and Young, 44–63.

Wang Ji 王琦 1993. '21 shiji – zhongyiyao de shiji' 二十一世紀 – 中醫藥的世紀 (The 21st Century – the Century of Chinese Medicine and Pharmaceutics). *Chuantong wenhua yu xiandaihua* 傳統文化與現代化 2, 64–7.

Wang Letao 王樂匋 (ed.) 1993. *Xu yi shu* 續醫書 (An Ongoing Medical Tradition). Anhui kexue jishu chubanshe, Hefei.

Wang Miqu 王米渠, Wang Keqin 王克勤, Zhu Wenfeng 朱文鋒 and Zhang Liutong 張六通 1986. *Zhongyi xinlixue* 中醫心理學 (Chinese Medical Psychology). Hubei kexue jishu chubanshe, Huanggang.

Wang Xudong 王旭東 1989. *Zhongyi meixue* 中醫美學 (Aesthetics of Chinese Medicine). Dongnan daxue chubanshe, Nanjing.

Wiseman, Nigel and Boss Ken, 1990. *Glossary of Chinese Medical Terms and Acupuncture Points*. Paradigm, Brookline, Mass.

Wu Dazhen 吳大真 and Wang Fengqi 王鳳岐 (eds.) 1983. *Qin Bowei yiwen ji* 秦伯未醫文集 (Collected Writings on Medicine by Qin Bowei). Hunan kexue jishu chubanshe, Changsha.

Xu Jiqun 許濟群 and Wang Mianzhi 王綿之 1995. *Fangjixue* 方濟學 (Formulas). Renmin weisheng chubanshe, Beijing.

Xu Xiaqun 1997. ' "National Essence" versus "Science": Chinese Native Physicians' Fight for Legitimacy 1912–32'. *Modern Asian Studies* 31, 847–78.

Yan Zhenghua 顏正華 (ed.) 1991. *Zhongyaoxue* 中藥學 (Chinese *Materia Medica*). Renmin weisheng chubanshe, Beijing.

Yang Yiya 楊醫亞 1994. *Fangjixue* 方濟學 (Formulas). Hebei kexue jishu chubanshe, Shijiazhuang.

Yu Junsheng 于俊生 (ed.) 1995. *Tanyu xiangguan xueshuo yu linchuang* 痰瘀相關學說與臨床 (A Theoretical and Clinical Guide to the Interrelation of Phlegm and Blood Stasis). Kexue jishu wenzhai chubanshe, Beijing.

Zang Kuntang 臧坤堂 and Wu Keqiang 吳克強 1990. *Zhongyao gujin yingyong zhidao* 中藥古今應用指導 (A Practical Guide to Traditional and Modern Uses of Chinese Medicinal Drugs). Guangdong keji chubanshe, Guangzhou.

Zhang Baiyu 張伯臾, Dong Jianhua 董建華 and Zhou Zhongying 周仲瑛 1988. *Zhongyi neikexue* 中醫內科學 (Chinese Internal Medicine). Renmin weisheng chubanshe, Beijing.

Zhang Enqin 張恩勤 (ed.) 1990. *Zhongyi linchuang geke* 中醫臨床各科 (Clinic of Traditional Chinese Medicine). Shanghai zhongyi xueyuan chubanshe, Shanghai.

Zhang Weiyao 張維耀 1994. *Zhongyide xianzai yu weilai* 中醫的現在與未來 (The Present and Future of Chinese Medicine). Tianjin kexue jishu chubanshe, Tianjin.

Zhang Xichun 張錫純 (1900–34) 1991. *Yixue zhong zhong can xi lu* 醫學衷中參西錄 (Records of a Sincere Search in Medicine with Reference to the West). 3 vols. Hebei kexue jishu chubanshe, Shijiazhuang.

Zhao Hongjun 趙洪鈞 1989. *Jindai zhongxiyi lunzheng shi* 近代中西醫論爭史 (History of the Polemics between Chinese and Western Medicine in Modern Times). Anhui kexue jishu chubanshe, Hefei.

Zhongyi dacidian: neike fence 中醫大辭典：內科分冊 1987. (Great Encyclopaedia of Chinese Medicine: Internal Medicine). 'Zhongyi dacidian' bianji weiyuanhui 《中醫大辭典》編輯委員會 (eds.) Renmin weisheng chubanshe, Beijing.

Zhongyi dacidian: zhongyao fence 中醫大辭典：中藥分冊 1982. (Great Encyclopaedia of Chinese Medicine: *Materia Medica*). 'Zhongyi dacidian' bianji weiyuanhui 《中醫大辭典》編輯委員會 (eds.) Renmin weisheng chubanshe, Beijing.

Zhongyi renming cidian 中醫人名詞典 1988. (Biographical Dictionary of Chinese Medicine). Li Yun 李雲 (ed.) Guoji wenhua chuban gongsi, Beijing.

Zhongguo yixue dacidian 中國醫學大辭典 (1921) 1988. (Great Dictionary of Chinese Medicine). Xie Guan 謝觀 (ed.) 4 vols. Zhongguo shudian, Beijing.

Zhongguo zhongyi yanjiuyuan 中國中醫研究院 (eds.) 1979. *Pu Fuzhou yiliao jingyan* 蒲輔周醫療經驗 (Pu Fuzhou's Experience of Medical Therapeutics). Renmin weisheng chubanshe, Beijing.

Zhonghua renmin gongheguo weishengbu zhongyisi 中華人民共和國衛生部中醫司 1985. *Zhongyi gongzuo wenjian huibian* 中醫工作文件匯編 (Collection of Documents Relating to Medical Work). Zhonghua Renmin Gongheguo weishengbu zhongyisi, Beijing.

Zhongshan yiyuan 'zhongyi fangji xuanjiang' bianxiezu 中山醫院《中醫方劑選講》編寫組 (eds.) 1983. *Zhongyi fangji xuanjiang* 中醫方劑選講 (Selected Lectures on Chinese Medical Formulas). Guangdong kexue chubanshe, Guangdong.

Zito, Angela and Barlow, Tania E. (eds.) 1994. *Body, Subject and Power in China*. University of Chicago Press, Chicago.

Index

Page numbers in *italics* refer to figures and tables.

quality 65, 84
rubbing 79
Western Han descriptions 46
yang 116
yin 115, 116
see also pulse diagnosis
Maifa (Model of the Vessels) 61, 99–100, 117
  mai 85
  pulse diagnostics 84–5
Maishu (Channel Document)
  body 33–5
  body description 39
  body piercing 39, 41
  channels 34–5, 46
  divisions 28
  mai 85
  pain 44n
  pulse diagnostics 84–5
  qi movement 41, 85
  symptoms 38
  Zhangjiashan tomb 27–31
malaria 60, 201–2
man, kinds (*zhong*) 233
Mao Zedong (1893–1976) 338, 343
  new democratic revolution 344
  support for Chinese medicine 345
marrow (*sui*) 378
martial arts 40
massage 35, 366
  body terminology 36–8, 39
  pre-coital 35–8, 42
Master Red Pine, Chi Song zi (immortal) 25
materia dietetica 168, 169, 173–87
  beginnings 174
  Meng Shen's 168–9, 184, 187
  Sun Simiao's 176
materia medica (*bencao*) 8, 143, 167–71, 216, 224–5
  categories (*lei*) 216–17, 224–5, 229, 251
  comparative description 247
  drug affinity with channels 155
  genre 8, 167–8
  government sponsored compilation 168, 178
  hierarchical structure of canonical *bencao* 224–5
  Li Shizhen's revision 223–4
  pishuang 202
  recipes 253
  symptomatic indications 154
  synthetic compound 199
  systemisation of correspondences 153
Mawangdui manuscripts 13, 14, 15, 19–22, 59n
  bing notion 83–5
  Cauterisation Canons 13, 14, 21, 84–5
  Confucius' apology for attachment to *Yijing* 101
  death vessels 115–16
  Fifty-two recipes 173, 194
  fruits 235
  He yinyang 35, 38–9, 42, 45, 46
  mai notion 74, 83
  medical knowledge 262
  sexual techniques 72n

vessel theory 116, 117
Year cycle 113
see also Maifa
Mawangdui tomb (168 BC) 13, 19–22
McCrae, Thomas 363–5
medical case histories/statements (*yi'an*) 56–63, 293–6
  biomedical interpretation 60–1, 62
  biomedical model 295
  Chunyu Yi 56–83, 304–5, 310
  cold damage disorders 308–9
  compilations 294–5
  consultation records 56–83, 310
  copying 373
  didactic use 327, 328
  disease names 333
  early written 9, 293–4, 302–9
  format prescription 295, 299, 311–14
  formulaic structure 63–83
  functions 295
  genre 295, 297–321
  Han Mao's 295, 310, 311–14
  He Lianchen's 331–2, 333–4
  Hua Tuo's 305–7
  identification of persons 63–4
  legal case records 64, 313, 316
  medical records 300–2
  Ming 299–300
  modernisation 324–35
  narrative 294
  non-medical advocates 316
  notebooks 327
  old-style 295–6
  prescriptions 332
  printed genre 309–21
  private documents of physicians 304–5
  publishing 309–10, 318–19, 325
  purpose of writing 319–21
  self-discipline 317
  student presentation 304
  therapy 332
  throat-rash 327–31
  Traditional Chinese Medicine 298
  Western style 296, 329–31, 334
  worldwide 300–2
  written records 302–9
medical encyclopaedia 136
medical ethics 55, 168
medical examinations 121, 154, 318
medical improvement schools 366
medical knowledge 10
medical lineages 6, 17, 62–3
  family tradition 294, 384
  internal factions 296
  Jin Yuan currents of thought 149n, 275n
  warmth factor disorder current of thought 274n, 276
medical practice
  generational oppositions 374
  as occupation 317–18, 319
  professional 337
  state control 169